The Human Complement System in Health and Disease

The Human Complement System in Health and Disease

Editor: Adah Blair

FOSTER ACADEMICS
www.fosteracademics.com

www.fosteracademics.com

FOSTER ACADEMICS

Cataloging-in-Publication Data

The human complement system in health and disease / edited by Adah Blair.
p. cm.
Includes bibliographical references and index.
ISBN 978-1-64646-606-1
1. Complement (Immunology). 2. Immunity. 3. Immunologic diseases. 4. Immune system.
5. Immunopathology. I. Blair, Adah.
QR185.8.C6 H86 2023
616.079--dc23

Foster Academics,
118-35 Queens Blvd., Suite 400,
Forest Hills, NY 11375, USA

ISBN 978-1-64646-606-1 (Hardback)

Contents

Preface

The part of the immune system, which improves the abilities of antibodies and phagocytic cells that eliminate microbes and destroyed cells from an organism, is known as the complement system. It also promotes inflammation and damages the pathogen's cell membrane. It is a continuous process and hence belongs to the innate immune system. It is non-adaptive and has a lifelong presence. The complement system can be used by antibodies, which are produced by the adaptive immune system. Various small proteins are included in the complement system which synthesize through the liver and circulate as inactive precursors in the blood. There are three biochemical pathways which contribute in the activation of complement system, namely, the alternative complement pathway, the classical complement pathway and the lectin pathway. Such selected concepts that redefine the study of the human complement system have been presented in this book. It aims to serve as a resource guide for students and experts alike and contribute to the growth of research in this area of study. Those in search of information to further their knowledge will be greatly assisted by this book.

All of the data presented henceforth, was collaborated in the wake of recent advancements in the field. The aim of this book is to present the diversified developments from across the globe in a comprehensible manner. The opinions expressed in each chapter belong solely to the contributing authors. Their interpretations of the topics are the integral part of this book, which I have carefully compiled for a better understanding of the readers.

At the end, I would like to thank all those who dedicated their time and efforts for the successful completion of this book. I also wish to convey my gratitude towards my friends and family who supported me at every step.

Editor

1

Complement Factor H and Apolipoprotein E Participate in Regulation of Inflammation in THP-1 Macrophages

Eija Nissilä [1], Pipsa Hakala [1†], Katarzyna Leskinen [1†], Angela Roig [1†], Shahan Syed [1†], Kok P. M. Van Kessel [2], Jari Metso [3], Carla J. C. De Haas [2], Päivi Saavalainen [1], Seppo Meri [1], Angeliki Chroni [4], Jos A. G. Van Strijp [2], Katariina Öörni [5], Matti Jauhiainen [3], T. Sakari Jokiranta [1] and Karita Haapasalo [1]*

[1] Department of Bacteriology and Immunology, and Research Programs Unit, Immunobiology, University of Helsinki, Helsinki, Finland, [2] Medical Microbiology, University Medical Center Utrecht, Utrecht, Netherlands, [3] Minerva Foundation Institute for Medical Research, Helsinki, Finland, [4] Institute of Biosciences and Applications, National Center for Scientific Research "Demokritos," Athens, Greece, [5] Wihuri Research Institute, Helsinki, Finland

***Correspondence:**
Karita Haapasalo
karita.haapasalo@helsinki.fi

† These authors have contributed equally to this work

The alternative pathway (AP) of complement is constantly active in plasma and can easily be activated on self surfaces and trigger local inflammation. Host cells are protected from AP attack by Factor H (FH), the main AP regulator in plasma. Although complement is known to play a role in atherosclerosis, the mechanisms of its contribution are not fully understood. Since FH via its domains 5–7 binds apoliporotein E (apoE) and macrophages produce apoE we examined how FH could be involved in the antiatherogenic effects of apoE. We used blood peripheral monocytes and THP-1 monocyte/macrophage cells which were also loaded with acetylated low-density lipoprotein (LDL) to form foam cells. Binding of FH and apoE on these cells was analyzed by flow cytometry. High-density lipoprotein (HDL)-mediated cholesterol efflux of activated THP-1 cells was measured and transcriptomes of THP-1 cells using mRNA sequencing were determined. We found that binding of FH to human blood monocytes and cholesterol-loaded THP-1 macrophages increased apoE binding to these cells. Preincubation of fluorescent cholesterol labeled THP-1 macrophages in the presence of FH increased cholesterol efflux and cholesterol-loaded macrophages displayed reduced transcription of proinflammatory/proatherogenic factors and increased transcription of anti-inflammatory/anti-atherogenic factors. Further incubation of THP-1 cells with serum reduced C3b/iC3b deposition. Overall, our data indicate that apoE and FH interact with monocytic cells in a concerted action and this interaction reduces complement activation and inflammation in the atherosclerotic lesions. By this way FH may participate in mediating the beneficial effects of apoE in suppressing atherosclerotic lesion progression.

Keywords: complement, complement system, Factor H, apolipoprotein E, atherosclerosis, inflammation

INTRODUCTION

Complement (C) system is part of the humoral innate immune response. It quickly attacks microbes and foreign particles invading the human body. Activation of complement through any of the three pathways, the classical, alternative (AP), and lectin pathways, leads to cleavage of C3 and covalent surface deposition of the C3b fragment that is capable of forming an enzyme with factor B. Surface deposited C3b and its fragments, inactive C3b (iC3b) and C3dg, are important opsonins that can be recognized by complement receptors expressed by phagocytes. Further activation of the C cascade leads to formation of membrane attack complexes and release of proinflammatory chemotactic and anaphylatoxic protein fragments C3a and C5a that mediate their effects by binding to receptors on phagocytes.

AP is constantly active in plasma leading to low grade challenge to all plasma-exposed particles and surfaces by spontaneous hydrolysis or enzymatic activation of C3. Activation proceeds rapidly through amplification on surfaces that are missing efficient regulatory mechanisms. Factor H (FH) is the main AP regulator as it keeps this spontaneous activation in control (1). This is obvious since depletion of plasma/serum from FH or blockage of FH by autoantibodies leads to activation of the AP leading to overconsumption and loss of active complement within <30 min (2, 3). FH is an elongated molecule composed of 20 domains. The N-terminal domains 1–4 are responsible for FH regulatory activity while domains 19–20 on the C-terminal end are responsible for the self surface recognition (4). Domain FH19 binds to surface-deposited C3b, while FH20 binds sialic acids and glycosaminoglycans (GAGs) present on self surfaces (5). In this way, FH discriminates host self surfaces from non-self ones. Also domains 6–7 of FH are important for self surface recognition. These mediate interaction with sulphated GAGs, heparin, and C-reactive protein (6, 7). When bound to C3b, the cofactor activity of FH helps in inactivation of C3b to iC3b by factor I and simultaneous inhibition of factor B binding to C3b (8, 9). Moreover, FH prevents further AP amplification by accelerating the decay of formed AP convertases (10). AP activation does not need a trigger as it is based on continuous low-grade activity. However, imbalance between activation and regulation e.g., when numerous C3b deposits are formed on protein complexes can lead to enhanced AP activation in serum/plasma (11). Recently, it has become clear that AP dysregulation is a central event in development of several complement-related diseases to which mutations or polymorphisms in domains FH5-7 and FH19-20 predispose. While mutations in FH19-20 cause atypical hemolytic uremic syndrome (aHUS), the Y402H polymorphism in domain 7 is associated with age-related macular degeneration (AMD) (12, 13) and dense deposit disease (DDD) (14).

Atherosclerosis is a chronic multifactorial inflammatory disease caused by the subendothelial accumulation of lipids, immune cells and fibrous elements in arteries leading to thickening and hardening of the arterial wall. Low-grade inflammation is a key mediator of the disease. Both adaptive and innate immune responses are crucial for initiation and progression of atherosclerosis, and these mechanisms have been exploited to develop new diagnostic biomarkers and therapies for patients recently (15). The hallmark of early atherosclerotic lesion is the formation of fatty streaks composed of cholesterol-laden macrophages, which are formed when low density lipoproteins (LDL) are modified by oxidation or proteolytic modification and accumulated in the subendothelium of arteries leading to monocyte recruitment and differentiation into macrophages (16). The balance between proinflammatory M1 type macrophages and anti-inflammatory M2 type macrophages plays a crucial role in the pathogenesis of atherosclerotic plaques.

The antiatherosclerotic activity of apoE is based on its ability to regulate lipoprotein metabolism and to promote cholesterol efflux from cells (17, 18). Endogenous production of apoE by macrophages in blood vessel walls has been shown to be critical in the prevention and healing of atherosclerotic plaques. Importantly, apoE modulates macrophage polarization into the anti-inflammatory M2 phenotype (17) and promotes reverse cholesterol transport from peripheral cells to high density lipoprotein (HDL) for further transportation of cholesterol to the liver for excretion (19).

Genetic variations in the *APOE* gene coding for apolipoprotein E constitute important risk factors both for AMD and atherosclerosis. Interestingly, similar underlining mechanisms including disturbances in lipid metabolism, oxidative stress and the inflammatory process are closely associated in the pathogenesis of both diseases. It has also been shown that in human eyes with AMD, FH co-localizes with and binds to oxidized lipids in drusen, fatty deposits under the retina. It seems that the common FH variant 402Y has a higher affinity for oxidized lipids than the risk allele 402H suggesting a stronger FH-mediated complement inhibition of the effects of oxidized lipids on macrophages (20).

We have shown before that FH binds both lipid-free and high density lipoprotein (HDL) associated apoE via domains 5–7 and thereby regulates AP activation in plasma (21). The present study was set up to investigate whether FH and apoE interaction could play a role in the induction and progression of atherosclerosis by macrophages. We show here that FH increases apoE binding to monocytes and THP-1 macrophages possibly via simultaneous interaction between cell surface sialic acids and apoE and thereby regulates local complement activation. Moreover, FH interaction with THP-1 macrophages and cholesterol-labeled cells increases macrophage-mediated cholesterol efflux and modulates the expression of inflammatory genes suggesting a yet unexplored anti-inflammatory mechanism for FH.

MATERIALS AND METHODS

Proteins

Cloning and *Pichia pastoris* expression of the recombinant fragments FH5-7, FH19-20, and FH1-4 has been described earlier (22, 23). If necessary, fragments were further purified by passing through a HiLoad 16/60 Superdex 200 prep-grade gel filtration column (GE healthcare) in phosphate buffered saline (NaCl 300mM, KCl 5.4 mM, Na2HPO4 20 mM, KH2PO4 3.6 mM, pH 7.4), and concentrated using heparin affinity chromatography. Labeling of proteins was performed using N-hydroxysuccinimide-reactive Red dye (NT647, catalog no. L001) following the manufacturer's instructions (NanoTemper).

Expression of apoE Proteins

The preparation of vectors, expression of recombinant apoE2, apoE3, and apoE4 in the *Escherichia coli* BL21-Gold (DE3) bacterial system following induction by IPTG, and purification by immobilized metal affinity chromatography has been described elsewhere (24–26).

Isolation of HDL and LDL and Acetylation of Human LDL

LDL (d = 1.019–1.050 g/mL) and HDL (d = 1.063–1.210 g/mL) were isolated from plasma of healthy volunteers obtained from the Finnish Red Cross Blood Service by sequential ultracentrifugation using KBr for density adjustment (27). LDL was acetylated by repeated additions of acetic anhydride (28). Briefly, LDL (10 mg as LDL protein) in 1.5 ml LDL buffer (150 mM NaCl, 1 mM EDTA, pH 7.4) was mixed 1:1 (vol/vol) with saturated sodium acetate and stirred in ice-water bath for 10 min. Next 30 μl acetic anhydride was added four times with 10 min stirring intervals. After the fourth addition of acetic anhydride, the incubation was continued for 60 min with continuous stirring. Finally, the mixture was dialysed for 24 h at 4°C against LDL buffer.

Isolation of Peripheral Blood Cells, Cell Cloning, and Culturing

For peripheral blood cell isolation blood was drawn to tubes containing hirudin (Roche Diagnostics, Mannheim, Germany) from healthy human volunteers after informed written and signed consent (Ethical Committee decision 406/13/03/00/2015, Hospital district of Helsinki and Uusimaa). The blood samples were diluted 1:1 (v/v) with PBS and centrifuged through a gradient (Histopaque® 1.119 and 1.077; Sigma-Aldrich) at 320 x g for 20 min at 22°C. The PBMC layer was collected, washed once with RPMI 1640 (Gibco®) containing 0.05% (w/v) HSA (RPMI-HSA) and diluted with RPMI-HSA. U937 human monocytic cells were obtained from the ATCC (American Type Culture Collection), cultured in RPMI medium supplemented with penicillin/streptomycin and 10% (v/v) FCS. CR3 was stably expressed in U937 cells using a lentiviral expression system as described (29). We cloned the CD11b (NM_001145808.1) and CD18 (NM_000211.4) cDNA in the dual promoter lentiviral vectors, RP137 (BIC-PGK-Zeo) and RP-139 (BIC-PGK-Puro), respectively. These vectors were constructed by replacing the Zeo-T2a-mAmetrine cassette from the BIC-PGK-Zeo-T2a-mAmetrine (RP172) vector (30) with either a Zeocin or Puromycin resistance gene. First CD11b was stably expressed in U937 cells, subsequently these cells were used for stable expression of CD18. THP-1 monocytes were transformed to macrophages by incubating the cells for 48–72 h in the presence of 100 nM phorbol 12-myristate 13-acetate (PMA) and for generating cholesterol loaded cells mimicking foam cells the macrophages were further incubated in the presence of 100 μg/ml (as LDL protein) acetylated LDL for 24–48 h in serum free media.

Detection of CR3 and Sialic Acid Expression on Cells and Binding of FH on Cell Surface Sialic Acids

The expression of CR3 was analyzed by incubating the cells in 50 μl RPMI-HSA at 5 × 10^6 cells/ml concentration for 45 min with FITC-conjugated anti-CD11b (sigma). The cells were washed once with RPMI-HSA and expression of CR3 was detected by flow cytometry. To detect the specificity of sialic acid expression on different cells and FH binding to cell surface sialic acids the cells were preincubated with 100U α2-3,6,8 Neuraminidase (New England biolabs) or PBS for 30 min at 37°C. Next, 45 nM NT647 labeled Maackia Amurensis Lectin II (MAL II*) or 200 nM NT647-FH was added to the wells and the plate was further incubated for 30 min at 37°C. The cells were washed once with 200 μl of icecold RPMI-HSA, centrifuged at 300 × g for 10 min, fixed with 100 μl of 1% (v/v) paraformaldehyde (Thermo) RPMI-HSA. Next, 2,000–10,000 cells were run by BD LSR Fortessa flow cytometer (Lazer 640 nm, filter 670/30) and analyzed using FlowJo V10 software, where the gating of the cells was performed by using forward scatter (FSC) and side scatter (SSC) to find viable, single cell events. Mean fluorescence intensities were calculated for the gated cells.

ApoE, FH5-7 and Factor H Binding to Cells

Binding of FH or FH5-7 to peripheral blood monocytic cells, U937 and THP-1 cells was studied by incubating 2 × 10^5 cells with 200 nM of NT647-FH or 1,3 μM of NT647 FH5-7 for 45 min at 4°C in round bottom 96-well plates. For inhibition assays, cells were incubated for 30 min at 4°C with 1.5 μM of apoE, FH1-4 or 9 and 3 μM of FH5-7 prior adding the labeled protein. The cells were washed once with 200 μl of icecold RPMI-HSA, centrifuged at 300 × g for 10 min and fixed with 100 μl of 1% (v/v) paraformaldehyde RPMI-HSA. To study the effect of apoE-FH interaction and their binding to monocytic cells a dilution series of FH (Complement technologies), FH19-20 or apoE was incubated in dark for 5 min at 37°C with a constant 200 nM concentration of NT647-labeled apoE or NT647-labeled FH. Then 40 μl of hirudin blood isolated monocytes were added in each well and incubated in dark for 25 min at 37°C. The incubation was stopped by adding 300 μl of ice-cold PBS to the tubes and the cells were run by flow cytometry and analyzed using the gating strategy described earlier.

FH5-7 Binding to a Panel of Leukocyte Receptors

Monocytes isolated from peripheral blood (PBMCs) cells (5 × 10^6 cells/ml) in RPMI-HSA 0.05% (w/v) were incubated in the presence of 14 μg/ml of FH5-7, or PBS for 15 min on ice followed by incubation with a panel of receptor specific FITC-, PE- or APC-labeled antibodies using a 96-well U-plate (greiner, Bio one) for 45 min at 4°C. The cells were washed with 200 μl of RPMI/HSA 0.05% (w/v) and fixed with 150 μl of 1% (v/v) paraformaldehyde in RPMI-HSA 0.05% for 30 min at 4°C before counting the fluorescence of 10,000 cells using on FACS flow cytometer (Lazers 405, 488, and 640 nm; filters 450/50, 525/50, and 670/30) and analyzed using the gating strategy described earlier. The inhibition value of FH5-7 on receptor specific antibody binding was calculated by dividing the mean fluorescence of FH5-7 treated cells by PBS treated cells.

C3b/iC3b Deposition on FH Incubated THP-1 Cells

Untreated THP-1 monocytes, PMA activated THP-1 macrophages, and PMA activated THP-1 macrophages loaded with cholesterol by using acLDL (100/ml μg of LDL protein) were incubated in the presence or absence of FH (320 nM) for 24 h in 24-well tissue culture plates at 37°C in 5% CO_2 in serum free THP-1 medium using 4 x 10^5 cells/well/200 μl. A 10 μl sample from the supernatant was taken at 0, 5 and 24 h timepoints after the media was centrifuged for 10 min at 300 x g to remove any cellular debris. These culture media aliquots were stored at −20 °C before analysis for the apoE ELISA method. After 24 h the cells were detached using 200 μl Cellstripper (Corning) for 45 min at 37°C, 5% CO_2, harvested by centrifugation as before and diluted with RPMI-HSA. Cells from this assay were used to analyze NT647-FH binding (described earlier), mRNA expression, apoE secretion (described later), ABCA1 protein expression and complement activation assays. To detect ABCA1 protein expression the cells were incubated with 0.3 μg/4 x 10^5 cells/well/150 μl mouse anti-ABCA1 antibody (abcam) washed once by centrifugation and incubated with 1:200 dilution of Alexa Fluor 488 conjugated goat anti-mouse IgG (Invitrogen). To compare serum complement activity in the presence or absence of preincubated FH 5 x 10^4 of THP-1 cells were incubated for 15 min in a 50 μl volume of 20% (v/v) serum. Cells were washed once by centrifugation and incubated with 2 μl of FITC conjugated anti-C3b (Cederlane) for 45 min at 4°C. The cells were washed, fixed, run by flow cytometry (Lazer 488, filter 525/50) and analyzed as described earlier.

Effect of FH on apoE Secretion and Binding to THP-1 Cells

The cells detached from the tissue culture 24-well plates were incubated in the presence of 2 μl of rabbit anti-human apoE (600 μg/ml, non affinity purified) in a 50 μl volume of RPMI-HSA 0.05% (w/v) for 45 min at 4°C. The cells were washed once by centrifugation and incubated in the presence of 1:100 diluted 488 goat anti-rabbit antibody (Life technologies) for 45 min at 4°C. After incubation the cells were washed, fixed and analyzed by flow cytometry as described earlier (Lazer 488, filter 525/50). Secretion of apoE by THP-1 cells was analyzed from 8 μl of culture media collected at different time points using apoE ELISA protocol as previously described (31).

Cholesterol Efflux Assay

The cholesterol efflux assay was performed according to manufacturer's instructions (Abcam) using THP-1 cells activated for 24 h with PMA. The cells were labeled overnight with fluorescently-labeled cholesterol in the presence or absence of 650 nM FH. After overnight labeling the PMA activated and cholesterol labeled THP-1 macrophages were washed gently with 200 μL of RPMI media and incubated then in the presence of 50 μg of HDL (as HDL protein) as cholesterol acceptor. After 5 h incubation the media and supernatant of lysed cells were measured separately for fluorescence (Ex/Em = 482/515 nm). The ratio between fluorescence intensity of media and fluorescence intensity of cell lysate plus media were calculated as percentage of cholesterol efflux.

RNA-Sequencing

RNA sequencing method was designed based on the Drop-seq protocol described earlier (32). Briefly, the cells were mixed with lysis buffer (0.3% (v/v) triton, 20 mM DTT, 2 mM dNTPs) in wells of U-bottomed 96-well plate. Magnetic Dynabeads (M-270 Streptavidin, Thermo Fisher Scientific) coated with Indexing Oligonucleotides (Integrated DNA Technologies, **Table 1**) were added to each well. After 5 min of incubation at ambient temperature the magnetic beads were separated from the supernatant and washed twice with 6X SSC buffer. Subsequently, the beads were combined with RT mix, containing 1 x Maxima RT buffer, 1 mM dNTPs, 10 U/μl Maxima H- RTase (all ThermoFisher Scientific), 1 U/μl RNase inhibitor (Lucigen), and 2.5 μM Template Switch Oligo (Integrated DNA Technologies). Samples were incubated in a T100 thermal cycler (BioRad) for 30 min at 22°C and 90 min at 52°C. The beads were washed twice with 6X SSC buffer and once in PCR-grade water. The constructed cDNA was amplified by PCR in a volume of 15 μl using 5 μl of RT mix as template, 1x HiFi HotStart Readymix (Kapa Biosystems) and 0.8 μM SMART PCR primer. The samples were thermocycled in a T100 thermocycler (BioRad) as follows: 95°C 3 min; subsequently four cycles of: 98°C for 20 s, 65°C for 45 s, 72°C for 3 min; following 13 cycles of: 98°C for 20 s, 67°C for 20 s, 72°C for 3 min; and with the final extension step of 5 min at 72°C. The PCR products were pooled together and purified with 0.6X Agencourt AMPure XP Beads (Beckman Coulter) according to the manufacturer's instructions. They were eluted in 10 μl of molecular grade water. The 3′-end cDNA fragments for sequencing were prepared using the Nextera XT (Illumina) tagmentation reaction with 600 pg of the PCR product serving as an input. The reaction was performed according to manufacturer's instruction, with the exception of the P5 SMART primer that was used instead of S5xx Nextera primer. Subsequently, the samples were PCR amplified as follows: 95°C for 30 s; 11 cycles of 95°C for 10 s, 55°C for 30 s, 72°C for 30 s; with the final extension step of 5 min at 72°C. Samples were purified twice using 0.6X and 1.0X Agencourt AMPure Beads (Beckman Coulter) and eluted in 10 μl of molecular grade water. The concentration of the libraries was measured using a Qubit 2 fluorometer (Invitrogen) and the Qubit DNA HS Assay Kit (ThermoFisher Scientific). The quality of the sequencing libraries was assessed using the LabChip GXII Touch HT electropheresis system (PerkinElmer), with the DNA High Sensitivity Assay (PerkinElmer) and the DNA 5K/RNA/Charge Variant Assay LabChip (PerkinElmer). Samples were stored at −20°C. The libraries were sequenced on Illumina NextSeq500, with a custom primer (**Table 1**) producing read 1 of 20 bp and read 2 (paired

TABLE 1 | Primers used in this study.

Name	Oligonucleotide sequence
DSbl 001	TTTTTTTAAGCAGTGGTATCAACGCAGAGTACACGTACGTACGTNNNNNNNNTTTTTTTTTTTTTTTTTTTTTTTTTTTTTT
DSbl 002	TTTTTTTAAGCAGTGGTATCAACGCAGAGTACCGTACGTACGTANNNNNNNNTTTTTTTTTTTTTTTTTTTTTTTTTTTTTT
DSbl 003	TTTTTTTAAGCAGTGGTATCAACGCAGAGTACGTACGTACGTACNNNNNNNNTTTTTTTTTTTTTTTTTTTTTTTTTTTTTT
DSbl 004	TTTTTTTAAGCAGTGGTATCAACGCAGAGTACTACGTACGTACGNNNNNNNNTTTTTTTTTTTTTTTTTTTTTTTTTTTTTT
DSbl 005	TTTTTTTAAGCAGTGGTATCAACGCAGAGTACACGTCGTACGTANNNNNNNNTTTTTTTTTTTTTTTTTTTTTTTTTTTTTT
DSbl 006	TTTTTTTAAGCAGTGGTATCAACGCAGAGTACCGTAGTACGTACNNNNNNNNTTTTTTTTTTTTTTTTTTTTTTTTTTTTTT
DSbl 007	TTTTTTTAAGCAGTGGTATCAACGCAGAGTACGTACTACGTACGNNNNNNNNTTTTTTTTTTTTTTTTTTTTTTTTTTTTTT
DSbl 008	TTTTTTTAAGCAGTGGTATCAACGCAGAGTACTACGACGTACGTNNNNNNNNTTTTTTTTTTTTTTTTTTTTTTTTTTTTTT
DSbl 009	TTTTTTTAAGCAGTGGTATCAACGCAGAGTACACGTGTACGTACNNNNNNNNTTTTTTTTTTTTTTTTTTTTTTTTTTTTTT
DSbl 010	TTTTTTTAAGCAGTGGTATCAACGCAGAGTACCGTATACGTACGNNNNNNNNTTTTTTTTTTTTTTTTTTTTTTTTTTTTTT
DSbl 011	TTTTTTTAAGCAGTGGTATCAACGCAGAGTACGTACACGTACGTNNNNNNNNTTTTTTTTTTTTTTTTTTTTTTTTTTTTTT
DSbl 012	TTTTTTTAAGCAGTGGTATCAACGCAGAGTACTACGCGTACGTANNNNNNNNTTTTTTTTTTTTTTTTTTTTTTTTTTTTTT
TSO	AAGCAGTGGTATCAACGCAGAGTGAATrGrGrG
SMART PCR primer	AAGCAGTGGTATCAACGCAGAGT
P5 SMART primer	AATGATACGGCGACCACCGAGATCTACACGCCTGTCCGCGGAAGCAGTGGTATCAACGCAGAGT*A*C
Sequencing read 1	GCCTGTCCGCGGAAGCAGTGGTATCAACGCAGAGTAC

** = phosphorothioate bond added*

end) of 55 bp (32). Sequencing was performed at the Functional Genomics Unit of the University of Helsinki, Finland.

Read Alignment and Generation of Digital Expression Data

Raw sequence data was filtered to remove reads shorter than 20 bp. Subsequently, the original pipeline suggested in Macosko et al. (32) for processing of drop-seq data was used. Briefly, reads were additionally filtered to remove polyA tails of length 6 or greater, then aligned to the human (GRCh38) genome using STAR aligner (33) with default settings. Uniquely mapped reads were grouped according to the 1–12 barcode, and gene transcripts were counted by their Unique Molecular Identifiers (UMIs) to reduce the bias emerging from the PCR amplification. Digital expression matrices (DGE) reported the number of transcripts per gene in a given sample (according to the distinct UMI sequences counted).

Statistical Methods

Statistical analyses between multiple samples were performed using one-way ANOVA supplemented with non-parametric Tamhane's multiple-comparison test. Statistical differences between two independent samples were calculated using non-parametric Mann-Whitney *U*-test (SPSS for Windows, Analytical Software).

RESULTS

Factor H Binds to Monocytic Cell CR3 via CD11b

FH interacts with human cell surfaces mainly via C3b and cell surface glycosaminoglycans, like heparan sulfate, and sialic acids. Previous studies have shown that especially on endothelial cells and platelets the presence of sialic acids is crucial for efficient FH-mediated complement regulation (34). In addition to surface sialic acids, FH has been shown to interact with CR3 (CD11b/CD18) on human neutrophils in the absence of C3b deposits (35). We studied binding of FH to different ligands on monocytes and monocytic cell lines to find out how these interactions could be altered by apoE that is known to be secreted by macrophages and to interact with FH domains 5–7 (21, 36). By using NT647-labeled FH we could detect clear binding of FH to monocytes even in the absence of C3b, while binding of FH to lymphocytes was closer to the background values (**Figure 1A**). To find out the receptor that interacts with the apoE binding domains FH5-7 (location of the apoE binding domains is shown in **Figure 1B**) on monocytes we performed a screening assay where the cells were preincubated with the recombinant FH5-7 fragment prior to adding the anti-receptor antibody. Incubation of the cells with FH5-7 resulted in a clear reduction in anti-CD11b binding that is the alpha-chain of the integrin-type CR3 receptor heterodimer (CD11b/18; **Figure 1C**). In addition, similar inhibition was also detected with antibodies against CD35 and CD89. Binding of FH5-7 on CR3 was further analyzed using CR3 overexpressing U937 monocytic cells (**Figure 1D**). Binding of NT647-labeled FH5-7 on these cells was reduced in the presence of increasing concentrations of non-labeled FH5-7 (3 and 9 μM) and on empty U937 cells that do not express CR3.

Binding of apoE to Monocytes Is Increased by Factor H

To study further the interaction between the apoE binding ligand FH and CR3 on human monocytes, we next performed an assay to see whether apoE could alter FH-CR3 interaction on U937 monocytic cells overexpressing the receptor. We found that on CR3 overexpressing U937 cells binding of NT647-FH was clearly inhibited by apoE2 to the level of binding of FH

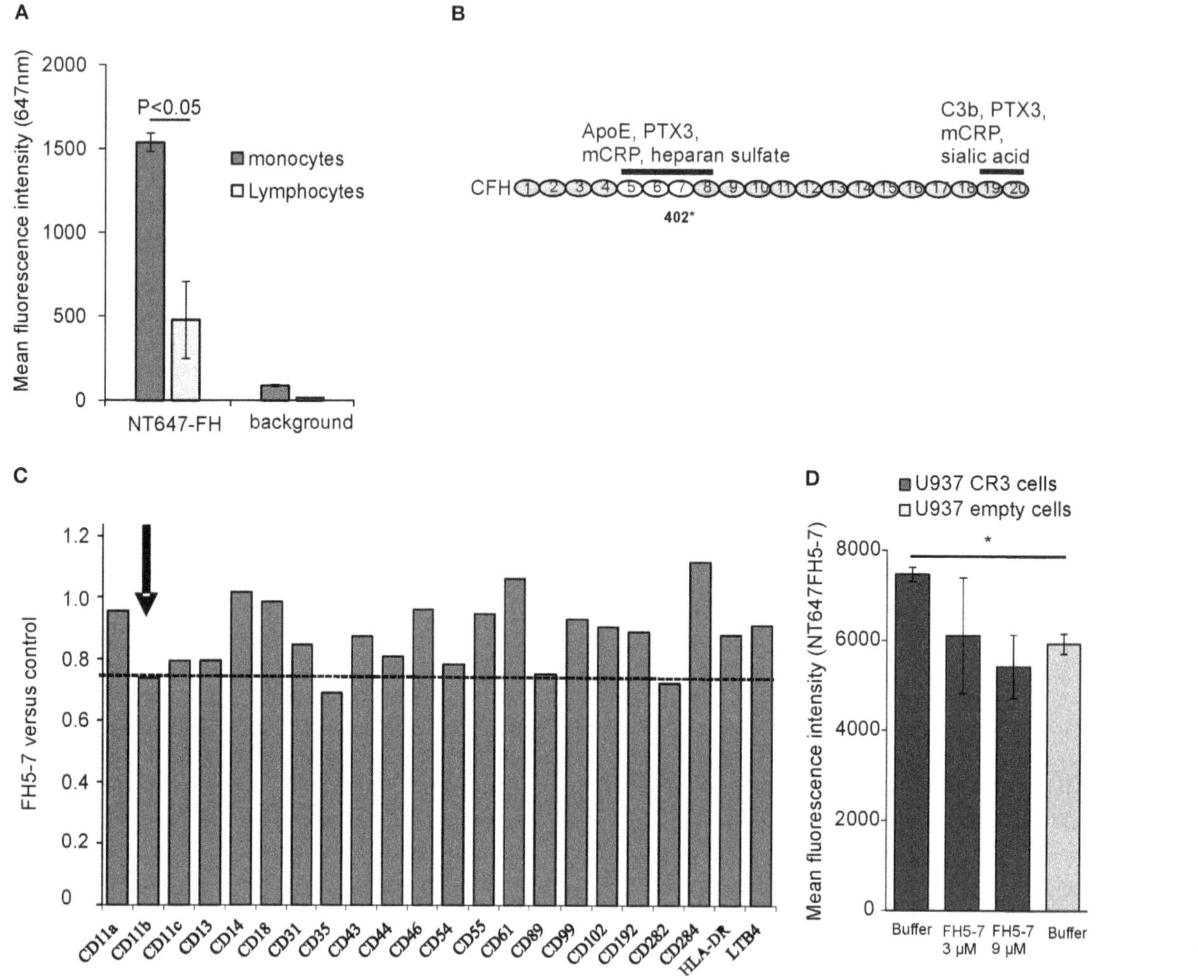

FIGURE 1 | Factor H binding to peripheral blood leukocytes. **(A)** Peripheral blood mononuclear cells were incubated with NT647-labeled FH and the mean fluorescence intensities were analyzed by flow cytometry ($n = 3$). **(B)** Schematic structure of the full length FH and the location of domains 5–7 that interact with apoE. The binding sites of different ligands, apoE, pentraxin3 (PTX3), monomeric C-reactive protein (mCRP) and heparin sulfate, and the common polymorphic Y402H site on domain 7 are shown. **(C)** Screening of FH5-7 binding by a panel of antibodies directed against various receptors and surface molecules on monocytes. Peripheral blood monocytic cells were preincubated for 30 min with or without 12 µg/ml of FH5-7 prior adding 2×10^5 cells cells/well in a 96-well plate with FITC-, APC- and/or PE-labeled antibody. Mean fluorescence intensities were calculated from the gated cells using flow cytometry. Inhibition of antibody binding was calculated by dividing the mean fluorescence of FH5-7 treated cells by PBS treated cells (FH5-7 vs. control). The CD11b part of CR3 dimer is marked. The dashed line shows the level of anti-CD11b binding in the presence of FH5-7 (< 0.8) compared to binding of the antibody without FH5-7 (1.0). **(D)** CR3 expressing and empty U937 mononuclear cells were incubated with NT647 labeled FH5-7 in the presence or absence of unlabeled FH5-7 (x-axis). Statistical significance between multiple samples was calculated using one-way ANOVA supplemented with non-parametric Tamhane's *post-hoc* multiple comparison test. Error bars indicate SD. * = $p < 0.05$.

to cells devoid of CR3. A slight inhibition was also detected by apoE3 and apoE4 but the levels of inhibition were not statistically significant (**Figure 2A**). As the apoE2 isotype showed significant inhibition we used the apoE2 isoform in the further assays. Surprisingly, when the same inhibition assay was performed using peripheral blood monocytes and lymphocytes we did not detect any inhibition of NT647-FH binding in the presence of increasing concentrations of unlabeled apoE (**Figure 2B**). On the contrary, a clear increase in binding of NT647-apoE was detected when the cells were incubated with increasing concentrations of unlabeled FH, while FH19-20 did not have the same effect. This indicates that FH increases rather than attenuates apoE binding to monocytes. To further study the cell surface receptors leading to increased binding of apoE to these cells, and because both apoE and FH are known to interact with cell surface heparan sulfate, we incubated monocytes with NT647-apoE and FH and increasing concentrations of anti-heparin antibody. Here, binding of NT647-apoE in the presence of anti-heparin antibody was reduced to the level of NT647-apoE only (**Figure 2C**) suggesting that increased binding of apoE to these cells is dependent on FH and cell surface heparan sulfate.

Because we could detect inhibition of FH binding by apoE only to U937 cells overexpressing CR3 but not to monocytes

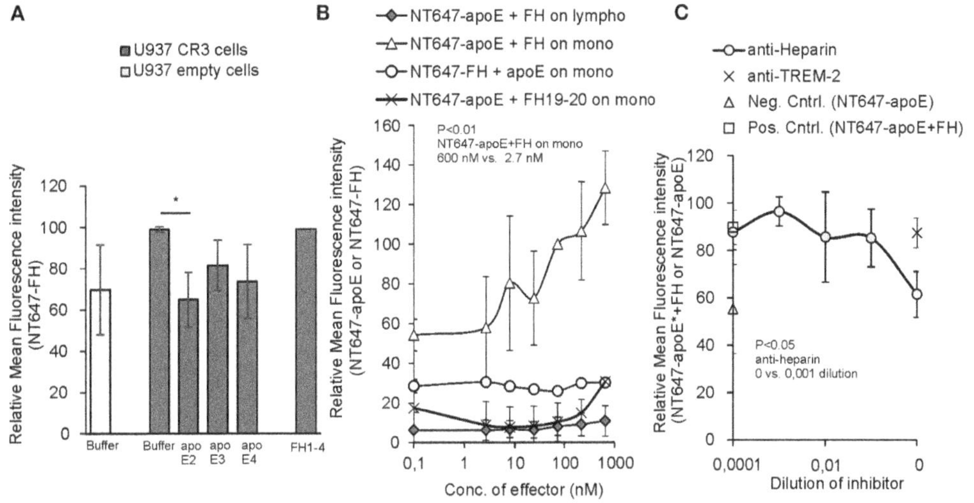

FIGURE 2 | Inhibition of Factor H/apoE binding to U937 and peripheral blood cells. **(A)** Binding of NT647-FH on U937 cells expressing CR3 in the absence (Buffer) or presence of 1.5 μM of apoE2, 3 and 4 ($n = 3$). Control cells without CR3 (empty cells) shows binding of FH without the receptor. Binding of NT647-FH in the presence of equal molarity of FH1-4 is shown. **(B)** Binding of NT647 labeled FH or apoE2 on peripheral blood cells with different concentrations of unlabeled inhibitor (FH or apoE). Levels are calculated as relative to apoE binding at 73 nM FH concentration ($n = 4$). **(C)** Inhibition of apoE+FH binding to monocytes in the presence of increasing concentrations of anti-heparin antibody. Anti-TREM-2 antibody was used as a negative control. Control (Neg. Cntrl. NT647-apoE) shows binding of apoE on the cells without FH incubation and Control (Pos. Cntrl. NT647-apoE+FH) binding of apoE in the presence of FH and apoE only ($n = 3$). Statistical significance was calculated using one-way ANOVA supplemented with non-parametric Tamhane's *post-hoc* multiple comparison test. Error bars indicate SD. Percentages of mean fluorescence intensities are shown as relative to the maximum intensity in each individual experiment. *= $p < 0.05$.

we hypothesized that on monocytes, where CR3 expression is lower, FH could simultaneously bind to apoE and cell surface sialic acids. This is because FH sialic acid binding domains are located within domains FH19-20 and not on apoE interacting domains FH5-7. This could also explain why apoE binding was increased by FH to monocytes. As expected, the human peripheral blood monocytes showed high sialic acid expression and low CR3 expression while the U937 cells showed very low expression of sialic acids and very high CR3 expression (**Figures 3A–C**). The high expression levels of CR3 and low levels of sialic acids on U937 cells may explain why inhibition of FH binding to CR3 in the presence of apoE could only be detected on these cells. To study the effect of sialic acids on binding of FH different cell types were preincubated with neuraminidase that removes cell surface sialic acids. All tested cells bound FH at different levels, but only monocytes showed significant reduction in FH binding after neuraminidase treatment. No decrease in FH binding was detected on other tested cell types with lower sialic acid expression (**Figures 3D,E**). These data suggest that FH interacts with several different ligands on cells but binding of FH to sialic acids via domains FH19-20 enables simultaneous binding of apoE via domains FH5-7 and cell surface heparan sulfate.

Binding of FH to THP-1 Cells Reduces Complement Activation

Since we found that FH interacts directly with human peripheral blood cells and because activation of complement is known to play a role in the induction and progression of atherosclerosis (37) we next studied whether FH binding to macrophages and cholesterol-loaded macrophages could have effect on local complement activation. To study this, we used THP-1 monocytes stimulated with PMA and acetyl LDL as model cells of early stage atherosclerosis. To avoid measuring FH binding to damaged cells the viability was determined using Trypan blue staining. These cell populations had cell viability of approximately 70%. When THP-1 monocytes, THP-1 macrophages and acLDL (i.e., cholesterol) loaded THP-1 macrophages were studied for NT647-FH binding in the absence of serum, a significant increase in FH binding was detected on activated cholesterol loaded THP-1 macrophages compared to THP-1 monocytes (**Figure 4A**). When the cells were incubated with NT647-FH in the presence of 20% serum a similar trend in FH binding could be detected indicating that the increase in FH binding due to THP-1 activation is independent from surface C3b deposition. Both THP-1 macrophages and cholesterol loaded macrophages showed a significant increase in FH binding compared to THP-1 monocytes (**Figures 4A,B**). To study whether increased FH binding to these cells has functional significance in reducing local complement activation, the serum incubated cells were also analyzed for C3b deposition. Surprisingly, preincubation of THP-1 cells in the presence of FH showed a clear reduction in cell surface C3b deposition only in the case of THP-1 macrophages (**Figure 4C**). Incubation of THP-1 monocytes or cholesterol-loaded THP-1 cells in 20% serum did not lead to an increase in cell surface C3b deposition. Therefore, the presence of additional FH had an effect on the cell targeted complement activity only on THP-1 macrophages.

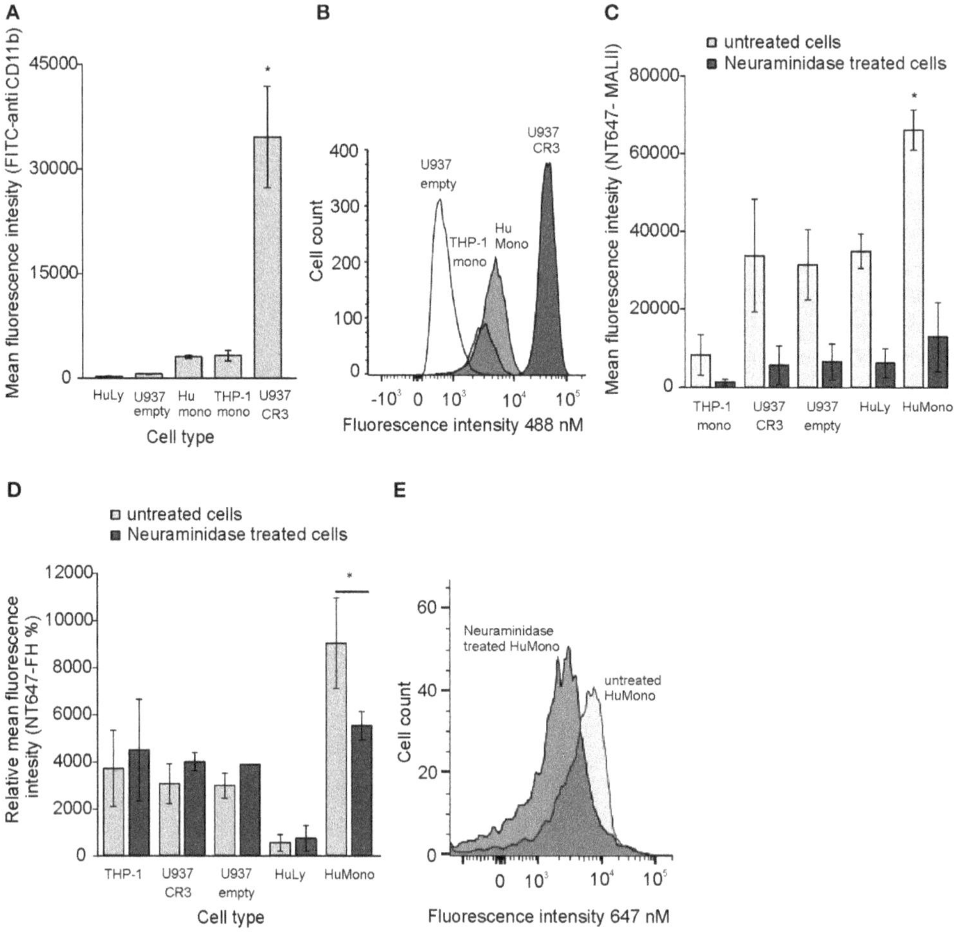

FIGURE 3 | CR3 and sialic acid expression and FH binding to neuraminidase treated cells. **(A)** The expression of CR3 in different cell types was tested using fluorescent labeled anti-CD11b antibody and flow cytometric analysis ($n = 4$). **(B)** Histogram showing distribution of CR3 receptors in different cell types. **(C)** Binding of NT647 labeled Maackia amurensis lectin I (MAL II) to cell surface sialic acids in the presence or absence of 100 U neuraminidase ($n = 3$). **(D)** Binding of NT647 labeled FH on cell surface sialic acids in the presence or absence of 100 U neuraminidase ($n = 3$). **(E)** Binding of NT647 labeled FH on monocyte surface sialic acids in the presence or absence of 100 U neuraminidase presented in a histogram. Percentages of mean fluorescence intensities is shown as relative to the intensity of neuraminidase treated U937 cells in each individual experiment. Histogram showing binding of NT647-FH on different cell types. Statistical significance between multiple samples was calculated using one-way ANOVA supplemented with Tamhane's *post-hoc* multiple comparison test. Statistical significance between two samples was calculated using Mann-Whiney *U*-test. Error bars indicate SD. * = $p < 0.05$.

FH Increases apoE Binding to THP-1 Cells and Macrophage-Mediated Cholesterol Efflux

We used anti-apoE antibody to detect surface bound apoE on THP-1 cells incubated with or without FH under cell culture conditions. Similarly to the human peripheral monocytes apoE binding was detected to activated THP-1 cells from which cholesterol loaded THP-1 macrophages demonstrated significant increase in apoE binding in the presence of FH, while binding of apoE on THP-1 monocytes was low (**Figure 5A**). This correlated well with the previous results, where cholesterol loading of the cells resulted in most significant FH binding. This indicates that FH binding to THP-1 cell surfaces increases apoE binding as well. Because endogenous production of apoE by macrophages in blood vessel wall has been suggested to promote healing of atherosclerotic plaques and efficient transport of cholesterol out from the cell (17), we analyzed the amount of secreted apoE in the culture media. After a 24 h incubation apoE secretion increased significantly from activated THP-1 cells among which cholesterol-loaded THP-1 cells showed highest apoE concentrations in the culture media (**Figure 5B**). These results also correlated well with the transcriptome data obtained from the apoE mRNA sequencing performed from the isolated cells after 24 h incubation (**Figure 5C**). No difference between cells incubated either in the presence or absence of FH could be observed in apoE expression. ApoE is a good cholesterol acceptor among many other apolipoproteins having the potential to bind phospholipids ensuring cholesterol removal (38). Therefore, we next studied whether elevated apoE binding via FH to THP-1 cells could affect cholesterol efflux. Here, a significant increase in cholesterol efflux could be detected from

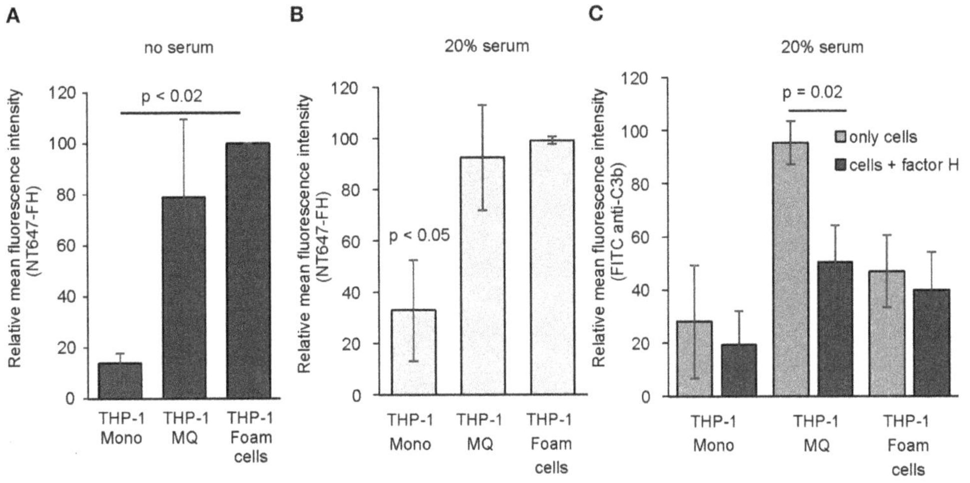

FIGURE 4 | Binding of FH and C3b deposition on THP-1 cells. Binding of NT647-labeled FH to THP-1 monocytes, THP-1 macrophages and cholesterol-loaded THP-1 macrophages (foam cells) in the **(A)** absence ($n = 3$) or **(B)** presence ($n = 3$) of 20% serum. **(C)** Deposition of serum C3b on THP-1 monocytes, THP-1 macrophages and THP-1 foam cells in the presence or absence of FH ($n = 3$). Statistical significance was calculated using using one-way ANOVA supplemented with Tamhane's *post-hoc* multiple comparison test. Error bars indicate SD. Percentages of mean fluorescence intensities are shown as relative to the maximum intensity in each individual experiment.

cholesterol-labeled THP-1 macrophages that were incubated in the presence of FH when compared to cells in the absence of FH (**Figure 5D**).

FH Increases Transcription of Anti-inflammatory Genes in Macrophages

While cholesterol loaded THP-1 macrophages showed highest apoE secretion FH did not have any effect on this. We, however, hypothesized that FH could display anti-inflammatory effects on macrophages as it interacts with both macrophages and cholesterol loaded cells, inhibits complement activity on macrophages, increases cholesterol efflux from cholesterol labeled THP-1 macrophages and increases apoE interaction with these cells as well. After 24 h incubation the THP-1 cell mRNAs were isolated and subjected to sequencing-based transcriptome analysis covering over 27,000 RNA sequences of different genes. Transcriptome analysis resulted in a selection of transcripts that are associated with inflammation, atherosclerosis and the complement system [**Table 2**, (18, 39–46)]. When these transcriptomes were compared between the FH and PBS incubated cells some clear effects/differences could be seen between THP-1 macrophages and cholesterol loaded THP-1 macrophages. As expected and based on the above FH and apoE binding assays THP-1 monocytes remained unresponsive to FH treatment. FH treatment resulted in increase of ABCA1 transcription in cholesterol loaded macrophages (foam cells) and in a significant increase in transcription of a regulator of ABCA1 expression, PPAR-α (40). Similarly, FH increased ABCA1 expression as well and correlated with the significantly increased transcription levels of the protein (**Figure 5E**). In THP-1 macrophages the expression of proinflammatory factors CX3CR1, CCL5, and SAAL1 was significantly decreased by FH. Moreover, a reduction in transcription of complement receptor C5aR2 by FH in macrophages was detected although this was not statistically significant ($p = 0.053$).

DISCUSSION

In the present study we showed that complement FH increases apoE binding to macrophages and leads to an increased cholesterol efflux and reduced inflammation. The FH/apoE interaction is hypothesized to limit the progression of atherosclerosis as complement regulation by FH is critical in the prevention self-cell damage and exacerbated inflammation.

We previously found that FH interacts with apoE and reduces complement activation in plasma HDL particles (21). The current study shows that this interaction apparently limits inflammation in the atherosclerotic lesions by affecting macrophage activation and cholesterol efflux. FH was found to interact with cell surface sialic acids and CR3 on monocytic cells in the absence of surface deposited C3b. In the presence of apoE the interaction between FH and CR3 was inhibited, while apoE had no effect on cells abundantly expressing sialic acids. In addition to CR3, our screening assay suggested that domains 5–7 of FH could also interact with CD35 (C3b/C4b receptor, CR1) and CD89. From these, CR3 and CR1 are receptors directly involved in C-mediated clearance and suppression of inflammation. We have previously shown that FH blocks binding of CR1 to C3b (47) as both molecules compete for the same binding site on C3b. Like FH, CR1 is also a C regulator and therefore should be separately analyzed for its role in C regulation during the atherosclerotic lesion development. CR1 is mostly present on cell surfaces but may also occur in soluble form. Its main function is the

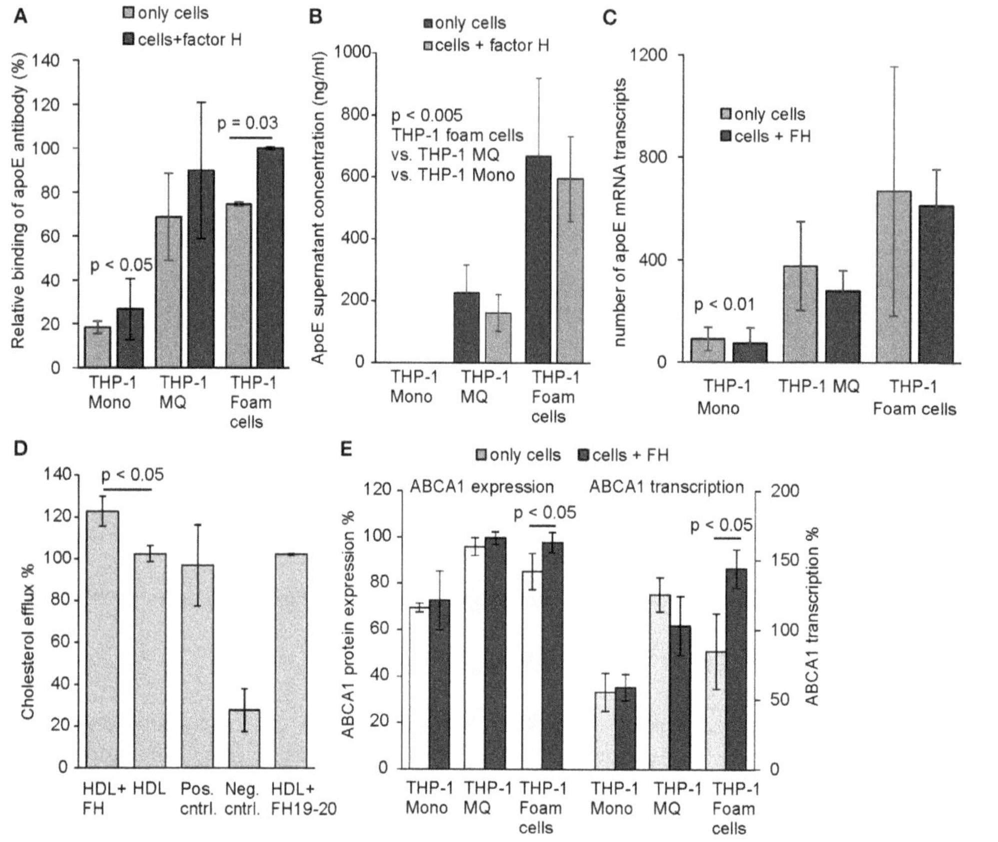

FIGURE 5 | Binding, secretion, and expression of apoE and cholesterol efflux by THP-1 cells. **(A)** Surface expression of and/or binding of apoE from culture supernatants to THP-1 monocytes, THP-1 macrophages and cholesterol-loaded THP-1 cells detected by anti-apoE antibody. Cells were incubated with and without FH for 24 h. Next, the cells were washed and detached from the tissue culture plates. Presence of apoE on cell surfaces were detected using anti-human apoE and Alexa 488 labeled goat anti-rabbit antibody in flow cytometry. ApoE binding is shown as relative to the maximum intensity in each individual experiment ($n = 3$). **(B)** Secretion of apoE to cell culture media by THP-1 monocytes, THP-1 macrophages and cholesterol-loaded THP-1 cells detected by ELISA ($n = 4$). **(C)** Number of apoE mRNA transcripts analyzed by sequencing the cell isolated mRNA ($n = 4$) **(D)** Cholesterol efflux from non-loaded THP-1 macrophages labeled with fluorescent cholesterol in the presence or absence of FH ($n = 3$). Cholesterol efflux in the presence of equal molarity of FH19-20 is shown. The positive (Pos. cntrl. from Abcam) and non HDL treated controls (Neg. cntrl.) were included in the assay. **(E)** Protein expression and transcription levels of ABCA1 in THP-1 monocytes, THP-1 macrophages and cholesterol-loaded THP-1 cells detected by anti-ABCA1 antibody and mRNA sequencing. Levels are calculated as relative to the protein expression and transcription in THP-1 macrophages ($n = 4$). Statistical significance calculated using Mann-Whiney *U*-test or one-way ANOVA supplemented with Tamhane's multiple comparison test. Error bars indicate SD.

transport of immune complexes and other unwanted materials for clearance by macrophages in the spleen and liver.

Factor H binding to cell surface C3b increases in the presence of self cell glycosaminoglycans and sialic acids. The binding of FH to CR3 has still been regarded as controversial, probably because of the possibility of C3b contamination in the sample. The novelty we show here in the regard of FH and CD11b interaction is that in the absence of C3b FH binding to CR3 expressing cells can be inhibited by apoE2 indicating a common binding site between apoE and CR3 on FH domains 5–7. Inhibition of FH binding to these cells by apoE3 and apoE4 was not that obvious indicating that the single amino acid differences (Cys and Arg in positions 112 and 158) between the apoE isotypes could alter binding to FH. Analogous differences between these isoforms have been observed earlier due to their structural variation. For instance, apoE3 and apoE4 protein isoforms bind well to LDL-receptors, whereas apoE2 displays defective binding (48). CR3 is known to interact with several ligands. A major ligand that promotes phagocytosis is iC3b on opsonised microbes and other particles. According to the mRNA expression data obtained from FH stimulated cells it is unlikely that FH could trigger CR3-mediated signaling, although a weak but not significant increase in CLEC7A (dectin-1) expression in cholesterol-loaded THP-1 macrophages could be detected in the presence of FH (**Table 2**). This C-type lectin is upregulated in anti-inflammatory M2 macrophages (49). However, earlier studies have shown that binding of FH on CD11b suppresses acute subretinal inflammation in mice indicating that FH-CR3 interaction could reduce inflammation in humans as well (50).

In contrast to the lacking inhibitory effect of apoE on FH-monocyte interaction, the presence of FH increased apoE binding to these cells significantly. This observation could be due to the

TABLE 2 | Changes in the transcriptome in response to FH in human THP-1 cells.

Immunological function	Up(+)/ down (–) regulation**	Function	Gene*	THP-1 Foam cells			THP-1 MQ			THP-1 Mono		
				FH	PBS	*p*-value	FH	PBS	*p*-value	FH	PBS	*p*-value
Anti-inflammatory	+	Nrf2 has a role in resistance to oxidant stress. Effect on atherogenesis may vary depending on the activator (39, 40)	NFE2L2	176.8	76.9	**0.013**	131.9	171.3	0.386	142.1	171.7	0.556
Antiatherogenic	+	Transporter that controls apoAI-mediated cholesterol efflux from macrophages (41)	ABCA1	832.8	555.1	**0.075**	598.9	742.6	0.270	340.4	324.7	0.835
Antiatherogenic	+	PPAR-α and PPAR-γ activators induce the expression ABCA1 (42)	PPARA	18.3	3.5	**0.032**	11.6	26.1	0.211	16.4	18.1	0.925
Clearance	+	The protein levels of RIPK1/3 are positively correlated with the extent of necroptosis (43)	RIPK1	39.8	3.5	**0.004**	20.3	43.7	0.053	25.4	9.2	0.071
Proinflammatory	±	Knockdown of SLC17A9 significantly suppres both M1-type polarization and IL-6 production (44)	SLC17A9	113.8	58.6	**0.039**	58.5	122.7	**0.033**	187.2	131.7	0.242
Proinflammatory	–	CX3CL1 is a chemokine involved in the adhesion and migration of leukocytes.	CX3CR1	0.0	3.5	0.356	0.0	13.0	**0.001**	6.8	12.4	0.633
Proinflammatory	–	CCL5 promotes macrophage recruitment and survival in human adipose tissue (45)	CCL5	32.9	32.7	0.990	5.3	27.8	**0.005**	31.1	10.1	0.145
Proinflammatory	–	promotes proliferation of fibroblasts upon inflammation (46)	SAAL1	8.8	0.0	**0.027**	1.9	16.4	**0.006**	3.8	2.0	0.618
Proinflammatory	+	receptor for IL-3 IL-5 GMCSF	CSF2RB	29.4	0.0	**0.000**	22.2	14.8	0.614	17.4	22.1	0.789
Proinflammatory	~	Binds C5a, involved in coronary artery disease and in pathogenesis of sepsis (18)	C5AR2	400.1	267.2	0.114	438.1	612.9	**0.053**	115.0	132.5	0.684
	No effect	Binds C5a	C5AR1	193.3	215.6	0.564	158.9	142.5	0.779	47.1	24.2	0.273
	No effect	apolipoprotein E	APOE	669.2	611.6	0.828	375.9	278.4	0.415	90.8	74.6	0.684
	No effect	factor H	CFH	0.0	0.0		0.0	5.1	0.214	0.0	0.0	

**Panel of genes known to play a role in inflammation or atherosclerosis with the description of their function in inflammation. The numbers show the amount of mRNA transcripts (=mRNA expression level). **Up- and downregulation marked as + and – and filled with dark or light gray colors, respectively. Statistical significance (p-values < 0.05 marked in bold numbers) calculated between cells incubated with or without FH using Student's t-test. Gray numbers = no statistical significance between FH and PBS treated cells.*

high abundance of sialic acids and low expression levels of CR3 on these cells. Sialic acids favor FH binding to the cell surface via domains 19–20 enabling simultaneous interaction with apoE via domains 5–7. The effect of sialic acids on FH binding was demonstrated by neuraminidase treatment of different cell types, where only monocytes showed a clear reduction in FH binding at different cell surface sialic acid densities. Moreover, binding of FH on THP-1 macrophages clearly reduced C3b deposition on these cells suggesting that FH binding to these cells prior to C3b deposition has an effect on local complement activation. As demonstrated by our mRNA expression data, FH expression on all THP-1 cell types was almost or completely absent, while apoE expression was clearly increased both by THP-1 macrophages and cholesterol-loaded cells.

We observed that FH did not induce secretion or expression of apoE by the studied cells but slightly reduced apoE concentrations in the culture media. However, FH significantly increased binding of apoE especially to cholesterol-loaded THP-1 cells that also showed the highest FH binding. According to trypan blue staining the increase in FH binding was not due to cell damage as the cell viabilities were the same in the absence and presence of FH. It is possible that this kind of rebinding or apoE capturing on the macrophage surfaces could promote apoE recycling that has been suggested to reduce intracellular

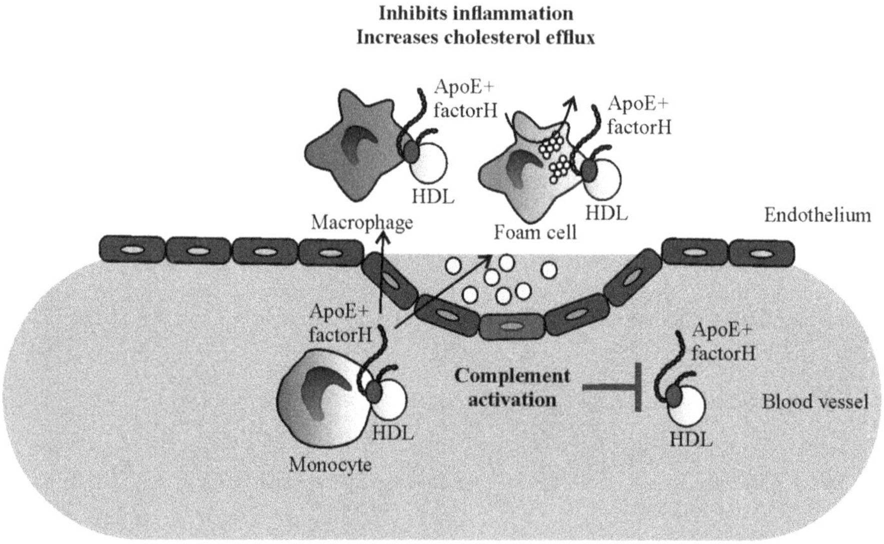

FIGURE 6 | Schematic illustrating the putative mechanism of the effect of factor H-apoE interaction in reducing inflammation in atherosclerotic lesions. Binding of factor H on apoE containing HDL particles reduces plasma complement activation (21) while elevated binding of apoE on monocytes/macrophages/foam cells via FH might reduce local inflammation and cholesterol efflux.

cholesterol accumulation and thereby prevent formation of foam cells. Previous studies have shown that apoE can be spared from degradation in lysosomes and recycled to the cell surface in order to maximize cholesterol removal from the cell (41). The intracellular ATP binding cassette transporter ABCA1 is an important regulator of cellular cholesterol homeostasis. It is involved in apoE secretion and in lipidating apoE-containing particles secreted by macrophages. ABCA1 is suggested to promote apoE recycling as well. Our results on the effect of FH on cholesterol efflux suggest that the increased binding of apoE caused by FH could promote apoE recycling and thereby maximize cholesterol efflux from macrophages. Importantly, the mRNA expression data showed increase in ABCA1 expression on FH-treated cholesterol-loaded THP-1 macrophages and a significant increase in the expression of PPAR-α transcription factor that is known to induce ABCA1 expression. This clearly suggests an anti-atherogenic function for FH-apoE interaction (42).

We found that treatment of THP-1 cells for 24 h clearly altered transcription of several genes associated with inflammation, atherosclerosis, and the complement system (**Table 2**). These changes occurred mainly within PMA-differentiated THP-1 macrophages and cholesterol loaded THP-1 macrophages while THP-1 monocytes as well as non-loaded THP-1 macrophages were less responsive to the treatment. These data did not suggest any clear M1/M2 polarization but general trend was that FH reduced significantly transcription of proinflammatory genes in macrophages (such as CXCR3, CCL5, SAAL1) but increased transcription of antiatherogenic genes that are involved in enhanced lipid metabolism (such as ABCA1, PPAR-α) mainly in cholesterol loaded cells. FH did not only result in increase in transcription of ABCA1 in cholesterol loaded macrophages but also in ABCA1 protein expression and PPAR-α transcription. This indicates that FH may affect in macrophage cholesterol efflux via this transcription factor known to activate ABCA1-mediated cholesterol efflux in human macrophages (42). Therefore, the difference between the transcription levels cannot be explained by the instability of mRNA transcripts that does not always correlate with the corresponding levels of protein expression (51).

Certain mutations and polymorphisms of FH are associated with AP dysregulation mediated diseases such as AMD, DDD, and aHUS. AMD and DDD are characterized by formation of deposits in the eye (drusen) or kidney (glomerular basement membrane) that are rich in complement activation products and, most importantly, also contain high amounts of apoE (52, 53). Therefore, in addition to atherosclerosis the pathogenesis of diseases such as AMD and DDD could be related to the FH and apoE-macrophage interactions. While FH interaction with apoE launches a concerted action leading to several anti-inflammatory responses on macrophages (**Figure 6**) genetic or acquired disturbances in this homeostatic mechanism could promote the progression of atherosclerotic and other analogous lesions.

AUTHOR CONTRIBUTIONS

EN helped in data interpretation and manuscript evaluation, wrote the paper, and performed analysis. PH, KL, AR, SS, and JM performed analysis. JvS, KVK, CDH, and PS contributed data or analysis tools. KÖ, MJ, AC, SM, and SJ helped in data interpretation, helped to evaluate and edit the manuscript, contributed data or analysis tools. KH supervised development of work, helped in data interpretation and manuscript evaluation, designed the analysis, wrote the paper, and performed analysis.

FUNDING

The work was supported by The Finnish Cultural Foundation (KH), Jane and Aatos Erkko Foundation (to MJ and JM) and Sigrid Juselius Foundation.

ACKNOWLEDGMENTS

We thank Bachelor student Mikael Gromyko for excellent technical assistance.

REFERENCES

1. Pangburn MK, Schreiber RD, Müller-Eberhard HJ. Formation of the initial C3 convertase of the alternative complement pathway. acquisition of C3b-like activities by spontaneous hydrolysis of the putative thioester in native C3. *J Exp Med.* (1981) 154:856–67.
2. Meri S, Koistinen V, Miettinen A, Tornroth T, Seppala IJ. Activation of the alternative pathway of complement by monoclonal lambda light chains in membranoproliferative glomerulonephritis. *J Exp Med.* (1992) 175:939–50. doi: 10.1084/jem.175.4.939
3. Jokiranta TS, Solomon A, Pangburn MK, Zipfel PF, Meri S. Nephritogenic lambda light chain dimer: a unique human miniautoantibody against complement factor H. *J Immunol.* (1999) 163:4590–6.
4. Pangburn MK. Cutting edge: localization of the host recognition functions of complement factor H at the carboxyl-terminal: implications for hemolytic uremic syndrome. *J Immunol.* (2002) 169:4702–6. doi: 10.4049/jimmunol.169.9.4702
5. Kajander T, Lehtinen MJ, Hyvarinen S, Bhattacharjee A, Leung E, Isenman DE, et al. Dual interaction of factor H with C3d and glycosaminoglycans in host-nonhost discrimination by complement. *Proc Natl Acad Sci USA.* (2011) 108:2897–902. doi: 10.1073/pnas.1017087108
6. Blackmore TK, Sadlon TA, Ward HM, Lublin DM, Gordon DL. Identification of a heparin binding domain in the seventh short consensus repeat of complement factor H. *J Immunol.* (1996) 157:5422–7.
7. Giannakis E, Jokiranta TS, Male DA, Ranganathan S, Ormsby RJ, Fischetti VA, et al. A common site within factor H SCR 7 responsible for binding heparin, C-reactive protein and streptococcal M protein. *Eur J Immunol.* (2003) 33:962–9. doi: 10.1002/eji.200323541
8. Pangburn MK, Schreiber RD, Muller-Eberhard HJ. Human complement C3b inactivator: isolation, characterization, and demonstration of an absolute requirement for the serum protein beta1H for cleavage of C3b and C4b in solution. *J Exp Med.* (1977) 146:257–70. doi: 10.1084/jem.146.1.257
9. Pangburn MK, Müller-Eberhard HJ. Complement C3 convertase: cell surface restriction of beta1H control and generation of restriction on neuraminidase-treated cells. *Proc Natl Acad Sci USA.* (1978) 75:2416–20.
10. Weiler JM, Daha MR, Austen KF, Fearon DT. Control of the amplification convertase of complement by the plasma protein beta1H. *Proc Natl Acad Sci USA.* (1976) 73:3268–72. doi: 10.1073/pnas.73.9.3268
11. Ramadass M, Ghebrehiwet B, Smith RJ, Kew RR. Generation of multiple fluid-phase C3b:plasma protein complexes during complement activation: possible implications in C3 glomerulopathies. *J Immunol.* (2014) 192:1220–30. doi: 10.4049/jimmunol.1302288
12. Richards A, Buddles MR, Donne RL, Kaplan BS, Kirk E, Venning MC, et al. Factor H mutations in hemolytic uremic syndrome cluster in exons 18-20, a domain important for host cell recognition. *Am J Hum Genet.* (2001) 68:485–90. doi: 10.1086/318203
13. Hageman GS, Anderson DH, Johnson LV, Hancox LS, Taiber AJ, Hardisty LI, et al. A common haplotype in the complement regulatory gene factor H (HF1/CFH) predisposes individuals to age-related macular degeneration. *Proc Natl Acad Sci USA.* (2005) 102:7227–32. doi: 10.1073/pnas.0501536102
14. Abrera-Abeleda MA, Nishimura C, Smith JL, Sethi S, McRae JL, Murphy BF, et al. Variations in the complement regulatory genes factor H (CFH) and factor H related 5 (CFHR5) are associated with membranoproliferative glomerulonephritis type II (dense deposit disease). *J Med Genet* (2006) 43:582–9. doi: 10.1136/jmg.2005.038315
15. Moriya J. Critical roles of inflammation in atherosclerosis. *J Cardiol.* (2018) S0914-5087(18)30145-X. doi: 10.1016/j.jjcc.2018.05.010
16. Hansson GK, Robertson AK, Soderberg-Naucler C. Inflammation and atherosclerosis. *Annu Rev Pathol.* (2006) 1:297–329. doi: 10.1146/annurev.pathol.1.110304.100100
17. Braesch-Andersen S, Paulie S, Smedman C, Mia S, Kumagai-Braesch M. ApoE production in human monocytes and its regulation by inflammatory cytokines. *PLoS ONE* (2013) 8:e79908. doi: 10.1371/journal.pone.0079908
18. Zhang T, Garstka MA Li K. The controversial C5a receptor C5aR2: its role in health and disease. *J Immunol Res.* (2017) 2017:8193932. doi: 10.1155/2017/8193932
19. Morton AM, Koch M, Mendivil CO, Furtado JD, Tjonneland A, Overvad K, et al. Apolipoproteins E and CIII interact to regulate HDL metabolism and coronary heart disease risk. *JCI Insight* (2018) 3:98045. doi: 10.1172/jci.insight.98045
20. Shaw PX, Zhang L, Zhang M, Du H, Zhao L, Lee C, et al. Complement factor H genotypes impact risk of age-related macular degeneration by interaction with oxidized phospholipids. *Proc Natl Acad Sci USA.* (2012) 109:13757–62. doi: 10.1073/pnas.1121309109
21. Haapasalo K, van Kessel K, Nissila E, Metso J, Johansson T, Miettinen S, et al. Complement factor H binds to human serum apolipoprotein E and mediates complement regulation on high density lipoprotein particles. *J Biol Chem.* (2015) 290:28977–87. doi: 10.1074/jbc.M115.669226
22. Haapasalo K, Jarva H, Siljander T, Tewodros W, Vuopio-Varkila J, Jokiranta TS. Complement factor H allotype 402H is associated with increased C3b opsonization and phagocytosis of Streptococcus pyogenes. *Mol Microbiol.* (2008) 70:583–94. doi: 10.1111/j.1365-2958.2008.06347.x
23. Jarva H, Janulczyk R, Hellwage J, Zipfel PF, Bjorck L, Meri S. *Streptococcus pneumoniae* evades complement attack and opsonophagocytosis by expressing the pspC locus-encoded Hic protein that binds to short consensus repeats 8-11 of factor H. *J Immunol.* (2002) 168:1886–94. doi: 10.4049/jimmunol.168.4.1886
24. Argyri L, Skamnaki V, Stratikos E, Chroni A. A simple approach for human recombinant apolipoprotein E4 expression and purification. *Protein Expr Purif.* (2011) 79:251–7. doi: 10.1016/j.pep.2011.06.011
25. Georgiadou D, Stamatakis K, Efthimiadou EK, Kordas G, Gantz D, Chroni A, et al. Thermodynamic and structural destabilization of apoE3 by hereditary mutations associated with the development of lipoprotein glomerulopathy. *J Lipid Res.* (2013) 54:164–76. doi: 10.1194/jlr.M030965
26. Dafnis I, Argyri L, Sagnou M, Tzinia A, Tsilibary EC, Stratikos E, et al. The ability of apolipoprotein E fragments to promote intraneuronal accumulation of amyloid beta peptide 42 is both isoform and size-specific. *Sci Rep.* (2016) 6:30654. doi: 10.1038/srep30654
27. Havel RJ, Eder HA, Bragdon JH. The distribution and chemical composition of ultracentrifugally separated lipoproteins in human serum. *J Clin Invest.* (1955) 34:1345–53. doi: 10.1172/JCI103182
28. Basu SK, Goldstein JL, Anderson GW, Brown MS. Degradation of cationized low density lipoprotein and regulation of cholesterol metabolism in homozygous familial hypercholesterolemia fibroblasts. *Proc Natl Acad Sci USA.* (1976) 73:3178–82. doi: 10.1073/pnas.73.9.3178
29. Tromp AT, Van Gent M, Abrial P, Martin A, Jansen JP, De Haas CJC, et al. Human CD45 is an F-component-specific receptor for the staphylococcal toxin Panton-Valentine leukocidin. *Nat Microbiol.* (2018) 2018:159. doi: 10.1038/s41564-018-0159-x
30. van de Weijer ML, Bassik MC, Luteijn RD, Voorburg CM, Lohuis MA, Kremmer E, et al. A high-coverage shRNA screen identifies TMEM129 as an

E3 ligase involved in ER-associated protein degradation. *Nat Commun.* (2014) 5:3832 doi: 10.1038/ncomms4832
31. Siggins S, Jauhiainen M, Olkkonen VM, Tenhunen J, Ehnholm C. PLTP secreted by HepG2 cells resembles the high-activity PLTP form in human plasma. *J Lipid Res.* (2003) 44:1698–704. doi: 10.1194/jlr.M300059-JLR200
32. Macosko EZ, Basu A, Satija R, Nemesh J, Shekhar K, Goldman M, et al. Highly parallel genome-wide expression profiling of individual cells using nanoliter droplets. *Cell* (2015) 161:1202–14. doi: 10.1016/j.cell.2015.05.002
33. Dobin A, Davis CA, Schlesinger F, Drenkow J, Zaleski C, Jha S, et al. STAR: ultrafast universal RNA-seq aligner. *Bioinformatics* (2013) 29:15–21. doi: 10.1093/bioinformatics/bts635
34. Hyvarinen S, Meri S, Jokiranta TS. Disturbed sialic acid recognition on endothelial cells and platelets in complement attack causes atypical hemolytic uremic syndrome. *Blood* (2016) 127:2701–10. doi: 10.1182/blood-2015-11-680009
35. Avery VM, Gordon DL. Characterization of factor H binding to human polymorphonuclear leukocytes. *J Immunol.* (1993) 151:5545–53.
36. Zuckerman SH, Evans GF, O'Neal L. Cytokine regulation of macrophage apo E secretion: opposing effects of GM-CSF and TGF-beta. *Atherosclerosis* (1992) 96:203–14. doi: 10.1016/0021-9150(92)90066-P
37. Vlaicu SI, Tatomir A, Rus V, Mekala AP, Mircea PA, Niculescu F, et al. The role of complement activation in atherogenesis: the first 40 years. *Immunol Res.* (2016) 64:1–13. doi: 10.1007/s12026-015-8669-6
38. Kockx M, Rye KA, Gaus K, Quinn CM, Wright J, Sloane T, et al. Apolipoprotein A-I-stimulated apolipoprotein E secretion from human macrophages is independent of cholesterol efflux. *J Biol Chem.* (2004) 279:25966–77. doi: 10.1074/jbc.M401177200
39. Ma Q. Role of nrf2 in oxidative stress and toxicity. *Annu Rev Pharmacol Toxicol.* (2013) 53:401–26. doi: 10.1146/annurev-pharmtox-011112-1 40320
40. Ruotsalainen AK, Lappalainen JP, Heiskanen E, Merentie M, Sihvola V, Napankangas J, et al. Nrf2 deficiency impairs atherosclerotic lesion development but promotes features of plaque instability in hypercholesterolemic mice. *Cardiovasc Res.* (2018) 2018:143. doi: 10.1093/cvr/cvy143
41. Hasty AH, Plummer MR, Weisgraber KH, Linton MF, Fazio S, Swift LL. The recycling of apolipoprotein E in macrophages: influence of HDL and apolipoprotein A-I. *J Lipid Res.* (2005) 46:1433–9. doi: 10.1194/jlr.M400418-JLR200
42. Chinetti G, Lestavel S, Bocher V, Remaley AT, Neve B, Torra IP, et al. PPAR-alpha and PPAR-gamma activators induce cholesterol removal from human macrophage foam cells through stimulation of the ABCA1 pathway. *Nat Med.* (2001) 7:53–8. doi: 10.1038/83348
43. Najjar M, Saleh D, Zelic M, Nogusa S, Shah S, Tai A, et al. RIPK1 and RIPK3 Kinases Promote Cell-Death-Independent Inflammation by Toll-like Receptor 4. *Immunity* (2016) 45:46–59. doi: 10.1016/j.immuni.2016.06.007
44. Sakaki H, Tsukimoto M, Harada H, Moriyama Y, Kojima S. Autocrine regulation of macrophage activation via exocytosis of ATP and activation of P2Y11 receptor. *PLoS ONE* (2013) 8:e59778. doi: 10.1371/journal.pone.0059778
45. Keophiphath M, Rouault C, Divoux A, Clement K, Lacasa D. CCL5 promotes macrophage recruitment and survival in human adipose tissue. *Arteriosclerosis Thrombosis Vasc Biol.* (2010) 30:39–45. doi: 10.1161/ATVBAHA.109.197442
46. Sato T, Fujii R, Konomi K, Yagishita N, Aratani S, Araya N, et al. Overexpression of SPACIA1/SAAL1, a newly identified gene that is involved in synoviocyte proliferation, accelerates the progression of synovitis in mice and humans. *Arthritis Rheum.* (2011) 63:3833–42. doi: 10.1002/art.30617
47. Amdahl H, Haapasalo K, Tan L, Meri T, Kuusela PI, van Strijp JA, et al. Staphylococcal protein Ecb impairs complement receptor-1 mediated recognition of opsonized bacteria. *PLoS ONE* (2017) 12:e0172675. doi: 10.1371/journal.pone.0172675
48. Mahley RW, Weisgraber KH, Huang Y. Apolipoprotein E: structure determines function, from atherosclerosis to Alzheimer's disease to AIDS. *J Lipid Res.* (2009) 50(Suppl):S183–8. doi: 10.1194/jlr.R800069-JLR200
49. Martinez FO, Helming L, Gordon S. Alternative activation of macrophages: an immunologic functional perspective. *Annu Rev Immunol.* (2009) 27:451–83. doi: 10.1146/annurev.immunol.021908.132532
50. Calippe B, Augustin S, Beguier F, Charles-Messance H, Poupel L, Conart JB, et al. Complement factor H inhibits CD47-mediated resolution of inflammation. *Immunity* (2017) 46:261–72. doi: 10.1016/j.immuni.2017.01.006
51. Vogel C, Marcotte EM. Insights into the regulation of protein abundance from proteomic and transcriptomic analyses. *Nat Rev Genet.* (2012) 13:227–32. doi: 10.1038/nrg3185
52. Sethi S, Gamez JD, Vrana JA, Theis JD, Bergen HR III, Zipfel PF, et al. Glomeruli of Dense Deposit Disease contain components of the alternative and terminal complement pathway. *Kidney Int.* (2009) 75:952–60. doi: 10.1038/ki.2008.657
53. Johnson LV, Forest DL, Banna CD, Radeke CM, Maloney MA, Hu J, et al. Cell culture model that mimics drusen formation and triggers complement activation associated with age-related macular degeneration. *Proc Natl Acad Sci USA.* (2011) 108:18277–82. doi: 10.1073/pnas.1109703108

2

Complement Component C1q as Serum Biomarker to Detect Active Tuberculosis

Rosalie Lubbers[1], Jayne S. Sutherland[2], Delia Goletti[3], Roelof A. de Paus[4], Coline H. M. van Moorsel[5], Marcel Veltkamp[5], Stefan M. T. Vestjens[6], Willem J. W. Bos[6,7], Linda Petrone[3], Franca Del Nonno[8], Ingeborg M. Bajema[9], Karin Dijkman[10], Frank A. W. Verreck[10], Gerhard Walzl[11], Kyra A. Gelderman[12], Geert H. Groeneveld[4], Annemieke Geluk[4], Tom H. M. Ottenhoff[4], Simone A. Joosten[4†] and Leendert A. Trouw[13†]*

[1] Department of Rheumatology, Leiden University Medical Center, Leiden, Netherlands, [2] Medical Research Council Unit The Gambia at the London School of Hygiene and Tropical Medicine, Banjul, Gambia, [3] Translational Research Unit, Department of Epidemiology and Preclinical Research, National Institute for Infectious Diseases, Rome, Italy, [4] Department of Infectious Diseases, Leiden University Medical Center, Leiden, Netherlands, [5] Department of Pulmonology, St. Antonius Hospital Nieuwegein, Nieuwegein, Netherlands, [6] Department of Internal Medicine, St. Antonius Hospital Nieuwegein, Nieuwegein, Netherlands, [7] Department of Nephrology, Leiden University Medical Center, Leiden, Netherlands, [8] Pathology Service, National Institute for Infectious Diseases, Rome, Italy, [9] Department of Pathology, Leiden University Medical Center, Leiden, Netherlands, [10] Section of TB Research & Immunology, Biomedical Primate Research Centre, Rijswijk, Netherlands, [11] Division of Molecular Biology and Human Genetics, Faculty of Medicine and Health Sciences, DST/NRF Centre of Excellence for Biomedical Tuberculosis Research, South African Medical Research Council Centre for Tuberculosis Research, Stellenbosch University, Cape Town, South Africa, [12] Sanquin Diagnostic Services, Amsterdam, Netherlands, [13] Department of Immunohematology and Blood Transfusion, Leiden University Medical Center, Leiden, Netherlands

***Correspondence:**
Simone A. Joosten
s.a.joosten@lumc.nl

† These authors have contributed equally to this work

Background: Tuberculosis (TB) remains a major threat to global health. Currently, diagnosis of active TB is hampered by the lack of specific biomarkers that discriminate active TB disease from other (lung) diseases or latent TB infection (LTBI). Integrated human gene expression results have shown that genes encoding complement components, in particular different C1q chains, were expressed at higher levels in active TB compared to LTBI.

Methods: C1q protein levels were determined using ELISA in sera from patients, from geographically distinct populations, with active TB, LTBI as well as disease controls.

Results: Serum levels of C1q were increased in active TB compared to LTBI in four independent cohorts with an AUC of 0.77 [0.70; 0.83]. After 6 months of TB treatment, levels of C1q were similar to those of endemic controls, indicating an association with disease rather than individual genetic predisposition. Importantly, C1q levels in sera of TB patients were significantly higher as compared to patients with sarcoidosis or pneumonia, clinically important differential diagnoses. Moreover, exposure to other mycobacteria, such as *Mycobacterium leprae* (leprosy patients) or BCG (vaccinees) did not result in elevated levels of serum C1q. In agreement with the human data, in non-human primates challenged with *Mycobacterium tuberculosis*, increased serum C1q levels were detected in animals that developed progressive disease, not in those that controlled the infection.

Conclusions: In summary, C1q levels are elevated in patients with active TB compared to LTBI in four independent cohorts. Furthermore, C1q levels from patients with TB were also elevated compared to patients with sarcoidosis, leprosy and pneumonia. Additionally, also in NHP we observed increased C1q levels in animals with active progressive TB, both in serum and in broncho-alveolar lavage. Therefore, we propose that the addition of C1q to current biomarker panels may provide added value in the diagnosis of active TB.

Keywords: complement, tuberculosis, C1q, infection, innate immunity, blood, mycobacterium

INTRODUCTION

Tuberculosis (TB) is a major global health threat, which is caused by infection by *Mycobacterium tuberculosis* (*M.tb*) (1). Current estimations indicate that a quarter of the global population is infected with *M.tb*, with a life-long risk to develop active TB disease. Particular regions, such as South-East Asia, Western-Pacific, and Africa regions account for more than 80% of infected individuals (2). Annually over 6 million people are diagnosed with TB disease, a serious and highly contagious condition, resulting in 1.3 million deaths in 2016 only (1). While most infected individuals remain asymptomatic latently infected (LTBI), a minority (5–10%) of these individuals progress to active TB. Given the high rate of infections with *M.tb* in some regions it is important to discriminate infection from disease, which is difficult with the currently available tests. At present, only *M.tb* detection in sputum using smear, PCR or culture is definitive proof of TB disease. Early diagnosis and treatment of TB disease is important to reduce transmission of infection and prevent disease associated mortality (1).

Diagnosis of active TB is made by microbiological or genetic detection of *M.tb* in sputum (or other specimens in case of extrapulmonary TB), but this can be expensive and time-consuming depending on bacterial burdens or requires complex methodology and infrastructure. Current immunological tests can detect infection with *M.tb* but often fail to discriminate active disease from latent infection (3). Therefore, there is an urgent need to identify biomarkers that can discriminate active and latent TB infection in order to promptly initiate treatment to prevent mortality and further spread of the pathogen, in particular in areas where *M.tb* is highly endemic. Ideally, such biomarkers should also be able to discriminate between TB and other respiratory infections that present with similar symptoms and abnormalities on chest X-rays.

Many studies have identified potential biomarkers that discriminate active TB from LTBI, or that are predictive of which individuals will progress to active TB (4–10). Differential gene expression profiles between patients with TB and LTBI or other (lung) diseases resulted in identification of an array of potential biomarkers, such as *FCGR1A* (11–13) and *GBP5* (5, 6, 14). Recently, complement has been highlighted as candidate biomarker for active TB disease (15–19) also in the presence of HIV co-infection (20). Most currently identified biomarkers have been identified at the transcriptomic level; however, easy, robust markers that can be measured at the protein level would be more ideal candidates for application in the field. Therefore, validation of markers previously identified at the mRNA level at the protein level would provide important insights into the applicability of such markers in clinical practice.

Next to biomarker studies in humans, there are various experimental models to study the host-pathogen interaction. The best available model is the non-human primate model (NHP), infection of rhesus macaques with *M.tb*, resulted in TB disease which closely resembles human TB as they experience similar lesions and clinical courses as humans, suggesting a common pathophysiology (21). The NHP model adds important information on kinetics of disease development following *M.tb* infection and can be manipulated with e.g., different dosages of infection, different infecting strains, but also with vaccines.

The complement system is an important part of the innate immune system and functions as a proteolytic cascade. The classical complement pathway is initiated by binding of C1q to ligands, such as immune complexes. Following the binding of C1q to ligands, enzymatic processes lead to the release of inflammation stimulating peptides, C3a and C5a, formation of the opsonin C3b and formation of the membrane attack complex, resulting in target cell lysis (22). Furthermore, C1q can bind several receptors that contribute to other important functions, such as phagocytosis or myeloid cell modulation, outside traditional complement system activation (23, 24). For instance, C1q is involved in neovascularization during pregnancy, coagulation processes and neurological synapse function (25). C1q is a 480 kDa protein composed of six arms, each comprising one A, B and C peptide chain (26). These three chains are encoded by individual genes, *C1QA*, *C1QB*, and *C1QC*, located on chromosome 1p. In contrast to most complement proteins, C1q is not produced by hepatocytes but mainly by monocyte derived cells, such as macrophages and immature dendritic cells (27–29) and by mast cells (30). Increased expression of mRNA for C1q has been associated with TB disease (16, 19).

Here, we analyzed differential expression of complement genes in patients with TB. Since in publicly available datasets, C1q expression was most pronouncedly upregulated, we validated C1q at the protein level in samples from various patient groups as a biomarker for active TB. Patients with active TB disease were compared to latently infected individuals, vaccinnees and to patients with clinical conditions that are important differential diagnoses in clinical practice. Finally, to obtain more insight in the pathophysiology, kinetic analyses were performed samples obtained from NHP animal models of TB.

MATERIALS AND METHODS

Patients and Controls

Demographic data and classification of the cohorts are presented in **Table 1**. Below we have specified the specific inclusion criteria per cohort.

Tuberculosis

Smear, GeneXpert or sputum culture positive pulmonary TB patients, LTBI patients and treated TB patients as well as endemic controls (in different combinations) were included from various demographic locations: Italy (31), the Gambia, Korea and South Africa (**Table 1**). Patients with active pulmonary TB disease, referred to as "TB" in the manuscript, were diagnosed based on local, routine methodology. Active pulmonary TB was sputum-culture confirmed (BACTEC^{TM}, Becton-Dickinson, USA), or based on positive Xpert Mtb/RIF assay (Cephaid Inc., Sunnyvale, CA, USA), patients were included within 7 days of TB treatment initiation. Latent TB infection, LTBI, was determined by Quantiferon TB Gold-in tube positivity (Qiagen, The Netherlands).

In the cohort from South Africa people suspected for TB were used as controls, these people were presenting with symptoms compatible with active TB but had negative X-ray and negative sputum cultures for TB. These suspected TB patients were seen again after 2 months and had recovered spontaneously or after appropriate (non-TB related) treatment. All TB patients were HIV-negative, as were the endemic controls. Additionally, from Italy both LTBI (QuantiFERON TB Gold-In-tube-positive individuals) and successfully treated TB patients (2–72 months after end of therapy) were included. TB patients from the Gambia were followed over time (1, 2, and 6 months after diagnosis), until completion of successful treatment.

TABLE 1 | Description of the cohorts.

Country	Classification	*N*	Age mean (range)	Sex (%male)
Italy	Control	15	38 (25–57)	40
	Latent TB	18	37 (21–77)	33
	Active TB	18	38 (23–67)	89
	Treated TB	17	39 (18–70)	35
The Gambia	Control	50	31 (15–60)	30
	Active TB	50	34 (17–62)	62
Korea	Control	10	23 (21–25)	90
	Active TB	10	51 (24–77)	40
South Africa	Suspect TB	31	32 (18–56)	26
	Active TB	20	32 (19–57)	65
Multiple*	Leprosy reactions	53	(18–69)	68
the Netherlands	Leprosy†	33	34 (18–57)	62
	Sarcoidosis	50	43 (26–57)	60
	Control	80	38 (21–67)	36
	BCG vaccinated	12	27 (23–57)	33
	Pneumonia (Leiden)	40	66 (23–93)	60
	Pneumonia (Nieuwegein)	28	73 (34–91)	57

In the table the different cohorts are described regarding the country of origin of the samples, the disease classification, and the total number of samples per group as well as the demographic info on age and sex.

**Nepal, Brasil, Ethiopia.*

†Diagnosis made in the Netherlands.

Other Mycobacterial Diseases and Vaccination

Leprosy patients (mostly immigrants with mixed ethnic backgrounds) at diagnosis of primary leprosy were included in the Netherlands. In addition, patients with type-1 reactions were enrolled in Brazil, Nepal and Ethiopia. Furthermore, we measured C1q in healthy Dutch individuals who were vaccinated with BCG Danish strain 1331 (Statens Serum Institut, Denmark) and followed over time (32).

Other Pulmonary Diseases

Patients with community acquired pneumonia were included in the Netherlands, one cohort comprised patients admitted to the intensive care unit in a tertiary care hospital in Leiden (one patient was HIV-infected with a normal CD4 count and one suffered from sarcoidosis) and the other cohort comprised patients admitted to a hospital ward of a non-academic teaching hospital in Nieuwegein. From both groups of pneumonia patients paired samples from the time of diagnosis and after recovery (10–124 days later) were available. Finally, samples were included prior to initiation of treatment from sarcoidosis patients in the Netherlands that had pulmonary involvement.

Additional Control Group

As a reference group we included a panel of Dutch healthy controls, not suffering from major infections or autoimmune disease.

Ethics Statement

Blood was obtained from individuals upon signing an informed consent. All studies comply with the Helsinki declaration. The use of the samples in this study was approved by local ethical committees. For Italy, Ethical Committee of the L. Spallanzani National Institute of Infectious diseases (02/2007 and 72/2015); The Gambia (SCC1333); Korea, Institutional Review Board for the Protection of Human Subjects at YUHS; South Africa, Health Research Ethics Committee of the Faculty of Medicine and Health Sciences at Stellenbosch University (N13/05/064); Brazil, National Council of Ethics in Research and UFU Research Ethics Committee (#499/2008); Nepal, Health Research Council (NHR#751); Ethiopia, Health Research Ethical Review committee Ethiopia (NERC#RDHE/127-83/08); The Netherlands leprosy patients, (MEC-2012-589); sarcoidosis patients, Medical research Ethics Committees United of the St Antonius (#R05.08A); BCG vaccinated individuals, Leiden University Medical Center Ethics Committee (P12.087); control group, (P237/94); pneumonia Leiden (P12.147); pneumonia Nieuwegein (C-04.03 and R07.12).

Gene Expression Analysis

Global transcriptomic analyses have been performed to compare patients with active TB disease with latently infected individuals. In addition, transcriptomes from patients with TB disease were compared with patients with other diseases, such as sarcoidosis, pneumonia or lung cancer (5–7, 33–37). Microarray data from these studies, publically available in Gene Expression Omnibus (GEO) (GSE37250, GSE19491, GSE39941, GSE28623, GSE73408, GSE34608, GSE42834, GSE83456), were retrieved from GEO and re-analyzed. Several of the studies described multiple independent cohorts, which we analyzed separately for each population [from Malawi (2), South Africa (3), United Kingdom (2), Kenya (only TB vs. LTBI), The Gambia (only TB vs. LTBI), USA and Germany (only TB vs. other diseases)]. All data were extracted from GEO and compared in the same way using GEO2R, thus not relying on the analysis performed in the original manuscript. GEO2R compared two or more groups of samples in order to identify genes that are differentially expressed across experimental or clinical conditions. Here, lists of differentially expressed genes between TB and LTBI or TB and other diseases (with a significance of $p > 0.05$ and a factorial change of >2 or <0.5) were generated. A list of complement genes and two reference genes was used to assess possible differential expression for each individual gene for each study population. All studies/populations with significant differential expression for a particular gene between patients with TB compared to LTBI/other diseases were enumerated and expressed as the percentage of the total number of comparisons investigated. E.g., differential expression of C1QA between TB and LTBI was observed in only 2/9 populations investigated (22%) whereas C1QB differed in 8/9 populations (88%). For all populations with significant differential expression, the factorial change (the difference between gene expression in TB patients compared to LTBI/other diseases) was calculated and plotted.

Animals

Non-human primate (NHP) serum was available from a biobank of samples collected from earlier TB studies in healthy, purpose-bred rhesus macaques (*Macaca mulatta*) for which ethical clearance was obtained from the independent ethical authority according to Dutch law. All housing and animal care procedures were in compliance with European directive 2010/63/EU, as well as the "Standard for Humane Care and Use of Laboratory Animals by Foreign Institutions" provided by the Department of Health and Human Services of the US National Institutes of Health (NIH, identification number A5539-01). Longitudinal banked serum samples were available for C1q analysis. Animals were non-vaccinated or vaccinated with BCG [BCG Danish 1331 (Statens Serum Institute, Denmark)] ($n = 23$) and experimentally infected via bronchoscopic instillation of 500 CFU of *M.* Erdman. Prior to infection and 3, 6, 12, 24, 36, and 52 weeks post-infection samples were collected and stored. Animals were sacrificed when reaching early humane endpoints (acute progressors) or after reaching the pre-defined end-point (52 weeks; non-progressors). Broncho-alveolar lavage (BAL) samples were available from six animals infected with 1–7 CFU of M. Erdman prior to infection and 6 or 12 weeks post-infection.

Detection of C1q by ELISA

C1q levels in sera were measured using an in-house developed ELISA. Maxisorp plates (nunc) were coated overnight with mouse anti-human C1q (2204) (38), Nephrology department, LUMC) in coating buffer (0.1 M Na_2CO_3, 0.1 M $NaHCO_3$, pH9.6). Plates were washed and blocked with PBS/1%BSA for 1 h at 37°C. After washing, a serial dilution of a pool of normal human serum (NHS) was applied as a standard and samples were added in dilution to the plate, all in duplicate, and incubated for 1 h at 37°C. Human sera were diluted 1:8,000 and NHP sera 1:4,000, the BAL fluids were diluted 1:1. After washing, plates were incubated with rabbit anti-human C1q (Dako cat#A0136) for 1 h at 37°C and for detection a goat anti-rabbit HRP (Dako cat#P0448) was used which was also incubated for 1 h at 37°C. All washing steps were performed with PBS/1%BSA/0.05%Tween. Plates were stained using ABTS and measured at absorbance of 415 nm, the measured C1q is expressed in μg/mL as compared to a C1q standard.

Immunohistochemical Staining of Lung Tissue for C1q

Samples were collected at autopsy from patients with fatal TB disease ($n = 3$), fatal pneumonia patients ($n = 4$) and a control that died of vascular disease ($n = 1$) at the National Institute for Infectious Diseases, Rome, Italy under local ethical approval (72/2015). Paraffin sections of 4 μm thickness were subjected to heat-induced antigen retrieval using tris/EDTA (pH 9.0) at 96°C for 30 min, and then stained with rabbit anti-human C1q (1:1,000; Dako cat#A0136) in PBS/1%BSA for 1 h at room temperature, followed by an anti-rabbit Envision (Dako) HRP conjugated antibody also for 1 h at room temperature, with DAB+ as the chromogen. Negative control rabbit immunoglobulin fraction (Dako) was used as a negative control in the same concentration as the primary antibody. Sections were counterstained with Haematoxylin (Klinipath; 4085.9001).

Statistics

Statistical analyses were carried out using SPSS statistics version 23 (IBM) or Graphpad Prism version 7. To compare C1q levels the Mann-Whitney U test, Kruskall-Wallis and Dunn's multiple comparisons test were used. In all graphs the median is shown unless indicated otherwise. Receiver operating characteristic (ROC) analysis was performed to assess the sensitivity and specificity of C1q as biomarker and was expressed as Area Under the Curve (AUC).

RESULTS

C1Q Expression Is Upregulated in Patients With Active TB Disease

Publically available microarray data from TB patients were retrieved from Gene Expression Omnibus, all data were ranked as differentially expressed between TB patients and either LTBI or other diseases (5, 7, 33–37). These studies contained information from diverse populations (Malawi, South Africa, United Kingdom, Kenya, The Gambia, USA, and Germany). A list of complement gene expression patterns was generated and the number of microarray studies that reported differential complement gene expression between patients with TB and LTBI (**Figure 1A**) or other diseases (**Figure 1B**) was enumerated. Complement genes *C1QB, SERPING1* were expressed at higher level (more than 2-fold) in 8/9 (88%) of studies comparing patients with active TB to LTBI (**Figure 1A**). C1QC was expressed at a higher level in TB patients in 7/9 studies (78%), whereas C1QA expression was only increased in TB patients in 2/9 studies (22%; **Figure 1A**). The observed factorial changes in the expression of these complement genes between TB patients and LTBI individuals were comparable with the changes as seen for *FCGR1A* and *GBP5*, which were previously described as promising and highly consistent biomarkers of active TB (**Figure 1C**). A similar pattern, although less pronounced, was seen when comparing TB patients with patients having another lung-disease (**Figures 1B,D**). As C1q is abundantly present, easy to measure and stable, therefore we continued to analyse C1q protein levels.

C1q Is Significantly Increased in Serum of TB Patients

C1q protein levels were measured in sera from TB patients and controls from independent and geographically distinct cohorts (**Figures 2A–D**). The levels of C1q were significantly higher in sera from patients with active TB as compared to their respective controls in all cohorts: Italy (**Figure 2A**), The Gambia (**Figure 2B**), Korea (**Figure 2C**) and South Africa (**Figure 2D**). LTBI individuals and successfully treated TB patients had serum C1q levels similar to controls (**Figure 2A**). Combined analysis of all TB patients, control groups, LTBI and the successfully treated TB patients from the different cohorts revealed that serum C1q protein levels are significantly ($p < 0.001$) increased in active TB (**Figure 2E**).

The Gambian TB patients were followed over time which allowed us to investigate C1q levels during successful treatment. At 1 month of treatment the median serum C1q level was still increased, however, the level of C1q began to decrease after 2 months ($p = 0.0650$), resulting in complete normalization compared to the TB contacts after 6 months of successful treatment ($p < 0.001$; **Figure 2F**). Thus, serum

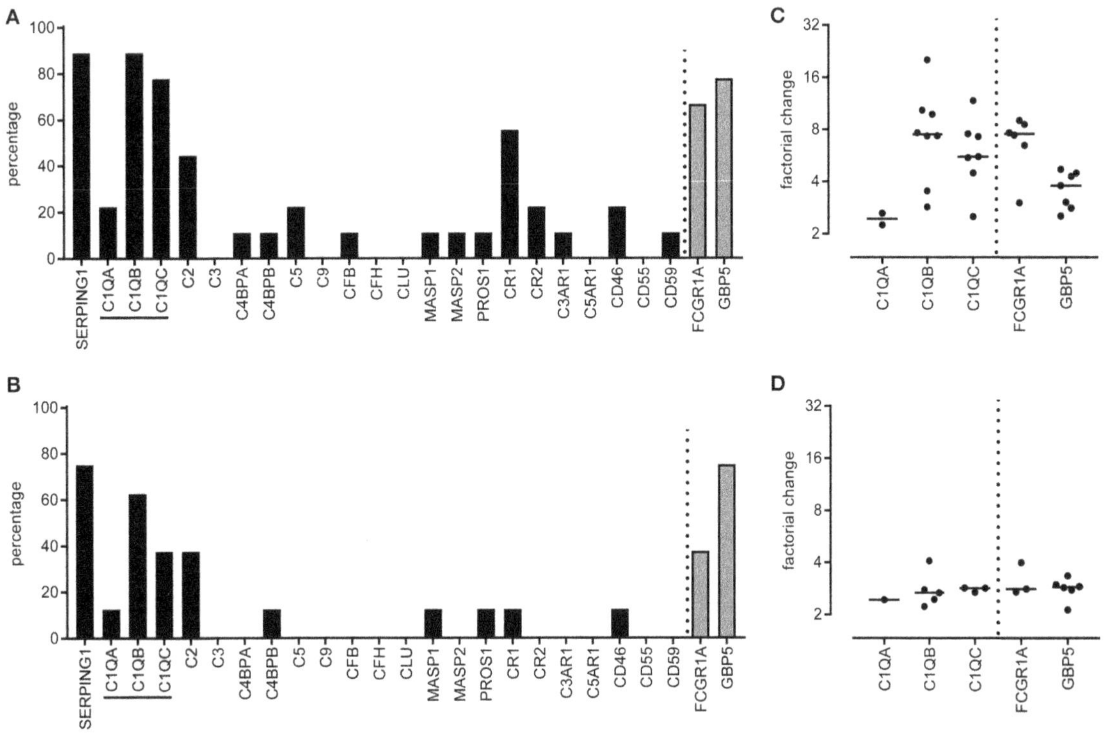

FIGURE 1 | Differentially expressed complement genes in whole blood tuberculosis transcript signatures. Tuberculosis specific transcript signatures, from various populations, were investigated for the presence of differentially expressed complement genes using a tuberculosis RNA biomarker database. Publically available transcriptome data was retrieved from Gene Expression Omnibus (5–7, 33–37) and analyzed using GEO2R. Data were available for nine populations comparing active TB with LTBI and for 8 populations comparing active TB with other diseases. For each population we determined if the complement family genes were differentially expressed between TB and LTBI or other diseases. Differential expression was defined as an adjusted *p*-value <0.05 and more than 2-fold change. Differential expression of a gene between TB and LTBI or other diseases was expressed as percentage of the total number of populations investigated. The differential expression of complement genes was scored **(A,B)** as well as the mean factorial change for the C1q genes, *C1QA, C1QB*, and *C1QC* **(C,D)** for the comparisons TB vs. LTBI **(A,C)** and TB vs. other diseases **(B,D)**. As a reference two other highly upregulated potential diagnostic TB markers, *FCGR1A*, and *GBP5*, were included in the analyses.

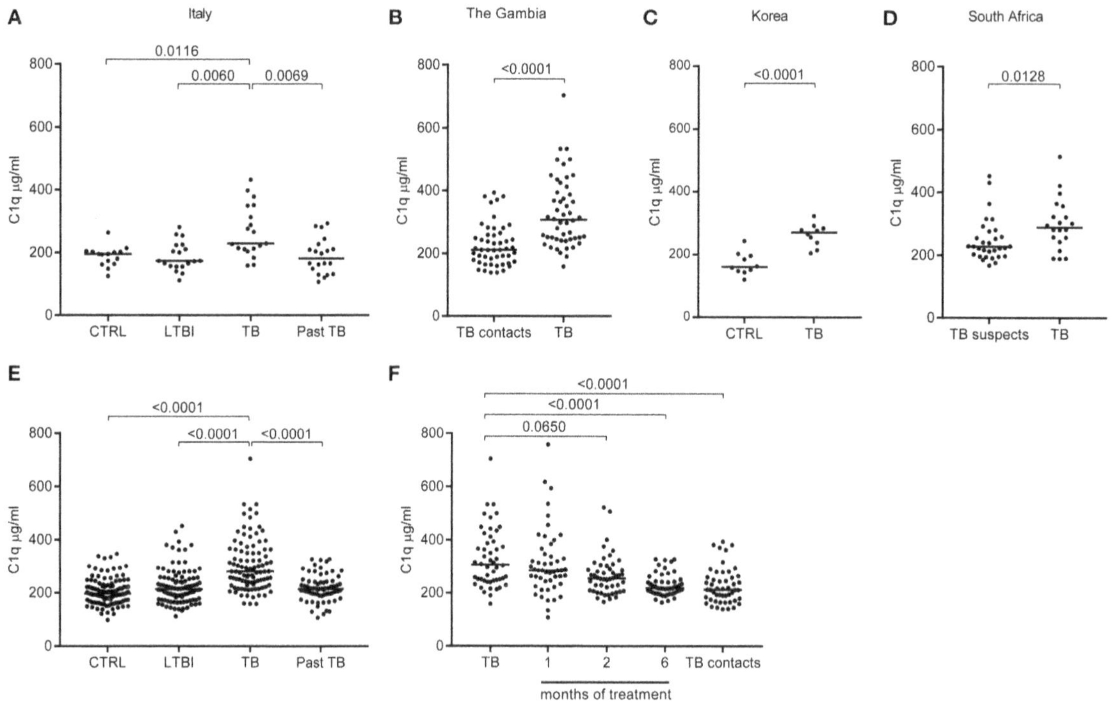

FIGURE 2 | C1q serum levels are increased in patients with pulmonary Tuberculosis. C1q levels (µg/ml) were measured with ELISA in sera from TB patients (active disease) and controls from different cohorts. First the results from the independent and geographically different cohorts are depicted. TB patients from Italy were compared to Latent TB infected (LTBI), to Past TB (patients that were successfully treated for TB) and to endemic controls **(A)**. TB patients from The Gambia were compared to TB contacts **(B)**. TB patients from Korea were compared to endemic controls **(C)**. From South Africa the TB patients were compared to patients suspected for TB but confirmed non-TB **(D)**. Subsequently, data from the cohorts were pooled: control (CTRL) comprises Dutch healthy controls, combined with the CTRL from Italy and Korea; moreover, healthy individuals prior to vaccination with BCG were included ($n = 117$). Latent TB infected (LTBI) comprises LTBI from Italy, TB suspects (confirmed non-TB) from South Africa and TB contacts from the Gambia ($n = 100$). Active tuberculosis (TB) from Italy, the Gambia, Korea and South Africa ($n = 99$); Past TB are patients that were successfully treated for TB and combined the past TB from Italy and the Gambia samples after 6 months of treatment ($n = 71$) **(E)**. From the Gambia the TB patients were followed over time during treatment, TB contacts are shown on the right ($n = 50$) **(F)**. Results were analyzed using the Mann-Whitney *U* test, >2 groups Kruskall-Wallis and Dunn's multiple comparisons test. The treatment months were compared to TB diagnosis with Friedman Test and Dunn's multiple comparisons test.

C1q protein levels were significantly elevated in patients with active TB, and levels decreased to the level of the control population during successful treatment. This further indicates that increased C1q levels are associated with active TB disease and do not reflect genetic variation in C1q expression.

Vaccination With BCG Does Not Increase C1q Levels in Serum

To investigate if vaccination with *M. bovis* BCG, a live replicating mycobacterium, induced a similar increase in serum C1q levels, samples were taken before and after BCG vaccination of healthy Dutch volunteers and C1q levels were measured (**Figure 3**). Samples taken at screening and directly before vaccination showed minimal variation in C1q levels, reflecting normal variation within individuals. BCG vaccination did not induce fluctuations in C1q levels larger than this naturally observed variation. Thus, BCG vaccination did not increase C1q levels in contrast to what was observed in TB disease, despite the presence of live, replicating mycobacteria.

C1q Levels Are Increased in Active TB Compared to Other Diseases

To investigate the specificity of increased C1q levels for active TB, sera from patients with other diseases with similar symptoms and radiological abnormalities (pneumonia, sarcoidosis) and sera from patients with other mycobacterial disease [leprosy, primary disease or type 1 (acute pro-inflammatory) reactions] were analyzed. C1q levels in sera from patients with TB were significantly higher compared to sera from patients with leprosy, pneumonia or sarcoidosis (**Figure 4A**, data from TB patients and controls same as used in **Figure 2E**). Some individual leprosy patients had C1q protein levels above the median of TB patients but this was not related to either primary disease or having type I reactions (**Supplementary Figure E1A**). Patients with sarcoidosis showed a slight increase in C1q levels compared to the controls. In contrast, patients with community acquired pneumonia showed a significant decrease in C1q levels compared to the control population. The reduced levels observed in patients with pneumonia at diagnosis was associated with the disease state since samples included from the same individuals at later time points had normal C1q levels (**Supplementary Figures E1B,C**).

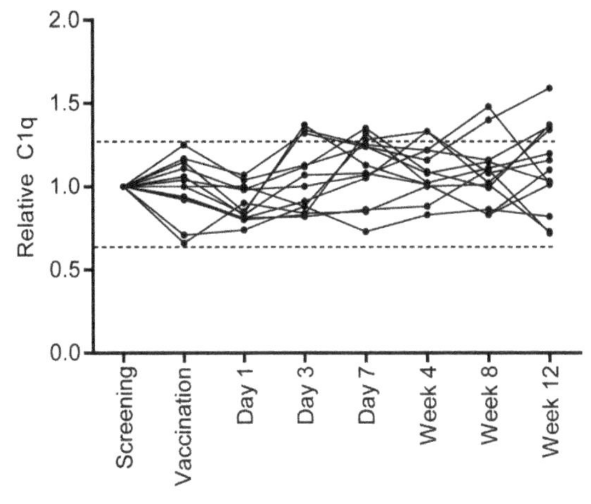

FIGURE 3 | BCG vaccination does not induce a similar C1q upregulation. Healthy individuals who were vaccinated with BCG ($n = 13$), were followed over time and C1q serum levels were measured. C1q levels were first calculated to μg/ml and for each individual set to 1 using the measurement of the C1q level before vaccination. The dotted lines indicate the variation that is present in C1q levels at the time of screening and prior to vaccination.

To assess the value of C1q as possible TB biomarker, the sensitivity, specificity and the positive likelihood ratio (LR+) were calculated from C1q concentration cut-offs (10). With a cut-off at the 95th percentile of the control population (300.2 μg/ml C1q) the sensitivity is 42% with a specificity of 91% resulting in a LR+ of 4.96. Application of a cut-off at the maximum of the control population (347.6 μg/ml) resulted in a sensitivity of 29% and a specificity of 97% resulting in a LR+ of 8.99. The capacity of serum C1q to discriminate active TB from LTBI, pneumonia and sarcoidosis was also analyzed using ROC analyses and expressed as AUC (**Figures 4B,C**). The AUC of C1q levels for TB vs. LTBI was 0.77, for TB vs. sarcoidosis 0.69, and for TB vs. pneumonia even an AUC of 0.93 was achieved.

C1q Is Locally Present in the Lungs of TB Patients

So far circulating RNA and protein levels of C1q have been analyzed, which reflect the systemic response to TB. Additionally, we analyzed the local C1q production or deposition in response to *M.tb* infection by staining lung tissue. Staining lung tissue from a control revealed scarce C1q staining with only few C1q positive macrophage-like cells in the lung parenchyma and in the intra-alveolar space (**Figure 5**). In contrast, lung tissue of fatal TB patients revealed, next to the intra-alveolar C1q positive cells also a pronounced C1q staining both in the necrotic centers of the granulomas and in the surrounding lung tissue with predominantly macrophage-like cells staining positive. Lung-tissue from patients that succumbed from pneumonia showed C1q staining predominantly in the intra-alveolar space. Staining of consecutive sections with an isotype control did not reveal any staining, also not in the necrotic centers, confirming specific staining for C1q. Thus, C1q protein is locally detected at an increased level in the lungs of TB patients ($n = 3$) compared to tissue samples from a non-pulmonary disease control ($n = 1$) or pneumonia patients ($n = 4$).

Non-human Primates With Active TB Disease Also Display Increased Serum C1q Levels

Non-human primate (NHP) *M.tb* infection models are widely used to study pathogen-host interactions and for pre-clinical evaluation of vaccine candidates (39). After infection, rhesus macaques develop TB disease which closely resembles human TB in most aspects. Sera banked over the course of a long-term follow-up study in rhesus macaques were used to determine C1q levels after experimental *M.tb* infection. 14 Out of 16 animals with active progressive disease, that had reached an early humane endpoint due to exacerbation of TB disease, had increased C1q levels compared to their baseline C1q levels before infection (**Figure 6A**). Such a rise in C1q levels was absent in six out of seven animals that did not develop overt disease, but controlled the infection over an extended period of time up to 1 year post-infection (**Figure 6A**). Additionally, in an separate cohort of *M.tb* infected NHPs we detected elevated C1q levels in five out of six broncho-alveolar lavage (BAL) fluid samples taken before necropsy, while no C1q could be detected in paired BAL fluids taken prior to infection (**Figure 6B**). The observed differences could not be explained by any differences in BAL volume recovery and thus these data reflect a true local increase in C1q after *M.tb* infection.

DISCUSSION

The accurate and fast identification of patients with active TB remains challenging, largely because of limitations in the current diagnostic tools to differentiate active TB from other diseases, as well as LTBI. Extensive searches for biomarkers that can discriminate active TB from other diseases with similar clinical presentation as well as from LTBI have been recently reported (3, 40). Several studies reported genes encoding for complement components to be upregulated in TB (15–19). Here, we compiled available genome wide gene expression data for TB compared to LTBI and TB compared to other lung diseases (5–7, 33–37) and observed that in particular C1q encoding genes were highly upregulated. Interestingly, these observations were made in studies using RNA from whole blood, indicating increased transcription of C1q genes in circulating blood cells, most likely monocytes/macrophages. Since C1q is not a typical acute-phase protein we were interested to confirm and validate these findings at the protein level. We have therefore measured C1q protein levels in serum and confirmed increased levels in patients with active TB, but not in other diseases with a similar clinical presentation, such as pneumonia or sarcoidosis, or mycobacterial exposure. C1q protein is also present in the lung tissue of deceased TB patients. The increased levels of local and circulating C1q in TB were replicated independently in a NHP TB infection model.

Literature suggests that expression of the three C1q genes *C1QA*, *C1QB*, and *C1QC* is regulated in a similar manner (41).

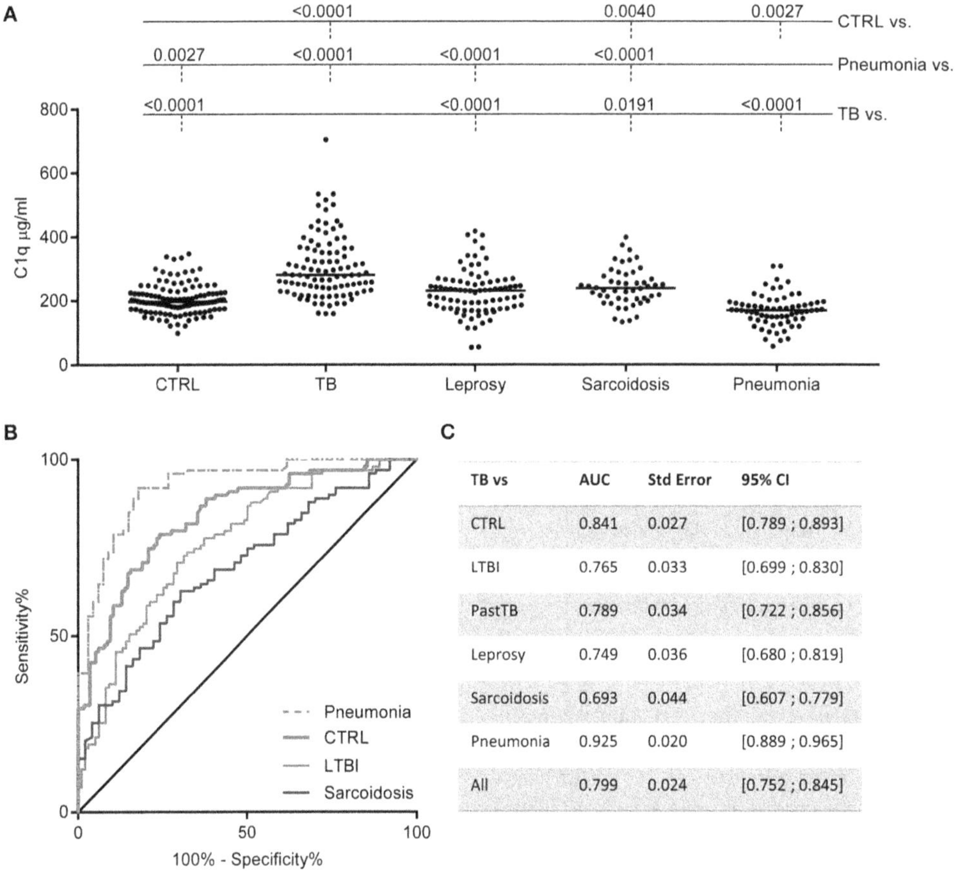

TB vs	AUC	Std Error	95% CI
CTRL	0.841	0.027	[0.789 ; 0.893]
LTBI	0.765	0.033	[0.699 ; 0.830]
PastTB	0.789	0.034	[0.722 ; 0.856]
Leprosy	0.749	0.036	[0.680 ; 0.819]
Sarcoidosis	0.693	0.044	[0.607 ; 0.779]
Pneumonia	0.925	0.020	[0.889 ; 0.965]
All	0.799	0.024	[0.752 ; 0.845]

FIGURE 4 | Increased C1q serum levels are associated with TB. C1q was measured in various cohorts by ELISA. The pooled data from **Figure 2E** control population (CTRL) and TB (active disease) is now compared to other diseases: leprosy ($n = 86$), sarcoidosis ($n = 50$), and community acquired pneumonia ($n = 68$) **(A)**. Differences between groups were analyzed using Kruskall-Wallis and Dunn's multiple comparisons test. Both the leprosy and the pneumonia cohort comprise two patient groups. The data for these individual groups is visualized in **Supplementary Figure E1**. ROC analysis of the ability of C1q to distinguish TB from CTRL, LTBI, sarcoidosis, and pneumonia are plotted together **(B)** and for all comparisons the Area Under the Curve (AUC) was calculated and summarized in the table **(C)**.

However, upon IFNγ-stimulation upregulation of *C1QB* is higher than *C1QC*, which is higher than *C1QA* (41). Similarly, our data also showed upregulated expression of *C1QB* and *C1QC* genes and *C1QA* was less frequently observed in active TB, also in the analysis from Cai et al. the extend of increase in the expression of *C1QA* was less pronounced as compared to the increase in expression of *C1QB* and *C1QC*. Since C1q protein production requires equal ratios of all three chains, the detected increase in C1q protein levels in TB patients indicates that all chains are expressed. The low detection of *C1QA* may thus be technical and reflect a poor capture of *C1QA* expression on the microarrays in general.

We measured C1q protein levels in four different geographical cohorts from Italy, The Gambia, Korea and South Africa. C1q levels were increased in patients with active TB compared to all relevant control populations. Importantly, treatment normalized serum C1q levels to those of endemic controls, indicating that the upregulation of C1q was associated with the disease and not intrinsic to the individuals. BCG vaccination, although being a live replicating mycobacterial vaccine, did not induce increased C1q levels. Although leucocytes of patients with leprosy reactions were reported to express increased levels of *C1QA*, *B*, and *C* (42), the cohorts analyzed here did not universal show increased serum C1q levels. Individual patients might have somewhat increased levels, both in this study (type 1 reaction) and a previous report (type 2 reaction) (43), which warrants more detailed analyses. We speculate that the different pathophysiologies of TB and leprosy, in particular the different levels of systemic inflammation and immune activation which are generally higher in active TB than in leprosy are responsible for the difference in C1q levels between the two diseases, even though both are caused by pathogenic mycobacteria.

To further evaluate the potential of C1q as a biomarker for active TB, C1q levels were compared to those of disease relevant controls as patients with untreated pulmonary sarcoidosis or pneumonia. Patients with TB had significantly higher circulating C1q levels as compared to patients with sarcoidosis or patients with pneumonia. Thus, the upregulation of C1q likely does not reflect a general response to inflammation. Patients with pneumonia rather had decreased C1q levels compared to

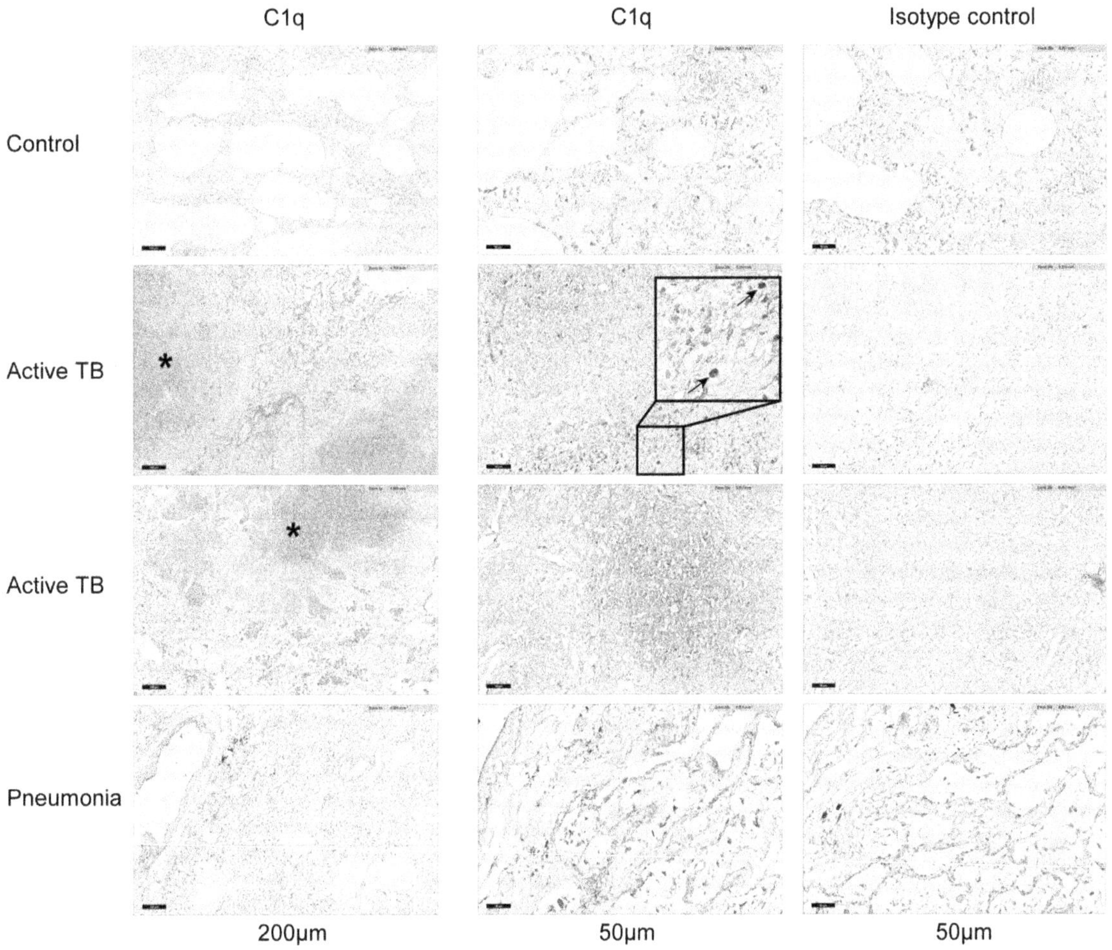

FIGURE 5 | C1q accumulates in lung tissue of patients with fatal pulmonary TB. Lung tissue, obtained at autopsy from a non-pulmonary disease control ($n = 1$), fatal active TB patients ($n = 3$), or patients with lethal pneumonia ($n = 3$) were stained for the presence of C1q. The left column shows the presence of C1q in a section of the control, two active TB patients and a pneumonia patient, scale bar at 200 μm. The middle column shows the same samples stained for C1q, while the right column shows consecutive tissue slides stained with a matched control antibody, scale bars at 50 μm. Necrotic areas that stain positive for C1q are highlighted with an asterisk (*) and individual cells that stain positive for C1q are highlighted with arrows.

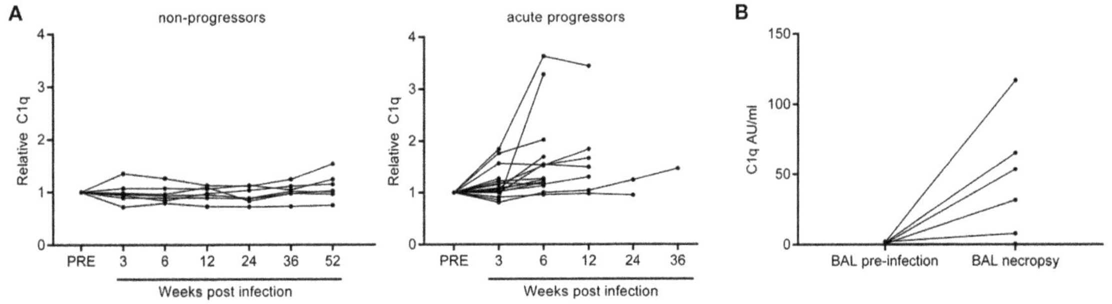

FIGURE 6 | Rhesus macaques infected with *Mycobacterium tuberculosis* display increased levels of C1q in serum and broncho-alveolar lavage fluid. C1q levels were measured in serum samples from rhesus macaques ($n = 23$) which were infected with *Mycobacterium tuberculosis* and followed over time. C1q levels were first calculated as Arbitrary Units (AU) per ml after which the C1q level of each animal at baseline was set as 1. Animals which controlled the infection are termed non-progressors and animals reaching a premature humane endpoint due to active disease progression are termed acute progressors **(A)**. Separately, C1q was measured in broncho-alveolar lavage (BAL) fluid obtained from animals before and 6 or 12 weeks after infection with *M.tb* ($n = 6$) and calculated as AU/ml **(B)**.

controls. Treatment of pneumonia normalized the levels of circulating C1q, suggesting that the observed decrease in C1q is non-genetic and likely associated with the disease process. ROC analysis indicated that C1q, even as a single marker, readily discriminated active TB from all other diseases investigated here. Furthermore, also in a setting of an experimental NHP model of TB disease we observed in both sera and BAL fluid increased C1q levels in animals with symptomatic TB disease compared to the level prior to infection with *M.tb*. This was not seen in animals that did not progress to TB disease, suggestion again an association with TB disease rather than infection only. These data fully agree with and support the observations described above in the human cohorts.

Longitudinal follow up of TB patients during treatment revealed that circulating C1q levels normalized to the level of endemic controls. However, here protein levels did not completely normalize until the 6 months time point. Previously published data showed a rapid decrease in C1q mRNA expression levels following treatment (16, 19). Cliff et al. show that already after 1 week of treatment the blood C1q gene expression decreased (16). Cai et al. reported a significant decrease in the expression of the C1q genes at 3 months of anti-TB chemotherapy whereas they also described a reduction in C1qc protein levels after 6 months (19). Our data presented here substantially expand the number of populations, including populations from different regions of the world. Transcriptomic analysis of genes encoding complement proteins were now assessed in 9 independent populations from different TB endemic as well as non-endemic regions, strongly supporting an increase in expression of C1Q as well as SERPING1 during active TB disease in cells present in peripheral blood. Moreover, 4 independent cohorts as well as the data obtained in the NHP model show increased circulating C1q plasma levels during active TB disease, but not infection. In addition to conforming the data previously published for a Chinese population (Cai et al.) in 4 different TB cohorts, we also showed the specificity for TB disease in comparison to clinically important differential diagnoses, such as sarcoidosis and pneumonia. As C1q is produced by cells of monocytic origin, it reflects another component of the immune space compared to most currently applied TB biomarkers, such as C-reactive protein and IP-10 (44–47). In addition, C1q levels are technically easy to measure and the C1q protein is not sensitive to degradation. Therefore, we hypothesize that addition of C1q to current biomarker panels or platforms, will have additive value in discrimination of TB patients.

Low levels of C1q have been reported in several inflammatory and autoimmune diseases, such as Systemic Lupus Erythematosus. This is largely the result of C1q consumption because of immune complex mediated disease and in some rare cases caused by genetic C1q deficiency (26). However, the increased levels of C1q, as occur in TB, are observed very rarely. So far the only other clinical condition in which increased levels of C1q have been reported is Kala Azar (48). The mechanism behind the increased C1q levels observed in TB patients, or the possible functional consequences for the host are unknown, and will need further investigation. The availability of the NHP model of tuberculosis for C1q research, as demonstrated for the first time in this study, should greatly accelerate and facilitate such work.

In conclusion, we show here that circulating C1q expression is increased in 9 different populations with TB disease, moreover, elevated C1q plasma levels were observed in 4 cohorts of TB patients compared to LTBI or endemic controls. Specifically, C1q levels in TB patients were significantly increased compared clinically relevant diseases, such as sarcoidosis, leprosy and pneumonia. Moreover, we show that increased C1q levels decreased to the level of the control population during successful treatment. In analogy with human TB, C1q also validated as a biomarker of TB disease in rhesus macaques, in both serum and BAL. Increased C1q levels were only observed in animals that progressed to active disease and not in those that controlled the infection, suggesting a direct association with disease rather than with infection. Therefore, we propose that the addition of C1q measurements to current biomarker panels may provide added value in the diagnosis of active TB.

AUTHOR CONTRIBUTIONS

RL, FV, AG, TO, SJ, and LT designed the study. RL, RdP, KD, IB, and KG performed analyses. JS, DG, CvM, MV, SV, WB, LP, FD, GW, and GG oversaw recruitment and collection of specimens. RL, SJ, and LT interpreted the data. All authors critically revised and approved the manuscript.

FUNDING

This study was supported by funding from the Italian Ministry of Health: Ricerca Corrente and a grant from the European Union EC HORIZON2020 TBVAC2020 (Grant Agreement No. 643381) and a grant from National Institutes of Health of USA (NIH 1R21AI127133-01). Additionally the work was supported by Zon-Mw TopZorg grant (842002001) (CvM and MV) and Zon-Mw Vidi grant (no. 91712334) (LT). The funders had no role in study design, data collection and analysis, decision to publish, or preparation of the manuscript.

ACKNOWLEDGMENTS

The authors are grateful to all the patients, the physicians, nurses that helped to perform the study. In particular we thank Gilda Cuzzi and Valentina Vanini (INMI, Rome, Italy) for the recruitment organization and lab work of the Italian cohort. Additionally, we would like to thank Sang-Nae Cho (Yonsei University, Seoul, South-Korea) for making available TB and control sera and Malu Zandbergen (Dept of Pathology, LUMC, Leiden, The Netherlands) for excellent support with immunohistochemistry. The IDEAL consortium is acknowledged for providing sera of leprosy patients.

SUPPLEMENTARY MATERIAL

Supplementary Figure E1 | C1q levels in leprosy and community acquired pneumonia. From leprosy two different cohorts were measured, one consists out of patients that were included in the Netherlands at the moment of diagnosis, the other out of sera samples from patients included at the moment they presented with a leprosy reaction. Reference C1q levels both the control groups as the pooled data from the active TB patients are depicted from **Figure 2E (A)**. For the community acquired pneumonia cohorts, samples were available from the moment the patientswere included and a follow up sample after recovery from both in Leiden **(B)** and in Nieuwegein **(C)**.

REFERENCES

1. WHO. *Global Tuberculosis Report* (2017). Available online at: http://www.who.int/tb/publications/global_report/en/
2. Houben RM, Dodd PJ. The global burden of latent tuberculosis infection: a re-estimation using mathematical modelling. *PLoS Med.* (2016) 13:e1002152. doi: 10.1371/journal.pmed.1002152
3. Goletti D, Lee MR, Wang JY, Walter N, Ottenhoff THM. Update on tuberculosis biomarkers: from correlates of risk, to correlates of active disease and of cure from disease. *Respirology* (2018) 23:455–66. doi: 10.1111/resp.13272
4. Zak DE, Penn-Nicholson A, Scriba TJ, Thompson E, Suliman S, Amon LM, et al. A blood RNA signature for tuberculosis disease risk: a prospective cohort study. *Lancet* (2016) 387:2312–22. doi: 10.1016/S0140-6736(15)01316-1
5. Berry MP, Graham CM, McNab FW, Xu Z, Bloch SA, Oni T, et al. An interferon-inducible neutrophil-driven blood transcriptional signature in human tuberculosis. *Nature* (2010) 466:973–7. doi: 10.1038/nature09247
6. Kaforou M, Wright VJ, Oni T, French N, Anderson ST, Bangani N, et al. Detection of tuberculosis in HIV-infected and -uninfected African adults using whole blood RNA expression signatures: a case-control study. *PLoS Med.* (2013) 10:e1001538. doi: 10.1371/journal.pmed.1001538
7. Anderson ST, Kaforou M, Brent AJ, Wright VJ, Banwell CM, Chagaluka G, et al. Diagnosis of childhood tuberculosis and host RNA expression in Africa. *New Engl J Med.* (2014) 370:1712–23. doi: 10.1056/NEJMoa1303657
8. Joosten SA, Fletcher HA, Ottenhoff TH. A helicopter perspective on TB biomarkers: pathway and process based analysis of gene expression data provides new insight into TB pathogenesis. *PLoS ONE* (2013) 8:e73230. doi: 10.1371/journal.pone.0073230
9. Ottenhoff TH, Dass RH, Yang N, Zhang MM, Wong HE, Sahiratmadja E, et al. Genome-wide expression profiling identifies type 1 interferon response pathways in active tuberculosis. *PLoS ONE* (2012) 7:e45839. doi: 10.1371/journal.pone.0045839
10. Petruccioli E, Scriba TJ, Petrone L, Hatherill M, Cirillo DM, Joosten SA, et al. Correlates of tuberculosis risk: predictive biomarkers for progression to active tuberculosis. *Eur Respir J.* (2016) 48:1751–63. doi: 10.1183/13993003.01012-2016
11. Sutherland JS, Loxton AG, Haks MC, Kassa D, Ambrose L, Lee JS, et al. Differential gene expression of activating Fcgamma receptor classifies active tuberculosis regardless of human immunodeficiency virus status or ethnicity. *Clin Microbiol Infect.* (2014) 20:O230–8. doi: 10.1111/1469-0691.12383
12. Jacobsen M, Repsilber D, Gutschmidt A, Neher A, Feldmann K, Mollenkopf HJ, et al. Candidate biomarkers for discrimination between infection and disease caused by Mycobacterium tuberculosis. *J Mol Med.* (2007) 85:613–21. doi: 10.1007/s00109-007-0157-6
13. Maertzdorf J, Repsilber D, Parida SK, Stanley K, Roberts T, Black G, et al. Human gene expression profiles of susceptibility and resistance in tuberculosis. *Genes Immun.* (2011) 12:15–22. doi: 10.1038/gene.2010.51
14. Sweeney TE, Braviak L, Tato CM, Khatri, P. Genome-wide expression for diagnosis of pulmonary tuberculosis: a multicohort analysis. *Lancet Respir Med.* (2016) 4:213–24. doi: 10.1016/S2213-2600(16)00048-5
15. Scriba TJ, Penn-Nicholson A, Shankar S, Hraha T, Thompson EG, Sterling D, et al. Sequential inflammatory processes define human progression from M. tuberculosis infection to tuberculosis disease. *PLoS Pathog.* (2017) 13:e1006687. doi: 10.1371/journal.ppat.1006687
16. Cliff JM, Lee JS, Constantinou N, Cho JE, Clark TG, Ronacher K, et al. Distinct phases of blood gene expression pattern through tuberculosis treatment reflect modulation of the humoral immune response. *J Infect Dis.* (2013) 207:18–29. doi: 10.1093/infdis/jis499
17. Wang C, Wei LL, Shi LY, Pan ZF, Yu XM, Li TY, et al. Screening and identification of five serum proteins as novel potential biomarkers for cured pulmonary tuberculosis. *Sci Rep.* (2015) 5:15615. doi: 10.1038/srep15615
18. Jiang TT, Shi LY, Wei LL, Li X, Yang S, Wang C, et al. Serum amyloid A, protein Z, and C4b-binding protein beta chain as new potential biomarkers for pulmonary tuberculosis. *PLoS ONE* (2017) 12:e0173304. doi: 10.1371/journal.pone.0173304
19. Cai Y, Yang Q, Tang Y, Zhang M, Liu H, Zhang G, et al. Increased complement C1q level marks active disease in human tuberculosis. *PLoS ONE* (2014) 9:e92340. doi: 10.1371/journal.pone.0092340
20. Esmail H, Lai RP, Lesosky M, Wilkinson KA, Graham CM, Horswell S, et al. Complement pathway gene activation and rising circulating immune complexes characterize early disease in HIV-associated tuberculosis. *Proc Natl Acad Sci USA.* (2018) 115:E964–73. doi: 10.1073/pnas.1711853115
21. Scanga CA, Flynn JAL. Modeling tuberculosis in nonhuman primates. *Cold Spring Harbor Perspect Med.* (2014) 4:a018564. doi: 10.1101/cshperspect.a018564
22. Ricklin D, Hajishengallis G, Yang K, Lambris JD. Complement: a key system for immune surveillance and homeostasis. *Nat Immunol.* (2010) 11:785–97. doi: 10.1038/ni.1923
23. Kishore U, Reid KB. C1q: structure, function, and receptors. *Immunopharmacology* (2000) 49:159–70. doi: 10.1016/S0162-3109(00)80301-X
24. Lu J, Kishore U. C1 complex: an adaptable proteolytic module for complement and non-complement functions. *Front Immunol.* (2017) 8:592. doi: 10.3389/fimmu.2017.00592
25. Nayak, Pednekar L, Reid KB, Kishore U. Complement and non-complement activating functions of C1q: a prototypical innate immune molecule. *Innate Immun.* (2012) 18:350–63. doi: 10.1177/1753425910396252
26. Beurskens FJ, van Schaarenburg RA, Trouw LA. C1q, antibodies and anti-C1q autoantibodies. *Mol Immunol.* (2015) 68:6-13. doi: 10.1016/j.molimm.2015.05.010
27. Gulati P, Lemercier C, Guc D, Lappin D, Whaley K. Regulation of the synthesis of C1 subcomponents and C1-inhibitor. *Behring Inst Mitt.* (1993) 196–203.
28. Castellano G, Woltman AM, Nauta AJ, Roos A, Trouw LA, Seelen MA, et al. Maturation of dendritic cells abrogates C1q production *in vivo* and *in vitro*. *Blood* (2004) 103:3813–20. doi: 10.1182/blood-2003-09-3046
29. Lubbers R, van Essen MF, van Kooten C, Trouw LA. Production of complement components by cells of the immune system. *Clin Exp Immunol.* (2017) 188:183–94. doi: 10.1111/cei.12952
30. van Schaarenburg RA, Suurmond J, Habets KL, Brouwer MC, Wouters D, Kurreeman FA, et al. The production and secretion of complement component C1q by human mast cells. *Mol Immunol.* (2016) 78:164–70. doi: 10.1016/j.molimm.2016.09.001
31. Joosten SA, van Meijgaarden KE, Del Nonno F, Baiocchini A, Petrone L, Vanini V, et al. Patients with tuberculosis have a dysfunctional circulating b-cell compartment, which normalizes following successful treatment. *PLoS Pathog.* (2016) 12:e1005687. doi: 10.1371/journal.ppat.1005687
32. Boer MC, Prins C, van Meijgaarden KE, van Dissel JT, Ottenhoff TH, Joosten SA. *Mycobacterium bovis* BCG vaccination induces divergent proinflammatory or regulatory T cell responses in adults. *Clin Vacc Immunol CVI* (2015) 22:778–88. doi: 10.1128/CVI.00162-15
33. Blankley S, Graham CM, Levin J, Turner J, Berry MP, Bloom CI, et al. A 380-gene meta-signature of active tuberculosis compared with healthy controls. *Eur Respir J.* (2016) 47:1873–6. doi: 10.1183/13993003.02121-2015

34. Bloom CI, Graham CM, Berry MP, Rozakeas F, Redford PS, Wang Y, et al. Transcriptional blood signatures distinguish pulmonary tuberculosis, pulmonary sarcoidosis, pneumonias and lung cancers. *PLoS ONE* (2013) 8:e70630. doi: 10.1371/journal.pone.0070630
35. Maertzdorf J, Ota M, Repsilber D, Mollenkopf HJ, Weiner J, Hill PC, et al. Functional correlations of pathogenesis-driven gene expression signatures in tuberculosis. *PLoS ONE* (2011) 6:e26938. doi: 10.1371/journal.pone.0026938
36. Maertzdorf J, Weiner J III, Mollenkopf HJ, Bauer T, Prasse A, Muller-Quernheim J, et al. Common patterns and disease-related signatures in tuberculosis and sarcoidosis. *Proc Natl Acad Sci USA.* (2012) 109:7853–8. doi: 10.1073/pnas.1121072109
37. Walter ND, Miller MA, Vasquez J, Weiner M, Chapman A, Engle M, et al. Blood transcriptional biomarkers for active tuberculosis among patients in the United States: a case-control study with systematic cross-classifier evaluation. *J Clin Microbiol.* (2016) 54:274–82. doi: 10.1128/JCM.01990-15
38. van Schaarenburg RA, Magro-Checa C, Bakker JA, Teng YK, Bajema IM, Huizinga TW, et al. C1q deficiency and neuropsychiatric systemic lupus erythematosus. *Front Immunol.* (2016) 7:647. doi: 10.3389/fimmu.2016.00647
39. Verreck AWF, Tchilian EZ, Vervenne RAW, Sombroek CC, Kondova I, Eissen OA, et al. Variable BCG efficacy in rhesus populations: pulmonary BCG provides protection where standard intra-dermal vaccination fails. *Tuberculosis* (2017) 104:46–57. doi: 10.1016/j.tube.2017.02.003
40. Goletti D, Sanduzzi A, Delogu G. Performance of the tuberculin skin test and interferon-gamma release assays: an update on the accuracy, cutoff stratification, and new potential immune-based approaches. *J Rheumatol. Suppl.* (2014) 91:24–31. doi: 10.3899/jrheum.140099
41. Chen G, Tan CS, Teh BK, Lu J. Molecular mechanisms for synchronized transcription of three complement C1q subunit genes in dendritic cells and macrophages. *J Biol Chem.* (2011) 286:34941–50. doi: 10.1074/jbc.M111.286427
42. Dupnik KM, Bair TB, Maia AO, Amorim FM, Costa MR, Keesen TS, et al. Transcriptional changes that characterize the immune reactions of leprosy. *J Infect Dis.* (2015) 211:1658–76. doi: 10.1093/infdis/jiu612
43. Negera E, Walker SL, Lemma T, Aseffa A, Lockwood DN, Dockrell HM. Complement C1q expression in Erythema nodosum leprosum. *PLoS Negl Trop Dis.* (2018) 12:e0006321. doi: 10.1371/journal.pntd.0006321
44. Awoniyi DO, Teuchert A, Sutherland JS, Mayanja-Kizza H, Howe R, Mihret A, et al. Evaluation of cytokine responses against novel *Mtb* antigens as diagnostic markers for TB disease. *J Infect.* (2016) 73:219–30. doi: 10.1016/j.jinf.2016.04.036
45. Chegou NN, Sutherland JS, Malherbe S, Crampin AC, Corstjens PL, Geluk A, et al. Diagnostic performance of a seven-marker serum protein biosignature for the diagnosis of active TB disease in African primary healthcare clinic attendees with signs and symptoms suggestive of TB. *Thorax* (2016) 71:785–94. doi: 10.1136/thoraxjnl-2015-207999
46. Jacobs R, Malherbe S, Loxton AG, Stanley K, van der Spuy G, Walzl G, et al. Identification of novel host biomarkers in plasma as candidates for the immunodiagnosis of tuberculosis disease and monitoring of tuberculosis treatment response. *Oncotarget* (2016) 7:57581–92. doi: 10.18632/oncotarget.11420
47. Petrone L, Cannas A, Vanini V, Cuzzi G, Aloi F, Nsubuga M, et al. Blood and urine inducible protein 10 as potential markers of disease activity. *Int J Tuberc Lung Dis.* (2016) 20:1554–61. doi: 10.5588/ijtld.16.0342
48. Kager PA, Hack CE, Hannema AJ, Rees PH, von dem Borne AE. High C1q levels, low C1s/C1q ratios, and high levels of circulating immune complexes in kala-azar. *Clin Immunol Immunopathol.* (1982) 23:86–93. doi: 10.1016/0090-1229(82)90073-3

3

Be on Target: Strategies of Targeting Alternative and Lectin Pathway Components in Complement-Mediated Diseases

*József Dobó, Andrea Kocsis and Péter Gál**

Institute of Enzymology, Research Centre for Natural Sciences, Hungarian Academy of Sciences, Budapest, Hungary

***Correspondence:**
Péter Gál
gal.peter@ttk.mta.hu

The complement system has moved into the focus of drug development efforts in the last decade, since its inappropriate or uncontrolled activation has been recognized in many diseases. Some of them are primarily complement-mediated rare diseases, such as paroxysmal nocturnal hemoglobinuria, C3 glomerulonephritis, and atypical hemolytic uremic syndrome. Complement also plays a role in various multifactorial diseases that affect millions of people worldwide, such as ischemia reperfusion injury (myocardial infarction, stroke), age-related macular degeneration, and several neurodegenerative disorders. In this review, we summarize the potential advantages of targeting various complement proteins with special emphasis on the components of the lectin (LP) and the alternative pathways (AP). The serine proteases (MASP-1/2/3, factor D, factor B), which are responsible for the activation of the cascade, are straightforward targets of inhibition, but the pattern recognition molecules (mannose-binding lectin, other collectins, and ficolins), the regulatory components (factor H, factor I, properdin), and C3 are also subjects of drug development. Recent discoveries about cross-talks between the LP and AP offer new approaches for clinical intervention. Mannan-binding lectin-associated serine proteases (MASPs) are not just responsible for LP activation, but they are also indispensable for efficient AP activation. Activated MASP-3 has recently been shown to be the enzyme that continuously supplies factor D (FD) for the AP by cleaving pro-factor D (pro-FD). In this aspect, MASP-3 emerges as a novel feasible target for the regulation of AP activity. MASP-1 was shown to be required for AP activity on various surfaces, first of all on LPS of Gram-negative bacteria.

Keywords: complement system, lectin pathway, alternative pathway, complement inhibitors, complement-related diseases

---

Abbreviations: 3MC syndrome, Malpuech–Michels–Mingarelli–Carnevale syndrome; aHUS, atypical hemolytic uremic syndrome; AMD, age-related macular degeneration; AP, alternative pathway; C4BP, C4b-binding protein; CARPA, complement activation-related pseudoallergy; CCP, complement control protein; CP, classical pathway; CNS, central nervous system; CR1, complement receptor 1; CR2, complement receptor 2; CRP, C-reactive protein; CUB, C1r/C1s, the sea urchin protein Uegf, and the human bone morphogenetic protein 1; CVF, cobra venom factor; EGF, epidermal growth factor; DAF, decay-accelerating factor; DAMP, damage-associated molecular pattern; FHL, FH-like protein; FHR, FH-related protein; FIMAC, FI membrane attack complex; GPI, glycosyl phosphatidylinositol; HAE, hereditary angioedema; HUVEC, human umbilical vein endothelial cell; LDLr, low-density lipoprotein receptor; LP, lectin pathway; MAC, membrane attack complex; MBL, mannose-binding lectin; MASP, MBL-associated serine protease; MCP, membrane cofactor protein; IGFBP-5, insulin-like growth factor-binding protein 5; IRI, ischemia–reperfusion injury; LPS, lipopolysaccharide; PAMP, pathogen-associated molecular pattern; PNH, paroxysmal nocturnal hemoglobinuria; PRM, pattern recognition molecule; SIRS, systemic inflammatory response syndrome; SP domain, serine protease domain; SLE, systemic lupus erythematosus; TAFI, thrombin-activatable fibrinolysis inhibitor; TSR, thrombospondin type repeat; TCC, terminal complement complex; VWA, Von Willebrand factor type-A.

BRIEF OVERVIEW OF THE COMPLEMENT SYSTEM

Initiation Phase

The complement system is a sophisticated network of serum proteins (recognition molecules, proteases, modulators, inhibitors) as well as cell-surface regulators and receptors that constitute a key part of the host defense machinery. The complement system is a powerful effector component of the innate immunity and a vital modulator of the adaptive immune response (1–3). The complement system recognizes, tags, and eliminates microbial intruders and other dangerous particles such as immune complexes, damaged, and altered self cells. The complement system is inactive (or at least shows a very low basic activity: "tickover") until it is activated by various danger signals. There are three canonical pathways through which the complement system can be activated: the classical pathway (CP), the lectin (LP), and the alternative pathways (AP) (**Figure 1**). CP and LP have several features in common. In both cases, pattern recognition molecules (PRMs) bind to the danger-associated structures. The PRMs, like the other complement components, are modular proteins, consisting of multiple structural domains (**Figure 2**). C1q, the single PRM of the CP binds primarily to immune complexes containing IgG or IgM, and to C-reactive protein (CRP) *via* its C-terminal globular domains (4). These globular domains are fused to N-terminal collagen-like arms forming the characteristic "bunch-of-six-tulips" structure. The structure of the PRMs of the LP resembles that of C1q; globular heads and collagen-like arms. However, the recognition domains of mannose-binding lectin (MBL), other collectins, and ficolins bind to different structures. The C-type lectin domains of MBL recognize the carbohydrate pattern of the bacterial surfaces. Ficolins (ficolin 1, 2, and 3) bind to acetylated compounds, typically to acetylated sugars of bacteria, *via* their fibrinogen-like domains (5). Collectins (CL-K1 and CL-L1) also recognize sugars and other potential danger signals. Unlike C1q, which has the well-established hexamer structure, MBL, ficolins, CL-K1, and CL-L1 exist in different oligomerization states, from dimer to hexamer; the tetramer being the dominant form at least for MBL. These PRMs circulate in complex with serine protease (SP) zymogens and monitor

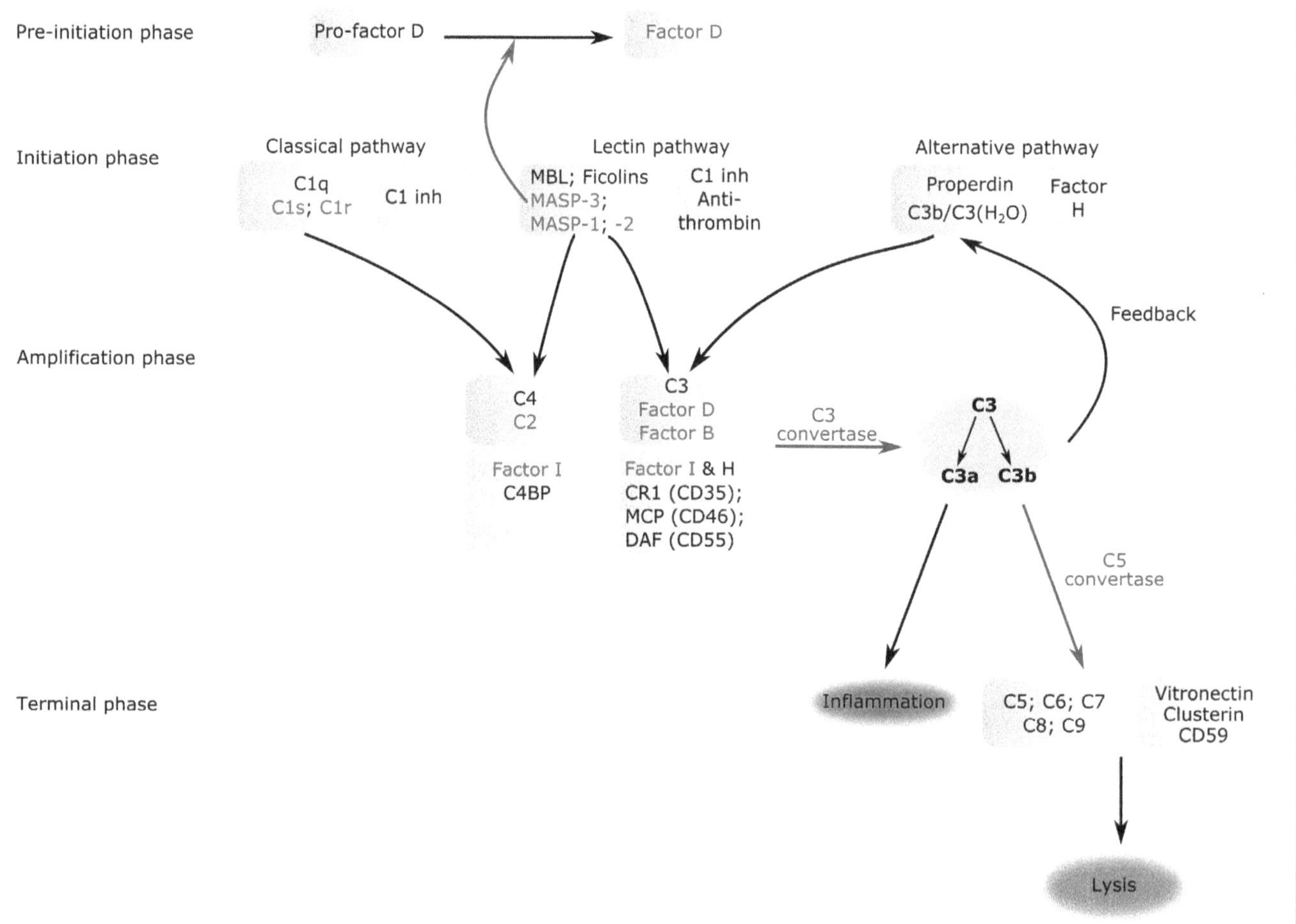

FIGURE 1 | Overview of the complement system. The components of all activation phases are listed in gray boxes, while their inhibitors in green boxes nearby. Serine proteases are indicated by red letters. Black arrows indicate the direction of the cascade. Certain enzymatic cleavages are emphasized by red arrows. The three activation routes merge at the cleavage of C3 highlighted by dark yellow background.

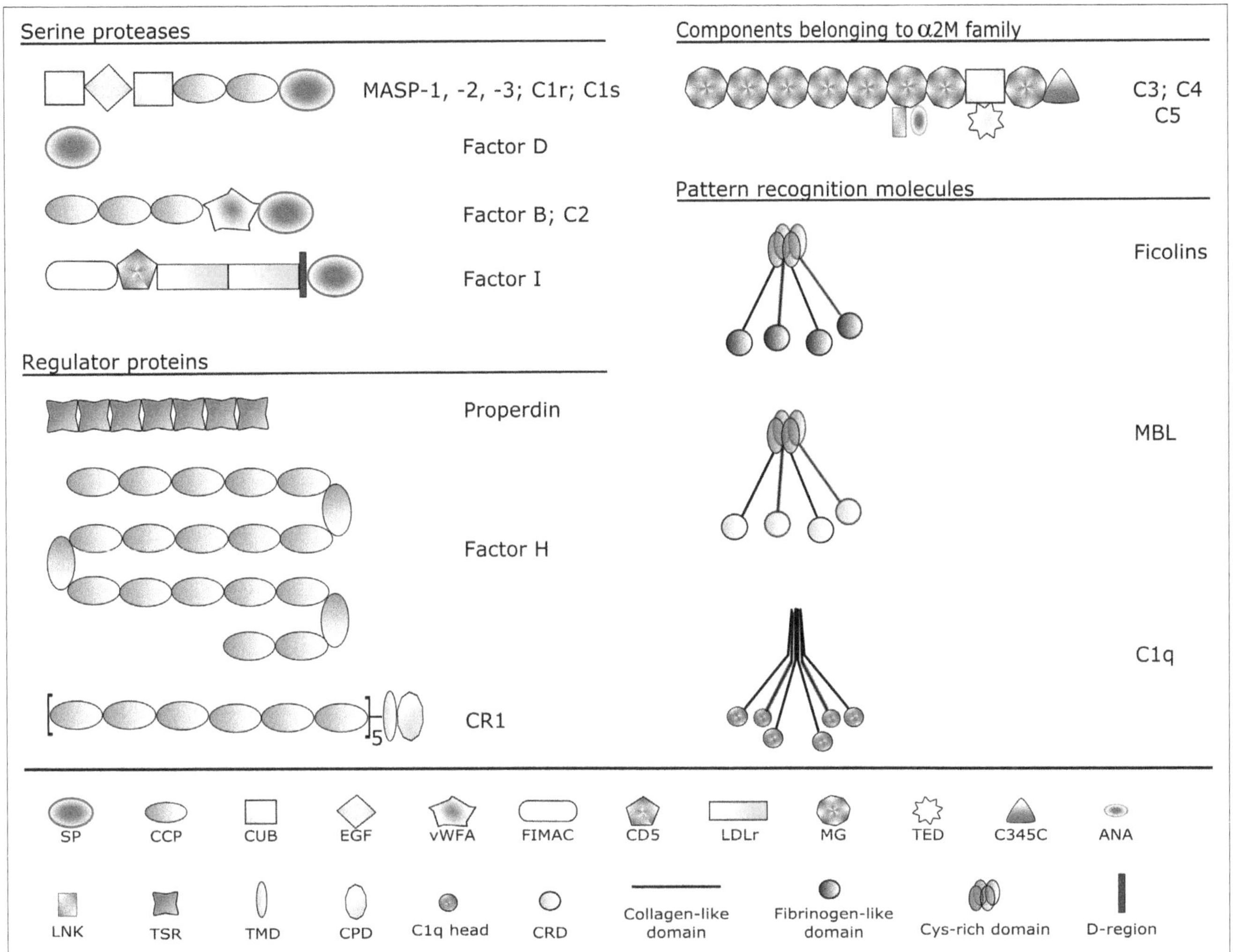

FIGURE 2 | Domain structures of the complement components discussed in the article. Each domain type is represented by a different symbol listed at the bottom. Domain abbreviations are as follows: SP, serine protease; CCP, complement control protein; CUB, complement C1r/C1s, sea urchin Uegf and bone morphogenetic protein-1; EGF, epidermal growth factor-like; vWFA, von Willebrand factor type A; FIMAC, factor I/membrane attack complex; CD5, scavenger receptor cysteine-rich domain; LDLr, low-density lipoprotein receptor; MG, α-macroglobulin; TED, thioester domain; ANA, anaphylatoxin; LNK, linker; TSR, thrombospondin-type 1 repeat; TMD, transmembrane domain; CPD, cytoplasmic domain; CRD, carbohydrate recognition domain.

continuously for dangerous particles the bloodstream. When the PRMs bind to the target surface, the associated SPs become activated and initiate a proteolytic cascade system, which amplifies the initial signal tremendously. C1q is associated with two C1r and two C1s proteases (the so-called "tetramer") to form the C1 complex of the CP (6). MBL/ficolin-associated serine protease 1 and 2 (MASP-1 and MASP-2) are the initial proteases of the LP (7, 8). These SPs, together with the third MBL/ficolin-associated SP (MASP-3) form a protease family with the same domain structure (**Figure 2**) and similar function. The activation of the CP and LP results in the formation of the same enzyme complex, a C3 convertase (C4b2a) that cleaves C3, the central component of the complement system. The first enzymatic step in the CP activation is the autoactivation of C1r. Activated C1r then cleaves zymogen C1s, which in turn cleaves C4 and C2. In the LP, MASP-1 autoactivates first and then cleaves MASP-2 (9). MASP-2 is the enzyme of the LP that cleaves C4 (10, 11), while C2 is cleaved by both MASP-1 and MASP-2. C3 and C4 are closely related thioester-containing proteins that form the basis of the convertase complexes (12, 13). Their function is to covalently attach the convertase to the activation surface and to capture the SP components of the enzyme complex. C2 is the SP component of the C3 convertase of the CP and LP. Activation of the AP is quite different from that of the CP and LP (14). When the CP/LP C3 convertase (C4b2a) cleaves C3, a smaller fragment is released (C3a). The larger fragment (C3b) covalently binds to the activation surface preferably through an ester or, less likely, through an amide bond due to the reaction of the exposed thioester bond (15, 16). The nascent C3b component binds factor B (FB), the SP component of the AP C3 convertase. FB is cleaved by FD, a SP which circulates predominantly in its cleaved form in the blood. The resulting C3bBb is the AP C3 convertase, which converts more C3 into C3b. The new C3b molecules serve as platforms for new C3 convertase complexes. In this way, a positive feedback loop amplifies the initial signal tremendously generated either by the CP or the LP (17). According to the C3 tickover hypothesis, the AP can also initiate on its own without involvement of CP or LP (18). The circulating C3 molecules hydrolyze slowly and spontaneously in the bloodstream. The resulting C3(H_2O) is a C3b-like molecule; it can bind FB and then form an "initiation" C3 convertase (C3(H_2O)Bb). If this fluid-phase C3 convertase emerges near a surface, the nascent C3b molecules can bind to the surface and initiate the positive feedback loop. In this way, the AP continuously monitors the different surfaces and if it finds an activator surface, it launches efficient complement activation. The self-tissues are protected from AP-mediated damage by cell-bound and fluid-phase inhibitors (**Figure 1**). These inhibitors dissociate the C3bBb complex and serve as cofactors for the serine protease factor I (FI) in the degradation of C3b (19). Decay-accelerating factor (DAF, CD55), membrane cofactor protein (MCP) (CD46), complement receptor 1 (CR1, CD35) are cell-surface-bound while the master regulator of the AP is the fluid-phase protein, factor H (FH). FH binds to cell-surface-deposited C3b and facilitates its degradation to iC3b, C3c, and C3dg by FI. On endogenous cell membranes, which expose sialic acid, binding of FH is tight and the degradation of C3b is rapid, while on the so-called "protected surfaces" (e.g., bacteria, fungi) binding is weak and the amplification loop of AP can build up. There is a positive regulator of the AP, properdin, which increases the half-life of the C3bBb complex. Originally, at its discovery, properdin was regarded as a pattern recognition-like initiator molecule of the AP (20). Later, it was considered as a positive regulator (21); however, recently, the pattern recognition function of properdin has been reconsidered (22, 23).

From the Central Phase to the Terminal Pathway

The cleavage of C3 by the C3 convertases is the turning point of complement activation. At this point, the three activation pathways (CP, LP, and AP) merge into a unified terminal pathway (**Figures 1** and **3**). When the density of surface-deposited C3b reaches a certain level, the substrate specificity of the C3 convertases switches to cleave the C5 component. The C4b2a(C3b)n and C3bBb(C3b)n convertases cleave the C5 component into a smaller (C5a) and larger (C5b) fragments. The C5a fragment, like the C3a fragment, is an anaphylatoxin. The anaphylatoxins bind to their receptors (C3aR and C5aR1/2) on leukocytes and endothelial cells and initiate inflammatory reactions (24). Structurally, C5 is similar to C3 and C4 (although it does not contain thioester bond) (25). The cleavage of C5 is the last enzymatic step in the complement cascade. From this point, conformational changes drive the formation of a self-organizing protein complex that damages the membrane of the attacked cells [membrane attack complex (MAC)]. After cleavage, the nascent C5b undergoes a conformational change that enables it to bind the C6 and C7 components (26). The resulting C5b–C7 complex binds to the cell membrane and captures C8. After conformational changes, C8 integrates into the membrane and pave the way to the integration of multiple copies of C9 molecules. The C9 molecules form a pore in the membrane, which results in the disintegration and destruction of the cell (27).

COMPLEMENT-MEDIATED DISEASES

The complement system is an extremely effective cell-killing and inflammation provoking machinery. To prevent excessive activation, the complement system is kept under strict control by the different inhibitory mechanisms. A delicate equilibrium between activation and inhibition is necessary to maintain the inflammatory homeostasis in the human body. When this equilibrium is disrupted by any reason, the self-tissues can be damaged and severe disease conditions can occur. There are many clinical disorders in which uncontrolled (or sometimes the insufficient) complement activation is involved. Usually, the etiology of these diseases is complex, and the unwanted complement activation is only one of the pathological factors. However, evidences obtained by using various disease models suggest that preventing or inhibiting the pathological complement activation can be a promising therapeutic approach.

Insufficient Complement Activation

Since the complement system provides a first line of defense against invading pathogen microorganisms, deficiency of a complement component can lead to severe infections. The consequences could be more severe during childhood, when the adaptive immune system is not developed enough. Deficiency of the initial SPs of CP and LP (C1r, C1s, MASP-2) can result in pyogenic infections (28). Deficiency of MBL is the most common immunodeficiency in humans, affecting approximately 30% of the human population (29). It predisposes to recurrent infections in infancy; however, it is not a major risk factor in the adult population. Deficiency of the alternative and the terminal pathway components can severely compromise the defense against Gram-negative bacterial infections (30). Deficiency of properdin or deficiencies in the components of MAC are associated with infections of *Neisseria* species causing meningococcal meningitis or sepsis (31–33). A very important function of the CP is the continuous removal of immune complexes and apoptotic cells. If this pathway is compromised in systemic lupus erythematosus (SLE) due to deficiency of C1q, or C4, or C1r/s, severe autoimmune reactions occur resulting in tissue injury in the kidneys.

Excess Complement Activation

The majority of complement-related diseases are associated with overwhelming complement activation due to inappropriate control. The kidney is especially vulnerable for complement-mediated attacks. In the case of C3 glomerulopathy, C3 deposition occurs in the glomeruli without immunoglobulin deposition (34, 35). C3 deposition in this case is likely the consequence of uncontrolled AP activation. In contrast to that, in the case of membranoproliferative glomerulonephritis, CP activation elicits C3 deposition, since immunoglobulins and C1q are also deposited (36, 37). The IgA nephropathy is characterized by deposition of polymeric IgA1, which triggers complement activation through the AP and the LP (38, 39). Atypical hemolytic uremic syndrome (aHUS) is also a complement-related disease, which can lead to end-stage renal failure (37, 40). The driving force behind aHUS is the inappropriate AP activation often due to variants of (41) or autoantibodies against (42) FH, the master regulator of the AP. aHUS is a form of thrombotic

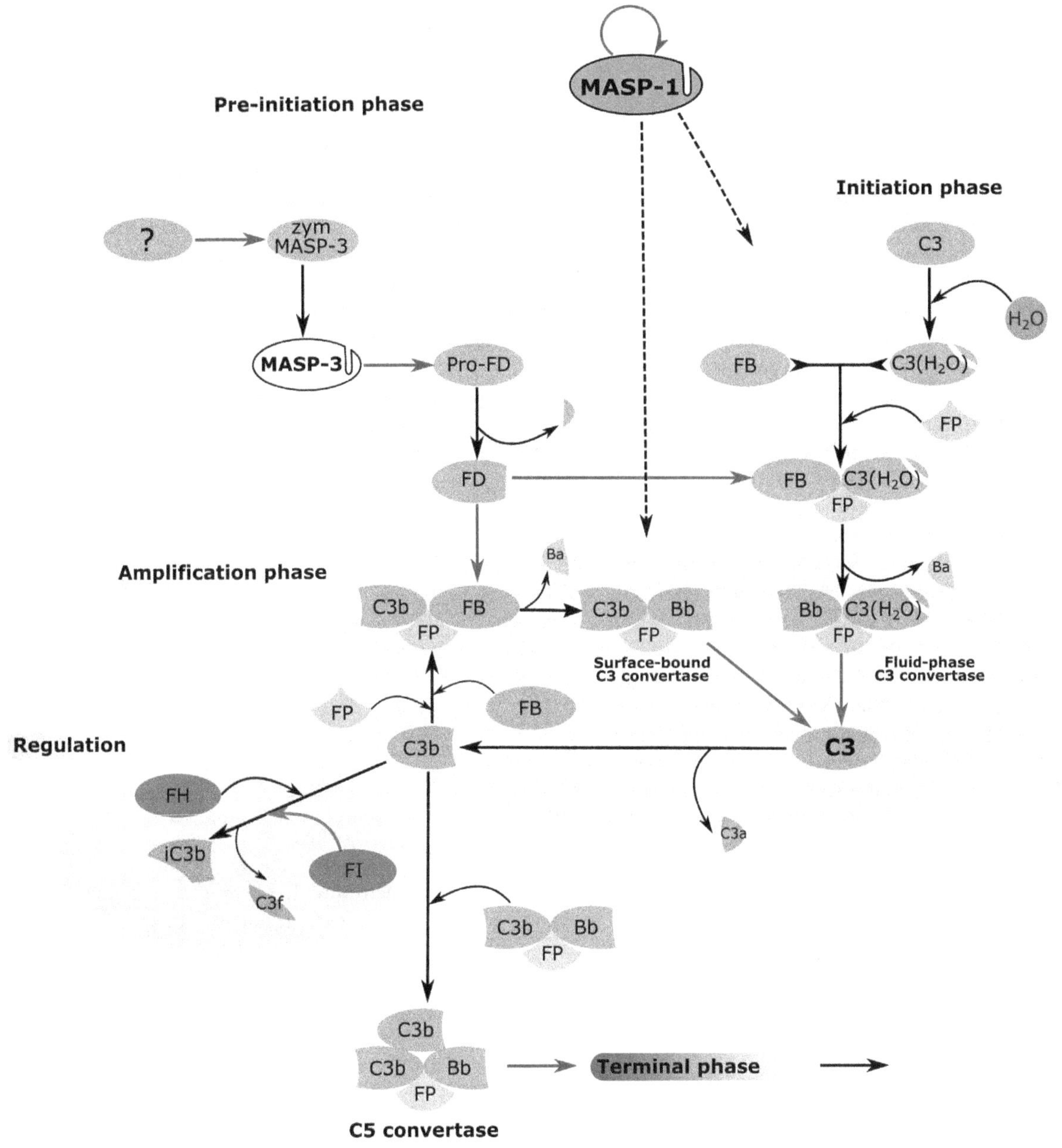

FIGURE 3 | MASP-1 and MASP-3 play roles in the activation of the alternative pathway (AP). The activation process of the AP is divided into several phases, which are indicated by differently colored backgrounds. MASP-3 is proved to be the professional activator of pro-factor D in blood, therefore, plays an important role in the pre-initiation phase. The physiological activator of zymogen MASP-3 (zym MASP-3) is hitherto undiscovered (shown by the question mark). MASP-1 is indispensable for efficient initiation and amplification of the AP on certain surfaces, although the mechanism is yet unknown (shown by dashed arrows). Black arrows represent conversion processes, while red arrows stand for enzymatic reactions pointing from the enzyme toward its substrate. The circle-shaped red arrow symbolizes the autoactivation of MASP-1.

microangiopathy accompanied with thrombocytopenia, hemolytic anemia, vascular damage, and thrombosis.

Another rare clinical condition associated with uncontrolled AP activation is paroxysmal nocturnal hemoglobinuria (PNH) (43, 44). In PNH patients, red blood cells are particularly prone to complement-mediated lysis due to the lack of two membrane-bound regulator proteins: DAF (CD55) and CD59. This is the consequence of the defect in glycosyl phosphatidylinositol (GPI) synthesis in the cells. GPI is responsible for anchoring various proteins to the cell membrane including these inhibitors that regulate the activation of the AP (CD55) and the formation of MAC (CD59).

Age-related macular degeneration (AMD) is a complement-related disease, which affects a large population (about 100 million AMD cases) worldwide. It is the leading cause of blindness among the elderly in the developed world (45). Genetic analyses strongly suggest that uncontrolled complement activation, especially that of the AP, plays a major role in the pathogenesis of AMD. Genetic variants of FH, C3, FB, FI, and C9 have been associated with AMD (46). In the center of the retina of AMD patients, the photoreceptor cells are gradually degraded due to a chronic inflammation, which manifests in the accumulation of immune deposits called drusen underneath the retinal pigment epithelium. The drusens (that contain activated complement components) compromise the transport of oxygen and nutrients to the photoreceptors facilitating their degeneration. Numerous attempts have been made to curb the unwanted AP activation in the eye with limited success (47). In order to efficiently influence complement activation in the eye, we have to reveal its exact mechanism, which could be different in the periphery than in the bloodstream.

Ischemia–reperfusion injury (IRI) can be considered as a severe autoimmune reaction (48), which plays a major role in a number of clinical conditions. When the blood flow in an organ stops temporarily for any reason, the deprivation of oxygen (hypoxia) induces changes in the tissues, which predisposes them for complement-mediated attack after reperfusion. The affected cells and tissues are recognized by the immune system as damaged self [damage-associated molecular pattern (DAMP)], and a complex inflammatory reaction is launched, in which the complement system plays a decisive role. IRI significantly contributes to the tissue damage in the case of myocardial infarction, stroke, transplant-induced inflammation, and it can cause a complication during coronary artery bypass graft surgery. Although the exact mechanism of complement activation in case of IRI is not fully clarified yet, a number of evidences suggest that inhibition of the LP could be therapeutically advantageous (49–53).

Artificial materials used in modern medicine, such as polymer plastics and metal alloys, can also activate the complement system and trigger inflammation (54). Nanoparticles used as contrast agents or drug carriers can also activate the complement system, sometimes causing a severe adverse reaction, called complement activation-related pseudoallergy (55, 56). In this type of hypersensitivity reaction, IgE is not involved. Liposomal drugs directly activate the complement system liberating C3a and C5a anaphylatoxins, which trigger mast cells and basophils.

If the immune system is exposed to an overwhelming amount of danger signals [pathogen-associated molecular patterns (PAMPs) or DAMPs], a systemic inflammatory reaction can occur, which could be more devastating than the original danger source. In the case of systemic inflammatory response syndrome, such as sepsis or polytrauma, the massive and systemic complement activation fuels a vicious cycle of hyperinflammatory events that can results in fatal tissue damage (57).

A growing number of evidences indicate that the complement system plays an important role in fundamental developmental processes. The lack of functional LP components (MASP-3, CL-K1, CL-L1) during embryogenesis results in the Malpuech–Michels–Mingarelli–Carnevale (3MC) syndrome that manifest in characteristic craniofacial dysmorphism and multiple other anomalies (58, 59). It was shown that an intact CP is essential for postnatal brain development. Contribution of C1, C4, and C3 was demonstrated to synaptic pruning essential for proper neuron circuit formation (60). These complement components tag synapses and mediate their elimination during a discrete window of postnatal brain development. C1q or C3 deficiency in mice results in improper central nervous system (CNS) synapse elimination. If these processes, essential during normal brain development, are pathologically upregulated during adulthood, they can contribute to the development of neurodegenerative diseases, such as Alzheimer disease and frontal temporal dementia (61). In addition to that, uncontrolled CP and LP activation in the CNS can also contribute to psychiatric disorders such as schizophrenia (62, 63).

CROSS-TALK BETWEEN THE AP AND THE LP

As described above, there are three canonical activation routes of the complement system. It is also obvious that the CP and the LP would not work efficiently without the amplification loop provided by the AP, hence, the three pathways are naturally interconnected. It is also possible that homologous proteins C4 and C3, or C2 and FB can substitute each other to a certain degree; at least *in vitro* experiments indicate a weak cross-reactivity between CP/LP an AP C3 convertase components (64). MASP-1 (65) and MASP-2 (66) have both been implicated to be able to directly cleave C3; however, the physiological relevance of these reactions is uncertain. MBL was also shown to be involved in AP activation without the requirement of C2, C4, and MASPs (67), but in the light of our recent results, the observed effect could be mediated by MASP-1 (68). In summary, the involvement of the LP or LP components in AP activation has been demonstrated in the literature before; however, some results still remain controversial. In the subsequent two sections, recent discoveries are presented regarding the role of MASP-3 during the very early stage of AP activation, and the requirement of MASP-1 for AP activation on various surfaces.

Active MASP-3 Is the Professional Pro-FD Maturase in Blood

The first evidence that MASP-1 or MASP-3 might have an essential role in AP function came from the group of T. Fujita (69). They created *MASP1* knock-out mice by replacing the second exon (8). Since this region encodes a common part of both MASP-1 and MASP-3, the final homozygous mouse strain lacked both proteins. Surprisingly, these mice had pro-FD in their sera and had no AP activity (69). They suggested that MASP-1 acts as an essential enzyme for pro-FD maturation. At the time, it seemed like a logical assumption to favor MASP-1 over MASP-3 since MASP-1 is a more active enzyme in general with a relatively broad substrate specificity (70). Later, the same group suggested that MASP-3 might be more important than MASP-1 in pro-FD activation and suggested that even the proenzyme form of MASP-3 can act as the activator (71).

Subsequent publications questioned the requirement of either MASP-1 or MASP-3 for AP activity. In the serum of a 3MC syndrome patient lacking both proteins, functional AP was observed (72), and in mice deficient for MASP-1, MASP-3, and FH extensive, AP activation was observed, just like in mice deficient for FH only (73).

To clarify the roles of MASPs in pro-FD activation, we set up a series of experiments. *In vitro* all active MASPs were shown to be able to cleave pro-FD efficiently to produce FD, whereas the MASP zymogens lacked such activity (74). We prepared fluorescently labeled pro-FD, added it to different types of human plasma and serum preparations and followed the conversion of pro-FD to FD. Pro-FD was efficiently cleaved in all types of blood preparations, even in citrated and EDTA plasma, where neither the complement nor the coagulation cascade is expected to be activated. This experiment established that at least one protease is present in normal human blood capable of converting pro-D to FD without the prior activation of the abovementioned proteolytic cascades. Using a MASP-1-specific and a MASP-2-selective inhibitor, these two enzymes could be excluded. After adding recombinant active catalytic fragments of MASPs to normal human plasma samples, the half-life of labeled pro-FD was markedly reduced upon the addition MASP-3, whereas the other two enzymes had no effect (74).

The final "killer" experiment that established MASP-3 as the professional (near exclusive) activator of pro-FD came using a MASP-3 specific inhibitor, TFMI-3 (75). TFMI-3 blocked the conversion of labeled pro-FD to FD in citrated plasma, EDTA plasma, and hirudin plasma completely, while in serum, the half-life was markedly increased. Another conclusion of our studies was that active MASP-3 must be present in the blood, since only the activated form of MASP-3 can convert pro-FD to FD. Later, we provided direct evidence for the extensive basal-level activation of MASP-3 in human blood by an unknown mechanism (76). Finally, the debate seems to have settled. A recent paper showed that in 3MC syndrome patients lacking MASP-3, predominantly pro-FD is present in their sera, and moreover, in healthy individuals, some pro-FD is also present beside the dominant active form (77).

The picture is now clear. Under normal circumstances, active MASP-3 is present in the blood, which activates pro-FD, therefore, continuously supplying active FD for the AP (**Figure 3**). However, MASP-3-deficient individuals are not completely defenseless. At least one coagulation enzyme can probably also provide low levels of FD for the AP, or when the LP is activated, MASP-1 or MASP-2 might also contribute. These backup mechanisms also need some consideration when targeting MASP-3 to control AP activity, as it will be discussed later.

MASP-1 Is Required for AP Initiation on Certain Activating Surfaces

Despite the fact that molecular mechanisms of the complement system have been thoroughly examined in the past decades, still many questions remained about the early steps of the activation. MASP-1 as a promiscuous enzyme with broad substrate specificity (70) has the potential to replace other SPs or amplify enzymatic reactions. It has been reported that MASP-1 is indeed involved in biological processes beyond LP or even the complement system.

Recently, we have found a novel function of MASP-1 in AP activation apart from its role in the LP (**Figure 3**). This function suggests an unexpected linkage between the two pathways and also highlights the differences between various activation surfaces (68). Previously, specific and highly selective small-protein inhibitors against all MASPs were developed from canonical inhibitor scaffolds using the phage-display technique. SGMI-1 is a specific MASP-1 inhibitor, whereas SGMI-2 inhibits MASP-2, and TFMI-3 is a specific inhibitor of MASP-3 (9, 75). Activation of the AP *in vitro* can be carried out on ELISA microtiter plates coated by bacterial lipopolysaccharide (LPS) or yeast zymosan. These materials serve as models of the pathogenic surfaces. In the absence of Ca^{2+} using Mg^{2+}-EGTA buffer, AP activation can be initiated without the involvement of CP and LP. Administration of the specific MASP-1 inhibitor, SGMI-1 in this system lead to surprising results. The activity of the AP was attenuated significantly through the inhibition of MASP-1. However, this effect was only seen on the bacterial surface represented by LPS, while zymosan-induced AP activation was not compromised. To rule out the possibility that SGMI-1 may impede other SPs, inhibitors of MASP-1 possessing different mode of action were also tested. Anti-MASP-1-SP antibody, N-terminal domains of MASP-1 (M1_D1-3) (78), and serpin domain of C1 inhibitor resulted in the same, considerable reduction of AP activity but only on LPS. The activity of AP in MASP-1-depleted serum remarkably decreased on LPS-coated surface while on zymosan-coated surface, it was only moderately affected. The mechanism of C3b deposition, which is followed in our assay, can be divided to initiation and amplification phases. Time-course measurement of C3b deposition in the presence of subsequently added SGMI-1 inhibitor indicated that MASP-1 contributes to both phases of C3b generation. Although we proved unambiguously that MASP-1 has an effect on AP activation, there are still many puzzling details to be solved. First, we tested the known components of AP as possible reaction partners of MASP-1. It was clarified earlier that MASP-1 cleaves C3 only at a very low rate (11) and now we confirmed that MASP-1 does not react significantly with C3b-bound FB. The contribution of FD was also excluded since SGMI-1 does not inhibit FD, and MASP-1 is not the physiological activator of pro-FD (74). Our results lead to the conclusion that the key player of MASP-1-driven AP activation is probably not among the core components of the AP.

Differences between the activating surfaces also need further investigations since it seems to be likely that AP initiation occurs by various mechanisms. Using specific antibodies in the ELISA system, neither MASP-1 nor MBL could be detected on LPS surface in Mg^{2+}-EGTA buffer (68). MASP-1 may be presented by some other PRMs, which do not necessarily require Ca^{2+} for binding (possibly ficolins). Another possible scenario is that MASP-1 forms a labile and transient complex with its reaction partners. One clue arises from the literature that properdin, which stabilizes C3bBb complex, is crucial for LPS-induced but not for zymosan-induced AP activation (79). Another coincidence is that LPS, rather than zymosan, binds FH with high affinity, which enhances the decay of C3 by FI activity. The ratio of these factors, which play a role in the regulation of AP, may be influenced by MASP-1 through a yet unknown mechanism.

These new findings draw attention to MASP-1 in the promotion of LPS-induced AP and, therefore, its role in the defense against Gram-negative bacteria.

COMPONENTS OF AP AND LP AS POTENTIAL DRUG TARGETS

Pattern Recognition Molecules

The PRM of the CP and LP recognize danger signals (PAMPs and DAMPs) and provide the framework of the initiation multimolecular complexes (the C1 complex, MBL–MASP complexes, ficolin–MASP complexes). They have similar overall domain architecture: N-terminal collagen-like domains and C-terminal globular domains. The structure of C1q is different from that of the other PRMs, since the basic trimeric subunit of C1q is composed of three different polypeptide chains (A, B, and C chains), while that of MBL and ficolins consist of only one kind of polypeptide chain. In the case of collectins, collectin kidney 1 (CL-K1) and collectin liver 1 (CL-L1), a heterotrimeric subunit was observed in human blood composed of one CL-L1 and two CL-K1 polypeptide chains (called CL-LK) (80). Another structural difference between C1q and the proteins of the collectin/ficolin family is that the latter contain a short N-terminal cysteine-rich region and an α-helical coiled-coil neck region between the collagen-like and the globular domains facilitating trimerization of the polypeptide chains. The collagen sequences (Gly-Xaa-Yaa repeats) are interrupted at one point in C1q and MBL generating a flexible kink region that may play an important role in binding to the danger patterns and activating the associated SPs. The PRMs bind the associated SPs in a Ca^{2+}-dependent manner. C1q binds the C1s-C1r-C1r-C1s tetramer, while MBL, ficolins, and CL-LK bind MASP dimers. It is probable that low oligomeric MBL and ficolins bind a single MASP dimer, while higher oligomers (pentamers, hexamers) can bind two MASP dimers simultaneously (81). There is a cross-interaction between the components of the CP and LP; MBL can bind the $C1r_2s_2$ tetramer and C1q can bind the MASP dimers, although with reduced affinity compared to the cognate pairs (82). It is unlikely that these interactions have a physiological relevance (except maybe in deficiencies); however, the existence of these cross-bindings proves that the interactions are analogous between the PRMs and the associated SPs among the components of the CP and LP. The binding of MBL and ficolins to their targets is Ca^{2+}-dependent. The affinity of a single carbohydrate-binding domain to its target sugar is low (Kd in the millimolar range), whereas the avidity of the whole oligomeric molecule is high with a Kd in the low nanomolar range. It is very likely that the PRMs of higher oligomeric state activate the LP more efficiently than the low oligomeric PRMs due to the stronger binding to both the target surface and to the MASPs (83). The mechanism of activation of the C1 and MBL–MASP complexes is not fully clarified yet.

Theoretically, if we want to prevent or inhibit improper complement activation in a pathological situation PRMs of the initiation complexes are ideal targets; since by inhibiting the PRMs, we can shut off the entire amplification machinery of the complement system at the very first step. There are three possibilities to inhibit the function of the PRMs: (1) to prevent the binding of the PRMs to their target; (2) to prevent the binding of the associated SPs to the PRMs; (3) to prevent the conformational changes of the PRMs that are necessary for the activation of the SPs. Monoclonal antibodies that bind to the globular domains of the PRMs can efficiently interfere with the ligand binding. Anti-C1q and anti-MBL antibodies were successfully used to block the CP and LP activation, respectively (84). An anti-MBL monoclonal antibody (3F8) attenuated myocardial IRI in mouse expressing human MBL (85).

Anti-C1q antibodies have been recently reported to greatly reduce the inflammatory demyelinating lesions in a mouse model of neuromyelitis optica (86) and also to attenuate injury with a consequent neuroprotective effect in acute Guillain–Barré syndrome mouse models (87). A peptide agent (called 2J) was selected from a peptide library on the basis of C1q binding (88). This peptide was shown to bind to the globular domain of C1q and prevented the binding of C1q to IgG. The 2J peptide efficiently inhibited CP-mediated C4 and C3 deposition and MAC formation *in vitro*. Although this peptide was a promising candidate for therapeutic complement inhibition, no further studies were reported about its *in vivo* application.

Another possibility for inhibiting the CP and the LP is to disassemble the initiation complexes. In this respect, it is worth noting that in *in vitro* experiments the C1 complex dissociates in the absence of Ca^{2+} (in the presence of EDTA), or at high ionic strength (1 M NaCl), whereas in the case of the MBL–MASP complexes, both conditions should apply at the same time (89). Moreover, C1 inhibitor, which makes covalent complexes with the SPs, dislodges C1r and C1s from C1q, while it cannot disassemble the MBL–MASP complexes (90). Nevertheless, it was shown that there is a dynamic equilibrium between the different MBL/ficolin–MASP complexes in human serum, in other words, MASPs can migrate between the complexes (91). Recently, it was shown that asparaginase, which is used in oncological treatments, inhibits the LP by reducing the amount of MBL–MASP complexes, very likely through dissociating the complexes (92). In this case, it is an adverse effect of the oncological treatment, but it indicates that a similar approach can be feasible in anticomplement therapy. An anti-MASP-2 monoclonal antibody (OMS721, Omeros), which binds to a non-catalytic complement control protein (CCP) domain of MASP-2, successfully inhibited the LP in *in vivo* experiments, and also it could disassemble the MBL-MASP-2 complexes.

There is a report about a viral-derived peptide (PIC1), which inhibits the classical pathway through binding to the collagen-like region of C1q in the C1 complex (93). This peptide might lock the conformation of C1q and/or displace the tetramer. There is no other report in the literature about an agent, which can block the conformational change necessary for the proper function of the initiation complexes. A deeper understanding of the activation mechanism of the C1 and MBL/ficolin–MASP complexes is needed to harness this possibility in the therapy.

MASP-1

MASP-1 is the most abundant protease of the LP, and it plays a central role in complement activation. Its average serum concentration is 143 nM (11 μg/mL), which is 24-times higher than the serum concentration of MASP-2 (6 nM, 0.4 μg/mL) (94). The members of the C1r/C1s/MASP protease family share the same domain organization (**Figure 2**). At the N-terminus, there is a CUB domain (initially recognized in C1r/C1s, sea urchin protein *U*egf, and human *b*one morphogenetic protein 1), followed by an epidermal growth factor-like (EGF) module and a second CUB domain. The MASPs are present as dimers in the circulation, and the N-terminal CUB1-EGF-CUB2 region is responsible for the dimerization. Another important function of this region is that it mediates the binding to the PRMs. The CUB and the EGF domains bind Ca^{2+}, and both the dimerization and the PRM binding are Ca^{2+}-dependent. The C-terminal region, which possesses the catalytic activity, consists of two CCP domains and a SP domain. The SP domain belongs to the chymotrypsin family (Family S1, MEROPS) and shows trypsin-like specificity cleaving after basic amino acids (Arg, Lys) in the polypeptide chain. The two CCP domains have at least two functions: they serve as spacers between the CUB1-EGF-CUB2 region and the SP domain and they provide additional binding sites (exosites) for the substrates (13). Both functions have essential roles in the activation of the PRM–MASP complexes and in the cleavage of the subsequent components (C2 and C4).

MASP-1 has multiple roles in the innate immune response. Zymogen MASP-1 has a high autoactivation capacity, which plays a key role in the activation of the lectin pathway (95). When PRM–MASP complexes bind to the activation surface, zymogen MASP-1 autoactivates and the active MASP-1 activates zymogen MASP-2 (9, 72). In this way, MASP-1 is the initiator protease of the LP. Recently, it has been demonstrated that MASP-1 significantly contributes to AP activation on LPS surface through an unknown mechanism (68). MASP-1 is also capable of activating endothelial cells by cleaving protease-activating receptor 4 (91, 96). The activated endothelial cells secrete cytokines (IL-6 and IL-8), and these cytokines promote the chemotaxis of neutrophil granulocytes (97). Moreover, MASP-1 treatment increased adhesion between neutrophils and endothelial cells by upregulating E-selectin expression in human umbilical vein endothelial cells (HUVECs) (98). A genome-wide gene expression profiling study on HUVECs corroborated the role of MASP-1 in triggering inflammation (99). The analysis showed that MASP-1 up- and downregulated numerous inflammation-related genes bridging complement activation and endothelial-cell-related inflammatory processes. It was also demonstrated that MASP-1 is able to cleave high-molecular-weight kininogen and liberate bradykinin (100). Bradykinin is a potent vasoactive, pro-inflammatory peptide, which is responsible for the swelling attacks in hereditary angioedema (HAE), a disease associated with C1 inhibitor deficiency (101). Uncontrolled activation of MASP-1 may contribute to the development of HAE attacks and worsening the symptoms of HAE patients. It was also recognized that MASP-1 serves as a link between the complement and the coagulation cascades. MASP-1 promotes coagulation by activating prothrombin, fXIII, and thrombin-activatable fibrinolysis inhibitor (102–104). The effect of MASP-1 on blood coagulation was confirmed by using a microvascular whole-blood-flow model (105). The physiological relevance of this phenomenon is not quite clear; however, it is very likely that the proteolytic activity of MASP-1 contributes to pro-inflammatory and pro-thrombotic events facilitating the development of thrombotic complications under pathological conditions (106). As the above examples highlight, MASP-1 has a relatively broad substrate specificity (it has about 10 known substrates), which is quite unusual among complement proteases. It should be noted, however, that all the known substrates of MASP-1 are related to the innate immune response. Evolutionary considerations indicate that MASP-1 is an ancient enzyme of the complement system compared to the other members of the MASP/C1r/C1s family (107). The relaxed substrate specificity of MASP-1 is reflected in its 3D structure (70). The substrate-binding groove of MASP-1 is broad and accessible resembling that of trypsin, rather than those of other early complement proteases. The physiological inhibitors of MASP-1 are serpins. C1 inhibitor, and in the presence of heparin antithrombin, attenuate very efficiently the activity of MASP-1 (108). Alpha$_2$-macroglubulin, a pan-specific protease inhibitor in the blood was suggested to inhibit MASP-1 and consequently the LP (109), but this issue is controversial (108, 110). Another potential physiological inhibitor of the LP is MAp44 (aka MAP-1), an alternative splice product of the *MASP1* gene (111, 112). MAp44 contains the CUB1-EGF-CUB2-CCP1 domains of MASP-1/3 plus a 17 amino-acid-long C-terminal peptide. Since MAp44 lacks the SP domain, it does not have proteolytic activity to initiate the LP, but it can dimerize and bind to the PRMs like the MASPs. MAp44 attenuates LP activity by competing with MASP-1 and MASP-2 for the PRMs and displacing them from the complexes. Recombinant MAp44 was shown to protect against myocardial IRI in mouse models, preserving cardiac function, decreasing the infarct size, and preventing thrombogenesis (113). Recombinant chimeric inhibitors were also designed and constructed by fusing MAp44 and the complement regulatory domains (1–5) of FH (114). One of these inhibitors showed simultaneous inhibition of the LP and AP.

Theoretically, the SPs are the most druggable targets in the complement system (115). The active sites of these enzymes can be easily targeted by small-molecule protease inhibitors. The main problem with this approach is the lack of specificity, since all the complement proteases and also the proteases of the other plasma cascade systems contain chymotrypsin-like SP domains (**Figure 4**). A small-molecule SP inhibitor, which blocks the activity of a particular complement SP, very likely will inhibit other complement proteases, as well as proteases of the coagulation, fibrinolysis, and kallikrein–kinin systems to some extent. For example, nafamostat mesilate (FUT-175 or Futhan) is a powerful inhibitor of the complement cascade, but it has a broad specificity. It was shown to attenuate renal and myocardial IRI (116, 117), but it also attenuates pancreatitis by inhibiting trypsin and other pancreatic enzymes (118), and also coagulation by inhibiting thrombin and other clotting enzymes (119). To enhance the specificity, the number of interactions should be increased between the SP and the inhibitor. A promising approach could be the fragment-based drug discovery, which generates highly specific molecules *via* linking small chemical fragments (Mw < 300 Da) together that

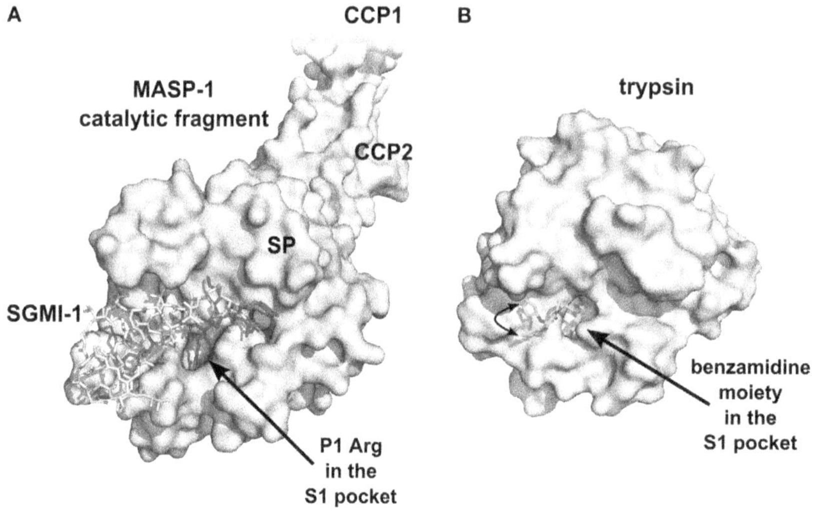

FIGURE 4 | Specific inhibition of proteases requires multiple favorable contacts in a large contact area with an inhibitor. **(A)** The structure of MASP-1 in complex with a specific small-protein inhibitor, SGMI-1 (PDB entry 4DJZ). SGMI-1 was developed by phage-display (122). Amino acid residues in the randomized positions are colored magenta (P4, P2, P1′, P2′, P4′) and blue (P1). All amino acid residues in the randomized positions have contacts with the protease body; moreover, SGMI-1 has other contact areas with MASP-1 in the non-randomized positions as well. **(B)** The structure of trypsin in complex with a non-specific small-molecule inhibitor (123) (PDB entry 3LJJ). The inhibitor is based on benzamidine. A two-headed arrow indicates the movement of the terminal cyclopentane moiety, which has two equivalent binding sites.

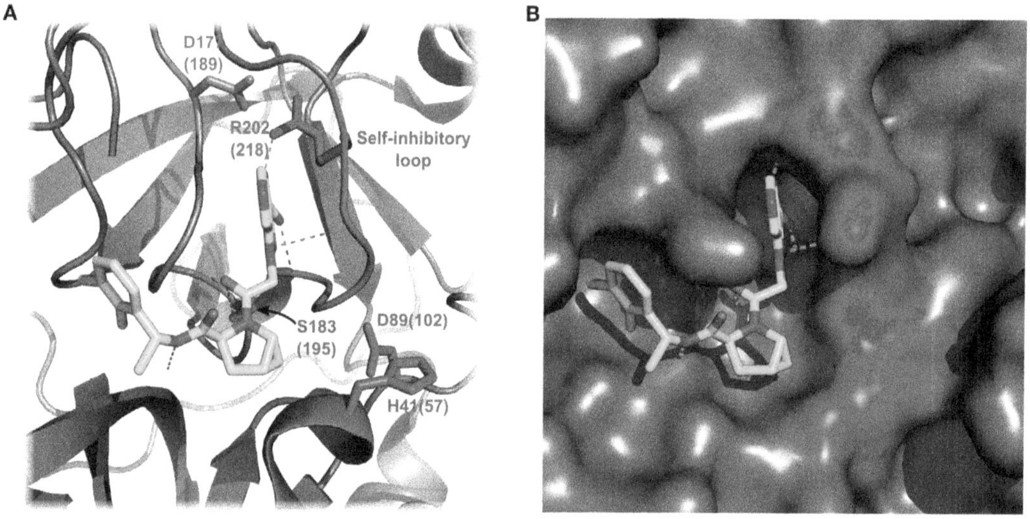

FIGURE 5 | Structure of factor D (FD) in complex with a selective small-molecule inhibitor. The figure is based on the structure of FD in complex with "inhibitor 6" described by Maibaum et al. (120) (PDB entry 5FCK). Inhibitor 6 has multiple polar and hydrophobic interactions with the protein body. It is notable that inhibitor 6 interacts with the self-inhibited conformation of FD, probably stabilizing FD in this form. Asp^{177} (blue) of the S1 pocket forms a salt bridge with Arg^{202} of the self-inhibitory loop (red). The catalytic triad is colored magenta. Numbers indicate amino acid positions in mature FD, while numbers in parenthesis reflect the traditional chymotrypsinogen numbering. Hydrogen bonds are indicated by yellow dashed lines. **(A)** FD shown by ribbon representation. **(B)** FD shown by surface representation.

bind only weakly on their own to the target. This approach was successfully used to develop specific small-molecule inhibitors against FD (120) (**Figure 5**), but there is no report about similar molecules against MASPs. Monoclonal antibodies and other biologics can also meet the specificity criterion. Highly selective MASP inhibitors were developed by the *in vitro* evolution of the interacting loop of canonical SP inhibitors. Sunflower trypsin inhibitor (SFTI) is a 14-amino acid-long cyclic peptide, which mimics the protease-interacting loop of the inhibitor scaffold of the Bowman–Birk inhibitor family. SFMI-1, an LP-selective peptide inhibitor was developed by phage-display selection of SFTI variants using MASP-1 as target (121). SFMI-1 proved to be a strong MASP-1 inhibitor (K_i = 65 nM), and a weak MASP-2 inhibitor (K_i = 1,030 nM). In order to further increase the specificity, a larger inhibitor scaffold was used in the phage-display selection. SGPI-2 (*S. gregaria* protease inhibitor-2) is a single domain small-protein inhibitor (35-amino acid-long) belonging to the Pacifastin family of canonical inhibitors. After randomizing six positions in the protease-interacting loop (P4, P2, P1, P1′, P2′, and P4′), a highly specific MASP-1 inhibitor (SGMI-1) was selected (122) (**Figure 4**). SGMI-1 inhibits MASP-1 very effectively (K_i = 7 nM), and very selectively. This inhibitor was used to clarify the function of MASP-1 in the innate immune response using numerous *in vitro* and *ex vivo* assays. Although MASP-1 is a tempting target to halt unwanted LP activation and to prevent various pro-inflammatory processes, no pharmaceutical development of a MASP-1 inhibitor has been reported to date.

MASP-2

MASP-2 is the only protease in the LP that can cleave C4. Its serum concentration is rather low (6 nM, 0.4 μg/mL), compared to the other complement proteases. These characteristics make MASP-2 an ideal target to inhibit pathological LP activation.

MASP-2 has identical domain organization with MASP-1 and MASP-3 (**Figure 2**). Isolated MASP-2 has a tendency to autoactivate in a concentrated solution (11, 124). This autoactivation capacity, however, cannot manifest in normal human serum, where the MASP-2 concentration is low, and each MASP-2 molecule is surrounded by MASP-1 molecules on the target surface. Under these circumstances, MASP-1 is the exclusive activator of MASP-2. The autoactivation ability of MASP-2 might be important in situations, where there is no MASP-1 present (e.g., MASP-1 deficiency). It should be noted, however, that in the serum of a 3MC syndrome patient, where there was neither MASP-1 nor MASP-3 present due to a mutation in the *MASP1* gene, no LP activity could be detected (72). On the other hand, birds lack MASP-1, but have functional LP, suggesting that MASP-2 can independently drive LP activation (125). In the sera of these animals, however, the autoactivation capacity of MASP-2 must be much higher than that of human MASP-2 in normal human serum. A recent publication shows that MASP-2 can directly cleave C3 in the absence of C4 and/or C2 on LP-activating surfaces (66). MASP-2 was also suggested to promote fibrin polymerization by cleaving prothrombin (126). The *MASP2* gene, like the *MASP1* gene, has an alternative splice product MAp19 (aka sMAP, MAP-2) (127, 128). This truncated gene product contains only the CUB1 and EGF domains plus 4 unique C-terminal residues. Since MAp19 can bind to the PRMs, it may regulate LP activity through displacing the MASPs from the complexes. Theoretically, the recombinant form of MAp19 could be suitable to attenuate LP activity, in practice, the larger MAp44 was used for this purpose since it binds to the PRMs with higher affinity.

The pathological relevance of MASP-2 was demonstrated in MASP-2 knock-out mice, where the animals were significantly protected against myocardial and gastrointestinal IRI (50). In the hearts of MASP-2-deficient mice, the infarct volume was significantly smaller than in those of the wild-type animals. Moreover, a recent study demonstrated that an inhibitory monoclonal anti-MASP-2 antibody successfully attenuated myocardial IRI in wild-type mice (129). An anti-MASP-2 antibody, OMS721, developed by Omeros Corporation, is under clinical trial for treating aHUS (130) and other thrombotic microangiopathies (131), IgA nephropathy, lupus nephritis, membranous nephropathy, and C3 glomerulopathy (132). The mechanism of the protecting effect of MASP-2 inhibition in these diseases is not clear, since AP activation is believed to be the main driver of these conditions. Selective canonical inhibitors against MASP-2 were also selected by phage-display using the SFTI and SGPI scaffolds (121, 122). Both inhibitors were highly specific: SFMI-2 (K_i = 180 nM) and SGMI-2 (K_i = 6 nM) prevented LP activation efficiently, while they did not compromise the activity of the other two pathways.

MASP-3

MASP-3 was discovered as the third SP component of the LP (133). It has the same domain organization (**Figure 2**) as MASP-1 and MASP-2, as described above; moreover, the amino acid sequence of its first five domains is identical with that of MASP-1. This feature is the consequence of the fact that MASP-1 and MASP-3 are the alternative splice products of the same *MASP1* gene, along with a third protein MAp44 (111, 112). Variants of the *MASP1* gene, resulting in the loss of the activity of MASP-3, cause the 3MC syndrome, characterized by serious craniofacial, genital, and often mental defects (58, 59, 134). The results indicate that MASP-3 is involved in neural crest cell migration in early embryonic development. Interestingly, the same phenotype is observed in patients carrying mutations in the *COLEC11* gene (58) or the *COLEC10* gene (135), both encoding LP components CL-K1 (aka collectin-11) and CL-L1 (aka collectin-10). It is possible that MASP-3 is in complex with CL-K1/L1 when it exerts its function during embryogenesis, and it is likely that the proteolytic activity of MASP-3 plays an important role.

MASP-3 is different from MASP-1 and MASP-2 in several ways. MASP-3 does not autoactivate, does not cleave downstream LP/CP components, C4 and C2, and the active form has very low activity on most synthetic substrates (136). *In vitro*, it was shown to cleave insulin-like growth factor-binding protein 5; however, the relevance of this reaction is uncertain (137). It has also no natural inhibitor in the blood; therefore, control of its activity is probably achieved simply by its very restricted substrate specificity. MASP-3 is present in the blood as the mixture of the proenzymic and the activated forms; moreover, the activated form seems to be the more dominant variant (76). In this aspect, it also differs from MASP-1 and MASP-2, which are proenzymic. On the other hand, in many regards, MASP-3 has similarities to FD, which circulates predominantly in the active form, has no natural inhibitor, and has very restricted substrate specificity.

The function of MASP-3 in the blood had been mysterious until recently. Initially, it was considered simply as a negative regulator of the LP since it competes with MASP-1 and MASP-2 for binding to PRMs (133). This function may still be valid; however, now, strong evidences exist that the active form of MASP-3 is the primary physiological activator of pro-FD, producing FD, a key enzyme of the AP. The story was detailed in a previous section; therefore, we jump to the functional consequences of this activity.

It seems logical that the activity of the AP can be downregulated by the inhibition of MASP-3. Inhibition of MASP-3 would result in the accumulation of pro-FD in the blood with only very low levels of active FD, hence greatly attenuating AP activity. A study presented at 16th European Meeting on Complement in Human Disease (138) provided a strong evidence for this assumption. A single dose of a monoclonal antibody inhibiting the activity of MASP-3 suppressed the activity of the AP and shifted the active to zymogen ratio of FD toward the proenzyme, pro-FD, both in mice and in cynomolgus monkey. So far, two specific inhibitors against MASP-3 were developed. One of them is a canonical Kunitz-type recombinant protein, which is based on the second domain of tissue factor pathway inhibitor (TFPI) and developed by phage-display (75). The other is the abovementioned monoclonal antibody by Omeros Corporation (138).

What are the potential advantages of MASP-3 inhibition over FD inhibition? Inhibition of both proteins is expected to result in similar systemic effects in the blood. The plasma concentration of both proteins is similar, around 60 nM. This relatively low value is attractive for drug development. On the other hand, FD has a very high turnover rate. Its half-life in humans is less than 1 h (139). The turnover rate of MASP-3 is not yet known, but because of its size, it is most certainly lower compared to FD. This could mean that a lower daily dose of a drug candidate inhibitor of MASP-3 would be required compared to a FD inhibitor.

Deficiency in the AP can result in potentially life-threatening meningococcal infections, and AP inhibition carries the same risk. Another potential benefit of MASP-3 inhibition would be that in this case, a pro-FD pool is still available. In case of a bacterial infection, the LP can be activated, and the resulting active MASP-1 and MASP-2 molecules could locally convert pro-FD to FD, making the AP amplification possible. Nonetheless, this mechanism needs experimental validation.

In all, based on MASP-3's requirement for the maturation of pro-FD, MASP-3 presents itself as a good target to attenuate the complement system, with several potential benefits over FD inhibition.

Factor D

Factor D (FD) is a single domain SP, which circulates in the blood predominantly in the active form (77, 140). It is synthesized mainly by adipocytes, hence the alternative name adipsin. In the 1970s, it was debated whether it is produced as a proenzyme or secreted in the active form (140, 141). Since only the active form could be isolated from blood (142), it was assumed that it might be activated even before secretion (143). Nevertheless, at the DNA level, after the signal sequence, an additional 5 to 7 amino acid long propeptide is encoded. Now the consensus is that active MASP-3 converts the pro from of FD to the active form constitutively (74, 75, 77).

Although it is an active SP, FD has an extremely restricted substrate specificity. It has very low activity toward synthetic substrates, basically, it cleaves only certain thioester compounds; however, its natural substrate, FB in complex with C3b or C3b-like molecules, is cleaved very efficiently (144). The free enzyme's very low activity is due to a unique self-inhibitory loop (145), which is displaced when FD binds to C3bB (146).

It has a relatively low mass concentration of 1–4 μg/mL in humans (147–149), which in combination with early reports showing that FD is the bottleneck of AP activity (140), led to the assumption that FD could be the best target to achieve AP inhibition. However, FD is a small protein of only 25 kDa, so, its molar concentration of 40–160 nM combined with its high turnover (139) suggest that high daily doses of a FD inhibitor would be required to achieve complete sustained inhibition. Recent results also suggest that FD may not even be the bottleneck of AP activity. In the serum of FD-deficient mice, the addition of FD corresponding to only about 1–2% of the normal FD level was sufficient for normal AP activity *in vitro* (147). In a 3MC syndrome patient, whose serum contained mostly pro-FD, some AP activity was still present (72), although lower than the normal level (134). These data together suggest that even if a potent and specific inhibitor is used, at least equimolar amount is required for AP inhibition, and even higher doses are necessary for sustained inhibition. A study with lampalizumab, a humanized monoclonal anti-FD IgG F_{ab} fragment, showed similar observations (150).

One must also consider that, at least *in vitro*, plasma kallikrein was shown to be able to cleave the C3bB pro-convertase (151), hence a residual, low-level AP activity might still be present even during complete FD inhibition, or FD deficiency; however, the *in vivo* relevance of this cleavage needs further validation.

Nevertheless, FD remains a prime target within the complement system. Several FD inhibitor molecules are under development, or in the clinical trial phase (152, 153) for PNH, aHUS, and AMD. Achillion developed several small molecule FD inhibitors that may be orally administered. A dose of 200 mg/kg of ACH-4471 per every 12 h resulted in complete AP inhibition in primates (154). An example of the combination of structure-based and fragment-based drug development targeting FD was published recently. Modifying the structure of a small-molecule kallikrein inhibitor several compounds were developed that selectively inhibit FD (120). **Figure 5** shows FD in complex with one of the compounds as an example.

Near complete inhibition of FD is expected to have a similar outcome as inhibition of MASP-3. Neisserial infection or other bacterial infections constitute a possible threat, which requires prophylactic treatment or treatment with antibiotics. This is actually valid for nearly all kinds of anticomplement drugs.

Factor B

Factor B (FB), a five-domain, 90 kDa glycoprotein, is composed of three CCP modules, a short connecting segment, a von Willebrand factor type A (vWFA) domain, and an SP domain (**Figure 2**). It circulates as a proenzyme, and its activation site (Arg^{234}-Lys^{235}) is hindered in the free enzyme from the cleavage by FD. FB can form a complex with C3b, or C3b-like molecules, to generate the AP pro-convertase, C3bB. The pro-convertase probably exists in two, closed and open conformations, in the latter, FB being accessible for FD cleavage (155). The FD-C3bB interaction facilitates both a shift toward the open conformation of C3bB, and a structural rearrangement in FD displacing its self-inhibitory loop (146). FD cleaves FB in the pro-convertase to release the Ba fragment. The other fragment, the catalytic

Bb itself is still just a marginally active enzyme (156), it has full activity only as part of labile C3bBb complex (157). Once Bb dissociates from the convertase complex, it cannot re-associate with C3b (157).

FB is absolutely essential for the AP; therefore, it is a prime target for AP inhibition, but because of its high concentration (about 200–250 μg/mL, or 2–3 μM), it might not seem to be ideal at first sight. On the other hand, in order to prevent AP activation, only the newly formed C3bBb complexes may have to be inhibited. Using a potent inhibitor with low Kd toward C3bBb could completely block the amplification phase, thereby halting the activation process. While C3bBb might be a difficult target for testing small-molecule inhibitors, because of the transient nature of this complex, the cobra venom factor (CVF)-Bb complex is more stable; therefore, it presents itself as a viable target for the development of such molecules. It is also notable that at high pH (proenzymic), FB alone has significant, easily detectable activity toward C3 and certain para-nitroanilide substrates (158). Several substrate-analog aldehyde FB inhibitors were developed along the way (158).

Inhibitory antibodies might be more easily obtained. They only need to prevent access to C3, the very large substrate of C3bBb, which is attainable by a bulky antibody molecule binding near the catalytic site. However, it is possible that such antibody would also bind to free FB; therefore, higher doses might be required. Optimally, a small-molecule inhibitor or an inhibitory antibody should only bind to Bb, or even better only to the C3bBb complex, so that a relatively low dose of the molecule be sufficient for complement inhibition. A blocking antibody, binding to free FB, which prevents the formation of the pro-convertase complex, is also a feasible option. In this case, also high doses would be required for optimal effect.

A set of small-molecule inhibitors are under development by Novartis against FB (CVF-Bb) for indications such as AMD and other complement-mediated diseases (159, 160). Neutralizing monoclonal antibodies against Bb by Novelmed Therapeutics are under development for various indications (161, 162). A monoclonal antibody to mouse FB has been shown to be protective in a mouse model of renal IRI (163). Other approaches using antisense oligonucleotides (164), or a phage-display selected cyclopeptides (165) are other feasible options to control AP activation through FB.

While FB is a promising target, so far, no therapeutic agent hit the market, or is in the advanced state in clinical trials. As with FD or MASP-3 inhibitors, bacterial infections manifest a potential risk when patients are treated with FB inhibitors.

C3 and CVF

C3 is the central molecule of complement; the three activation routes are merged at the generation of C3b and continue together as the terminal phase (**Figures 1** and **3**). C3 circulates in the serum at high concentration (4–7 μM; 0.75–1.35 mg/mL). Native C3 is a 185 kDa protein containing 13 domains (**Figure 2**). C3 is composed of two chains, α and β. The core is built up of 8 domains belonging to the α2-macroglobulin family. The thioester domain carries a buried thioester bond, which is prone to suffer hydrolysis or other nucleophilic attack.

Primary C3 deficiencies were described in a few families over the world. Mutation in C3 gene caused impaired C3 synthesis or secretion, which produced a low C3 level in the blood. These individuals are extremely susceptible to recurrent pyogenic bacterial infections, especially to Gram-negative but also to Gram-positive bacteria (166). Moreover, C3 deficiency impairs maturation of immune cells (dendritic cells, memory B cells, certain T cells) (166, 167). Furthermore, SLE and various renal diseases were also observed; however, their mechanism is not fully understood. Secondary C3 deficiency is due to malfunctioning of the complement regulatory proteins, typically FI and FH (168).

Complement activation can be blocked completely at the level of C3. On the other hand, C3 is the most abundant protein in the complement cascade; therefore, a large amount of an inhibitor would be needed to achieve a substantial effect. Compstatin, a promising complement-based therapeutic agent, was developed against C3 by phage-display using naïve library in 1996 (169). Compstatin is a cyclic peptide of 13 amino acids with a single disulfide bond. It blocks the access of the convertase to C3 through steric hindrance. Crystal structure with C3c showed that compstatin forms expansive H-bonds with its partner (170) (**Figure 6**). Neither complement regulator proteins nor other structurally related proteins (C4, C5) bind compstatin. In the past 20 years, the compstatin family has been constantly developed. New generations of compstatin analogs possess better

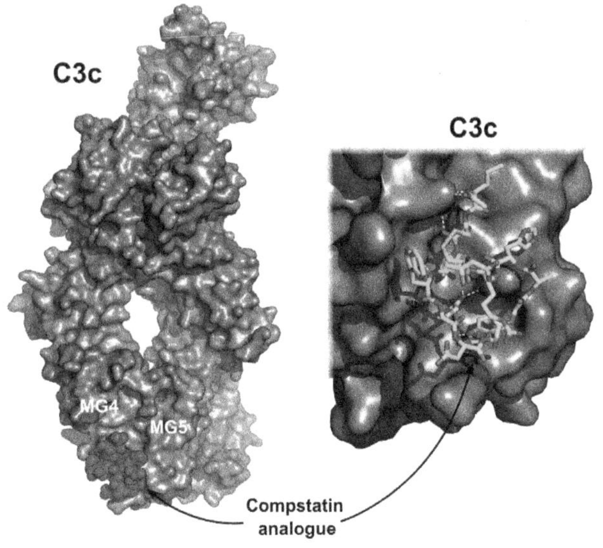

FIGURE 6 | C3c in complex with a compstatin analog. Compstatin, a cyclic peptide, was developed by phage-display. Since its discovery, several modified compstatin analogs have been developed. Compstatin and its analogs bind to C3, C3b, or C3c between the MG4 and MG5 domains. Compstatin sterically prevents the C3-convertase (C3bBb) to access its substrate C3. The depicted structure was determined using the Ac-V4W/H9A-NH2 variant of the original peptide. The figure was prepared based on the structure by Janssen et al. (170) (PDB entry 2QKI). On the left, the whole structure is shown with C3c (brown) in surface representation and compstatin (magenta) with spheres. On the right, a close-up of the binding site is shown with compstatin represented by sticks. Hydrogen bonds are indicated by yellow dashed lines.

pharmacokinetic and pharmacodynamic features. Compstatin derivatives were investigated in many complement-related animal diseases models and showed promising results (171). Just to mention a few, compstatins are efficient in primates in inflammatory diseases induced by cardiac surgery, cardiopulmonary bypass, or *E. coli* infection, in treatment of organ transplantation to reduce the possibility of xenograft rejection, and in sepsis. One of the compstatin derivatives (APL-2) already completed a Phase II clinical trial in treatment of AMD by Apellis Pharmaceuticals, and another one (AMY-101) started in 2017, the "first-in-human" clinical study against PNH by Amyndas Pharmaceuticals. Certainly, compstatins, as a peptide drug candidates, have their limitations especially considering oral administration. The rapid proteolytic degradation and poor biocompatibility make drug formulation challenging. On the other hand, the high specificity, the relatively low cost of production, and high variability gives the compstatin family members great potential to become widely used, effective, and safe complement therapeutics (171).

There are some other approaches to target complement activation through C3. Since 1970s, CVF is widely applied to deplete complement and to gain knowledge about its role in diseases. CVF is a structural and functional analog of C3, forms an AP convertase with Bb; however, it is resistant to the activity of FI and FH. Since decay of the convertase is abolished, C3 and C5 are rapidly exhausted from the blood. Nevertheless, CVF is immunogenic; therefore, it can be used only once to avoid antibody response. In the last decade, interesting results have been published about a chimeric protein, humanized CVF (172). It is a C3 derivative obtained by simply replacing the C-terminal part with the homologous sequence from CVF. This protein is safe and proved to be efficient in various animal disease models (AMD, collagen-induced arthritis, PNH, myasthenia gravis, etc.), and furthermore, no neutralizing antibody effect was detected in mice after prolonged usage (173).

Properdin

The only known positive regulator of the AP is properdin, also referred to as factor P. Properdin circulates in the plasma at 20–125 nM (4–25 μg/mL) concentration as a cyclic polymeric glycoprotein. In contrast to most complement proteins, it is synthesized primarily by leukocytes and shows different activity depending on the type of producing cells. The properdin monomer comprises six complete and one truncated thrombospondin type 1 repeat (TSR) domain in tandem connection. The 53 kDa monomer is able to form dimers, trimers, and even tetramers in a head-to-tail arrangement. Physiologically, the most abundant form is the trimer; however, properdin shows tendency to self-aggregate into higher oligomers under conditions used for its preparation. It has an extremely high positive charge, hence it tends to bind *via* ionic interactions to polyanion structures.

Properdin has a significant and well-established role in the AP of complement by stabilizing the very labile C3bB and C3bBb complexes offering binding sites to C3b, and FB or Bb. Extending the half-life of the AP convertase by 5- to 10-fold is essential for the effective AP activity (174). Another role of properdin, serving as a PRM, was proposed about 10 years ago. A similar function was originally suggested by Pillemer, who discovered the "properdin pathway." However, findings of this subject are controversial. Caution must be taken since repeated freezing and thawing resulted in highly polymerized, therefore, non-physiological, aggregated properdin, which binds non-specifically to surfaces. Experiments using unfractionated properdin could have led to physiologically not relevant observations (175). The binding abilities of properdin are also influenced by the contact surface and the presence of specific ligands. Experiments in properdin knock-out mice demonstrated that in the absence of properdin, bacterial LPS- and lipooligosaccharide-induced AP activation was absent, while zymosan or CVF-induced activation was only partially affected (79). Using compstatin and anti-FP antibody in ELISA assays, it has been shown that properdin does not attach directly to zymosan or *Escherichia coli* surfaces, but it contributes only to the stabilization of C3bBb complex (176). Recent studies showed that the binding of properdin to activating surfaces is always preceded by deposition of C3b (23), concluding that properdin can act as an initiator of AP only in a C3b-dependent manner.

Properdin deficiency especially in combination with the lack of other complement components (MBL, C2, etc.) causes unequivocal susceptibility to bacterial infections. Disorder in properdin and one of the late complement components (C5–C9) increases the risk of *Neisseria meningitidis* infection by 1,000- to 10,000-fold (28). Interestingly, the lack of IgG G2m(n) allotype in properdin-deficient persons also increased the susceptibility to meningococcal disease (177).

Therapeutic application of properdin emerged recently. In mouse model, it has been shown that a highly polymerized form of recombinant properdin gives protection against *N. meningitidis* and *Streptococcus pneumoniae*. A single low-dose treatment was enough to boost complement-activated lysis, which significantly reduced bacteremia and increased survival rates (178). We should note, however, that the recombinant properdin had histidine tag, which could influence its antimicrobial activity (179). Newly developed mouse monoclonal antibody against properdin was proved to be useful in sandwich-ELISA system to determine serum level of properdin in human samples (180). This antibody also successfully blocked AP activation in human sera.

The lack of properdin can efficiently abolish physiological or even unwanted AP activity. Inhibiting the AP through properdin can abate the amplification of deposited C3, hereby, the activity of the complement cascade. In contrast to C3, properdin is present at a relatively low concentration. Consequently, as an important regulator of the AP, it may turn out to be a promising therapeutic target to block complement activation. Novelmed is developing new drug candidates against the components of the AP, which do not interfere with the CP, as part of their effors, they evolved a new monoclonal antibody against the N-terminal fragment of properdin (181).

Factor I

Factor I has an outstanding role in the control of the complement system. Along with its cofactors, FI belongs to the regulators of complement activation. Although it possesses a low catalytic activity on its own, FI can downregulate all activation routes by dismantling the central component of the complement cascade: C3b (and also C4b). FI contributes to the self-defense of host tissues against complement damage through the acceleration of the decay of fluid-phase and surface-bound C3b to iC3b. Degradation products of C3b initiate the cellular immune response *via* their interaction with various receptors on immune cells.

FI is an 88 kDa glycoprotein synthesized as a single polypeptide chain by hepatocytes. It is a trypsin-like SP consisting of five domains; some of them are common in the components of the terminal pathway. The heavy chain contains the first four domains: FI membrane attack complex domain, CD5-like domain, low-density lipoprotein receptor 1 and 2 (LDLr 1 and 2) domains, and a small section called D-region with unknown homology (**Figure 2**). The light chain, which is attached to the heavy chain by a disulfide bond consists of the catalytically active SP domain.

FI has several unusual characteristics: it circulates as an "active" enzyme in the blood and does not have an inhibitor (19). These and some other features of FI resemble that of two other proteases of complement, Factor D (182) and MASP-3. FI has an extremely low catalytic activity toward synthetic substrates and also toward free C3b and C4b. In order to cleave C3b and C4b efficiently, FI needs cofactors. C4b-binding protein (C4BP) and FH are soluble cofactors of FI, while MCP (CD46) and CR1 (CD31) are membrane-bound cofactors. Since no natural inhibitor of FI is known, it is regulated by other mechanisms. First of all, the type of the substrate and also the type of its cofactor influences the activity of FI, and also the cleavage site on C3b or C4b and their degradation products. Second, structural data has proven recently that many crucial loops of the SP domain are disordered without the interacting partners (183). As the ternary complex of C3b-FH-FI is formed, ligand binding induces stabilization of the SP domain and, therefore, FI obtains full proteolytic activity. After the cleavage of the first bond in C3b (**Figure 7**), the substrates rearranges and the second or third cleavage site becomes accessible, while the SP domain of FI endures only minor movements (184).

According to its important role in complement regulation, the absence of FI causes dangerous, even life-threatening conditions. Due to the lack of decay acceleration, increased amounts of C3b lead to uncontrolled AP activation. The more C3b molecules are present, the more C3 convertases are generated, which results in the rapid exhaustion of C3 from the plasma. Individuals with FI deficiency are prone to suffer from recurring bacterial infections, severe kidney diseases, and most of all AMD (185, 186). Recent studies show that identifying rare CR1 variants in combination with low serum level of FI can enable therapist to find patients, who are the most likely candidates to develop AMD (187). FI deficiency is often associated with aHUS. Symptoms frequently appear in early childhood after a severe infection or in young females shortly after pregnancy. Large international cohorts have been established to characterize all genetic variants and clinical outcomes. The prognosis of FI-associated aHUS is quite poor, in half of the cases, end-stage renal failure developed rapidly. Treatment with eculizumab, which is the major therapeutic for aHUS, resulted in partial remission in patients having FI-associated aHUS (188).

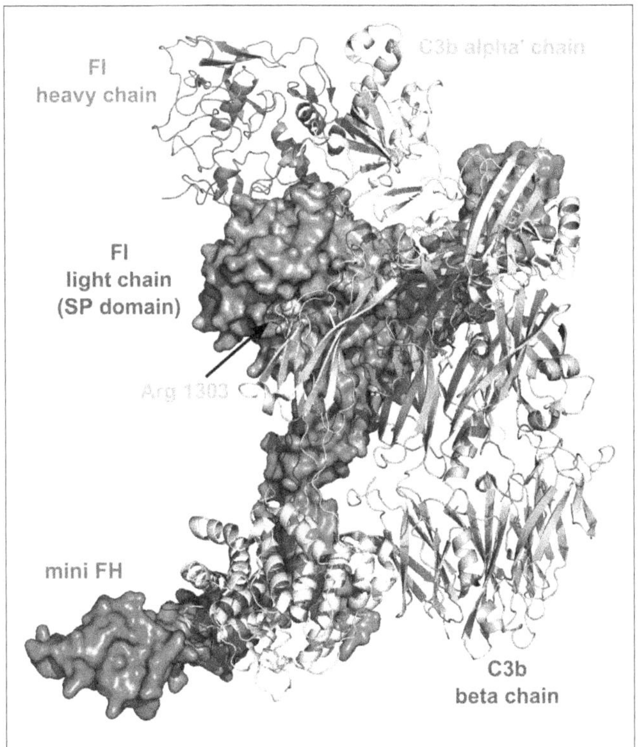

FIGURE 7 | Structure of the complex of C3b, mini factor H (FH), and factor I (FI). Mini FH is a potential drug candidate. *In vitro*, it is more effective than full-length FH in accelerating the decay of C3b by FI. The structure shows extensive contacts between the three proteins. The figure was made based on the structure of ternary complex of C3b-mini FH-FI (S525A) (184) (PDB entry 5O32). The colors of the legends match the depicted protein chains. The P1 residue (Arg^{1303}) of the primary cleavage site in C3b by FI is indicated by sphere representation. Mini FH and the light chain of FI are shown by surface representation, whereas C3b and the heavy chain of FI are shown by ribbon representation.

Another aspect that makes FI a potential drug candidate is the phenomenon of multiple polymorphisms in complement components that can affect the delicate balance between activation and regulation of an individual's complement system. The inherited repertoire of the complement gene variants was dubbed complotype (189). Some variant alleles can result a more reactive complement, which usually appears in the increased activity of C3b feedback cycle. Hyperactive complotypes raise significantly the risk of complement-related diseases at later age. Lower serum level of FI compared to FH (along with FH-related proteins) is advantageous to produce an effect. Moreover, the administration of FI in the presence of cofactor CR1 also enhances the conversion of inflammatory product iC3b to C3dg (190). Experimental data prove that increasing the amount of FI in serum of different complotypes can convert higher-risk to lower-risk activity. The extra amount of FI needed is approximately 50% of normal level, which would be a useful therapy in such patients (191). Comprehensive characterization of the complement regulatory genes in patients already suffering from complement-related disorders would enhance developments of personal and successful therapies.

Factor H, FH-Like, and FH-Related Proteins

Factor H (FH) is the major regulator of the AP. It is a fluid-phase molecule; however, it can bind to surface-deposited C3b and regulate the AP C3 convertase by several ways. By binding to C3b, it can prevent the capture of FB, consequently, the formation of the pro-convertase (C3bB). It has also a convertase decay-accelerating activity by facilitating the irreversible dissociation of the C3bBb complex. Probably, the most important function of FH is the cofactor activity, which is necessary for the FI-mediated cleavage of C3b to iC3b, through which it prevents the build-up of the amplification feedback loop of the AP. FH is a glycoprotein of 115 kDa and it consists of 20 CCP (aka short consensus repeat or sushi) domains (**Figure 2**). These domains, which are about 60 residues in length and contain two highly conserved disulfide bonds, are widespread among the complement proteins. Many complement regulatory proteins, such as FH and the FH-related proteins, CR1, CR2, MCP, DAF, C4BP, are composed predominantly or exclusively of these repeating structural motifs. The four N-terminal CCP domains of FH are responsible for the convertase decay-accelerating and cofactor activity. The other CCP domains take place in the interaction with different ligands. The C-terminal CCP 19–20 domains are indispensable for binding to self-surface deposited C3b. According to the current knowledge, FH recognizes the juxtaposition of C3b and carbohydrates containing sialic acid or glycosaminoglycan on the surface and binds strongly through the CCP 19–20 domains. The other domains may contribute to the binding to several ligands (e.g., heparin/CCP 7), but they are not indispensable for the function of FH. Based on this knowledge, minimal-size FH molecules were designed by combining the N- and C-terminal regions. Two constructs contain only six domains (CCP1-4 and 19-20) (192, 193). These mini FH molecules (**Figure 7**) showed more effective complement inhibition in different assay systems than the full-length FH molecule (192). Another, slightly extended construct containing CCP1–5 and 18–20 domains effectively inhibited complement activation *in vivo* and reduced abnormal glomerular C3 deposition in a FH-deficient mouse model of C3 glomerulopathy (194). Recently, a monoclonal anti-FH antibody has been found that could inhibit AP activation by potentiating FH (195). This potentiating antibody increases the affinity of FH for C3b and facilitates the degradation of the convertase by FH. There is an alternative splice product of the FH gene, which consists of only the CCP1-7 domains plus a four-amino-acid long C-terminus (196). This FH-like protein 1 (FHL-1) has complement-inhibitory activity, and it may have important function in the periphery. It is supposed that FHL-1 is able to penetrate through the Bruch's membrane beneath the retinal pigment epithelial cells in the eye, while FH cannot. In this way, FHL-1 may have a crucial role in the protection of retinal cells against complement-mediated attack and prevention of the development of AMD (197). Besides FH and FHL-1, there are five FH-related proteins (FHR) in the human serum. These proteins are encoded by separate genes situated next to the FH gene, and these genes arouse very probably through partial gene duplications. These proteins are shorter than FH and usually consist of CCP domains homologs to CCP6-9 and CCP18-20 of FH. Since the FHRs lack the complement regulatory CCP1-4 domains, their physiological relevance was underestimated at the time of their discovery (198). Since then, increasing number of evidences have been accumulated demonstrating the physiological role of FHRs, although this area is still controversial. Since the FHRs contain domains sharing high sequence identity with CCP18-20 of FH, these proteins can bind to ligands of FH (e.g., C3b, heparin, CRP).

TABLE 1 | Potential drug targets of the complement system discussed in this review.

Protein	Role in complement activation	Expected effects of inhibition	Potential diseases	Type of the drug candidate molecules	Reference
C1q	Pattern recognition molecule (PRM) of the classical pathway (CP)	Blocking the CP	Neurodegenerative diseases	Antibody, peptide	(84, 86–88)
MBL, ficolins	PRM of the lectin pathway (LP)	Blocking the LP	Ischemia–reperfusion injury (IRI)	Antibody	(84, 85)
MASP-1	LP initiation, boosting the alternative pathway (AP)	Attenuation of the LP and LPS-driven AP	IRI	Protein, small protein	(113, 121, 122)
MASP-2	LP initiation	Attenuation of the LP	IRI, renal diseases, atypical hemolytic uremic syndrome (aHUS)	Antibody, small protein	(121, 122, 129–132)
MASP-3	AP pre-initiation	Attenuation of the AP	AP-driven diseases	Antibody, small protein	(75, 138)
FD	AP initiation	Attenuation of the AP	Age-related macular degeneration (AMD), renal diseases	Antibody, small molecule	(120, 150, 154)
FB	Driving the AP	Attenuation of the AP	AMD, renal diseases	Small molecule, antibody	(158–165)
C3/C3b	Component of the AP C3 convertase and both C5 convertases	Blocking of AP and TP	AMD, paroxysmal nocturnal hemoglobinuria (PNH), renal diseases, transplantation	Peptide, protein	(169, 171–173)
Properdin	AP C3/C5 convertase stabilization	Attenuation of the AP	AMD, PNH	Antibody	(160, 181)
FI	Regulation of all pathways *via* degradation of C3b and C4b	NA	AMD, aHUS	Protein (FI for replacement therapy)	(191)
FH	AP regulation	NA	AMD, aHUS, transplantation	Antibody, proteins (rec. FH constructs for replacement therapy)	(192–195)

NA, not applicable, because inhibition of negative regulators is generally not desirable; however, potentiation could be a feasible approach (195).

However, these molecules cannot efficiently inhibit the AP since they lack the N-terminal regulatory domains of FH (CCP1-4).

FHR-1 was reported to enhance, rather than to inhibit complement activation through binding to CRP (199). This phenomenon could explain the protective effect of FHR-1 deficiency in AMD (200). FHR-4 was able to facilitate AP and CP activation by binding to C3b and CRP, respectively (201). FHR-5 was also shown to promote complement activation by binding to pentraxin 3 (PTX3) and extracellular matrix and by enhancing C1q deposition (202). It is also possible that FHRs compete with FH on the surface of bacteria, thereby compromising the ability of the microorganism to evade complement-mediated attack (203). It has been demonstrated that FHR-3 acts as a decoy, being captured by *N. meningitidis* cells instead of FH (204). The level of protection against *N. meningitidis* infection may depend on the FH/FHR-3 ratio in the serum. In general, the serum concentration of FH and the FHRs, and their affinity to various ligands may be a key factor in the fine tuning of complement-mediated opsonization and inflammation. If the delicate balance between FH and FHRs is disturbed due to genetic variations, or the amount and the composition of the ligands changes in the course of a disease (infection, oxidative stress), improper complement activation can take place resulting in self-tissue damage.

CONCLUDING REMARKS

The complement system was an appealing drug target even in the 1970s. However, the early drug development efforts failed mainly because of two reasons. The first reason was the lack of specificity of the anticomplement compounds. At that time, there was no technology to design or select highly specific agents against the individual complement components. The advance of structure-based and fragment-based drug design approaches made possible to generate selective and efficient small-molecule drugs. In addition to that, the modern biotechnological methods have provided highly specific biologics [monoclonal antibodies, recombinant proteins, nucleic-acid aptamers (205, 206), etc.] developed for anticomplement therapy. The most successful anticomplement drug so far, eculizumab, is a monoclonal antibody, and many antibodies are in preclinical or clinical phase in the pipeline. The second reason, which hindered the introduction of anticomplement drugs in the clinical practice in the past, was the insufficient knowledge about the mechanism of action of complement in both health and disease. In the recent years, the mechanism of activation and regulation of the LP and AP has been revealed in more detail, and we got insight into the cross-talks between the individual pathways inside the complement system and also the cross-talks between the complement and other proteolytic cascade systems (e.g., coagulation). New discoveries have also been made about the role of complement in the regulation of the adaptive immune system. Based on all of the above mentioned scientific and technical advances, essentially, all components of the LP and AP became targets of drug development (**Table 1**). It is likely that new drugs with more efficiency and less adverse effect will be approved for treating complement-related disorders in the near future.

AUTHOR CONTRIBUTIONS

All authors contributed equally to this article.

FUNDING

The study was supported by the National Research, Development and Innovation Office (NKTH) OTKA grants K108642 and K119374, and by the MedInProt program of the Hungarian Academy of Sciences.

REFERENCES

1. Ricklin D, Hajishengallis G, Yang K, Lambris JD. Complement: a key system for immune surveillance and homeostasis. *Nat Immunol* (2010) 11:785–97. doi:10.1038/ni.1923
2. Merle NS, Church SE, Fremeaux-Bacchi V, Roumenina LT. Complement system part I – molecular mechanisms of activation and regulation. *Front Immunol* (2015) 6:262. doi:10.3389/fimmu.2015.00262
3. Merle NS, Noe R, Halbwachs-Mecarelli L, Fremeaux-Bacchi V, Roumenina LT. Complement system part II: role in immunity. *Front Immunol* (2015) 6:257. doi:10.3389/fimmu.2015.00257
4. Thielens NM, Tedesco F, Bohlson SS, Gaboriaud C, Tenner AJ. C1q: a fresh look upon an old molecule. *Mol Immunol* (2017) 89:73–83. doi:10.1016/j.molimm.2017.05.025
5. Degn SE, Thiel S. Humoral pattern recognition and the complement system. *Scand J Immunol* (2013) 78:181–93. doi:10.1111/sji.12070
6. Gaboriaud C, Thielens NM, Gregory LA, Rossi V, Fontecilla-Camps JC, Arlaud GJ. Structure and activation of the C1 complex of complement: unraveling the puzzle. *Trends Immunol* (2004) 25:368–73. doi:10.1016/j.it.2004.04.008
7. Matsushita M, Thiel S, Jensenius JC, Terai I, Fujita T. Proteolytic activities of two types of mannose-binding lectin-associated serine protease. *J Immunol* (2000) 165:2637–42. doi:10.4049/jimmunol.165.5.2637
8. Takahashi M, Iwaki D, Kanno K, Ishida Y, Xiong J, Matsushita M, et al. Mannose-binding lectin (MBL)-associated serine protease (MASP)-1 contributes to activation of the lectin complement pathway. *J Immunol* (2008) 180:6132–8. doi:10.4049/jimmunol.180.9.6132
9. Héja D, Kocsis A, Dobó J, Szilágyi K, Szász R, Závodszky P, et al. Revised mechanism of complement lectin-pathway activation revealing the role of serine protease MASP-1 as the exclusive activator of MASP-2. *Proc Natl Acad Sci U S A* (2012) 109:10498–503. doi:10.1073/pnas.1202588109
10. Thiel S, Vorup-Jensen T, Stover CM, Schwaeble W, Laursen SB, Poulsen K, et al. A second serine protease associated with mannan-binding lectin that activates complement. *Nature* (1997) 386:506–10. doi:10.1038/386506a0
11. Ambrus G, Gál P, Kojima M, Szilágyi K, Balczer J, Antal J, et al. Natural substrates and inhibitors of mannan-binding lectin-associated serine protease-1 and -2: a study on recombinant catalytic fragments. *J Immunol* (2003) 170:1374–82. doi:10.4049/jimmunol.170.3.1374
12. Janssen BJC, Huizinga EG, Raaijmakers HCA, Roos A, Daha MR, Nilsson-Ekdahl K, et al. Structures of complement component C3 provide insights into the function and evolution of immunity. *Nature* (2005) 437:505–11. doi:10.1038/nature04005
13. Kidmose RT, Laursen NS, Dobó J, Kjaer TR, Sirotkina S, Yatime L, et al. Structural basis for activation of the complement system by component C4 cleavage. *Proc Natl Acad Sci U S A* (2012) 109:15425–30. doi:10.1073/pnas.1208031109
14. Harrison RA. The properdin pathway: an "alternative activation pathway" or a "critical amplification loop" for C3 and C5 activation? *Semin Immunopathol* (2018) 40:15–35. doi:10.1007/s00281-017-0661-x
15. Gadjeva M, Dodds AW, Taniguchi-Sidle A, Willis AC, Isenman DE, Law SK. The covalent binding reaction of complement component C3. *J Immunol* (1998) 161:985–90.
16. Law SK, Minich TM, Levine RP. Covalent binding efficiency of the third and fourth complement proteins in relation to pH, nucleophilicity, and

availability of hydroxyl groups. *Biochemistry* (1984) 23:3267–72. doi:10.1021/bi00309a022
17. Lachmann PJ. The amplification loop of the complement pathways. *Adv Immunol* (2009) 104:115–49. doi:10.1016/S0065-2776(08)04004-2
18. Nilsson B, Nilsson Ekdahl K. The tick-over theory revisited: is C3 a contact-activated protein? *Immunobiology* (2012) 217:1106–10. doi:10.1016/j.imbio.2012.07.008
19. Nilsson SC, Sim RB, Lea SM, Fremeaux-Bacchi V, Blom AM. Complement factor I in health and disease. *Mol Immunol* (2011) 48:1611–20. doi:10.1016/j.molimm.2011.04.004
20. Pillemer L, Blum L, Lepow IH, Ross OA, Todd EW, Wardlaw AC. The properdin system and immunity. I. Demonstration and isolation of a new serum protein, properdin, and its role in immune phenomena. *Science* (1954) 120:279–85. doi:10.1126/science.120.3112.279
21. Fearon DT, Austen KF. Properdin: binding to C3b and stabilization of the C3b-dependent C3 convertase. *J Exp Med* (1975) 142:856–63. doi:10.1084/jem.142.4.856
22. Spitzer D, Mitchell LM, Atkinson JP, Hourcade DE. Properdin can initiate complement activation by binding specific target surfaces and providing a platform for de novo convertase assembly. *J Immunol* (2007) 179:2600–8. doi:10.4049/jimmunol.179.4.2600
23. Harboe M, Johnson C, Nymo S, Ekholt K, Schjalm C, Lindstad JK, et al. Properdin binding to complement activating surfaces depends on initial C3b deposition. *Proc Natl Acad Sci U S A* (2017) 114:E534–9. doi:10.1073/pnas.1612385114
24. Verschoor A, Karsten CM, Broadley SP, Laumonnier Y, Köhl J. Old dogs-new tricks: immunoregulatory properties of C3 and C5 cleavage fragments. *Immunol Rev* (2016) 274:112–26. doi:10.1111/imr.12473
25. Fredslund F, Laursen NS, Roversi P, Jenner L, Oliveira CLP, Pedersen JS, et al. Structure of and influence of a tick complement inhibitor on human complement component 5. *Nat Immunol* (2008) 9:753–60. doi:10.1038/ni.1625
26. Aleshin AE, DiScipio RG, Stec B, Liddington RC. Crystal structure of C5b-6 suggests structural basis for priming assembly of the membrane attack complex. *J Biol Chem* (2012) 287:19642–52. doi:10.1074/jbc.M112.361121
27. Serna M, Giles JL, Morgan BP, Bubeck D. Structural basis of complement membrane attack complex formation. *Nat Commun* (2016) 7:10587. doi:10.1038/ncomms10587
28. Grumach AS, Kirschfink M. Are complement deficiencies really rare? Overview on prevalence, clinical importance and modern diagnostic approach. *Mol Immunol* (2014) 61:110–7. doi:10.1016/j.molimm.2014.06.030
29. Heitzeneder S, Seidel M, Förster-Waldl E, Heitger A. Mannan-binding lectin deficiency – good news, bad news, doesn't matter? *Clin Immunol Orlando Fla* (2012) 143:22–38. doi:10.1016/j.clim.2011.11.002
30. Fijen CA, Kuijper EJ, Hannema AJ, Sjöholm AG, van Putten JP. Complement deficiencies in patients over ten years old with meningococcal disease due to uncommon serogroups. *Lancet Lond Engl* (1989) 2:585–8. doi:10.1016/S0140-6736(89)90712-5
31. Petersen BH, Lee TJ, Snyderman R, Brooks GF. *Neisseria meningitidis* and *Neisseria gonorrhoeae* bacteremia associated with C6, C7, or C8 deficiency. *Ann Intern Med* (1979) 90:917–20. doi:10.7326/0003-4819-90-6-917
32. Gulati S, Agarwal S, Vasudhev S, Rice PA, Ram S. Properdin is critical for antibody-dependent bactericidal activity against *Neisseria gonorrhoeae* that recruit C4b-binding protein. *J Immunol* (2012) 188:3416–25. doi:10.4049/jimmunol.1102746
33. Genel F, Atlihan F, Gulez N, Sjöholm AG, Skattum L, Truedsson L. Properdin deficiency in a boy with fulminant meningococcal septic shock. *Acta Paediatr* (2006) 95:1498–500. doi:10.1080/08035250600603008
34. Fakhouri F, Frémeaux-Bacchi V, Noël L-H, Cook HT, Pickering MC. C3 glomerulopathy: a new classification. *Nat Rev Nephrol* (2010) 6:494–9. doi:10.1038/nrneph.2010.85
35. Pickering MC, D'Agati VD, Nester CM, Smith RJ, Haas M, Appel GB, et al. C3 glomerulopathy: consensus report. *Kidney Int* (2013) 84:1079–89. doi:10.1038/ki.2013.377
36. Marinozzi MC, Roumenina LT, Chauvet S, Hertig A, Bertrand D, Olagne J, et al. Anti-factor B and Anti-C3b autoantibodies in C3 glomerulopathy and Ig-associated membranoproliferative GN. *J Am Soc Nephrol* (2017) 28:1603–13. doi:10.1681/ASN.2016030343
37. Noris M, Remuzzi G. Glomerular diseases dependent on complement activation, including atypical hemolytic uremic syndrome, membranoproliferative glomerulonephritis, and C3 glomerulopathy: core curriculum 2015. *Am J Kidney Dis* (2015) 66:359–75. doi:10.1053/j.ajkd.2015.03.040
38. Maillard N, Wyatt RJ, Julian BA, Kiryluk K, Gharavi A, Fremeaux-Bacchi V, et al. Current understanding of the role of complement in IgA nephropathy. *J Am Soc Nephrol* (2015) 26:1503–12. doi:10.1681/ASN.2014101000
39. Daha MR, van Kooten C. Role of complement in IgA nephropathy. *J Nephrol* (2016) 29:1–4. doi:10.1007/s40620-015-0245-6
40. Kaartinen K, Martola L, Meri S. Atypical hemolytic-uremic syndrome. *Duodecim Laaketieteellinen Aikakauskirja* (2017) 133:539–47.
41. Neumann HPH, Salzmann M, Bohnert-Iwan B, Mannuelian T, Skerka C, Lenk D, et al. Haemolytic uraemic syndrome and mutations of the factor H gene: a registry-based study of German speaking countries. *J Med Genet* (2003) 40:676–81. doi:10.1136/jmg.40.9.676
42. Hofer J, Giner T, Józsi M. Complement factor H-antibody-associated hemolytic uremic syndrome: pathogenesis, clinical presentation, and treatment. *Semin Thromb Hemost* (2014) 40:431–43. doi:10.1055/s-0034-1375297
43. Hill A, DeZern AE, Kinoshita T, Brodsky RA. Paroxysmal nocturnal haemoglobinuria. *Nat Rev Dis Primer* (2017) 3:17028. doi:10.1038/nrdp.2017.28
44. Risitano AM, Marotta S. Therapeutic complement inhibition in complement-mediated hemolytic anemias: past, present and future. *Semin Immunol* (2016) 28:223–40. doi:10.1016/j.smim.2016.05.001
45. Geerlings MJ, de Jong EK, den Hollander AI. The complement system in age-related macular degeneration: a review of rare genetic variants and implications for personalized treatment. *Mol Immunol* (2017) 84:65–76. doi:10.1016/j.molimm.2016.11.016
46. Fritsche LG, Igl W, Bailey JNC, Grassmann F, Sengupta S, Bragg-Gresham JL, et al. A large genome-wide association study of age-related macular degeneration highlights contributions of rare and common variants. *Nat Genet* (2016) 48:134–43. doi:10.1038/ng.3448
47. Dolgin E. Age-related macular degeneration foils drugmakers. *Nat Biotechnol* (2017) 35:1000–1. doi:10.1038/nbt1117-1000
48. Carroll MC, Holers VM. Innate autoimmunity. *Adv Immunol* (2005) 86:137–57. doi:10.1016/S0065-2776(04)86004-8
49. Hart ML, Ceonzo KA, Shaffer LA, Takahashi K, Rother RP, Reenstra WR, et al. Gastrointestinal ischemia-reperfusion injury is lectin complement pathway dependent without involving C1q. *J Immunol* (2005) 174:6373–80. doi:10.4049/jimmunol.174.10.6373
50. Schwaeble WJ, Lynch NJ, Clark JE, Marber M, Samani NJ, Ali YM, et al. Targeting of mannan-binding lectin-associated serine protease-2 confers protection from myocardial and gastrointestinal ischemia/reperfusion injury. *Proc Natl Acad Sci U S A* (2011) 108:7523–8. doi:10.1073/pnas.1101748108
51. Walsh MC, Bourcier T, Takahashi K, Shi L, Busche MN, Rother RP, et al. Mannose-binding lectin is a regulator of inflammation that accompanies myocardial ischemia and reperfusion injury. *J Immunol* (2005) 175:541–6. doi:10.4049/jimmunol.175.1.541
52. La Bonte LR, Dokken B, Davis-Gorman G, Stahl GL, McDonagh PF. The mannose-binding lectin pathway is a significant contributor to reperfusion injury in the type 2 diabetic heart. *Diab Vasc Dis Res* (2009) 6:172–80. doi:10.1177/1479164109336051
53. Asgari E, Farrar CA, Lynch N, Ali YM, Roscher S, Stover C, et al. Mannan-binding lectin-associated serine protease 2 is critical for the development of renal ischemia reperfusion injury and mediates tissue injury in the absence of complement C4. *FASEB J* (2014) 28:3996–4003. doi:10.1096/fj.13-246306
54. Ekdahl KN, Lambris JD, Elwing H, Ricklin D, Nilsson PH, Teramura Y, et al. Innate immunity activation on biomaterial surfaces: a mechanistic model and coping strategies. *Adv Drug Deliv Rev* (2011) 63:1042–50. doi:10.1016/j.addr.2011.06.012
55. Szebeni J. Complement activation-related pseudoallergy: a new class of drug-induced acute immune toxicity. *Toxicology* (2005) 216:106–21. doi:10.1016/j.tox.2005.07.023
56. Chen F, Wang G, Griffin JI, Brenneman B, Banda NK, Holers VM, et al. Complement proteins bind to nanoparticle protein corona and undergo dynamic exchange in vivo. *Nat Nanotechnol* (2017) 12:387–93. doi:10.1038/nnano.2016.269
57. Rittirsch D, Redl H, Huber-Lang M. Role of complement in multiorgan failure. *Clin Dev Immunol* (2012) 2012:962927. doi:10.1155/2012/962927
58. Rooryck C, Diaz-Font A, Osborn DPS, Chabchoub E, Hernandez-Hernandez V, Shamseldin H, et al. Mutations in lectin complement pathway genes

COLEC11 and MASP1 cause 3MC syndrome. *Nat Genet* (2011) 43:197–203. doi:10.1038/ng.757

59. Sirmaci A, Walsh T, Akay H, Spiliopoulos M, Sakalar YB, Hasanefendioğlu-Bayrak A, et al. MASP1 mutations in patients with facial, umbilical, coccygeal, and auditory findings of Carnevale, Malpuech, OSA, and Michels syndromes. *Am J Hum Genet* (2010) 87:679–86. doi:10.1016/j.ajhg.2010.09.018
60. Presumey J, Bialas AR, Carroll MC. Complement system in neural synapse elimination in development and disease. *Adv Immunol* (2017) 135:53–79. doi:10.1016/bs.ai.2017.06.004
61. Hong S, Beja-Glasser VF, Nfonoyim BM, Frouin A, Li S, Ramakrishnan S, et al. Complement and microglia mediate early synapse loss in Alzheimer mouse models. *Science* (2016) 352:712–6. doi:10.1126/science.aad8373
62. Sekar A, Bialas AR, de Rivera H, Davis A, Hammond TR, Kamitaki N, et al. Schizophrenia risk from complex variation of complement component 4. *Nature* (2016) 530:177–83. doi:10.1038/nature16549
63. Mayilyan KR, Weinberger DR, Sim RB. The complement system in schizophrenia. *Drug News Perspect* (2008) 21:200–10. doi:10.1358/dnp.2008.21.4.1213349
64. Laich A, Sim RB. Complement C4bC2 complex formation: an investigation by surface plasmon resonance. *Biochim Biophys Acta* (2001) 1544:96–112. doi:10.1016/S0167-4838(00)00208-9
65. Matsushita M, Fujita T. Cleavage of the third component of complement (C3) by mannose-binding protein-associated serine protease (MASP) with subsequent complement activation. *Immunobiology* (1995) 194:443–8. doi:10.1016/S0171-2985(11)80110-5
66. Yaseen S, Demopulos G, Dudler T, Yabuki M, Wood CL, Cummings WJ, et al. Lectin pathway effector enzyme mannan-binding lectin-associated serine protease-2 can activate native complement C3 in absence of C4 and/or C2. *FASEB J* (2017) 31:2210–9. doi:10.1096/fj.201601306R
67. Selander B, Mårtensson U, Weintraub A, Holmström E, Matsushita M, Thiel S, et al. Mannan-binding lectin activates C3 and the alternative complement pathway without involvement of C2. *J Clin Invest* (2006) 116:1425–34. doi:10.1172/JCI25982
68. Paréj K, Kocsis A, Enyingi C, Dani R, Oroszlán G, Beinrohr L, et al. Cutting edge: a new player in the alternative complement pathway, MASP-1 is essential for LPS-Induced, but not for Zymosan-induced, alternative pathway activation. *J Immunol* (2018) 200:2247–52. doi:10.4049/jimmunol.1701421
69. Takahashi M, Ishida Y, Iwaki D, Kanno K, Suzuki T, Endo Y, et al. Essential role of mannose-binding lectin-associated serine protease-1 in activation of the complement factor D. *J Exp Med* (2010) 207:29–37. doi:10.1084/jem.20090633
70. Dobó J, Harmat V, Beinrohr L, Sebestyén E, Závodszky P, Gál P. MASP-1, a promiscuous complement protease: structure of its catalytic region reveals the basis of its broad specificity. *J Immunol* (2009) 183:1207–14. doi:10.4049/jimmunol.0901141
71. Iwaki D, Kanno K, Takahashi M, Endo Y, Matsushita M, Fujita T. The role of mannose-binding lectin-associated serine protease-3 in activation of the alternative complement pathway. *J Immunol* (2011) 187:3751–8. doi:10.4049/jimmunol.1100280
72. Degn SE, Jensen L, Hansen AG, Duman D, Tekin M, Jensenius JC, et al. Mannan-binding lectin-associated serine protease (MASP)-1 is crucial for lectin pathway activation in human serum, whereas neither MASP-1 nor MASP-3 is required for alternative pathway function. *J Immunol* (2012) 189:3957–69. doi:10.4049/jimmunol.1201736
73. Ruseva MM, Takahashi M, Fujita T, Pickering MC. C3 dysregulation due to factor H deficiency is mannan-binding lectin-associated serine proteases (MASP)-1 and MASP-3 independent in vivo. *Clin Exp Immunol* (2014) 176:84–92. doi:10.1111/cei.12244
74. Oroszlán G, Kortvely E, Szakács D, Kocsis A, Dammeier S, Zeck A, et al. MASP-1 and MASP-2 do not activate pro-factor D in resting human blood, whereas MASP-3 is a potential activator: kinetic analysis involving specific MASP-1 and MASP-2 inhibitors. *J Immunol* (2016) 196:857–65. doi:10.4049/jimmunol.1501717
75. Dobó J, Szakács D, Oroszlán G, Kortvely E, Kiss B, Boros E, et al. MASP-3 is the exclusive pro-factor D activator in resting blood: the lectin and the alternative complement pathways are fundamentally linked. *Sci Rep* (2016) 6:31877. doi:10.1038/srep31877
76. Oroszlán G, Dani R, Szilágyi A, Závodszky P, Thiel S, Gál P, et al. Extensive basal level activation of complement mannose-binding lectin-associated serine protease-3: kinetic modeling of lectin pathway activation provides possible mechanism. *Front Immunol* (2017) 8:1821. doi:10.3389/fimmu.2017.01821
77. Pihl R, Jensen L, Hansen AG, Thøgersen IB, Andres S, Dagnaes-Hansen F, et al. Analysis of factor D isoforms in Malpuech-Michels-Mingarelli-Carnevale patients highlights the role of MASP-3 as a Maturase in the alternative pathway of complement. *J Immunol* (2017) 199:2158–70. doi:10.4049/jimmunol.1700518
78. Paréj K, Hermann A, Donáth N, Závodszky P, Gál P, Dobó J. Dissociation and re-association studies on the interaction domains of mannan-binding lectin (MBL)-associated serine proteases, MASP-1 and MASP-2, provide evidence for heterodimer formation. *Mol Immunol* (2014) 59:1–9. doi:10.1016/j.molimm.2013.12.003
79. Kimura Y, Miwa T, Zhou L, Song W-C. Activator-specific requirement of properdin in the initiation and amplification of the alternative pathway complement. *Blood* (2008) 111:732–40. doi:10.1182/blood-2007-05-089821
80. Henriksen ML, Brandt J, Andrieu J-P, Nielsen C, Jensen PH, Holmskov U, et al. Heteromeric complexes of native collectin kidney 1 and collectin liver 1 are found in the circulation with MASPs and activate the complement system. *J Immunol* (2013) 191:6117–27. doi:10.4049/jimmunol.1302121
81. Degn SE, Jensen L, Olszowski T, Jensenius JC, Thiel S. Co-complexes of MASP-1 and MASP-2 associated with the soluble pattern-recognition molecules drive lectin pathway activation in a manner inhibitable by MAp44. *J Immunol* (2013) 191:1334–45. doi:10.4049/jimmunol.1300780
82. Phillips AE, Toth J, Dodds AW, Girija UV, Furze CM, Pala E, et al. Analogous interactions in initiating complexes of the classical and lectin pathways of complement. *J Immunol* (2009) 182:7708–17. doi:10.4049/jimmunol.0900666
83. Kjaer TR, Jensen L, Hansen A, Dani R, Jensenius JC, Dobó J, et al. Oligomerization of Mannan-binding lectin dictates binding properties and complement activation. *Scand J Immunol* (2016) 84:12–9. doi:10.1111/sji.12441
84. Roos A, Bouwman LH, Munoz J, Zuiverloon T, Faber-Krol MC, Fallaux-van den Houten FC, et al. Functional characterization of the lectin pathway of complement in human serum. *Mol Immunol* (2003) 39:655–68. doi:10.1016/S0161-5890(02)00254-7
85. Pavlov VI, Tan YS, McClure EE, La Bonte LR, Zou C, Gorsuch WB, et al. Human mannose-binding lectin inhibitor prevents myocardial injury and arterial thrombogenesis in a novel animal model. *Am J Pathol* (2015) 185:347–55. doi:10.1016/j.ajpath.2014.10.015
86. Phuan P-W, Zhang H, Asavapanumas N, Leviten M, Rosenthal A, Tradtrantip L, et al. C1q-targeted monoclonal antibody prevents complement-dependent cytotoxicity and neuropathology in in vitro and mouse models of neuromyelitis optica. *Acta Neuropathol* (2013) 125:829–40. doi:10.1007/s00401-013-1128-3
87. McGonigal R, Cunningham ME, Yao D, Barrie JA, Sankaranarayanan S, Fewou SN, et al. C1q-targeted inhibition of the classical complement pathway prevents injury in a novel mouse model of acute motor axonal neuropathy. *Acta Neuropathol Commun* (2016) 4:23. doi:10.1186/s40478-016-0291-x
88. Roos A, Nauta AJ, Broers D, Faber-Krol MC, Trouw LA, Drijfhout JW, et al. Specific inhibition of the classical complement pathway by C1q-binding peptides. *J Immunol* (2001) 167:7052–9. doi:10.4049/jimmunol.167.12.7052
89. Thiel S, Petersen SV, Vorup-Jensen T, Matsushita M, Fujita T, Stover CM, et al. Interaction of C1q and mannan-binding lectin (MBL) with C1r, C1s, MBL-associated serine proteases 1 and 2, and the MBL-associated protein MAp19. *J Immunol* (2000) 165:878–87. doi:10.4049/jimmunol.165.2.878
90. Keizer MP, Kamp AM, Brouwer N, van de Wetering MD, Wouters D, Kuijpers TW. Plasma-derived mannose-binding lectin shows a direct interaction with C1-inhibitor. *Mol Immunol* (2014) 58:187–93. doi:10.1016/j.molimm.2013.11.022
91. Megyeri M, Jani PK, Kajdácsi E, Dobó J, Schwaner E, Major B, et al. Serum MASP-1 in complex with MBL activates endothelial cells. *Mol Immunol* (2014) 59:39–45. doi:10.1016/j.molimm.2014.01.001
92. Keizer MP, Aarts C, Kamp AM, Caron HN, van de Wetering MD, Wouters D, et al. Asparaginase inhibits the lectin pathway of complement activation. *Mol Immunol* (2018) 93:189–92. doi:10.1016/j.molimm.2017.11.027
93. Sharp JA, Whitley PH, Cunnion KM, Krishna NK. Peptide inhibitor of complement c1, a novel suppressor of classical pathway activation: mechanistic studies and clinical potential. *Front Immunol* (2014) 5:406. doi:10.3389/fimmu.2014.00406

94. Thiel S, Jensen L, Degn SE, Nielsen HJ, Gál P, Dobó J, et al. Mannan-binding lectin (MBL)-associated serine protease-1 (MASP-1), a serine protease associated with humoral pattern-recognition molecules: normal and acute-phase levels in serum and stoichiometry of lectin pathway components. *Clin Exp Immunol* (2012) 169:38–48. doi:10.1111/j.1365-2249.2012.04584.x
95. Megyeri M, Harmat V, Major B, Végh Á, Balczer J, Héja D, et al. Quantitative characterization of the activation steps of mannan-binding lectin (MBL)-associated serine proteases (MASPs) points to the central role of MASP-1 in the initiation of the complement lectin pathway. *J Biol Chem* (2013) 288:8922–34. doi:10.1074/jbc.M112.446500
96. Megyeri M, Makó V, Beinrohr L, Doleschall Z, Prohászka Z, Cervenak L, et al. Complement protease MASP-1 activates human endothelial cells: PAR4 activation is a link between complement and endothelial function. *J Immunol* (2009) 183:3409–16. doi:10.4049/jimmunol.0900879
97. Jani PK, Kajdácsi E, Megyeri M, Dobó J, Doleschall Z, Futosi K, et al. MASP-1 induces a unique cytokine pattern in endothelial cells: a novel link between complement system and neutrophil granulocytes. *PLoS One* (2014) 9:e87104. doi:10.1371/journal.pone.0087104
98. Jani PK, Schwaner E, Kajdácsi E, Debreczeni ML, Ungai-Salánki R, Dobó J, et al. Complement MASP-1 enhances adhesion between endothelial cells and neutrophils by up-regulating E-selectin expression. *Mol Immunol* (2016) 75:38–47. doi:10.1016/j.molimm.2016.05.007
99. Schwaner E, Németh Z, Jani PK, Kajdácsi E, Debreczeni ML, Doleschall Z, et al. Transcriptome analysis of inflammation-related gene expression in endothelial cells activated by complement MASP-1. *Sci Rep* (2017) 7:10462. doi:10.1038/s41598-017-09058-8
100. Dobó J, Major B, Kékesi KA, Szabó I, Megyeri M, Hajela K, et al. Cleavage of kininogen and subsequent bradykinin release by the complement component: mannose-binding lectin-associated serine protease (MASP)-1. *PLoS One* (2011) 6:e20036. doi:10.1371/journal.pone.0020036
101. Csuka D, Veszeli N, Varga L, Prohászka Z, Farkas H. The role of the complement system in hereditary angioedema. *Mol Immunol* (2017) 89:59–68. doi:10.1016/j.molimm.2017.05.020
102. Hess K, Ajjan R, Phoenix F, Dobó J, Gál P, Schroeder V. Effects of MASP-1 of the complement system on activation of coagulation factors and plasma clot formation. *PLoS One* (2012) 7:e35690. doi:10.1371/journal.pone.0035690
103. Jenny L, Dobó J, Gál P, Schroeder V. MASP-1 of the complement system promotes clotting via prothrombin activation. *Mol Immunol* (2015) 65:398–405. doi:10.1016/j.molimm.2015.02.014
104. Jenny L, Dobó J, Gál P, Schroeder V. MASP-1 induced clotting – the first model of prothrombin activation by MASP-1. *PLoS One* (2015) 10:e0144633. doi:10.1371/journal.pone.0144633
105. Jenny L, Dobó J, Gál P, Pál G, Lam WA, Schroeder V. MASP-1 of the complement system enhances clot formation in a microvascular whole blood flow model. *PLoS One* (2018) 13:e0191292. doi:10.1371/journal.pone.0191292
106. La Bonte LR, Pavlov VI, Tan YS, Takahashi K, Takahashi M, Banda NK, et al. Mannose-binding lectin-associated serine protease-1 is a significant contributor to coagulation in a murine model of occlusive thrombosis. *J Immunol* (2012) 188:885–91. doi:10.4049/jimmunol.1102916
107. Gál P, Barna L, Kocsis A, Závodszky P. Serine proteases of the classical and lectin pathways: similarities and differences. *Immunobiology* (2007) 212:267–77. doi:10.1016/j.imbio.2006.11.002
108. Paréj K, Dobó J, Závodszky P, Gál P. The control of the complement lectin pathway activation revisited: both C1-inhibitor and antithrombin are likely physiological inhibitors, while α2-macroglobulin is not. *Mol Immunol* (2013) 54:415–22. doi:10.1016/j.molimm.2013.01.009
109. Gulati S, Sastry K, Jensenius JC, Rice PA, Ram S. Regulation of the mannan-binding lectin pathway of complement on *Neisseria gonorrhoeae* by C1-inhibitor and alpha 2-macroglobulin. *J Immunol* (2002) 168:4078–86. doi:10.4049/jimmunol.168.8.4078
110. Petersen SV, Thiel S, Jensen L, Vorup-Jensen T, Koch C, Jensenius JC. Control of the classical and the MBL pathway of complement activation. *Mol Immunol* (2000) 37:803–11. doi:10.1016/S0161-5890(01)00004-9
111. Degn SE, Hansen AG, Steffensen R, Jacobsen C, Jensenius JC, Thiel S. MAp44, a human protein associated with pattern recognition molecules of the complement system and regulating the lectin pathway of complement activation. *J Immunol* (2009) 183:7371–8. doi:10.4049/jimmunol.0902388
112. Skjoedt M-O, Hummelshoj T, Palarasah Y, Honore C, Koch C, Skjodt K, et al. A novel mannose-binding lectin/ficolin-associated protein is highly expressed in heart and skeletal muscle tissues and inhibits complement activation. *J Biol Chem* (2010) 285:8234–43. doi:10.1074/jbc.M109.065805
113. Pavlov VI, Skjoedt M-O, Siow Tan Y, Rosbjerg A, Garred P, Stahl GL. Endogenous and natural complement inhibitor attenuates myocardial injury and arterial thrombogenesis. *Circulation* (2012) 126:2227–35. doi:10.1161/CIRCULATIONAHA.112.123968
114. Nordmaj MA, Munthe-Fog L, Hein E, Skjoedt M-O, Garred P. Genetically engineered fusion of MAP-1 and factor H domains 1-5 generates a potent dual upstream inhibitor of both the lectin and alternative complement pathways. *FASEB J* (2015) 29:4945–55. doi:10.1096/fj.15-277103
115. Ricklin D, Lambris JD. Complement-targeted therapeutics. *Nat Biotechnol* (2007) 25:1265–75. doi:10.1038/nbt1342
116. Na K-R, Choi H, Jeong JY, Lee KW, Chang Y-K, Choi DE. Nafamostat mesilate attenuates ischemia-reperfusion-induced renal injury. *Transplant Proc* (2016) 48:2192–9. doi:10.1016/j.transproceed.2016.03.050
117. Schwertz H, Carter JM, Russ M, Schubert S, Schlitt A, Buerke U, et al. Serine protease inhibitor nafamostat given before reperfusion reduces inflammatory myocardial injury by complement and neutrophil inhibition. *J Cardiovasc Pharmacol* (2008) 52:151–60. doi:10.1097/FJC.0b013e318180188b
118. Marotta F, Fesce E, Rezakovic I, Chui DH, Suzuki K, Idéo G. Nafamostat mesilate on the course of acute pancreatitis. Protective effect on peritoneal permeability and relation with supervening pulmonary distress. *Int J Pancreatol* (1994) 16:51–9. doi:10.1007/BF02925610
119. Inagaki H, Nonami T, Kurokawa T, Takeuchi Y, Okuda N, Nakao A, et al. Effects of nafamostat mesilate, a synthetic protease inhibitor, on immunity and coagulation after hepatic resection. *Hepatogastroenterology* (1999) 46:3223–8.
120. Maibaum J, Liao S-M, Vulpetti A, Ostermann N, Randl S, Rüdisser S, et al. Small-molecule factor D inhibitors targeting the alternative complement pathway. *Nat Chem Biol* (2016) 12:1105–10. doi:10.1038/nchembio.2208
121. Kocsis A, Kékesi KA, Szász R, Végh BM, Balczer J, Dobó J, et al. Selective inhibition of the lectin pathway of complement with phage display selected peptides against mannose-binding lectin-associated serine protease (MASP)-1 and -2: significant contribution of MASP-1 to lectin pathway activation. *J Immunol* (2010) 185:4169–78. doi:10.4049/jimmunol.1001819
122. Héja D, Harmat V, Fodor K, Wilmanns M, Dobó J, Kékesi KA, et al. Monospecific inhibitors show that both mannan-binding lectin-associated serine protease-1 (MASP-1) and -2 are essential for lectin pathway activation and reveal structural plasticity of MASP-2. *J Biol Chem* (2012) 287:20290–300. doi:10.1074/jbc.M112.354332
123. Brandt T, Holzmann N, Muley L, Khayat M, Wegscheid-Gerlach C, Baum B, et al. Congeneric but still distinct: how closely related trypsin ligands exhibit different thermodynamic and structural properties. *J Mol Biol* (2011) 405:1170–87. doi:10.1016/j.jmb.2010.11.038
124. Gál P, Harmat V, Kocsis A, Bián T, Barna L, Ambrus G, et al. A true autoactivating enzyme. Structural insight into mannose-binding lectin-associated serine protease-2 activations. *J Biol Chem* (2005) 280:33435–44. doi:10.1074/jbc.M506051200
125. Lynch NJ, Khan S-H, Stover CM, Sandrini SM, Marston D, Presanis JS, et al. Composition of the lectin pathway of complement in *Gallus gallus*: absence of mannan-binding lectin-associated serine protease-1 in birds. *J Immunol* (2005) 174:4998–5006. doi:10.4049/jimmunol.174.8.4998
126. Krarup A, Wallis R, Presanis JS, Gál P, Sim RB. Simultaneous activation of complement and coagulation by MBL-associated serine protease 2. *PLoS One* (2007) 2:e623. doi:10.1371/journal.pone.0000623
127. Stover CM, Thiel S, Thelen M, Lynch NJ, Vorup-Jensen T, Jensenius JC, et al. Two constituents of the initiation complex of the mannan-binding lectin activation pathway of complement are encoded by a single structural gene. *J Immunol* (1999) 162:3481–90.
128. Takahashi M, Endo Y, Fujita T, Matsushita M. A truncated form of mannose-binding lectin-associated serine protease (MASP)-2 expressed by alternative polyadenylation is a component of the lectin complement pathway. *Int Immunol* (1999) 11:859–63. doi:10.1093/intimm/11.5.859
129. Clark JE, Dudler T, Marber MS, Schwaeble W. Cardioprotection by an anti-MASP-2 antibody in a murine model of myocardial infarction. *Open Heart* (2018) 5:e000652. doi:10.1136/openhrt-2017-000652
130. *Safety and Efficacy Study of OMS721 in Patients With Atypical Hemolytic Uremic Syndrome – Full Text View – ClinicalTrials.gov*. Available from: https://clinicaltrials.gov/ct2/show/NCT03205995 (Accessed: May 25, 2018).

131. *Safety and Efficacy Study of OMS721 in Patients With Thrombotic Microangiopathies - Full Text View - ClinicalTrials.gov*. Available from: https://clinicaltrials.gov/ct2/show/NCT02222545 (Accessed: May 25, 2018).
132. *Safety Study of IgAN, LN, MN, & C3 Glomerulopathy Including Dense Deposit Disease Treated With OMS721 - Full Text View - ClinicalTrials.gov*. Available from: https://clinicaltrials.gov/ct2/show/NCT02682407 (Accessed: May 25, 2018).
133. Dahl MR, Thiel S, Matsushita M, Fujita T, Willis AC, Christensen T, et al. MASP-3 and its association with distinct complexes of the mannan-binding lectin complement activation pathway. *Immunity* (2001) 15:127–35. doi:10.1016/S1074-7613(01)00161-3
134. Atik T, Koparir A, Bademci G, Foster J, Altunoglu U, Mutlu GY, et al. Novel MASP1 mutations are associated with an expanded phenotype in 3MC1 syndrome. *Orphanet J Rare Dis* (2015) 10:128. doi:10.1186/s13023-015-0345-3
135. Munye MM, Diaz-Font A, Ocaka L, Henriksen ML, Lees M, Brady A, et al. COLEC10 is mutated in 3MC patients and regulates early craniofacial development. *PLoS Genet* (2017) 13:e1006679. doi:10.1371/journal.pgen.1006679
136. Zundel S, Cseh S, Lacroix M, Dahl MR, Matsushita M, Andrieu J-P, et al. Characterization of recombinant mannan-binding lectin-associated serine protease (MASP)-3 suggests an activation mechanism different from that of MASP-1 and MASP-2. *J Immunol* (2004) 172:4342–50. doi:10.4049/jimmunol.172.7.4342
137. Cortesio CL, Jiang W. Mannan-binding lectin-associated serine protease 3 cleaves synthetic peptides and insulin-like growth factor-binding protein 5. *Arch Biochem Biophys* (2006) 449:164–70. doi:10.1016/j.abb.2006.02.006
138. Cummings WJ, Wood C, Yabuki M, Li Y, Dudler T, Yaseem S, et al. *MASP-3 Antibody Treatment Blocks Pro-Df Maturation, Reduces AP Activity, and Prevents Collagen Antibody-Induced Arthritis. Late-Breaking Abstract. 16th European Meeting on Complement in Human Disease, Copenhagen*. (2017).
139. Pascual M, Steiger G, Estreicher J, Macon K, Volanakis JE, Schifferli JA. Metabolism of complement factor D in renal failure. *Kidney Int* (1988) 34:529–36. doi:10.1038/ki.1988.214
140. Lesavre PH, Müller-Eberhard HJ. Mechanism of action of factor D of the alternative complement pathway. *J Exp Med* (1978) 148:1498–509. doi:10.1084/jem.148.6.1498
141. Fearon DT, Austen KF, Ruddy S. Properdin factor D: characterization of its active site and isolation of the precursor form. *J Exp Med* (1974) 139:355–66. doi:10.1084/jem.139.2.355
142. Johnson DM, Gagnon J, Reid KB. Factor D of the alternative pathway of human complement. Purification, alignment and N-terminal amino acid sequences of the major cyanogen bromide fragments, and localization of the serine residue at the active site. *Biochem J* (1980) 187:863–74. doi:10.1042/bj1870863
143. Volanakis JE, Narayana SV. Complement factor D, a novel serine protease. *Protein Sci Publ Protein Soc* (1996) 5:553–64. doi:10.1002/pro.5560050401
144. Taylor FR, Bixler SA, Budman JI, Wen D, Karpusas M, Ryan ST, et al. Induced fit activation mechanism of the exceptionally specific serine protease, complement factor D. *Biochemistry* (1999) 38:2849–59. doi:10.1021/bi982140f
145. Narayana SV, Carson M, el-Kabbani O, Kilpatrick JM, Moore D, Chen X, et al. Structure of human factor D. A complement system protein at 2.0 A resolution. *J Mol Biol* (1994) 235:695–708. doi:10.1006/jmbi.1994.1021
146. Forneris F, Ricklin D, Wu J, Tzekou A, Wallace RS, Lambris JD, et al. Structures of C3b in complex with factors B and D give insight into complement convertase formation. *Science* (2010) 330:1816–20. doi:10.1126/science.1195821
147. Wu X, Hutson I, Akk AM, Mascharak S, Pham CTN, Hourcade DE, et al. Contribution of adipose-derived factor D/adipsin to complement alternative pathway activation: lessons from lipodystrophy. *J Immunol* (2018) 200:2786–97. doi:10.4049/jimmunol.1701668
148. Reynolds R, Hartnett ME, Atkinson JP, Giclas PC, Rosner B, Seddon JM. Plasma complement components and activation fragments: associations with age-related macular degeneration genotypes and phenotypes. *Invest Ophthalmol Vis Sci* (2009) 50:5818–27. doi:10.1167/iovs.09-3928
149. Pomeroy C, Mitchell J, Eckert E, Raymond N, Crosby R, Dalmasso AP. Effect of body weight and caloric restriction on serum complement proteins, including Factor D/adipsin: studies in anorexia nervosa and obesity. *Clin Exp Immunol* (1997) 108:507–15. doi:10.1046/j.1365-2249.1997.3921287.x
150. Loyet KM, Good J, Davancaze T, Sturgeon L, Wang X, Yang J, et al. Complement inhibition in cynomolgus monkeys by anti-factor d antigen-binding fragment for the treatment of an advanced form of dry age-related macular degeneration. *J Pharmacol Exp Ther* (2014) 351:527–37. doi:10.1124/jpet.114.215921
151. DiScipio RG. The activation of the alternative pathway C3 convertase by human plasma kallikrein. *Immunology* (1982) 45:587–95.
152. Ricklin D, Barratt-Due A, Mollnes TE. Complement in clinical medicine: clinical trials, case reports and therapy monitoring. *Mol Immunol* (2017) 89:10–21. doi:10.1016/j.molimm.2017.05.013
153. Ricklin D, Mastellos DC, Reis ES, Lambris JD. The renaissance of complement therapeutics. *Nat Rev Nephrol* (2018) 14:26–47. doi:10.1038/nrneph.2017.156
154. Achillion Pharmaceuticals, Inc. *Factor D: A Trigger Point for Complement Activity*. (2017). Available from: http://www.achillion.com/science-and-technology/complement-factor-d/ (Accessed: April 19, 2018).
155. Torreira E, Tortajada A, Montes T, Rodríguez de Córdoba S, Llorca O. Coexistence of closed and open conformations of complement factor B in the alternative pathway C3bB(Mg2+) proconvertase. *J Immunol* (2009) 183:7347–51. doi:10.4049/jimmunol.0902310
156. Fishelson Z, Müller-Eberhard HJ. Residual hemolytic and proteolytic activity expressed by Bb after decay-dissociation of C3b,Bb. *J Immunol* (1984) 132:1425–9.
157. Pangburn MK, Müller-Eberhard HJ. The C3 convertase of the alternative pathway of human complement. Enzymic properties of the bimolecular proteinase. *Biochem J* (1986) 235:723–30. doi:10.1042/bj2350723
158. Le GT, Abbenante G, Fairlie DP. Profiling the enzymatic properties and inhibition of human complement factor B. *J Biol Chem* (2007) 282:34809–16. doi:10.1074/jbc.M705646200
159. Adams CM. Complement factor B inhibitors and uses there of. United States Patent Application 20160024079. (2016).
160. Risitano AM, Marotta S. Toward complement inhibition 2.0: next generation anticomplement agents for paroxysmal nocturnal hemoglobinuria. *Am J Hematol* (2018) 93:564–77. doi:10.1002/ajh.25016
161. Bansal R. Method of inhibiting complement activation with factor Bb specific antibodies. United States Patent 8981060. (2015).
162. Bansal R. Humanized anti-factor C3b antibodies and uses there of. United States Patent 9243060. (2016).
163. Thurman JM, Royer PA, Ljubanovic D, Dursun B, Lenderink AM, Edelstein CL, et al. Treatment with an inhibitory monoclonal antibody to mouse factor B protects mice from induction of apoptosis and renal ischemia/reperfusion injury. *J Am Soc Nephrol* (2006) 17:707–15. doi:10.1681/ASN.2005070698
164. Grossman TR, Hettrick LA, Johnson RB, Hung G, Peralta R, Watt A, et al. Inhibition of the alternative complement pathway by antisense oligonucleotides targeting complement factor B improves lupus nephritis in mice. *Immunobiology* (2016) 221:701–8. doi:10.1016/j.imbio.2015.08.001
165. Kadam AP, Sahu A. Identification of Complin, a novel complement inhibitor that targets complement proteins factor B and C2. *J Immunol* (2010) 184:7116–24. doi:10.4049/jimmunol.1000200
166. Ghannam A, Pernollet M, Fauquert J-L, Monnier N, Ponard D, Villiers M-B, et al. Human C3 deficiency associated with impairments in dendritic cell differentiation, memory B cells, and regulatory T cells. *J Immunol* (2008) 181:5158–66. doi:10.4049/jimmunol.181.7.5158
167. Ghannam A, Fauquert J-L, Thomas C, Kemper C, Drouet C. Human complement C3 deficiency: Th1 induction requires T cell-derived complement C3a and CD46 activation. *Mol Immunol* (2014) 58:98–107. doi:10.1016/j.molimm.2013.11.010
168. Reis SE, Falcão DA, Isaac L. Clinical aspects and molecular basis of primary deficiencies of complement component C3 and its regulatory proteins factor I and factor H. *Scand J Immunol* (2006) 63:155–68. doi:10.1111/j.1365-3083.2006.01729.x
169. Sahu A, Kay BK, Lambris JD. Inhibition of human complement by a C3-binding peptide isolated from a phage-displayed random peptide library. *J Immunol* (1996) 157:884–91.
170. Janssen BJC, Halff EF, Lambris JD, Gros P. Structure of compstatin in complex with complement component C3c reveals a new mechanism of complement inhibition. *J Biol Chem* (2007) 282:29241–7. doi:10.1074/jbc.M704587200
171. Huang Y. Evolution of compstatin family as therapeutic complement inhibitors. *Expert Opin Drug Discov* (2018) 13:435–44. doi:10.1080/17460441.2018.1437139
172. Fritzinger DC, Hew BE, Thorne M, Pangburn MK, Janssen BJC, Gros P, et al. Functional characterization of human C3/cobra venom factor hybrid proteins for therapeutic complement depletion. *Dev Comp Immunol* (2009) 33:105–16. doi:10.1016/j.dci.2008.07.006

173. Ing M, Hew BE, Fritzinger DC, Delignat S, Lacroix-Desmazes S, Vogel C-W, et al. Absence of a neutralizing antibody response to humanized cobra venom factor in mice. *Mol Immunol* (2018) 97:1–7. doi:10.1016/j.molimm.2018.02.018
174. Medicus RG, Götze O, Müller-Eberhard HJ. Alternative pathway of complement: recruitment of precursor properdin by the labile C3/C5 convertase and the potentiation of the pathway. *J Exp Med* (1976) 144:1076–93. doi:10.1084/jem.144.4.1076
175. Blatt AZ, Pathan S, Ferreira VP. Properdin: a tightly regulated critical inflammatory modulator. *Immunol Rev* (2016) 274:172–90. doi:10.1111/imr.12466
176. Harboe M, Garred P, Lindstad JK, Pharo A, Müller F, Stahl GL, et al. The role of properdin in zymosan- and *Escherichia coli*-induced complement activation. *J Immunol* (2012) 189:2606–13. doi:10.4049/jimmunol.1200269
177. Späth PJ, Sjöholm AG, Fredrikson GN, Misiano G, Scherz R, Schaad UB, et al. Properdin deficiency in a large Swiss family: identification of a stop codon in the properdin gene, and association of meningococcal disease with lack of the IgG2 allotype marker G2m(n). *Clin Exp Immunol* (1999) 118:278–84. doi:10.1046/j.1365-2249.1999.01056.x
178. Ali YM, Hayat A, Saeed BM, Haleem KS, Alshamrani S, Kenawy HI, et al. Low-dose recombinant properdin provides substantial protection against *Streptococcus pneumoniae* and *Neisseria meningitidis* infection. *Proc Natl Acad Sci U S A* (2014) 111:5301–6. doi:10.1073/pnas.1401011111
179. Zimmer J, Hobkirk J, Mohamed F, Browning MJ, Stover CM. On the functional overlap between complement and anti-microbial peptides. *Front Immunol* (2014) 5:689. doi:10.3389/fimmu.2014.00689
180. Pauly D, Nagel BM, Reinders J, Killian T, Wulf M, Ackermann S, et al. A novel antibody against human properdin inhibits the alternative complement system and specifically detects properdin from blood samples. *PLoS One* (2014) 9:e96371. doi:10.1371/journal.pone.0096371
181. McGeer PL, Lee M, McGeer EG. A review of human diseases caused or exacerbated by aberrant complement activation. *Neurobiol Aging* (2017) 52:12–22. doi:10.1016/j.neurobiolaging.2016.12.017
182. Sim RB, Laich A. Serine proteases of the complement system. *Biochem Soc Trans* (2000) 28:545–50. doi:10.1042/bst0280545
183. Roversi P, Johnson S, Caesar JJE, McLean F, Leath KJ, Tsiftsoglou SA, et al. Structural basis for complement factor I control and its disease-associated sequence polymorphisms. *Proc Natl Acad Sci U S A* (2011) 108:12839–44. doi:10.1073/pnas.1102167108
184. Xue X, Wu J, Ricklin D, Forneris F, Di Crescenzio P, Schmidt CQ, et al. Regulator-dependent mechanisms of C3b processing by factor I allow differentiation of immune responses. *Nat Struct Mol Biol* (2017) 24:643–51. doi:10.1038/nsmb.3427
185. Alba-Domínguez M, López-Lera A, Garrido S, Nozal P, González-Granado I, Melero J, et al. Complement factor I deficiency: a not so rare immune defect: characterization of new mutations and the first large gene deletion. *Orphanet J Rare Dis* (2012) 7:42. doi:10.1186/1750-1172-7-42
186. Alexander P, Gibson J, Cree AJ, Ennis S, Lotery AJ. Complement factor I and age-related macular degeneration. *Mol Vis* (2014) 20:1253–7.
187. Kavanagh D, Yu Y, Schramm EC, Triebwasser M, Wagner EK, Raychaudhuri S, et al. Rare genetic variants in the CFI gene are associated with advanced age-related macular degeneration and commonly result in reduced serum factor I levels. *Hum Mol Genet* (2015) 24:3861–70. doi:10.1093/hmg/ddv091
188. Kavanagh D, Richards A, Fremeaux-Bacchi V, Noris M, Goodship T, Remuzzi G, et al. Screening for complement system abnormalities in patients with atypical hemolytic uremic syndrome. *Clin J Am Soc Nephrol* (2007) 2:591–6. doi:10.2215/CJN.03270906
189. Harris CL, Heurich M, Rodriguez de Cordoba S, Morgan BP. The complotype: dictating risk for inflammation and infection. *Trends Immunol* (2012) 33:513–21. doi:10.1016/j.it.2012.06.001
190. Lay E, Nutland S, Smith JE, Hiles I, Smith RA, Seilly DJ, et al. Complotype affects the extent of down-regulation by Factor I of the C3b feedback cycle in vitro. *Clin Exp Immunol* (2015) 181:314–22. doi:10.1111/cei.12437
191. Lachmann PJ, Lay E, Seilly DJ, Buchberger A, Schwaeble W, Khadake J. Further studies of the down-regulation by factor I of the C3b feedback cycle using endotoxin as a soluble activator and red cells as a source of CR1 on sera of different complotype. *Clin Exp Immunol* (2016) 183:150–6. doi:10.1111/cei.12714
192. Hebecker M, Alba-Domínguez M, Roumenina LT, Reuter S, Hyvärinen S, Dragon-Durey M-A, et al. An engineered construct combining complement regulatory and surface-recognition domains represents a minimal-size functional factor H. *J Immunol* (2013) 191:912–21. doi:10.4049/jimmunol.1300269
193. Schmidt CQ, Bai H, Lin Z, Risitano AM, Barlow PN, Ricklin D, et al. Rational engineering of a minimized immune inhibitor with unique triple-targeting properties. *J Immunol* (2013) 190:5712–21. doi:10.4049/jimmunol.1203548
194. Nichols E-M, Barbour TD, Pappworth IY, Wong EKS, Palmer JM, Sheerin NS, et al. An extended mini-complement factor H molecule ameliorates experimental C3 glomerulopathy. *Kidney Int* (2015) 88:1314–22. doi:10.1038/ki.2015.233
195. Kuijpers TW, Wouters D, Brouwer N, Pouw RB. *Factor h Potentiating Antibodies and Uses Thereof.* (2016). Available from: https://patents.google.com/patent/WO2016028150A1/en (Accessed: July 23, 2018).
196. Zipfel PF, Skerka C. FHL-1/reconectin: a human complement and immune regulator with cell-adhesive function. *Immunol Today* (1999) 20:135–40. doi:10.1016/S0167-5699(98)01432-7
197. Clark SJ, Schmidt CQ, White AM, Hakobyan S, Morgan BP, Bishop PN. Identification of factor H-like protein 1 as the predominant complement regulator in Bruch's membrane: implications for age-related macular degeneration. *J Immunol* (2014) 193:4962–70. doi:10.4049/jimmunol.1401613
198. Zipfel PF, Skerka C. Complement factor H and related proteins: an expanding family of complement-regulatory proteins? *Immunol Today* (1994) 15:121–6. doi:10.1016/0167-5699(94)90155-4
199. Csincsi ÁI, Szabó Z, Bánlaki Z, Uzonyi B, Cserhalmi M, Kárpáti É, et al. FHR-1 binds to C-reactive protein and enhances rather than inhibits complement activation. *J Immunol* (2017) 199:292–303. doi:10.4049/jimmunol.1600483
200. Hughes AE, Orr N, Esfandiary H, Diaz-Torres M, Goodship T, Chakravarthy U. A common CFH haplotype, with deletion of CFHR1 and CFHR3, is associated with lower risk of age-related macular degeneration. *Nat Genet* (2006) 38:1173–7. doi:10.1038/ng1890
201. Hebecker M, Okemefuna AI, Perkins SJ, Mihlan M, Huber-Lang M, Józsi M. Molecular basis of C-reactive protein binding and modulation of complement activation by factor H-related protein 4. *Mol Immunol* (2010) 47:1347–55. doi:10.1016/j.molimm.2009.12.005
202. Csincsi ÁI, Kopp A, Zöldi M, Bánlaki Z, Uzonyi B, Hebecker M, et al. Factor H-related protein 5 interacts with pentraxin 3 and the extracellular matrix and modulates complement activation. *J Immunol* (2015) 194:4963–73. doi:10.4049/jimmunol.1403121
203. Józsi M, Tortajada A, Uzonyi B, Goicoechea de Jorge E, Rodríguez de Córdoba S. Factor H-related proteins determine complement-activating surfaces. *Trends Immunol* (2015) 36:374–84. doi:10.1016/j.it.2015.04.008
204. Caesar JJE, Lavender H, Ward PN, Exley RM, Eaton J, Chittock E, et al. Competition between antagonistic complement factors for a single protein on *N. meningitidis* rules disease susceptibility. *Elife* (2014) 3:e04008. doi:10.7554/eLife.04008
205. Biesecker G, Dihel L, Enney K, Bendele RA. Derivation of RNA aptamer inhibitors of human complement C5. *Immunopharmacology* (1999) 42:219–30. doi:10.1016/S0162-3109(99)00020-X
206. Hoehlig K, Maasch C, Shushakova N, Buchner K, Huber-Lang M, Purschke WG, et al. A novel C5a-neutralizing mirror-image (l-)aptamer prevents organ failure and improves survival in experimental sepsis. *Mol Ther* (2013) 21:2236–46. doi:10.1038/mt.2013.178

4

Complement in the Initiation and Evolution of Rheumatoid Arthritis

*V. Michael Holers and Nirmal K. Banda**

Division of Rheumatology, Department of Medicine, University of Colorado Anschutz Medical Campus, Aurora, CO, United States

***Correspondence:**
Nirmal K. Banda
nirmal.banda@ucdenver.edu

The complement system is a major component of the immune system and plays a central role in many protective immune processes, including circulating immune complex processing and clearance, recognition of foreign antigens, modulation of humoral and cellular immunity, removal of apoptotic and dead cells, and engagement of injury resolving and tissue regeneration processes. In stark contrast to these beneficial roles, however, inadequately controlled complement activation underlies the pathogenesis of human inflammatory and autoimmune diseases, including rheumatoid arthritis (RA) where the cartilage, bone, and synovium are targeted. Recent studies of this disease have demonstrated that the autoimmune response evolves over time in an asymptomatic preclinical phase that is associated with mucosal inflammation. Notably, experimental models of this disease have demonstrated that each of the three major complement activation pathways plays an important role in recognition of injured joint tissue, although the lectin and amplification pathways exhibit particularly impactful roles in the initiation and amplification of damage. Herein, we review the complement system and focus on its multi-factorial role in human patients with RA and experimental murine models. This understanding will be important to the successful integration of the emerging complement therapeutics pipeline into clinical care for patients with RA.

Keywords: complement, arthritis, classical pathway, lectin pathway, alternative pathway, mannose-binding protein-associated serine proteases, inflammation

COMPLEMENT SYSTEM AND ITS ACTIVATION

It was Buchner who, at the University of Munich, discovered a blood born substance that was able to destroy bacteria. He named it "alexin." The term "complement" was subsequently introduced by Ehrlich as part of his grand model of the immune system (1–6). Although initially considered primarily in the context of resistance to infection, the complement system, as an important arm of

---

Abbreviations: CP, classical pathway; LP, lectin pathway; MBL, mannose-binding lectin; AP, alternative pathway; CICs, circulating immune complexes; CRDs, carbohydrate recognition domains; FLS, fibroblast-like synoviocytes; CII, bovine type II collagen; PAD2 or PAD4, peptidyl arginine deiminase type 2 or 4; CDA, clinical disease activity; RF, rheumatoid factor; ACPA, anti-citrullinated protein antibodies; anti-CarP, anti-carbamylated protein; CIA, collagen-induced arthritis; PIA, pristane-induced arthritis; ZIA, zymosan-induced arthritis; PGIA, proteoglycan-induced arthritis; SCWA, streptococcal cell wall arthritis; CAIA, collagen antibody-induced arthritis; mBSA, methylated bovine serum-induced arthritis; KBxN STA, KBxN serum transfer model of arthritis; Crry, mouse complement receptor-related gene y; MASP-1, mannose-binding lectin-associated serine protease-1; MASP-2, mannose-binding lectin-associated serine protease-2; MASP-3, mannose-binding lectin-associated serine protease-3; MAp44, mannose-binding lectin-associated protein of 44 kDa a.k.a. MBL/ficolin/CL-11-associated protein-1 (MAP-1); FCNs, ficolins; FCN A, ficolin A; FCN B, ficolin B; CL-11, collectin liver 11; mAb, monoclonal antibody; MAC, membrane attack complex.

the innate immune system, has been long recognized to play an important role in tissue damage in many autoimmune diseases, including rheumatoid arthritis (RA). Thus, the complement system responds not only to microorganisms but also mediates inflammation through the orderly activation of a cascade of multi-protein enzymes and proteases.

Key functions of the complement system include clearance of foreign microorganisms through specific recognition, opsonization, and lysis (7). The system also plays major roles in the clearance of circulating immune complexes (CICs), apoptotic cells, apoptotic bodies, and dead cells (8, 9). Out of three different types of CICs (small, intermediate, and large), intermediate CICs typically cause the most damage as they get trapped in the tissues or in the joints. These protective functions provide potent properties for the benefit of the host, even in the absence of an adaptive immune response.

Although the complement system limits its pro-inflammatory and anti-inflammatory activities, through action of many inhibitors under normal physiological conditions, these natural complement inhibitors are not enough when the complement system gets over-activated during acute inflammatory conditions and thereby causes more damage than good. The functions of the complement system are not only limited to serum or plasma where these are found in abundance but to each and every tissue or organ of the body which are the direct target of various complement components.

Most proteins of the complement system are normally present in the circulation in an inactive (zymogen) form to be activated *via* proteolytic processing upon the recognition of danger. Interestingly, there exists multiple pathways by which the complement system may be activated, each employing different recognition molecules, which underscores its great complexity. The complement system is activated by three different major pathways: the classical pathway (CP), the lectin pathway (LP), and the alternative pathway (AP) and one minor pathway, the C2/C4 bypass (10) (**Figure 1**). All of these pathways are activated by various antibodies, ICs, molecules or microorganisms, or spontaneously as discussed below.

Classical Pathway Activation

The CP is activated by binding of C1q to the heavy-chain crystallizable fragment (Fc) domain of immunoglobulin (Ig). In mice, IgM, IgG1, IgG2a, and IgG2b all have complement activation sites, and these can form CICs when combined with an antigen and complement. C1q leads to the activation of C1r, followed by activation of C1s. C1s cleaves and activates C4 into C4a and C4b and also C2 into C2a and C2b, leading to the formation of C4b2a (CP C3 convertase), which itself cleaves C3 into C3a and C3b (11). C3b further binds to C4b2a to generate the C5 convertase of the CP. This initiates the formation of C5b-9, the membrane attack complex (MAC) (12).

Through its recognition mechanisms, C1 can help to distinguish self from non-self, which is important for the maintenance of self-tolerance and homeostasis (13). Conversely, its pathologic activation has been implicated in many inflammatory and autoimmune diseases, and its activation is limited by C1 esterase

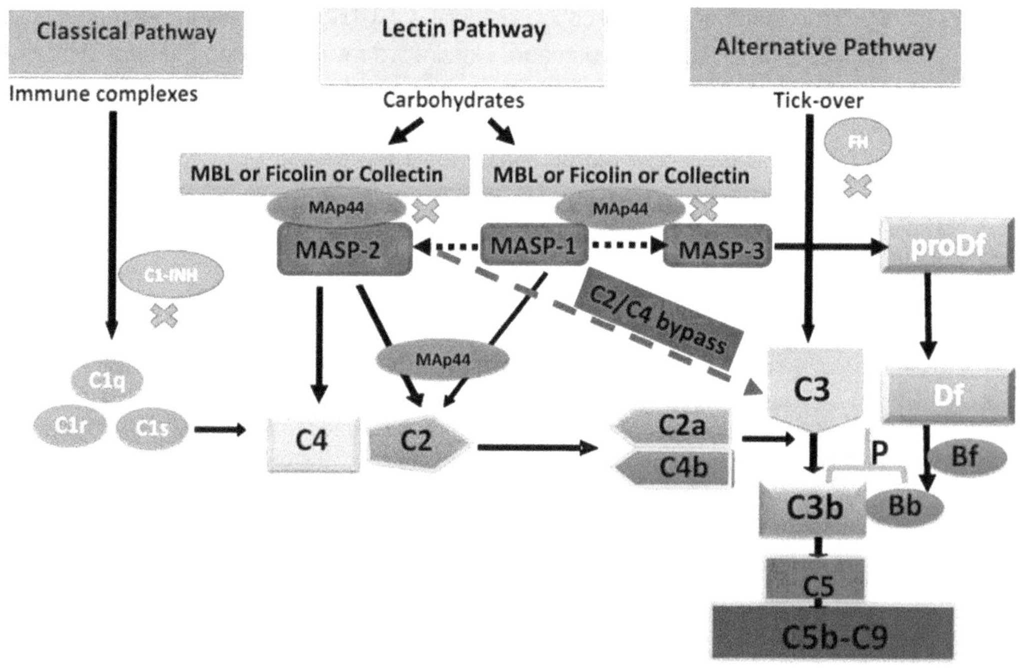

FIGURE 1 | Complement system with four different activating pathways, i.e., classical, lectin, alternative, and C2/C4 bypass. Only major complement inhibitors of the classical pathway, lectin pathway, and alternative pathway, i.e., Cl-INH, mannose-binding lectin-associated protein of 44 kDa a.k.a. MBL/ficolin/CL-11-associated protein-1, and FH, respectively, have been shown. All pathways converse to cleave C3 and C5 to initiate the terminal pathway of the complement system, i.e., membrane attack complex (C5b-9).

inhibitor (C1-INH) (14). Recently, it has been shown that C4a is a ligand for protease-activated receptor (PAR) 1 and PAR4, extending the direct link between the complement and coagulation systems (15). In addition, MAC assembly has been shown on the surface of parasites, and to eliminate Gram-negative bacteria and unwanted host cells (16–18). The MAC can rupture cells with varied composition of lipids and once MAC assembly initiates on cell surfaces other factors can still block it (16). Interestingly, sublytic levels of MAC either causes the release of pro-inflammatory mediators or in other circumstances acts to increases the protection of cells to avoid further innocent bystander cell lysis (19, 20).

Lectin Pathway Activation

The recognition components of the LP, mannose-binding lectins (MBLs), ficolins (FCNs), and collectins (CLs) bind directly to microbial and other surfaces with exposed carbohydrates and *N*-acetyl groups and activate complement *via* MBL-associated serine proteases (MASPs) (21–23).

Ficolins, which contain a carbohydrate recognition domain (CRD), consist of collagen-like and fibrinogen-like domains and preferentially bind to *N*-acetylglucosamine (GlcNAc) (24–26). There are two mouse FCNs: ficolin A (FCN A) (27) and ficolin B (FCN B) (28); by contrast, humans express three FCNs; ficolin M (FCN-M a.k.a. FCN 1), ficolin L (FCN-L a.k.a. FCN 2), and ficolin H (FCN-H a.k.a. FCN 3) (29–33). Mouse FCN A, but not FCN B, exhibits a splice variant known as FCN A variant (34). FCN A is present in the serum and expressed in liver hepatocytes (35). Mouse FCN B was originally found in the lysosomes of macrophages, similar to human FCN-M, which is also found in the secretary granules of monocytes and neutrophils (36, 37). We have reported that FCN B is also present in the circulation of mice suggesting that it is secreted from macrophages (38).

Mannose-binding lectin is a C-type lectin containing a CRD as well as a collagen-like domain (21, 22). MBL binds to mannose-containing molecules as well as *N*-acetylglucosamine (21, 22). There are two types of mouse MBLs, i.e., MBL-A and MBL-C, whereas there is only one type in human (39). Four different types of MASPs called mannose-binding lectin-associated serine protease-1 (MASP-1), mannose-binding lectin-associated serine protease-2 (MASP-2), mannose-binding lectin-associated serine protease-3 (MASP-3), and sMAP (also called Map19) (small MBL-associated protein) circulate complexed with MBL, FCNs, and CL (40). Although no specific function has been assigned to sMAP by generating *sMAP*$^{-/-}$ mice, it was shown that the expression of MASP-2 was also decreased in the sera of these mice because of the MASP-2 gene disruption (41). These authors have also shown by using sera from *sMAP*$^{-/-}$ mice that sMAP plays a regulatory role in the activation of the LP but it is not clear whether sMAP plays a regulatory role before or after the LP activation. sMAP and MASP-2 compete to bind to MBL, and sMAP has the ability to downregulate the LP (41). MAp44 (also called MAP-1), an alternatively spliced product of the *MASP-1/3* gene, is a natural inhibitor of the interactions between MBLs and FCNs and serves as a major regulator of the LP (42, 43). MASP-1, MASP-2, and MASP-3 consist of an A chain (1CUB, EGF, 2CUB, 1CCP, 2CCP, and the linker region) linked by a disulfide bond to a B-chain (serine protease domain).

Both the CP and LP share C2 and C4 complement components. Similar to the CP, the LP forms the C3 and C5 convertases leading to the formation of MAC. A recent additional breakthrough has been the finding that MASP-3, which is an alternative spliced form of *MASP-1/3* gene, is a positive regulator of the AP of the complement system (44) and MASP-3 exclusively enables FD maturation (45). It has been shown that both MASP-1 and MASP-2 can activate MASP-3, but MASP-3 in resting human blood is also present in an active form (46). *In vitro*, not *in vivo* studies, have shown that MASP-1 is essential for bacterial LPS but not Zymosan-induced AP activation (47), indicating that MASP-1 can regulate a specific AP activation mechanism but not the entire AP.

The third class of LP initiators, designated CLs, are similarly C-type lectins containing CRDs (48). Three different human CLs have been identified: Collectin-10 (a.k.a. collectin liver 1, CL-L1, or CL-10), Collectin 11 (a.k.a. collectin kidney 1, CL-K1, or CL-11), and Collectin-12 (collectin placenta 1, CL-P1, or CL-12) (49–52). CL-K1 is present in various human and mouse tissues (49, 53). It has also been shown that CL-K1 acts as a soluble pattern recognition receptor for *Mycobacterium tuberculosis* (54). Additionally, it binds to L-fucose beside other potential ligands (55). In a renal injury model, CL-11 expression was rapidly upregulated and recognized the abnormal presentation of L-fucose leading to complement activation and tissue injury (56). Interestingly, both CL-11 and MASP-2 have been shown to generate C3d on injured cells (56). All of the abovementioned collectins play an important role in an innate immunity because these can bind to the LPS from various species of bacteria (57–60).

Alternative Pathway Activation

The original properdin-dependent pathway, now called the AP of the complement system, was discovered in the 1950s (61). The AP consists of four proteins, factor B (FB), factor D (FD), Properdin (Pf or P), and C3. In contrast to the CP and LP, the AP is activated spontaneously through hydrolysis of C3, thereby generating C3(H_2O), which can associate with FB, resulting in the cleavage of FB into Ba and Bb by FD. Therefore, the AP does not require a specific recognition molecule in order to be activated. Nevertheless, as C3 hydrolysis (a.k.a. C3 "tick over") is always happening regardless of the presence of FB or FD (62), the system is always poised for activation. In that process, FB binds to C3(H_2O), and can be cleaved by FD to generate C3(H_2O)Bb (C3 convertase). The cleavage is much slower without properdin, which is a positive regulator of the AP convertase and can also independently promote the activation of the AP on certain surfaces (63). C3b bound to Bb on a surface is a potent C3 convertase and can cleave C3 to generate more C3b and C3a. The C3 convertase can also combine with another C3b molecule forming an AP C5 convertase. The latter can start the formation of the MAC after cleaving complement component C5 into C5b and C5a. In contrast to activation, complement factor H (FH) is the natural regulator of the AP, and in addition to solution phase AP blockade the binding of this molecule to one or more of the host marker recognition sites enables it to control surface activation of the AP (64). There are also several membrane-bound inhibitory proteins described below which determine the location and activity of the complement system (65). Finally, regardless of the activation route, all of these pathways generate two major potent pro-inflammatory molecules; C3a and C5a, *via* C3 and C5 convertases, respectively, which play a vital role in the pathogenesis of arthritis.

C4/C2 Bypass Pathway Activation

A fourth pathway has also been found to be important in the generation of complement pro-inflammatory mediators and termed the "C4/C2 bypass pathway" or "C2-independent" pathway (66). Initially, it was shown that C4 and C2 complement components were not necessary to lyse cells by the CP (67–69) despite the fact that C4 and C2 are important constituents of the C3 convertase. More recently, it was shown that the components of the LP such as MBL in the absence of C2, C4, or MASP-2 induce C3 deposition (70). This could be mediated by LP ligands such as MBL or FCNs. These could activate the AP directly *via* MASP-3, which cleaves proFD into FD (10). C3 activation in the absence of C2, C4, or MASP-2 requires FB as well as a high concentration of serum (70). C3 activation on adherent anti-collagen (anti-CII) antibodies, was also reported at a high concentration using sera from mice lacking C4 by an unknown mechanism (71). This C3 activation on adherent anti-CII antibodies was fully inhibited by an anti-FB inhibitory antibody (71), confirming specific AP activation in the absence of C4. Even in human serum lacking C4, MASP-2-dependent C3 activation was reported *via* a C4 bypass route (72). So, this C4/C2 bypass pathway is operative without forming conventional CP or LP C3 convertases. It has been shown that thrombin is capable of generating the complement activation product C5a in the complete absence of C3 (73), which represents another bypass mechanism to generate C5a and C5b. Recently it has been shown that in the absence of C4, the CP cannot be activated however, LP still retains the capacity to cleave C3 into C3a and C3b. This residual C4/C2 bypass is dependent on MASP-2 (74). This study further demonstrated that MASP-2 dependent cleavage of C3 was inhibited by MASP-2-specific inhibitors. All of these studies are consistent with the presence of a backup or bypass complement pathway that works *in vivo* in the absence of C4 or C2. Whether this pathway, like CP, LP, and AP, is controlled by the well-described complement regulators is not known. Importantly, the relative importance of the C4/C2 bypass pathway in relation to arthritis models has recently been shown (10), and other studies have revealed its importance in some ischemia/reperfusion-related models (72).

Complement Mediators of Inflammation and Their Receptors

Regardless of the activation pathway, cleavage of C3 is followed by generation of C3a, C3b, iC3b, C3d, C5a, C5b, and MAC (75, 76). Recently, it has been shown that human plasma kallikrein directly cleaves C3 into C3a and C3b and triggers an amplification loop (77). Interestingly, the cleavage site within C3 is identical to that recognized by C3 convertase and is also inhibited by FH. The cleavage of C3 and C5 by kallikrein or thrombin appears to represent a coordination between the complement system and the coagulation pathways (78). C4 cleavage leads to the generation of C4a, another anaphylatoxin but it is not clear whether it is a chemoattractant. C3a, C4a, and C5a are called anaphylatoxins because they are able to carry out pro-inflammatory activities even at a very low concentration. Thus, complement can contribute to the inflammatory injury through many mechanisms.

Previously, it has been shown that C3a is less potent than C5a while C3a desArg (a.k.a. acylation-stimulating protein) has no inflammatory activity. It has also been shown that C3a is not a chemoattractant for neutrophils but can cause migration of eosinophils (79). But this view has shifted based on new findings. C3a binds C3aR expressed on the surface of neutrophils, eosinophils, and basophils, monocytes/macrophages, and mast cells (80, 81). C3a and C5a can bind and equally activate through their receptors C3aR and C5aR, respectively, present on the surface of basophils and mast cells (82).

C4a is very weak anaphylatoxin which is formed by the cleavage of C4 into C4a and C4b. The view whether or not C4a is a classical anaphylatoxin has been recently questioned because evidence has been provided that C4a is a ligand for PAR1 and PAR4 (15). These authors have shown that C4a showed no activity toward known anaphylatoxin receptors but it acted as a non-traditional agonist for both PAR1 and PAR4.

C5a is a cleaved by-product of C5 after complement activation. C5a is rapidly converted by carboxypeptidases to less potent C5a desArg but still has biological activity, and the view regarding C5a desArg potency has also been challenged. Most of the C5a found in the circulation is in the C5a desArg form (83). The binding affinity of C5a to C5aR been reported 100-fold higher than that of C5a desArg for C5aR (84). Although C5a is considered as the triggering molecule but it has been shown that C5a desArg also acts as an important molecule triggering of local inflammation and also maintain blood surveillance and homeostatic status. This study has elegantly shown that C5a desArg induce cell activation in even higher than C5a, which was dependent on the C5aR because it was inhibited by PMX-53, a C5aR antagonist (85). C5a acts as a chemotactic factor of neutrophils and increases neutrophil adhesion to endothelium (86, 87). C5a binds to C5aR (C5aR1 or CD88) and C5L2 (C5aR2 or GPR77) present on many cells leading to chemotaxis of inflammatory cells, vascular permeability, phagocytosis, and release of pro-inflammatory cytokines and chemokines. C5a amplifies tissue injury and inflammation by triggering release of oxygen free radicals and arachidonic acid metabolities (88). C5a is an essential component of the inflammatory response to bacterial infection. *Porphyromonas gingivalis* expresses a peptidyl arginine deiminase (PAD) with a strong preference for the C-terminal arginine of C5a, disabling protein function resulting in decreased chemotaxis of human neutrophils (89). It has been shown that C5a, released at sites of inflammation, upregulates FcγRIIIa and downregulates FcγRIIb simultaneously (90, 91).

The biological and pathological role of the second C5a receptor, C5L2 is controversial. C5L2 does not bind C3a or ASP/C3adesArg. C5L2 also binds to C5a and C5a desArg. C5a desArg binds 20-fold to 30-fold with higher affinity with C5L2 than C5aR (84, 92). Although C5L2 binds to C5a with the same high affinity as C5aR but function may depend on the cell type, species, and disease context (93). While C5aR is a G protein-coupled receptor, C5L2 is not which led to the hypothesis that C5L2 functions as a decoy receptor. This view is not universally accepted, however. Evidence has been generated linking C5L2 to both anti-inflammatory and pro-inflammatory functions (93). We have found no evidence for C5L2 playing a role in RA; however, so we will leave this fascinating topic for others to review.

Membrane attack complex formation is the final step of the terminal pathway after cleavage of C5 by C5 convertases of the CP/LP or of the AP leading to the formation of the pore consisting of C5b–C9 complement proteins (94). MAC formation may lead either to necrosis or apoptosis, in part depending on the number of pores formed. The choice of necrosis vs. apoptosis is clinically relevant as necrosis is invariably pro-inflammatory, while apoptosis can lead to the resolution of an inflammatory response (95, 96). In general, eukaryotic cells require more pores than prokaryotic cells to induce death. Interestingly, low numbers of MAC, rather than leading to cell death, induce inflammatory signaling events such as the release of TNF-α and IL-1 (97).

Additionally, complement receptor 1 (CR1 or CD35), complement receptor 2 (CR2 or CD21), complement receptor 3 (CR3 or CD11b/CD18), complement receptor 4 (or CD11c/CD18), and complement inhibitors such as FH, decay-accelerating factor (DAF or CD55), membrane cofactor protein (or CD46), and protectin (CD59) have been shown to play an important role in the complement-mediated injury and also, as we will discuss below, in the pathogenesis of arthritis.

Measurement of Complement Activation in Inflammation

Classical pathway activity is commonly measured using the CH50 test. Here, serum can be used to lyse sheep erythrocytes coated with anti-sheep antibodies, and degree of hemolysis is measured. By contrast, the AH50 is the best screening test used to measure the proper functioning of the AP. Low levels in either test indicate a deficiency of one or more components of the CP or AP of the complement system, respectively (98). Function of the LP can be measured by enzyme-linked immunosorbent assay pre-coated with mannan particles, and here C4d bound to mannan can be measured. Furthermore, the CP component C4d has been used as a measure to explore the activation of the CP. Bb levels have been used to as a measure to explore the activation of the AP. Tissue bound or soluble MAC levels have been used as measure of the activation of all pathways of the complement system thus as the most important indicator of complement activation within a microenvironment. To measure complement activation and its split products in serum or plasma, there are excellent standard protocols. Conversely, results can be obtained by using fee for services complement focused laboratories and commercially available kits (99–102).

Most of the stable complement components are measured in serum whereas activated split products are measured in plasma (EDTA-anticoagulated blood) due to the interference of the coagulation system enzymes leading to erroneous results. Furthermore, most measurements of complement activity are focused on serum or plasma with no attention paid to specific cells or tissues (e.g., synovial fluid). Since, in clinical disease, complement causes damage locally, more work must be done to assess complement activity on tissue surfaces and within sequestered regions such as synovial fluid. Measurements of CICs along with complement products such as C1q, C3b, C3d, C3dg, and MASPs levels in the serum and synovial fluid of RA patients along with rheumatoid factor (RF), anti-citrullinated protein antibodies (ACPA), and anti-carbamylated protein (anti-CarP) antibodies can provide a better picture of the local production and their role in the RA pathogenesis. Sometimes it is hard to make any conclusion from measuring C3 or C4 levels alone using serum or plasma or synovial fluid because excessive production due to inflammation masks their consumption and results are confounded by the coagulation pathway. Furthermore, endogenous complement inhibitors of the CP, LP, and AP work only under normal physiological conditions but these are ineffective under pathophysiological conditions due to the hyper-activation of complement. Therefore, their measurement provides less useful information.

INITIATION OF RHEUMATOID ARTHRITIS

Rheumatoid arthritis is a chronic inflammatory systemic disease that primarily affects peripheral joints, thereby leading to synovial inflammation followed by cartilage and bone destruction. During the development of the disease, the synovium undergoes proliferation, thickens, and incorporates a large number of infiltrating immune cells to become a new tissue called pannus that causes cartilage and bone damage (103–105). Although the exact origin or initiation or development of RA is unknown, studies have shown associations in patients with active RA with infections in the temporomandibular joints (106, 107) or in the gums due to severe periodontitis (108). Dysbiosis of the microbiome in the oral or gut regions has also been strongly associated with onset of RA (109). Furthermore, interstitial lung disease (110), infections by alphaviruses (mosquito-transmitted viruses) such as Ross River virus (111), Chikungunya virus (112), and HBV (113) are also associated with a risk for the development of RA. RA also exhibits a genetic predisposition, with approximately 50% of this genetic risk contributed by certain HLA-DR alleles (114). Many other genes have been shown to contribute to RA pathogenesis (115). Additionally, environmental exposures such as air pollution, occupational exposure to silica, active smoking, wood burning, and mineral oil have been shown to acts a risk factor for initiating and/or developing RA (116, 117). The hypothesis that smoking and pollution lead to an increased risk of RA paved the way to the hypothesis that initial inflammation and production of RA-related autoantibodies (called ACPA anti-citrullinated protein/peptide antibodies) in the lungs may lead to RA (116, 118). So far, there are no studies showing the direct migration of ACPA from lungs to the peripheral joints to precipitate disease. ACPA is the most reliable and specific biological marker to diagnose RA and these antibodies are increased in RA patients sera almost 10 years prior to clinical diagnosis (116, 118–121). Hundreds of citrullinated proteins have been found in the synovial fluid of RA patients which might contribute to the RA pathology (122–125) but why only few autoantigens such as enolase, fibrinogen, and vimentin generate autoantibodies is not clear. How these citrullinated proteins present locally in the synovial fluid interact directly with various complement proteins and activate the complement system is also unknown.

It has been shown that there is a relationship between ACPA, RF, and systemic bone loss in early RA patients (101). The presence of citrullinated antigens on the surface of osteoclastic linage cells makes these cells the main targets of circulating ACPA leading to pro-osteoclastic events (126, 127). There is an argument for complement involvement in this process. Bacterial antigens, perforin, and the MAC cause calcium influx leading to cytolysis. PAD enzymes that convert peptidylarginine into peptidyl citrulline are calcium-dependent (128–131). Interestingly, perforin and the MAC have been shown to reproduce identical patterns of hypercitrullination seen in the neutrophils present in the synovial fluid of RA patients (132). A huge number of neutrophils are present in the synovial fluid of RA patients and are the major source of intracellular citrullination and PADs for extracellular citrullination (132–136). These data suggest that citrullinated proteins along with activation of the complement system might be contributing to the initiation of RA.

Complement Activation on Articular Cartilage Surface and in Synovium in Rheumatoid Arthritis

Earlier studies have shown that autoantibodies to type II collagen present in the serum of RA patients bind to the cartilage components or to antigen present on the surface of articular cartilage (137). Articular cartilage is a hyaline cartilage and connective tissue of the joints. The main cellular component of adult articular cartilage is the chondrocyte. These cells, which make up approximately 1% of the tissue, function to organize collagen into ordered structures and secrete extracellular matrix (ECM) components. The ECM is composed of water, collagen type II, proteoglycans, non-collagenous proteins, and glycoproteins (138, 139). Complement activation due to antibody–cartilage surface interaction in RA patients have shown the abundant co-deposition of IgGs and activated complement components (140). Interestingly chondrocytes can also synthesize complement components including C1 and C1 inhibitor (141, 142).

An important piece of evidence linking complement activation to pathogenesis in RA was that C1 staining was negative in normal articular cartilage and positive in degenerating cartilage biopsies from all RA patients examined (143). This study strongly implicated the involvement of the CP in the pathogenesis of RA. C3b was also present on the cartilage surface of RA patients; thus, this study clearly showed that C1s can activate the downstream complement cascade thereby causing irreversible damage. It has also been shown that the level of C1q in serum correlates with clinical disease activity (CDA) in RA patients (144–146). In mouse model of RA, C3b gets deposited first on the surface of cartilage vs. synovium and increased rapidly from 4 to 120 h (**Figure 2**). Interestingly, during this time, there is not enough FH availability on the surface of cartilage as well as in the synovium to protect them from complement-mediated damage (**Figure 2**). The presence of C2, C3, C4, and C5 in rheumatoid synovial fluid had been shown previously (147). Levels of properdin and FB of the AP were depressed. An increase in the levels of C3d, C4d, Ba, and MAC has been found in the synovial fluid of RA patients (148, 149). Normally, IgG containing ICs and also C3 split fragments can be found in the joints of more than 90% of RA patients (140, 150) and mediate complement activation. IgG with C3d has been present in the synovial fluid of RA patients and also MAC and Bb levels are elevated in the synovial fluid of RA patients (151, 152). No statistical differences in the levels of C3c and C4 in serum and in the synovial fluid of RA patients have been seen in a cross-sectional study although significant differences were seen in the CICs in both biological fluids (153). DAF expression is increased in RA synovium, while the expression of CD59 significantly decreased in the synovial lining (154, 155). The presence of split components of the complement system on the cartilage surface and in the synovium of RA patients indicate that local complement presence/and or synthesis and activation can attract macrophages for phagocytosis of chondrocytes which can further damage the cartilage and synovium.

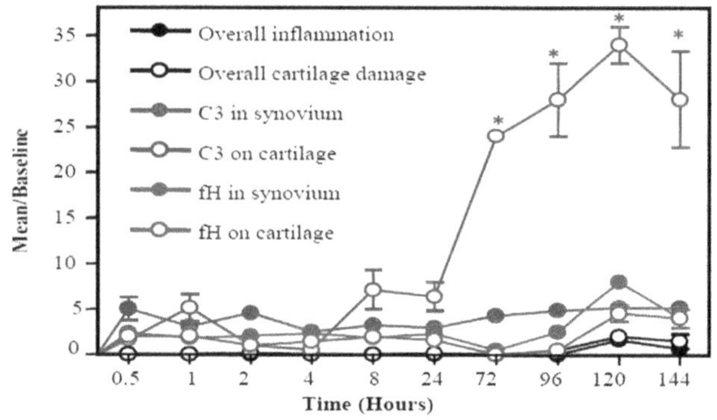

FIGURE 2 | A slow snapshot of the early histopathological analysis from the knee joints of wild-type (WT) mice with collagen antibody-induced arthritis (CAIA) for C3 and FH deposition on the surface of cartilage and in the synovium. A mixture of four monoclonal antibody (mAb) to CII (8 mg/mouse) was injected i.p. to induce arthritis, and mice were sacrificed at 0.5, 1, 2, 4, 8, 24, 72, 96, 120, and 144 h later. A low level of FH was present on the surface the cartilage and in the synovium at all time points with slight non-significant increases at 72, 96, 120, and 144 h. By contrast, C3 deposition on the cartilage surface showed a large increase over baseline beginning at 8 h after injection of the anti-CII mAbs and peaking at 120 h. Thus, an imbalance exists between FH deposition and C3 deposition in the early stages of disease leading to failure to protect the knee joints in mice with CAIA. Histopathologic scoring for inflammation (black solid circle) and cartilage damage (white empty circle) from the knee joints (right and left) was performed following tissue processing and Toluidine-blue staining of sections. C3 deposition in knee joints in the synovium (red solid circle) and on the surface of cartilage (red empty circle) is illustrated, as is FH deposition in the synovium (blue solid circle) and on the surface of cartilage (blue empty circle). The data are expressed as mean of disease/baseline ± SEM (n = 3 each time point). Baseline = background levels of inflammation, cartilage damage, and C3 and FH deposition in the knee joints of WT mice without treatment with mAb to CII (n = 3).

Complement Activation due to Glycosylation, Citrullination, and/or Carbamylation in Rheumatoid Arthritis

It has been documented that IgG is the most abundant immunoglobulin isotype comprising ~75% of the total serum immunoglobulins (157). IgG triggers its effector function (i.e., complement activation *via* its Fc). Therefore, any change due to posttranslational modification in the Fc region such as glycosylation will influence the effector function of IgG mediated by the FcγR (158–162). The glycosylation of the Fc is characterized by presence of a single chain N-linked glycan attached to each heavy chain at asparagine 297. It has been shown that the lack of fucose, sialic acid, and galactose residues on the Fc-N-linked glycans increases the inflammatory capacity of IgG in mice (163–166). IgG in RA patients contains less galactose and sialic acid (167). Interestingly, the glycosylation pattern of ACPA changes before the onset of RA skewing toward more inflammation (168, 169). Pregnancy-induced spontaneous improvement of RA as well as flares after delivery has been linked to pregnancy-related changed in the glycosylation of IgGs (170–172). This study was the first natural evidence of that changes in IgG galactosylation can cause disease pathogenicity in humans. Later on, it was shown that agalactosyl IgG is pathogenic in mice and arthritis could be transferred in mice by injecting agalactosyl IgG (173). The LP pathway component, MBL was shown to be associated with the pathogenicity of agalactosyl IgG (159). Not only the Fc but also the Fab domains of IgG has also been reported to contain N-glycosylation consensus sequences (174). It has been reported that more than 90% of ACPA-IgG molecules carry Fab glycans that are highly sialylated (175). More interestingly, ACPA-IgG purified from synovial fluid of RA patients, could even exceed 100% Fab glycosylation implying that multiple glycans can be attached to the variable domain (176). What role Fab-glycan plays in the functionality of ACPA-IgGs is unknown so far, but studies have shown that ACPA-IgG in RA have a pro-inflammatory Fc glycosylation pattern with reduced galactosylation and sialylation levels (177, 178). It has been shown that ACPA have the capacity to activate the CP and AP of the complement system (179). Thus, ACPA reduced galactosylation and sialylation have more capacity to activate the complement system to generate more vigorous effector response.

Citrullination is a normal physiological process which occurs inside apoptotic cells. Normally, apoptotic cells are scavenged by macrophages. If this system is defective, then PAD enzymes and citrullinated proteins can become externalized to influence the immune system (180).

There are five PAD isoenzymes (PAD1–4 and 6) that regulate key cellular processes (181). The PAD enzymes will citrullinate proteins by converting arginine into citrulline. Cl-amidine is the most widely used pan-PAD inhibitor (182, 183). During inflammation many cells die, and it is common to find citrullinated proteins at the inflamed sites such as in the inflamed synovium of RA patients, suggesting that ACPA could be generated as part of an immune response to self-proteins (184). In filaggrin, fibrin, and vimentin, anti-cyclic citrullinated peptide antibody (ACPA a.k.a. anti-CCP) recognizes the arginine residues modified by PAD enzymes to citrulline (185, 186). The presence of citrullinated proteins, as mentioned above, does not always mean generation of ACPA, however (180). The combination of high specificity (90–99%) and high sensitivity (66–88%) of anti-CPP for diagnosing RA, and above all, correlation with radiological damage has led to the conclusion that these antibodies have a pathological connection to the initiation of RA (185, 187–192). The clinical measure of above 20 U/ml suggests the possibility of RA. Additionally, approximately 20% RA patients are anti-CCP negative. Despite the radiological damage association with anti-CCP antibodies, the levels are not being used to determine the progression of disease since even during remission most of the subjects remains anti-CCP positive. This raises question regarding the direct pathogenicity of these antibodies in RA. It is not clear whether anti-CCP antibodies are the cause or the result of inflammation in RA patients. Whether anti-CCP antibodies are the result of defective coagulation system in RA patients is also not clear. Defective coagulation can in principle modulate the generation of anti-CCP autoantibodies. This is due to the fact that thrombin cleaves fibrinogen into fibrin followed by a clot formation but if fibrinogen is citrullinated then thrombin cannot cleave it resulting in anti-CCP immune response. The target protein is not one citrullinated protein but hundreds of citrullinated proteins as mentioned above.

One study has shown that anti-CCP antibodies activate the complement system *in vitro via* the CP and the AP but not by the LP in RA (179). In this study, anti-CCP antibodies from all 60 patients activated the complement system. This important observation leads to the evidence that complement activation can play very important role in the pathogenesis of RA in ACPA-positive patients but not all RA patients are ACPA-positive. Later on, it has been shown that citrullination locally in the joints can increase inflammation indicating the direct target of ACPA (193) and it will be consistent with the accepted paradigm that complement activation at the site of antibody recognition of citrullinated antigens can cause damage.

Furthermore, IgM RF and IgA RF amplify complement activation mediated by ACPA-IC (194). These authors concluded that ACPA-IC incorporating IgM or IgA RF participate in the triggering of the inflammation-promoting activation of complement cascades occurring in RA joints. The ACPA test has been used to classify the RA into two disease subsets, i.e., ACPA-positive (which includes the HLA-DR shared epitope subset) and ACPA-negative (no HLA shared epitope association is present) (195). These authors concluded that ACPA-positive RA is genetically different from the ACPA-negative RA. The possibility remains that ACPA-positive and ACPA-negative RA patients have differential level of IgG galactoyslation and carbamylation patterns, thereby activating different pathways of the complement system. This area has not been explored in-depth and it could provide some clues regarding the direct role of complement system in the pathogenesis of ACPA-negative patients.

Recently, anti-CarP antibodies have been described in 16% ACPA-negative RA patients (196) and up to 46% patients with RA in various clinical studies. This led to the hypothesis that anti-CarP are closely related ACPA. ACPA recognize targets that are the result of the enzymatic process whereby arginine is converted into citrulline, while anti-CarP antibodies are the result of a chemical process in which lysine have been converted into homocitrulline (196). A few studies have shown that, similar to ACPA, anti-CarP antibodies are found before the onset of clinical symptoms of arthritis (119, 196). Anti-CarP antibodies have been found even in animal models of arthritis prior to the onset of disease, and its relevance will be discussed later (197). Furthermore, the significant association with radiological progression of anti-CarP IgG in ACPA-negative RA patients strongly suggested that anti-CarP antibody can also be used as a biological marker to diagnose a high risk RA population (196). Anti-CarP antibodies recognize many carbamylated antigens including human serum albumin, fibrinogen, and alpha-1 antitrypsin (196, 198–201). The comparative importance of anti-CarP vs. ACPA in the initiation of RA is unknown.

MOUSE MODELS OF HUMAN RHEUMATOID ARTHRITIS

Mouse models are commonly used to study human autoimmune diseases, including RA. Although mice do not develop arthritis naturally, arthritis that shares phenotypic, biochemical, physiological, and immunological properties similar to human RA can be induced in mice. Human RA often develops rapidly as an inflammation in one or more joints which is then followed by the development of the pannus. This acute inflammatory response to some extent has been replicated in some mouse models of inflammatory arthritis such as pristane-induced arthritis (202), zymosan-induced arthritis (203), proteoglycan-induced arthritis (204), streptococcal cell wall arthritis (205), the SKG mouse model of arthritis (206), and methylated bovine serum-induced arthritis (207). Several models are more adaptive immune-mediated or related, and include collagen-induced arthritis (CIA) (208), collagen antibody-induced arthritis (CAIA) (209), and the KBxN serum transfer model of arthritis (KBxN STA) (210, 211). Others are induced entirely by cytokines and include TNF-α transgenic mice (212) and IL-1Ra knockout mice (213). While some of these models are quite similar, in aggregate they possess different clinical, pathological, and mechanistic features that each representing a subset of the different aspects of human RA. With that caveat, here we will discuss the initiation and evolution of disease in three mouse models of human RA which are dependent on the complement system.

Collagen-Induced Arthritis and Complement Activation

Approximately 50 years ago, CIA was first reported in rats following an intradermal injection of CII emulsified in Freund adjuvant (214), and later on in many susceptible strains of mice (208) as well as in non-human primates (215, 216). At present, CIA has become one gold standard mouse model of human RA and is used in many laboratories to examine the effect of therapeutics for treatment of RA. Immunization with bovine type II collagen/Freund's complete adjuvant (CFA) or with chicken CII/CFA results in a severe polyarthritis disease after 3 weeks. Often a second injection is given on day 21, in some cases consisting of a second dose of CII/CFA and in some cases simply CII. The re-exposure to CII antigen continues to activate T and B cells and, in mice with the appropriate H2 alleles, creates an autoimmune disease attacking self-CII. In joints, CIA like human RA is characterized by the presence of activated synovial fibroblast like cells, pannus formation (multi-layered synovium), periosteal bone formation, cartilage surface damage, fibrin deposition, infiltration of macrophages and neutrophils, and finally ankylosis of one or more joints (208, 214). Similar to the anti-CII antibodies generated due to the presence of CII autoantigens in mice, similar antibodies to native or citrullinated CII are also present in human RA and appear to have pathophysiological significance (137, 140, 217).

In CIA, recombinant TNF-α induced an increase in anti-CII antibody levels indicating TNF-α contributes to disease development by both initiation of inflammation and production of autoantibodies (218). Anti-CII autoantibodies are generated in CIA mouse model arthritis and accumulated before the initiation of clinical signs of disease after the booster injection (219). This is somewhat similar situation in human RA where ACPA are present in the early evolution of RA before clinical signs of the disease, thereby suggesting that anti-CII or ACPA first accumulates to initiate the arthritis. In this regard, it has been observed that ACPA levels show an increase 3–5 years before the onset of clinical disease and then stabilize at a high levels (220). Perhaps, a certain threshold level of autoantibodies must be reached in a preclinical stage both in CIA and in human RA to develop disease. Additionally, in RA anti-CII autoantibodies were significantly associated with increased radiographic damage at the time of diagnosis (221).

It is interesting that not all strains of mice are equally susceptible to the CIA. Mice with the *H-2q* allele (MHC class II molecule) are highly susceptible to CIA, for example. It is thought that a particular immunodominant CII peptide region binds to this particular MHC allele with high affinity leading to a powerful anti-CII response (222–225). It is possible that a similar immunodominant CII peptide region binds to human RA associated allele HLA-DR (DR1*0401) (222, 226). The efficacy of abatacept (Orencia®), a fusion recombinant protein consisting of extracellular domain of T lymphocyte-associated antigen 4 linked to modified Fc of human IgG1, in human RA, clearly implicates T cell activity as important for disease progression, which is mirrored by the requirement for T cell help in CIA. Abatacept selectively inhibits T cell activation by two mechanisms, i.e., by blocking the specific interaction of CD80/CD86 receptors to CD28 and also by binding to CD80 and CD86 receptors on the antigen-presenting cells, thereby inhibiting B cell immune response. Immunization of mice with CII results in activation of CII-specific B cells followed by generation of IgG2a as a part of the humoral response (227, 228). The induction phase of CIA through activation of the CP leads to the activation of the adaptive immune response and the generation of anti-CII antibodies. These anti-CII antibodies then bind to cartilage, thereby leading to the effector phase *via* ICs formation and the activation of complement on the cartilage surface. So CIA pathology like human RA is dependent on both humoral and cell-mediated immunity (224, 229).

A vital role for complement in CIA was first suggested by studies in rats, in which injection of cobra venom factor (CVF), inducing marked activation followed by depletion of complement components, led to a delay in the onset of arthritis until serum C3 levels returned to normal (230). Both IgG and C3 are deposited on the cartilage surface in CIA (231), and C3 depletion (a.k.a. de-complementation) of recipient rats with CVF also prevented passive transfer of CIA with anti-collagen Ig (232). Pretreatment of rats with soluble complement receptor type 1 (sCR1), an inhibitor of the classical and AP C3 convertases, led to a delay in the development and progression of CIA (233). Whereas CVF could not alter the course of established CIA, sCR1 injections attenuated inflammation during active disease. Soluble CR1 binds to both C3b and C4b, leading to inhibition of C3 and C5 convertases and decreased activation of both C3 and C5. Furthermore, in CII-immunized mice, gene therapy with sCR1 delayed the development of CIA and decreased its severity (234). In addition, those mice expressing sCR1 exhibited decreased levels of anti-CII as well as markedly reduced lymph node and splenocyte proliferative responses to CII *in vitro*. Recent studies have shown that human TT32 (CR2-CR1), a potent CP and AP inhibitor, compared with human sCR1-10 attenuated CDA in mice with CIA (235). Normally, CR1 is expressed on many cells but a soluble form of CR1 is also present in human plasma therefore synthesized lacking the transmembrane and cytoplasmic domains (236). CR1 consists of four long homologous repeats (A–D), each containing seven SCR repeats (237). The first 10 SCR domains (1–10) of CR1 contain all important modalities required for pan-complement inhibition, acting as cofactors for irreversible proteolytic cleavage of C3b or C4b as well as decay accelerators for AP and CP convertases.

At that point, the relative importance of the CP or LP or AP of the complement system was not clear. One study clearly showed that complement activation by both the CP and the AP plays a deleterious role in CIA (224). Here, it was shown that $C3^{-/-}$ and $FB^{-/-}$ mice were highly resistant to CIA and demonstrated decreased CII-specific IgG Ab response. Repeated injection of CII for 3 weeks in $C3^{-/-}$ mice eventually resulted in the development of a low level of arthritis. Thus, C3 and FB deficiency ameliorate CIA, but do not fully protect against the development (224). Mouse complement receptor-related 1 gene/protein y (Crry), a C3 convertase inhibitor, plays a somewhat similar complement regulatory role as CR1. Transgenic mice overexpressing soluble Crry were generated and used for various complement related studies (238). Nonetheless, the AP activity in Crry-Tg mice was not inhibited as originally expected (238).

There was a suppression of CIA in Crry-Tg mice due to enhanced synthesis of Crry locally in the joint with decreased production of pro-inflammatory cytokines (239). The mice transgenic for Crry exhibited more inhibition of CIA than was recently observed in mice treated with a recombinant Crry-Ig fusion protein (219). It was concluded from these studies that the effects of Crry in CIA may be due both to inhibition of B cell function as well as to local blockade of production of pro-inflammatory cytokines.

More effective suppression of the complement system in disease may result from enhanced levels of complement regulatory proteins locally (knee joints) in tissues. Endogenous expression of complement regulatory proteins appears to be important in resistance to inflammatory disease as blockade of both Crry and CD59 led to more severe CIA in rats (240). These studies show that inhibition of an up-stream complement C3 or its C3 convertase can demonstrate profound effects on the initiation of CIA.

To show the role of downstream complement components such as C5 or C5a-C5aR axis in CIA, administration of anti-C5 inhibitory (BB5.1) antibody was used and was found to both prevent the initiation and decrease the severity of arthritis (219, 241). This inhibitory anti-C5 antibody prevented the cleavage of C5 into C5a and C5b, thereby blocking the terminal pathway. Furthermore, mice lacking C5 were partially resistant to CIA (242). However, in other studies, C5-deficient mice were not resistant to the CIA (243–245). So which component of the complement system C3 or C5 is important for the development of arthritis? Of the several components of complement, current evidence still points to the component C5-generated C5a as the strongest inducer of inflammation (246).

The greater inhibitory effects on CIA of an inhibitory anti-C5 antibody in comparison with Crry-Ig may be attributable to decreased levels of IL-1β and TNF α mRNA in the joints (219). To support ongoing clinical development and clinical trials, an inhibitory anti-C5aR monoclonal antibody not only completely inhibited the disease progression including reduced cartilage and bone destruction but also reduced TNF-α, IL-6, and IL-17A (247). Attempts have been made to design a recombinant vaccine to prevent CIA and also other mouse models of RA by inducing C5a-specific neutralizing antibodies without effecting C5/C5b (248). Injection of anti-rat CD59 induced spontaneous complement-dependent arthritis (240) and mice lacking CD59 are susceptible to antigen-induced arthritis (249). Thus, CIA is a valuable model of human RA to examine therapeutic intervention to block the upstream and downstream pathological by-products of the complement activation.

Collagen Antibody-Induced Arthritis and Complement Activation

Collagen antibody-induced arthritis can be induced in mice by injecting a mixture of five monoclonal antibodies known as ArthritoMab™ or Arthrogen-CIA® to different epitopes of the CII (250, 251). These antibodies binds to CII epitopes C11b, J1, D3, and U1 and spread across the entire CII region such as CB8, CB10, and CB11 fragments for better immune complex on the surface of cartilage to initiate arthritis.[1,2] To induce CAIA in certain strains of mice and to get a 90–100% penetrance rate, the immunization with LPS following a mixture of four or five ArhritoMabs is essential (156). CAIA, like CIA, does not require the involvement of T and B cells for the priming phase and thus represents only the effector phase (252). There is evolving consensus that ACPAs predict the development of human RA (197, 253–255). It has been shown that arthritis can be introduced in mice by injecting a panel of mouse ACPAs (ACC1, ACC3, and ACC4) directed against citrullinated CII epitope (253, 256, 257). In a subset of human patients, ACPAs appears many years before the onset of disease. Furthermore, ACPAs from RA patients have been shown to activate complement *via* both the CP and the AP (179), but serum from RA patients failed to induce arthritis in mice. A somewhat similar experiment also failed to induce arthritis in DBA mice by transferring mouse mAbs against citrullinated fibrinogen (258). Nonetheless, these anti-citrullinated fibrinogen mAbs enhanced the suboptimal disease already established by

[1] www.mdbioproducts.com (Accessed: March 26, 2018).
[2] www.chondrex.com (Accessed: March 26, 2018).

the development of citrullinated antigens in the joint that are induced by the mixture of anti-CII (258). Thus, mouse models of RA clearly shows the importance of B cell generating anti-CII Abs or ACPAs which trigger the effector phase by activating the complement system. There is no mouse model of RA yet developed showing that anti-CarP autoantibodies such as anti-CII Abs can induce arthritis in mice through complement dependence. Nonetheless, similar to ACPA, their presence has been shown in mice and rhesus monkeys with arthritis (197, 200). Although the presence of ACPA in mice with arthritis is controversial, nonetheless the effector functions of anti-CII antibodies in mouse models have provided a clear picture of the pathophysiological processes or events likely to be involved in the initiation of human RA. One study has shown, using a rabbit arthritis model, that first anti-CarP antibodies might be generated from homocitrulline followed by ACPA (259). This observation alone related to the presence of anti-CarP before ACPA can have a huge impact to understanding the initiation of RA in ACPA-positive and ACPA-negative subset of patients.

It has been debated which pathway of the complement system is relevant in RA and how this pathway gets activated in human RA. CAIA using complement component gene-deficient mice has proven very useful to answer many of these questions. Some previous studies have shown that AP of the complement system is the main contributor because there were correlations between Bb and ICs levels (260, 261). The AP can be activated by IgA (261, 262) consistent with the current views regarding the mucosal (gut or lung) origin of the RA. Studies in CAIA mice have shown that the AP of complement is necessary and sufficient for the development of arthritis (263). In this study, C57BL/6 mice genetically deficient in either the AP protein FB (*FB*$^{-/-}$) or in the CP component C4 (*C4*$^{-/-}$) were used. CDA was markedly decreased in *FB*$^{-/-}$ compared with wild-type (WT) mice. Conversely, disease activity scores were not different between *C4*$^{-/-}$ and WT mice. Analyses of joints showed that C3 deposition, inflammation, pannus, cartilage, and bone damage scores were all significantly less in *FB*$^{-/-}$ as compared with WT mice. There were significant decreases in mRNA levels of C3, C4, CR2, CR3, C3aR, and C5aR in the knees of *FB*$^{-/-}$ as compared with *C4*$^{-/-}$ and WT mice with arthritis; mRNA levels for complement regulatory proteins did not differ between the three strains. The authors concluded that the AP is absolutely required for the induction of arthritis following injection of anti-CII Abs (263). In a subsequent study, it was shown that arthritis was not altered in *C1q*$^{-/-}$ or *MBL A/C*$^{-/-}$ or in *C1q*$^{-/-}$/*MBL A/C*$^{-/-}$ (no CP no LP) mice. These *in vivo* CAIA results proved the ability of the AP to carry out pathologic complement activation in the combined absence of intact CP and LP (71). In this study, C3 activation results confirmed the ability of the AP to mediate IC-induced C3 activation using sera from *C4*$^{-/-}$ or *C1q*$^{-/-}$/*MBL A/C*$^{-/-}$ or both *C1q*$^{-/-}$/*MBL A/C*$^{-/-}$ mice (71).

From these studies, it was concluded that the AP amplification loop, with its ability to greatly enhance C3 activation, is necessary to mediate inflammatory arthritis induced by adherent ICs. Then, it was questioned whether CP or LP alone mediate CAIA. Later on, it was reported that *FD*$^{-/-}$ (CP and LP), *C1q*$^{-/-}$/*FD*$^{-/-}$ (no CP no AP), and *MBL A/C*$^{-/-}$/*FD*$^{-/-}$ (no LP no AP) mice all these gene-deficient mice failed to develop to CAIA (264). One thing was common among these gene-deficient mice that there was lack of the AP of complement system. But whether AP is sufficient to initiate and sustain RA in humans is unknown. The AP alone on adherent anti-CII antibodies was capable of generating C5a to a level equal to that observed with WT sera. However, the CP alone, in the absence of the AP, generated 71% less C5a than was observed with WT sera; the LP alone generated minimal C5a (264). Huge activation of C5a using sera from *C1q*$^{-/-}$/*MBL A/C*$^{-/-}$ (only AP) equivalent to sera from WT mice and their huge susceptibility to CAIA further suggested that enzymes/and or proteases independent from the MBL might be activating or regulating the AP (264). To this end, it was also confirmed by using *MBL A/C*$^{-/-}$/*FCN A*$^{-/-}$, and FCN A$^{-/-}$ mice that these ligands plays no role in CAIA (38). Mice lacking FCN B were partially protected while mice lacking Collectin 11 were susceptible to CAIA (10). FCN B is generated by the macrophages and macrophages infiltrate in the joints in mice with CAIA. These data solidify the role of LP as does the FCN B and MASP-1/3 in regulating the AP of the complement system.

While we have demonstrated that the AP plays a critical role in CAIA, we do not yet understand how it is activated in any molecular detail. Given our data, we suspect that factors independently from the LP ligands (MBL, FCN, and Collectins) such as such as MASPs might be activating the AP in CAIA.

Almost a decade ago, a landmark discovery was made regarding a LP enzyme, MASP-1/3 that entirely shifted the paradigm to the in-depth understanding of the interaction between the LP and AP of complement (265–267). It was shown by using *in vitro* studies that MASP-1/3 can cleave proFD (inactive) into FD (active). In this fashion, it seems that a MASP involved with the recognition of pathogens *via* the LP is also a critical activator of FD, a major component of the AP (265). Consistent with this observation, mice lacking the *MASP-1/3* gene have no LP and also have a defective AP (265, 266). Relating this to CAIA, we found that both *FD*$^{-/-}$ and *MASP1/3*$^{-/-}$ mice were resistant to CAIA (268) and there was no change in the status of proFD in *MASP-1/3*$^{-/-}$ mice before or after the induction of CAIA (38), confirming the *in vivo* role of MASP-1/3 in the cleavage of proFD into FD. *In vitro*, adherent anti-CII antibodies failed to fully restore C3 activation using AP-defective sera from *MASP-1/3*$^{-/-}$ or *FD*$^{-/-}$ mice (268) consistent with the *in vivo* CAIA resistance. It was further shown, using *ex vivo* cartilage microparticles (CMP), that MASP-1/3 proteases can cleave proFD in the knee joint microenvironment (269). Here, cultured differentiated 3T3 adipocytes were used as a surrogate for synovial adipose tissue. They produce proFD but not mature FD. On the other hand, fibroblast-like synoviocytes (FLS) derived from CIA synovium, were the main source of MASP-1/3 and were expected to process proFD to mature FD. Using CMP coated with anti-CII mAb and serum from *MASP-1/3*$^{-/-}$ mice as a source of FB, proFD in 3T3 supernatants was cleaved into mature FD by MASP-1/3 in FLS supernatants. The mature FD was eluted from the CMP and was not present in the supernatants from the incubation with CMP, indicating that cleavage of proFD into mature FD by MASP-1/3 occurred on the CMP. These results demonstrated that pathogenic activation of the AP may occur in the joint through

IC adherent to cartilage along with the local production of necessary AP proteins by adipocytes and FLS (269). To provide another proof-of-concept experiment, *in vivo* reconstitution of MASP-1 or MASP-3, by liver derived from *FD*$^{-/-}$ mice, transplanted under the kidney capsule of *MASP-1/3*$^{-/-}$ mice and restored the cleavage of proFD into FD in the circulation of *MASP-1/3*$^{-/-}$ mice (270). Consistent with this, we found that sera from *MASP-1/3*$^{-/-}$ mice, which have defective AP, only after transplantation restored the full AP activity (270). These data confirmed that MASP-1/3 proteases of the LP are essential for the activation of the AP in mice. A new concept evolved from these studies that liver (generating MASPs) and adipose tissue (generating proFD) might acts in concert to activate the AP, thereby playing a vital role in the development of CAIA in mice (38, 43, 264, 270).

There are a number of ligands which can activate the LP. Presumably, the LP contribution to CAIA involves a subset of ligand interactions. Known candidates include MBL A, MBL C, FCN A, FCN B, and collectin 11. To address this, we examined CAIA in *FCN A*$^{-/-}$, *FCN B*$^{-/-}$, and *CL-11*$^{-/-}$ mice as mentioned earlier (10). These studies showed the important role of FCN B ligand of the LP in directly activating MASP-1 or MASP-3 to activate the AP. By contrast, we also observed partial protection in *MASP-2/sMAp*$^{-/-}$ mice. This was likely due to the involvement of the C4/C2 bypass pathway in CAIA (10). Given that MASP-1 and MASP-3 are splice variants derived from a single MASP-1/3 gene, it has been difficult to separate the two functionally. Nonetheless, our most recent data suggest that MASP-3, compared with MASP-1 or MASP-2, is the main driver of the AP and thus CAIA (271). In these studies, MASP-3 siRNA inhibited CAIA compared with MASP-1 or MASP-2 siRNAs (271). All of the above, *in vivo* CAIA studies, show that MASP-3 proteases of the LP regulate the AP, a finding that has also been confirmed by using *in vitro* studies by various research groups (44, 45, 265, 268, 272). There is a possibility that this amplification driven phenomena is surface-specific or disease specific as MASP-1/3 deficiency did affect kidney pathology in *MASP-1/3*$^{-/-}$/*FH*$^{-/-}$ mice (273) whether this kidney pathology is different from *FD*$^{-/-}$ mice is unknown. It has been reported that mechanism of AP activation depends on the activator surface (47). Here, it was shown that MASP-1 inhibition prevent AP activation as well as prevent already initiated AP activity on the LPS surface but not for zymosan-induced AP activation (47). Overall, it appears that AP is not one holistic linear pathway as previously thought but it is an interwoven network of multiple pathways regulated by the LP enzymes.

Using CAIA, the effector roles of C3aR and the C3a–C3aR axis, C5aR, and the C5a–C5aR axis, and MAC deposition have also been dissected. Mice lacking C5aR were more resistant to CAIA than C3aR- or MAC-deficient mice, confirming the pivotal role C5–C5aR axis (274). These results are consistent with the concept of the predominant role of C5 over the role of C3 in the pathogenesis of CAIA and that the C5–C5aR axis is essential for CAIA, although C3aR and the MAC also played important roles. Consistent with this conclusion, *C3*$^{-/-}$ mice were partially protected from CAIA (71) while *C5*$^{-/-}$ failed to develop CAIA (242).

By contrast, why the inhibitory anti-human C5 antibody (Eculizimab, Soliris®) was not effective against RA in clinical trials is not known. There is a possibility that C5 is generated in high quantities in RA, so even high doses of antibody do not prevent C5a generation in the joints. Alternatively, it may be the case that complement plays a more important role early in disease and that eventually RA evolves to a state where complement is only one of several drivers that can each compensate for the other. In this scenario, it might be the case that only certain RA patients would be effectively treated by Eculizimab. While the liver is the major source of C5, neutrophils, macrophages, and T cells are all known to be sources of C5. Blocking of C5aR in human neutrophils using the small molecule inhibitor; PMX-53, resulted in a dose-dependent block of C5a-mediated activation but why it was unsuccessful and very disappointing in RA clinical trial is unknown (275). Possibly, the drug was cleared rapidly and never reached the joints. No doubt that preclinical studies support targeting C5aR in RA because C5a and C5aR are elevated in the joints of RA and psoriatic arthritis patients and their blockade attenuate leukocyte migration to the synovial fluid (276). Almost complete inhibition of CIA was reported using anti-mC5aR inhibitory antibody (247). Based on these preclinical studies, a fully human antibody that blocks the binding of C5a to C5aR was developed and tested in RA patients by Novo Nordisk, a pharmaceutical company. This company has conducted two Phase I clinical trials in Europe with anti-C5aR in patients with RA, where a good drug safety profile was demonstrated.[3] Further results regarding the success or failure related to the phase II clinical trials by Novo Nordisk using anti-C5aR therapeutic antibody in RA patients are unknown at this points. Therefore, it is too early to make any conclusions regarding the therapeutic use of anti-C5aR antibody in the clinical settings. Furthermore, mice treated with GalNAc C5siRNAs targeting liver C5 are resistant to arthritis (277). Recently, with a new approach, CAIA mice injected with anti-C5aR antibody conjugated with C5siRNA inhibited arthritis in mice identical to the *C5aR*$^{-/-}$ mice with an inhibition of more than 80% of the disease (278). These results in CAIA are promising, showing selective and simultaneous inhibition of both C5aR activity and C5 mRNA production within the C5a–C5aR axis can dampen inflammatory response and attenuate arthritis in mice. Intriguingly, it has been shown in an experimental mouse model of autoimmune hemolytic anemia that C5aR activation does not necessarily involve C5 and C5a (279). This striking observation suggests that we must also consider the coordinate modulation of the FcγR system when interpreting the role of C5aR in RA.

Factor H is known to regulate the AP and due to the concurrent absence of C3 through uncontrolled complement activation in the fluid phase, *FH*$^{-/-}$ mice are resistant to CAIA (156). There is a variant of human FH gene, i.e., factor H-like-1 (FHL-1). There are five different forms of FHR proteins in humans (FHR-1 to FHR-5) (a.k.a. complement factor H-related proteins). Of these, FHL-1 and FHR are believed to counteract the effects of FH. At present, little is known of the effect of FHL-1 or FHR on CAIA due to the lack of experimental models. FH and FHL-1 have been shown to be expressed and secreted by synovial fibroblasts and were present

[3]http://ClinicalTrials.gov Identifier: NCT02151409 (Accessed: March 26, 2018).

in synovial fluid derived from patients suffering from rheumatoid or reactive arthritis (280). Endogenous FH is capable of inhibiting activation of the AP of complement on cartilage and synovium in joints *in vivo* exposed to a submaximal level of anti-CII mAb (156). This conclusion was derived from experiments in CAIA, with mice treated with rFH19-20 to prevent engagement of full-length endogenous FH. This takes advantage of the observation that domains 19 and 20 of rFH bind to cartilage. By treating with rFH19-20, the interaction of FH with cartilage is inhibited. To evaluate the *in vivo* importance, it was found that competitive blockade by murine rFH19-20 of the binding of endogenous fluid phase FH to either cartilage or an injured FLS surface significantly increased CAIA in WT mice. Further support for the conclusion that FH plays a key role in regulating AP-induced complement deposition on cartilage and cell surfaces in the joint is derived from studies with $FH^{\pm}$ heterozygous-deficient mice. These mice exhibit lower circulating levels of FH but are not more susceptible to CAIA unless they are treated with rFH19-20 to disrupt tissue binding of endogenous FH. Recombinant fH19-20 impairs only surface control of the AP by FH and does not influence the systemic activation of the complement system as indicated by unchanged serum levels of C5a. Thus, FH controls AP activation on cartilage and injured FLS *in vivo* in a manner dependent on the FH SCR19-20 domain, indicating that the AP can be regulated on these joint surfaces. Mice lacking FH do not develop arthritis due to the lacking of C3 present in the circulation (156).

In contrast to FH, there are no studies showing the direct role of mouse FHR proteins which shows some sequence homologies to FH in the pathogenesis of inflammatory arthritis in mice. In mice, various transcripts of FHR proteins have been reported such as FHR-A, FHR-B, and FHR-C (278, 281, 282). One study has shown that recombinant mouse FHR-B bound to human C3b and was able to compete with human FH for C3b binding. FHR-B supported the assembly of AP convertase *via* its interaction with C3b. The authors concluded that mouse FHR-B similar to human FHR-1 and FHR-5 promoted complement activation *via* interaction with C3b and *via* competition with mouse FH (283). Similarly, it has been shown that mouse FHR-A and mouse FHR-B proteins antagonize the protective function of FH using sheep erythrocyte hemolytic assays and in two cell lines, kidney proximal tubular cell line and a human retinal pigment epithelial cell line (ARPE-19) (284). Lack of mouse FHR-C has been linked to an autoimmune disease (278). Still none of these above FHR studies have shown the direct role mouse FHR-A, FHR-B and FHR-C in mice with arthritis for $FH^{-/-}$ are resistance to CAIA and depletion of C3 in these mice occurs in $FH^{-/-}$ mice even in the presence of all mouse FHR proteins when there is no absolute competition.

These findings related to the role of AP in CAIA are very likely to be relevant to the initiation and perpetuation of arthritis in humans (103). Recent preclinical studies have shown that human TT32 (CR2-CR1), a potent CP and AP inhibitor, compared with control human sCR1-10 also significantly attenuated CDA in mice with CAIA (235). In man, circulating autoantibodies, including anti-CII Abs, are present for several years prior to the onset of clinically apparent arthritis (221). Substantial evidence suggests that in RA joint-based inflammation is initiated through Ag/Ab complexes that are present on the cartilage surface (285). The observation that only injured FLS, but not normal FLS expressing complement regulatory proteins, could exhibit C3 binding suggests that cartilage damage may precede injury to the synovium. Initial complement activation by solid phase immune complexes in the cartilage may lead to secondary damage to the FLS and thus to subsequent development of synovitis. Therefore, potent CP and AP inhibitors might be helpful clinically to attenuate cartilage damage seen in human RA. This strategy of using complement inhibitors can be very useful during the early development of RA because once ACPA antibodies are present in subjects without clinical signs of joints damage then there are 50% chances of developing RA with 3-year period. Such clinical trials "Strategy for the Prevention of Onset of Clinically-Apparent RA" or a.k.a. StopRA[4] are already in progress.

K/BxN Serum Transfer Mouse Model of Arthritis and Complement Activation

About 20 years ago, an additional mouse model of RA, i.e., K/BxN serum transfer arthritis (STA) was discovered (210). It is also being used extensively to examine the role of effector pathways of the autoantibodies. This RA mouse model is different from the CIA and CAIA models as disease is driven by activation of T cells that recognize a self-peptide (i.e., glucose-6-phosphate isomerase, G6PI) (286). These T cells then help B cells to generate IgG antibodies against G6PI which induces arthritis. Furthermore, either purified IgGs or serum alone from K/BxN arthritic mice, when injected into naïve mice, is capable of inducing severe arthritis (287). So G6PI autoantibodies target the G6PI antigen in the joints thereby inducing arthritis by binding to cartilage. In this model, a pooled serum from several arthritic K/BxN mice is transferred into naïve mice to induce arthritis. The isotype of G6PI autoantibodies is IgG1 which does not activate complement as compared to the anti-CII antibodies used for CAIA (288). Whether G6PI antibodies present in RA patients have any practical diagnostic value is unknown. One study has shown the presence of anti-G6PI antibodies in sera but there were no marked differences in the levels of anti-G6PI antibodies among RA, non-RA patients, and healthy controls. Also, there was no significant difference G6PI antibody levels between the active phase and the inactive phase in RA patients (289). It is also controversial as to whether synovial fibroblasts from RA patients can secrete G6PI. One study has been published showing the presence of a distinct population of cells at the surface of the synovial lining of inflamed RA joints that has a high concentration of G6PI (290). This cell population could be T cells present in the RA synovium (291). Interestingly, serum G6PI concentration, C1q/G6PI-CIC, and G6PI mRNA levels within peripheral blood mononuclear cells were significantly higher in active RA than that in non-active RA (292). This is controversial for it has been shown that G6PI is not a specific autoantigen in RA and only few autoimmune sera contains G6PI (293, 294).

Using the K/BxN STA mouse model, the severity of inflammation has been correlated with the expression of PAD2 and PAD4 in the close proximity of citrullinated fibrinogen (295).

[4]http://ClinicalTrials.gov NCT02603146 (Accessed: March 26, 2018).

Two isotypes of PAD2 and PAD4 have been shown to be highly expressed in the synovium of RA patients (295) and infiltrating cells neutrophils, macrophages, and mast cells are the major source these enzymes indicating local citrullination in the joints can take place. Moreover, anti-PAD4 autoantibodies are present in a subset of RA patients (296). Perhaps these autoantibodies are generated to inhibit the excessive conversion of arginine to citrulline as a defensive mechanism. Interestingly, although PAD4 is required for citrullination, PAD4-deficient mice were not protected from arthritis in the K/BxN STA model (295). Once again, human RA clinical studies reflect a different picture of the GPI autoantibodies and also the role PAD4 than the mouse models of K/BxN STA.

Despite the lack of activation of complement by anti-G6PI antibodies, it is fascinating to note that complement activation is still required for K/BxN mice to progress to RA. Studies have examined mice lacking complement components, C3 or FB or C5 in the context of the K/BxN model and have established that these genes are required for disease development (287, 297, 298), thereby showing that the AP of complement is required. Mice lacking C1q, C4, CR1, and CR2 remained susceptible to disease development in the context of K/BxN STA (287, 297, 299). These studies have shown that CP is not required for disease progression in K/BxN STA. Properdin deficiency rescued mice from complement-mediated injury and ameliorated disease in K/BxN STA and Ab neutralization of properdin in WT mice similarly protected mice from arthritis (300). Mice lacking MAC also were not protected using K/BxN STA (287) showing that MAC is not a significant mediator of disease in this model. By contrast, C6 deficiency has been shown to partially protect mice from CAIA (274) indicating MAC, i.e., the terminal pathways of the complement can play important role. Overall, K/BxN STA have provided very important information regarding the role complement in RA and illustrates the complex nature of human RA. Furthermore, most of the data in K/BxN STA are consistent with CAIA regarding the role of AP in the initiation of arthritis.

MOUSE MODELS OF HUMAN RHEUMATOID ARTHRITIS AND COMPLEMENT IN THE PRESENT AND FUTURE

Human RA is a complex disease. This becomes readily apparent when one considers that some patients respond well to TNF-α blockade while others do not and instead respond to T or B cell inhibition. In this regard then, it is useful to have multiple mouse models, each of which uses a different driver to ultimately produce synovitis. Given that all three models require a functional complement system, it suggests that the actions of complement are fundamental components of disease progression.

We might divide the process of disease progression in RA into two general subprocesses: initiation and the effector phase. During initiation, autoantibodies find their way to the cartilage and synovial space. These may be generated in response to a pathogen such as *P. gingivalis* or as a response to altered self (i.e., citrullination). ACPA or anti-CarP antibodies in human patients are detected years before disease becomes apparent. In CIA, bovine CII is introduced causing the production initially of anti-bovine CII and then of anti-self-CII. In CAIA, anti-self-CII antibodies are directly introduced. We believe that these autoantibodies serve to initiate the complement cascade either through the CP or the LP. This early activation of complement then initiates an inflammatory response *via* the production of C3a and C5a. As the autoantibodies are located in the joint space, the response is synovitis. The epitope to which the antibody is directed appears to be mutable. Thus, CIA mouse model replicate somewhat an identical chain of early events mostly in RA patients in the initial phases of arthritis. While, ACPA is present in many RA patients, there exist a population of ACPA-negative RA patients which presumably have initiated disease *via* a different mechanism. Although this finding challenges a universal pathogenic model for a key role of autoantibodies in all types of RA, but our preliminary data from CAIA show that even a tiny amount of anti-CII autoantibodies can still bind to the cartilage surface when these autoantibodies are completely absent in the circulation. Therefore, one cannot rule out the presence of a very low levels, i.e., below threshold levels of ACPA or anti-CarP or anti-CII autoantibodies in other body secretions such as nasal secretions or sputum or gingival crevicular fluid or saliva, when autoantibodies are completely absent in the circulation.

Once other immune cells have infiltrated the joint, synoviocytes have proliferated, and pannus has formed, RA has entered into the effector phase. Here, pannus secretes matrix metalloproteinases which act to destroy bone and cartilage while also secreting a complex mixture of cytokines, prostaglandins, and complement components to maintain the inflammatory state. Complement can play a role here as well, although this may be less prominent. Such a later stage role can be seen in the K/BxN STA model of RA. Anti-G6PD antibodies are of the IgG1 type which do not serve to activate complement. Thus here, RA is initiated by a different mechanism. However, as discussed above, components of the AP appear to be necessary for disease in this model. We suspect that in this model complement is required for the formation of pannus and thus acts in the effector phase of RA. Indeed, we find that components of the AP are essential for CAIA to progress as well.

Considering commonalities among the various mouse models of RA, it seems that the AP of complement is universally shared. Here FD cleaves and activates FB, which in turn is necessary for the formation of the C3 convertase on surfaces to amplify the complement response. MASP-3 generated by the liver has recently been identified as the protease critical for the cleavage of proFD and thus for the activation of the AP. In this regard, it we believe that MASP-3 may serve as an important clinical target for the treatment of human RA.

AUTHOR CONTRIBUTIONS

Both authors listed have made a substantial, direct, and intellectual contribution to the work and approved it for publication.

FUNDING

This study was supported by National Institutes of Health grant R01AR51749 to VMH (PI) and NKB (Co-I).

REFERENCES

1. Ehrlich P, Morgenroth J. Zur Theorie der Lysenwirkung. *Berlin Klin Woch* (1899) 36:6–9.
2. Buchner H. Zur Nomenklatur der schutzenden Eiweisskorper. *Centr Bakteriol Parasitenk* (1891) 10:699–701.
3. Kaufmann SH. Immunology's foundation: the 100-year anniversary of the Nobel Prize to Paul Ehrlich and Elie Metchnikoff. *Nat Immunol* (2008) 9:705–12. doi:10.1038/ni0708-705
4. Nesargikar PN, Spiller B, Chavez R. The complement system: history, pathways, cascade and inhibitors. *Eur J Microbiol Immunol (Bp)* (2012) 2:103–11. doi:10.1556/EuJMI.2.2012.2.2
5. Skarnes RC, Watson DW. Antimicrobial factors of normal tissues and fluids. *Bacteriol Rev* (1957) 21:273–94.
6. BP M. *Complement: Clinical Aspects and Relevance to Disease*. UK: Academic Press (1990).
7. Schifferli JA, Ng YC, Peters DK. The role of complement and its receptor in the elimination of immune complexes. *N Engl J Med* (1986) 315:488–95. doi:10.1056/NEJM198608213150805
8. Davies KA, Schifferli JA, Walport MJ. Complement deficiency and immune complex disease. *Springer Semin Immunopathol* (1994) 15:397–416. doi:10.1007/BF01837367
9. Mevorach D, Mascarenhas JO, Gershov D, Elkon KB. Complement-dependent clearance of apoptotic cells by human macrophages. *J Exp Med* (1998) 188:2313–20. doi:10.1084/jem.188.12.2313
10. Banda NK, Acharya S, Scheinman RI, Mehta G, Takahashi M, Endo Y, et al. Deconstructing the lectin pathway in the pathogenesis of experimental inflammatory arthritis: essential role of the lectin ficolin B and mannose-binding protein-associated serine protease 2. *J Immunol* (2017) 199:1835–45. doi:10.4049/jimmunol.1700119
11. Arumugam TV, Magnus T, Woodruff TM, Proctor LM, Shiels IA, Taylor SM. Complement mediators in ischemia-reperfusion injury. *Clin Chim Acta* (2006) 374:33–45. doi:10.1016/j.cca.2006.06.010
12. Morgan BP. Regulation of the complement membrane attack pathway. *Crit Rev Immunol* (1999) 19:173–98. doi:10.1615/CritRevImmunol.v19.i3.10
13. Botto M, Walport MJ. C1q, autoimmunity and apoptosis. *Immunobiology* (2002) 205:395–406. doi:10.1078/0171-2985-00141
14. Ricklin D, Lambris JD. Complement in immune and inflammatory disorders: pathophysiological mechanisms. *J Immunol* (2013) 190:3831–8. doi:10.4049/jimmunol.1203200
15. Wang H, Ricklin D, Lambris JD. Complement-activation fragment C4a mediates effector functions by binding as untethered agonist to protease-activated receptors 1 and 4. *Proc Natl Acad Sci U S A* (2017) 114:10948–53. doi:10.1073/pnas.1707364114
16. Bayly-Jones C, Bubeck D, Dunstone MA. The mystery behind membrane insertion: a review of the complement membrane attack complex. *Philos Trans R Soc Lond B Biol Sci* (2017) 372:1–9. doi:10.1098/rstb.2016.0221
17. Berends ET, Dekkers JF, Nijland R, Kuipers A, Soppe JA, van Strijp JA, et al. Distinct localization of the complement C5b-9 complex on Gram-positive bacteria. *Cell Microbiol* (2013) 15:1955–68. doi:10.1111/cmi.12170
18. Hoover DL, Berger M, Nacy CA, Hockmeyer WT, Meltzer MS. Killing of *Leishmania tropica* amastigotes by factors in normal human serum. *J Immunol* (1984) 132:893–7.
19. Reiter Y, Ciobotariu A, Fishelson Z. Sublytic complement attack protects tumor cells from lytic doses of antibody and complement. *Eur J Immunol* (1992) 22:1207–13. doi:10.1002/eji.1830220515
20. Reiter Y, Ciobotariu A, Jones J, Morgan BP, Fishelson Z. Complement membrane attack complex, perforin, and bacterial exotoxins induce in K562 cells calcium-dependent cross-protection from lysis. *J Immunol* (1995) 155:2203–10.
21. Matsushita M, Fujita T. Cleavage of the third component of complement (C3) by mannose-binding protein-associated serine protease (MASP) with subsequent complement activation. *Immunobiology* (1995) 194:443–8. doi:10.1016/S0171-2985(11)80110-5
22. Matsushita M, Fujita T. Ficolins and the lectin complement pathway. *Immunol Rev* (2001) 180:78–85. doi:10.1034/j.1600-065X.2001.1800107.x
23. Hansen S, Selman L, Palaniyar N, Ziegler K, Brandt J, Kliem A, et al. Collectin 11 (CL-11, CL-K1) is a MASP-1/3-associated plasma collectin with microbial-binding activity. *J Immunol* (2010) 185:6096–104. doi:10.4049/jimmunol.1002185
24. Endo Y, Iwaki D, Ishida Y, Takahashi M, Matsushita M, Fujita T. Mouse ficolin B has an ability to form complexes with mannose-binding lectin-associated serine proteases and activate complement through the lectin pathway. *J Biomed Biotechnol* (2012) 2012:105891. doi:10.1155/2012/105891
25. Garlatti V, Belloy N, Martin L, Lacroix M, Matsushita M, Endo Y, et al. Structural insights into the innate immune recognition specificities of L- and H-ficolins. *EMBO J* (2007) 26:623–33. doi:10.1038/sj.emboj.7601500
26. Garlatti V, Martin L, Gout E, Reiser JB, Fujita T, Arlaud GJ, et al. Structural basis for innate immune sensing by M-ficolin and its control by a pH-dependent conformational switch. *J Biol Chem* (2007) 282:35814–20. doi:10.1074/jbc.M705741200
27. Fujimori Y, Harumiya S, Fukumoto Y, Miura Y, Yagasaki K, Tachikawa H, et al. Molecular cloning and characterization of mouse ficolin-A. *Biochem Biophys Res Commun* (1998) 244:796–800. doi:10.1006/bbrc.1998.8344
28. Ohashi T, Erickson HP. Oligomeric structure and tissue distribution of ficolins from mouse, pig and human. *Arch Biochem Biophys* (1998) 360:223–32. doi:10.1006/abbi.1998.0957
29. Endo Y, Sato Y, Matsushita M, Fujita T. Cloning and characterization of the human lectin P35 gene and its related gene. *Genomics* (1996) 36:515–21. doi:10.1006/geno.1996.0497
30. Lu J, Tay PN, Kon OL, Reid KB. Human ficolin: cDNA cloning, demonstration of peripheral blood leucocytes as the major site of synthesis and assignment of the gene to chromosome 9. *Biochem J* (1996) 313(Pt 2):473–8. doi:10.1042/bj3130473
31. Matsushita M, Endo Y, Fujita T. Cutting edge: complement-activating complex of ficolin and mannose-binding lectin-associated serine protease. *J Immunol* (2000) 164:2281–4. doi:10.4049/jimmunol.164.5.2281
32. Matsushita M, Endo Y, Taira S, Sato Y, Fujita T, Ichikawa N, et al. A novel human serum lectin with collagen- and fibrinogen-like domains that functions as an opsonin. *J Biol Chem* (1996) 271:2448–54. doi:10.1074/jbc.271.5.2448
33. Sugimoto R, Yae Y, Akaiwa M, Kitajima S, Shibata Y, Sato H, et al. Cloning and characterization of the Hakata antigen, a member of the ficolin/opsonin p35 lectin family. *J Biol Chem* (1998) 273:20721–7. doi:10.1074/jbc.273.33.20721
34. Endo Y, Nakazawa N, Liu Y, Iwaki D, Takahashi M, Fujita T, et al. Carbohydrate-binding specificities of mouse ficolin A, a splicing variant of ficolin A and ficolin B and their complex formation with MASP-2 and sMAP. *Immunogenetics* (2005) 57:837–44. doi:10.1007/s00251-005-0058-1
35. Endo Y, Takahashi M, Iwaki D, Ishida Y, Nakazawa N, Kodama T, et al. Mice deficient in ficolin, a lectin complement pathway recognition molecule, are susceptible to *Streptococcus pneumoniae* infection. *J Immunol* (2012) 189:5860–6. doi:10.4049/jimmunol.1200836
36. Liu Y, Endo Y, Iwaki D, Nakata M, Matsushita M, Wada I, et al. Human M-ficolin is a secretory protein that activates the lectin complement pathway. *J Immunol* (2005) 175:3150–6. doi:10.4049/jimmunol.175.5.3150
37. Runza VL, Hehlgans T, Echtenacher B, Zahringer U, Schwaeble WJ, Mannel DN. Localization of the mouse defense lectin ficolin B in lysosomes of activated macrophages. *J Endotoxin Res* (2006) 12:120–6. doi:10.1177/09680519060120020801
38. Banda NK, Takahashi M, Takahashi K, Stahl GL, Hyatt S, Glogowska M, et al. Mechanisms of mannose-binding lectin-associated serine proteases-1/3 activation of the alternative pathway of complement. *Mol Immunol* (2011) 49:281–9. doi:10.1016/j.molimm.2011.08.021
39. Hansen S, Holmskov U. Structural aspects of collectins and receptors for collectins. *Immunobiology* (1998) 199:165–89. doi:10.1016/S0171-2985(98)80025-9
40. Diepenhorst GM, van Gulik TM, Hack CE. Complement-mediated ischemia-reperfusion injury: lessons learned from animal and clinical studies. *Ann Surg* (2009) 249:889–99. doi:10.1097/SLA.0b013e3181a38f45
41. Iwaki D, Kanno K, Takahashi M, Endo Y, Lynch NJ, Schwaeble WJ, et al. Small mannose-binding lectin-associated protein plays a regulatory role in the lectin complement pathway. *J Immunol* (2006) 177:8626–32. doi:10.4049/jimmunol.177.12.8626
42. Pavlov VI, Skjoedt MO, Siow Tan Y, Rosbjerg A, Garred P, Stahl GL. Endogenous and natural complement inhibitor attenuates myocardial injury and arterial thrombogenesis. *Circulation* (2012) 126:2227–35. doi:10.1161/CIRCULATIONAHA.112.123968

43. Banda NK, Mehta G, Kjaer TR, Takahashi M, Schaack J, Morrison TE, et al. Essential role for the lectin pathway in collagen antibody-induced arthritis revealed through use of adenovirus programming complement inhibitor MAp44 expression. *J Immunol* (2014) 193:2455–68. doi:10.4049/jimmunol.1400752
44. Dobo J, Szakacs D, Oroszlan G, Kortvely E, Kiss B, Boros E, et al. MASP-3 is the exclusive pro-factor D activator in resting blood: the lectin and the alternative complement pathways are fundamentally linked. *Sci Rep* (2016) 6:31877. doi:10.1038/srep31877
45. Pihl R, Jensen L, Hansen AG, Thogersen IB, Andres S, Dagnaes-Hansen F, et al. Analysis of factor D isoforms in Malpuech-Michels-Mingarelli-Carnevale patients highlights the role of MASP-3 as a maturase in the alternative pathway of complement. *J Immunol* (2017) 199:2158–70. doi:10.4049/jimmunol.1700518
46. Oroszlan G, Dani R, Szilagyi A, Zavodszky P, Thiel S, Gal P, et al. Extensive basal level activation of complement mannose-binding lectin-associated serine protease-3: kinetic modeling of lectin pathway activation provides possible mechanism. *Front Immunol* (2017) 8:1821. doi:10.3389/fimmu.2017.01821
47. Parej K, Kocsis A, Enyingi C, Dani R, Oroszlan G, Beinrohr L, et al. Cutting edge: a new player in the alternative complement pathway, MASP-1 is essential for LPS-induced, but not for zymosan-induced, alternative pathway activation. *J Immunol* (2018) 200:2247–52. doi:10.4049/jimmunol.1701421
48. Drickamer K. Two distinct classes of carbohydrate-recognition domains in animal lectins. *J Biol Chem* (1988) 263:9557–60.
49. Keshi H, Sakamoto T, Kawai T, Ohtani K, Katoh T, Jang SJ, et al. Identification and characterization of a novel human collectin CL-K1. *Microbiol Immunol* (2006) 50:1001–13. doi:10.1111/j.1348-0421.2006.tb03868.x
50. Ma YJ, Hein E, Munthe-Fog L, Skjoedt MO, Bayarri-Olmos R, Romani L, et al. Soluble collectin-12 (CL-12) is a pattern recognition molecule initiating complement activation via the alternative pathway. *J Immunol* (2015) 195:3365–73. doi:10.4049/jimmunol.1500493
51. Nakamura K, Funakoshi H, Miyamoto K, Tokunaga F, Nakamura T. Molecular cloning and functional characterization of a human scavenger receptor with C-type lectin (SRCL), a novel member of a scavenger receptor family. *Biochem Biophys Res Commun* (2001) 280:1028–35. doi:10.1006/bbrc.2000.4210
52. Ohtani K, Suzuki Y, Eda S, Kawai T, Kase T, Yamazaki H, et al. Molecular cloning of a novel human collectin from liver (CL-L1). *J Biol Chem* (1999) 274:13681–9. doi:10.1074/jbc.274.19.13681
53. Motomura W, Yoshizaki T, Ohtani K, Okumura T, Fukuda M, Fukuzawa J, et al. Immunolocalization of a novel collectin CL-K1 in murine tissues. *J Histochem Cytochem* (2008) 56:243–52. doi:10.1369/jhc.7A7312.2007
54. Troegeler A, Lugo-Villarino G, Hansen S, Rasolofo V, Henriksen ML, Mori K, et al. Collectin CL-LK is a novel soluble pattern recognition receptor for *Mycobacterium tuberculosis*. *PLoS One* (2015) 10:e0132692. doi:10.1371/journal.pone.0132692
55. Selman L, Hansen S. Structure and function of collectin liver 1 (CL-L1) and collectin 11 (CL-11, CL-K1). *Immunobiology* (2012) 217:851–63. doi:10.1016/j.imbio.2011.12.008
56. Farrar CA, Tran D, Li K, Wu W, Peng Q, Schwaeble W, et al. Collectin-11 detects stress-induced L-fucose pattern to trigger renal epithelial injury. *J Clin Invest* (2016) 126:1911–25. doi:10.1172/JCI83000
57. Devyatyarova-Johnson M, Rees IH, Robertson BD, Turner MW, Klein NJ, Jack DL. The lipopolysaccharide structures of *Salmonella enterica* serovar Typhimurium and *Neisseria gonorrhoeae* determine the attachment of human mannose-binding lectin to intact organisms. *Infect Immun* (2000) 68:3894–9. doi:10.1128/IAI.68.7.3894-3899.2000
58. Matsushita M, Endo Y, Fujita T. MASP1 (MBL-associated serine protease 1). *Immunobiology* (1998) 199:340–7. doi:10.1016/S0171-2985(98)80038-7
59. Swierzko AS, Cedzynski M, Kirikae T, Nakano M, Klink M, Kirikae F, et al. Role of the complement-lectin pathway in anaphylactoid reaction induced with lipopolysaccharide in mice. *Eur J Immunol* (2003) 33:2842–52. doi:10.1002/eji.200323949
60. Thiel S, Vorup-Jensen T, Stover CM, Schwaeble W, Laursen SB, Poulsen K, et al. A second serine protease associated with mannan-binding lectin that activates complement. *Nature* (1997) 386:506–10. doi:10.1038/386506a0
61. Hinz CF Jr, Jordan WS Jr, Pillemer L. The properdin system and immunity. IV. The hemolysis of erythrocytes from patients with paroxysmal nocturnal hemoglobinuria. *J Clin Invest* (1956) 35:453–7. doi:10.1172/JCI103296
62. Lachmann PJ, Halbwachs L. The influence of C3b inactivator (KAF) concentration on the ability of serum to support complement activation. *Clin Exp Immunol* (1975) 21:109–14.
63. Hourcade DE. The role of properdin in the assembly of the alternative pathway C3 convertases of complement. *J Biol Chem* (2006) 281:2128–32. doi:10.1074/jbc.M508928200
64. Pangburn MK. Host recognition and target differentiation by factor H, a regulator of the alternative pathway of complement. *Immunopharmacology* (2000) 49:149–57. doi:10.1016/S0162-3109(00)80300-8
65. Noris M, Remuzzi G. Overview of complement activation and regulation. *Semin Nephrol* (2013) 33:479–92. doi:10.1016/j.semnephrol.2013.08.001
66. Matsushita M, Okada H. Alternative complement pathway activation by C4b deposited during classical pathway activation. *J Immunol* (1986) 136:2994–8.
67. May JE, Frank MM. A new complement-mediated cytolytic mechanism – the C1-bypass activation pathway. *Proc Natl Acad Sci U S A* (1973) 70:649–52. doi:10.1073/pnas.70.3.649
68. May JE, Frank MM. Hemolysis of sheep erythrocytes in guinea pig serum deficient in the fourth component of complement. I. Antibody and serum requirements. *J Immunol* (1973) 111:1671–7.
69. May JE, Frank MM. Hemolysis of sheep erythrocytes in guinea pig serum deficient in the fourth component of complement. II. Evidence for involvement of C1 and components of the alternate complement pathway. *J Immunol* (1973) 111:1668–76.
70. Selander B, Martensson U, Weintraub A, Holmstrom E, Matsushita M, Thiel S, et al. Mannan-binding lectin activates C3 and the alternative complement pathway without involvement of C2. *J Clin Invest* (2006) 116:1425–34. doi:10.1172/JCI25982
71. Banda NK, Takahashi K, Wood AK, Holers VM, Arend WP. Pathogenic complement activation in collagen antibody-induced arthritis in mice requires amplification by the alternative pathway. *J Immunol* (2007) 179:4101–9. doi:10.4049/jimmunol.179.6.4101
72. Schwaeble WJ, Lynch NJ, Clark JE, Marber M, Samani NJ, Ali YM, et al. Targeting of mannan-binding lectin-associated serine protease-2 confers protection from myocardial and gastrointestinal ischemia/reperfusion injury. *Proc Natl Acad Sci U S A* (2011) 108:7523–8. doi:10.1073/pnas.1101748108
73. Huber-Lang M, Sarma JV, Zetoune FS, Rittirsch D, Neff TA, McGuire SR, et al. Generation of C5a in the absence of C3: a new complement activation pathway. *Nat Med* (2006) 12:682–7. doi:10.1038/nm1419
74. Yaseen S, Demopulos G, Dudler T, Yabuki M, Wood CL, Cummings WJ, et al. Lectin pathway effector enzyme mannan-binding lectin-associated serine protease-2 can activate native complement C3 in absence of C4 and/or C2. *FASEB J* (2017) 31:2210–9. doi:10.1096/fj.201601306R
75. Bhole D, Stahl GL. Therapeutic potential of targeting the complement cascade in critical care medicine. *Crit Care Med* (2003) 31:S97–104. doi:10.1097/00003246-200301001-00014
76. Chenoweth DE, Cooper SW, Hugli TE, Stewart RW, Blackstone EH, Kirklin JW. Complement activation during cardiopulmonary bypass: evidence for generation of C3a and C5a anaphylatoxins. *N Engl J Med* (1981) 304:497–503. doi:10.1056/NEJM198102263040901
77. Irmscher S, Doring N, Halder LD, Jo EAH, Kopka I, Dunker C, et al. Kallikrein cleaves C3 and activates complement. *J Innate Immun* (2017) 10:94–105. doi:10.1159/000484257
78. Markiewski MM, Nilsson B, Ekdahl KN, Mollnes TE, Lambris JD. Complement and coagulation: strangers or partners in crime? *Trends Immunol* (2007) 28:184–92. doi:10.1016/j.it.2007.02.006
79. Daffern PJ, Pfeifer PH, Ember JA, Hugli TE. C3a is a chemotaxin for human eosinophils but not for neutrophils. I. C3a stimulation of neutrophils is secondary to eosinophil activation. *J Exp Med* (1995) 181:2119–27. doi:10.1084/jem.181.6.2119
80. Martin U, Bock D, Arseniev L, Tornetta MA, Ames RS, Bautsch W, et al. The human C3a receptor is expressed on neutrophils and monocytes, but not on B or T lymphocytes. *J Exp Med* (1997) 186:199–207. doi:10.1084/jem.186.2.199
81. Zwirner J, Gotze O, Begemann G, Kapp A, Kirchhoff K, Werfel T. Evaluation of C3a receptor expression on human leucocytes by the use of novel monoclonal antibodies. *Immunology* (1999) 97:166–72. doi:10.1046/j.1365-2567.1999.00764.x
82. Stone KD, Prussin C, Metcalfe DD. IgE, mast cells, basophils, and eosinophils. *J Allergy Clin Immunol* (2010) 125:S73–80. doi:10.1016/j.jaci.2009.11.017

83. Mueller-Ortiz SL, Wang D, Morales JE, Li L, Chang JY, Wetsel RA. Targeted disruption of the gene encoding the murine small subunit of carboxypeptidase N (CPN1) causes susceptibility to C5a anaphylatoxin-mediated shock. *J Immunol* (2009) 182:6533–9. doi:10.4049/jimmunol.0804207
84. Cain SA, Monk PN. The orphan receptor C5L2 has high affinity binding sites for complement fragments C5a and C5a des-Arg. *J Biol Chem* (2002) 277:7165–9. doi:10.1074/jbc.C100714200
85. Reis ES, Chen H, Sfyroera G, Monk PN, Kohl J, Ricklin D, et al. C5a receptor-dependent cell activation by physiological concentrations of desarginated C5a: insights from a novel label-free cellular assay. *J Immunol* (2012) 189:4797–805. doi:10.4049/jimmunol.1200834
86. Mulligan MS, Schmid E, Till GO, Hugli TE, Friedl HP, Roth RA, et al. C5a-dependent up-regulation in vivo of lung vascular P-selectin. *J Immunol* (1997) 158:1857–61.
87. Tonnesen MG, Anderson DC, Springer TA, Knedler A, Avdi N, Henson PM. Adherence of neutrophils to cultured human microvascular endothelial cells. Stimulation by chemotactic peptides and lipid mediators and dependence upon the Mac-1, LFA-1, p150,95 glycoprotein family. *J Clin Invest* (1989) 83:637–46. doi:10.1172/JCI113928
88. Sacks T, Moldow CF, Craddock PR, Bowers TK, Jacob HS. Oxygen radicals mediate endothelial cell damage by complement-stimulated granulocytes. An in vitro model of immune vascular damage. *J Clin Invest* (1978) 61: 1161–7. doi:10.1172/JCI109031
89. Bielecka E, Scavenius C, Kantyka T, Jusko M, Mizgalska D, Szmigielski B, et al. Peptidyl arginine deiminase from *Porphyromonas gingivalis* abolishes anaphylatoxin C5a activity. *J Biol Chem* (2014) 289:32481–7. doi:10.1074/jbc.C114.617142
90. Shushakova N, Skokowa J, Schulman J, Baumann U, Zwirner J, Schmidt RE, et al. C5a anaphylatoxin is a major regulator of activating versus inhibitory FcgammaRs in immune complex-induced lung disease. *J Clin Invest* (2002) 110:1823–30. doi:10.1172/JCI16577
91. Tsuboi N, Ernandez T, Li X, Nishi H, Cullere X, Mekala D, et al. Regulation of human neutrophil Fcgamma receptor IIa by C5a receptor promotes inflammatory arthritis in mice. *Arthritis Rheum* (2011) 63:467–78. doi:10.1002/art.30141
92. Okinaga S, Slattery D, Humbles A, Zsengeller Z, Morteau O, Kinrade MB, et al. C5L2, a nonsignaling C5A binding protein. *Biochemistry* (2003) 42:9406–15. doi:10.1021/bi034489v
93. Li R, Coulthard LG, Wu MC, Taylor SM, Woodruff TM. C5L2: a controversial receptor of complement anaphylatoxin, C5a. *FASEB J* (2013) 27:855–64. doi:10.1096/fj.12-220509
94. Pangburn MK, Rawal N. Structure and function of complement C5 convertase enzymes. *Biochem Soc Trans* (2002) 30:1006–10. doi:10.1042/bst030a098c
95. Huynh ML, Fadok VA, Henson PM. Phosphatidylserine-dependent ingestion of apoptotic cells promotes TGF-beta1 secretion and the resolution of inflammation. *J Clin Invest* (2002) 109:41–50. doi:10.1172/JCI0211638
96. Majno G, La Gattuta M, Thompson TE. Cellular death and necrosis: chemical, physical and morphologic changes in rat liver. *Virchows Arch Pathol Anat Physiol Klin Med* (1960) 333:421–65. doi:10.1007/BF00955327
97. Nicholson-Weller A, Halperin JA. Membrane signaling by complement C5b-9, the membrane attack complex. *Immunol Res* (1993) 12:244–57. doi:10.1007/BF02918256
98. Costabile M. Measuring the 50% haemolytic complement (CH50) activity of serum. *J Vis Exp* (2010) 1–3. doi:10.3791/1923
99. Lachmann PJ. Preparing serum for functional complement assays. *J Immunol Methods* (2010) 352:195–7. doi:10.1016/j.jim.2009.11.003
100. Banda NK, Takahashi K. Analysis of the complement activation in mice. *Methods Mol Biol* (2014) 1100:365–71. doi:10.1007/978-1-62703-724-2_31
101. Bugatti S, Bogliolo L, Vitolo B, Manzo A, Montecucco C, Caporali R. Anti-citrullinated protein antibodies and high levels of rheumatoid factor are associated with systemic bone loss in patients with early untreated rheumatoid arthritis. *Arthritis Res Ther* (2016) 18:226. doi:10.1186/s13075-016-1116-9
102. Prohaszka Z, Nilsson B, Frazer-Abel A, Kirschfink M. Complement analysis 2016: clinical indications, laboratory diagnostics and quality control. *Immunobiology* (2016) 221:1247–58. doi:10.1016/j.imbio.2016.06.008
103. Arend WP, Firestein GS. Pre-rheumatoid arthritis: predisposition and transition to clinical synovitis. *Nat Rev Rheumatol* (2012) 8:573–86. doi:10.1038/nrrheum.2012.134
104. Feldmann M, Brennan FM, Maini RN. Rheumatoid arthritis. *Cell* (1996) 85:307–10. doi:10.1016/S0092-8674(00)81109-5
105. Firestein GS. Evolving concepts of rheumatoid arthritis. *Nature* (2003) 423:356–61. doi:10.1038/nature01661
106. Bayar N, Kara SA, Keles I, Koc MC, Altinok D, Orkun S. Temporomandibular joint involvement in rheumatoid arthritis: a radiological and clinical study. *Cranio* (2002) 20:105–10. doi:10.1080/08869634.2002.11746198
107. Lin YC, Hsu ML, Yang JS, Liang TH, Chou SL, Lin HY. Temporomandibular joint disorders in patients with rheumatoid arthritis. *J Chin Med Assoc* (2007) 70:527–34. doi:10.1016/S1726-4901(08)70055-8
108. Bingham CO III, Moni M. Periodontal disease and rheumatoid arthritis: the evidence accumulates for complex pathobiologic interactions. *Curr Opin Rheumatol* (2013) 25:345–53. doi:10.1097/BOR.0b013e32835fb8ec
109. Zhang X, Zhang D, Jia H, Feng Q, Wang D, Liang D, et al. The oral and gut microbiomes are perturbed in rheumatoid arthritis and partly normalized after treatment. *Nat Med* (2015) 21:895–905. doi:10.1038/nm.3914
110. Kim EJ, Collard HR, King TE Jr. Rheumatoid arthritis-associated interstitial lung disease: the relevance of histopathologic and radiographic pattern. *Chest* (2009) 136:1397–405. doi:10.1378/chest.09-0444
111. Suhrbier A, La Linn M. Clinical and pathologic aspects of arthritis due to Ross River virus and other alphaviruses. *Curr Opin Rheumatol* (2004) 16:374–9. doi:10.1097/01.bor.0000130537.76808.26
112. Schilte C, Staikowsky F, Couderc T, Madec Y, Carpentier F, Kassab S, et al. Chikungunya virus-associated long-term arthralgia: a 36-month prospective longitudinal study. *PLoS Negl Trop Dis* (2013) 7:e2137. doi:10.1371/journal.pntd.0002137
113. Wands JR, Mann E, Alpert E, Isselbacher KJ. The pathogenesis of arthritis associated with acute hepatitis-B surface antigen-positive hepatitis. Complement activation and characterization of circulating immune complexes. *J Clin Invest* (1975) 55:930–6. doi:10.1172/JCI108022
114. Gregersen PK, Silver J, Winchester RJ. The shared epitope hypothesis. An approach to understanding the molecular genetics of susceptibility to rheumatoid arthritis. *Arthritis Rheum* (1987) 30:1205–13. doi:10.1002/art.1780301102
115. Plenge RM, Padyukov L, Remmers EF, Purcell S, Lee AT, Karlson EW, et al. Replication of putative candidate-gene associations with rheumatoid arthritis in >4,000 samples from North America and Sweden: association of susceptibility with PTPN22, CTLA4, and PADI4. *Am J Hum Genet* (2005) 77:1044–60. doi:10.1086/498651
116. Essouma M, Noubiap JJ. Is air pollution a risk factor for rheumatoid arthritis? *J Inflamm (Lond)* (2015) 12:48. doi:10.1186/s12950-015-0092-1
117. Klareskog L, Padyukov L, Ronnelid J, Alfredsson L. Genes, environment and immunity in the development of rheumatoid arthritis. *Curr Opin Immunol* (2006) 18:650–5. doi:10.1016/j.coi.2006.06.004
118. Ruiz-Esquide V, Sanmarti R. Tobacco and other environmental risk factors in rheumatoid arthritis. *Reumatol Clin* (2012) 8:342–50. doi:10.1016/j.reuma.2012.02.011
119. Gan RW, Deane KD, Zerbe GO, Demoruelle MK, Weisman MH, Buckner JH, et al. Relationship between air pollution and positivity of RA-related autoantibodies in individuals without established RA: a report on SERA. *Ann Rheum Dis* (2013) 72:2002–5. doi:10.1136/annrheumdis-2012-202949
120. Hart JE, Kallberg H, Laden F, Bellander T, Costenbader KH, Holmqvist M, et al. Ambient air pollution exposures and risk of rheumatoid arthritis: results from the Swedish EIRA case-control study. *Ann Rheum Dis* (2013) 72:888–94. doi:10.1136/annrheumdis-2012-201587
121. Nogueira L, Cornillet M, Singwe-Ngandeu M, Viatte S, Bas S, Gabay C, et al. In Black Africans with rheumatoid arthritis, ACPA recognize citrullinated fibrinogen and the derived peptides alpha36-50Cit38,42 and beta60-74Cit60,72,74, like in Caucasians. *Clin Immunol* (2014) 152:58–64. doi:10.1016/j.clim.2014.02.011
122. Darrah E, Andrade F. Rheumatoid arthritis and citrullination. *Curr Opin Rheumatol* (2018) 30:72–8. doi:10.1097/BOR.0000000000000452
123. Tutturen AE, Fleckenstein B, de Souza GA. Assessing the citrullinome in rheumatoid arthritis synovial fluid with and without enrichment of citrullinated peptides. *J Proteome Res* (2014) 13:2867–73. doi:10.1021/pr500030x
124. van Beers JJ, Schwarte CM, Stammen-Vogelzangs J, Oosterink E, Bozic B, Pruijn GJ. The rheumatoid arthritis synovial fluid citrullinome reveals novel citrullinated epitopes in apolipoprotein E, myeloid nuclear differentiation

antigen, and beta-actin. *Arthritis Rheum* (2013) 65:69–80. doi:10.1002/art.37720
125. Wang F, Chen FF, Gao WB, Wang HY, Zhao NW, Xu M, et al. Identification of citrullinated peptides in the synovial fluid of patients with rheumatoid arthritis using LC-MALDI-TOF/TOF. *Clin Rheumatol* (2016) 35:2185–94. doi:10.1007/s10067-016-3247-4
126. Harre U, Georgess D, Bang H, Bozec A, Axmann R, Ossipova E, et al. Induction of osteoclastogenesis and bone loss by human autoantibodies against citrullinated vimentin. *J Clin Invest* (2012) 122:1791–802. doi:10.1172/JCI60975
127. Malmstrom V, Catrina AI, Klareskog L. The immunopathogenesis of seropositive rheumatoid arthritis: from triggering to targeting. *Nat Rev Immunol* (2017) 17:60–75. doi:10.1038/nri.2016.124
128. Fujisaki M, Sugawara K. Properties of peptidylarginine deiminase from the epidermis of newborn rats. *J Biochem* (1981) 89:257–63. doi:10.1093/oxfordjournals.jbchem.a133189
129. Rogers GE. Occurrence of citrulline in proteins. *Nature* (1962) 194:1149–51. doi:10.1038/1941149a0
130. Rogers GE, Harding HW, Llewellyn-Smith IJ. The origin of citrulline-containing proteins in the hair follicle and the chemical nature of trichohyalin, an intracellular precursor. *Biochim Biophys Acta* (1977) 495:159–75. doi:10.1016/0005-2795(77)90250-1
131. Rogers GE, Simmonds DH. Content of citrulline and other amino-acids in a protein of hair follicles. *Nature* (1958) 182:186–7. doi:10.1038/182186a0
132. Romero V, Fert-Bober J, Nigrovic PA, Darrah E, Haque UJ, Lee DM, et al. Immune-mediated pore-forming pathways induce cellular hypercitrullination and generate citrullinated autoantigens in rheumatoid arthritis. *Sci Transl Med* (2013) 5:209ra150. doi:10.1126/scitranslmed.3006869
133. Darrah E, Rosen A, Giles JT, Andrade F. Peptidylarginine deiminase 2, 3 and 4 have distinct specificities against cellular substrates: novel insights into autoantigen selection in rheumatoid arthritis. *Ann Rheum Dis* (2012) 71:92–8. doi:10.1136/ard.2011.151712
134. Konig MF, Abusleme L, Reinholdt J, Palmer RJ, Teles RP, Sampson K, et al. Aggregatibacter actinomycetemcomitans-induced hypercitrullination links periodontal infection to autoimmunity in rheumatoid arthritis. *Sci Transl Med* (2016) 8:369ra176. doi:10.1126/scitranslmed.aaj1921
135. Malinin TI, Pekin TJ Jr, Zvaifler NJ. Cytology of synovial fluid in rheumatoid arthritis. *Am J Clin Pathol* (1967) 47:203–8. doi:10.1093/ajcp/47.2.203
136. Spengler J, Lugonja B, Ytterberg AJ, Zubarev RA, Creese AJ, Pearson MJ, et al. Release of active peptidyl arginine deiminases by neutrophils can explain production of extracellular citrullinated autoantigens in rheumatoid arthritis synovial fluid. *Arthritis Rheumatol* (2015) 67:3135–45. doi:10.1002/art.39313
137. Beard HK, Ryvar R, Skingle J, Greenbury CL. Anti-collagen antibodies in sera from rheumatoid arthritis patients. *J Clin Pathol* (1980) 33:1077–81. doi:10.1136/jcp.33.11.1077
138. Buckwalter JA, Mankin HJ. Articular cartilage: tissue design and chondrocyte-matrix interactions. *Instr Course Lect* (1998) 47:477–86.
139. Buckwalter JA, Hunzinker E, Rosenberg L. Articular cartilage: composition and structure. In: Woo SLY, Buckwalter JA, editors. *Injury and Repair of the Musculoskeletal Soft Tissues*. Park Ridge, IL: American Academy of Orthopaedic Surgeons (1988). p. 405–25.
140. Cooke TD, Hurd ER, Jasin HE, Bienenstock J, Ziff M. Identification of immunoglobulins and complement in rheumatoid articular collagenous tissues. *Arthritis Rheum* (1975) 18:541–51. doi:10.1002/art.1780180603
141. Bradley K, North J, Saunders D, Schwaeble W, Jeziorska M, Woolley DE, et al. Synthesis of classical pathway complement components by chondrocytes. *Immunology* (1996) 88:648–56.
142. Gulati P, Lemercier C, Guc D, Lappin D, Whaley K. Regulation of the synthesis of C1 subcomponents and C1-inhibitor. *Behring Inst Mitt* (1993) 93:196–203.
143. Nakagawa K, Sakiyama H, Tsuchida T, Yamaguchi K, Toyoguchi T, Masuda R, et al. Complement C1s activation in degenerating articular cartilage of rheumatoid arthritis patients: immunohistochemical studies with an active form specific antibody. *Ann Rheum Dis* (1999) 58:175–81. doi:10.1136/ard.58.3.175
144. Ochi T, Iwase R, Yonemasu K, Matsukawa M, Yoneda M, Yukioka M, et al. Natural course of joint destruction and fluctuation of serum C1q levels in patients with rheumatoid arthritis. *Arthritis Rheum* (1988) 31:37–43. doi:10.1002/art.1780310106
145. Ochi T, Yonemasu K, Iwase R, Sasaki T, Tsuyama K, Ono K. Serum C1q levels as a prognostic guide to articular erosions in patients with rheumatoid arthritis. *Arthritis Rheum* (1984) 27:883–7. doi:10.1002/art.1780270807
146. Olsen NJ, Ho E, Barats L. Clinical correlations with serum C1q levels in patients with rheumatoid arthritis. *Arthritis Rheum* (1991) 34:187–91. doi:10.1002/art.1780340209
147. Ruddy S, Colten HR. Rheumatoid arthritis. Biosynthesis of complement proteins by synovial tissues. *N Engl J Med* (1974) 290:1284–8. doi:10.1056/NEJM197406062902304
148. Morgan BP, Daniels RH, Williams BD. Measurement of terminal complement complexes in rheumatoid arthritis. *Clin Exp Immunol* (1988) 73:473–8.
149. Perrin LH, Nydegger UE, Zubler RH, Lambert PH, Miescher PA. Correlation between levels of breakdown products of C3, C4, and properdin factor B in synovial fluids from patients with rheumatoid arthritis. *Arthritis Rheum* (1977) 20:647–52. doi:10.1002/art.1780200202
150. Holers VM. Complement and its receptors: new insights into human disease. *Annu Rev Immunol* (2014) 32:433–59. doi:10.1146/annurev-immunol-032713-120154
151. Bedwell AE, Elson CJ, Carter SD, Dieppe PA, Hutton CW, Czudek R. Isolation and analysis of complement activating aggregates from synovial fluid of patients with rheumatoid arthritis using monoclonal anti-C3d antibodies. *Ann Rheum Dis* (1987) 46:55–64. doi:10.1136/ard.46.1.55
152. Brodeur JP, Ruddy S, Schwartz LB, Moxley G. Synovial fluid levels of complement SC5b-9 and fragment Bb are elevated in patients with rheumatoid arthritis. *Arthritis Rheum* (1991) 34:1531–7. doi:10.1002/art.1780341209
153. Mijuskovic Z, Rackov L, Pejovic J, Zivanovic S, Stojanovic J, Kovacevic Z. Immune complexes and complement in serum and synovial fluid of rheumatoid arthritis patients. *J Med Biochem* (2009) 28:166–71. doi:10.2478/v10011-009-0016-9
154. Konttinen YT, Ceponis A, Meri S, Vuorikoski A, Kortekangas P, Sorsa T, et al. Complement in acute and chronic arthritides: assessment of C3c, C9, and protectin (CD59) in synovial membrane. *Ann Rheum Dis* (1996) 55:888–94. doi:10.1136/ard.55.12.888
155. Tarkowski A, Trollmo C, Seifert PS, Hansson GK. Expression of decay-accelerating factor on synovial lining cells in inflammatory and degenerative arthritides. *Rheumatol Int* (1992) 12:201–5. doi:10.1007/BF00302153
156. Banda NK, Mehta G, Ferreira VP, Cortes C, Pickering MC, Pangburn MK, et al. Essential role of surface-bound complement factor H in controlling immune complex-induced arthritis. *J Immunol* (2013) 190:3560–9. doi:10.4049/jimmunol.1203271
157. Koro C, Bielecka E, Dahl-Knudsen A, Enghild JJ, Scavenius C, Brun JG, et al. Carbamylation of immunoglobulin abrogates activation of the classical complement pathway. *Eur J Immunol* (2014) 44:3403–12. doi:10.1002/eji.201444869
158. Brady LJ, Velayudhan J, Visone DB, Daugherty KC, Bartron JL, Coon M, et al. The criticality of high-resolution N-linked carbohydrate assays and detailed characterization of antibody effector function in the context of biosimilar development. *MAbs* (2015) 7:562–70. doi:10.1080/19420862.2015.1016692
159. Malhotra R, Wormald MR, Rudd PM, Fischer PB, Dwek RA, Sim RB. Glycosylation changes of IgG associated with rheumatoid arthritis can activate complement via the mannose-binding protein. *Nat Med* (1995) 1:237–43. doi:10.1038/nm0395-237
160. Nose M, Wigzell H. Biological significance of carbohydrate chains on monoclonal antibodies. *Proc Natl Acad Sci U S A* (1983) 80:6632–6. doi:10.1073/pnas.80.21.6632
161. Thomann M, Schlothauer T, Dashivets T, Malik S, Avenal C, Bulau P, et al. In vitro glycoengineering of IgG1 and its effect on Fc receptor binding and ADCC activity. *PLoS One* (2015) 10:e0134949. doi:10.1371/journal.pone.0134949
162. Vestrheim AC, Moen A, Egge-Jacobsen W, Bratlie DB, Michaelsen TE. Different glycosylation pattern of human IgG1 and IgG3 antibodies isolated from transiently as well as permanently transfected cell lines. *Scand J Immunol* (2013) 77:419–28. doi:10.1111/sji.12046
163. Anthony RM, Nimmerjahn F. The role of differential IgG glycosylation in the interaction of antibodies with FcgammaRs in vivo. *Curr Opin Organ Transplant* (2011) 16:7–14. doi:10.1097/MOT.0b013e328342538f
164. Banda NK, Wood AK, Takahashi K, Levitt B, Rudd PM, Royle L, et al. Initiation of the alternative pathway of murine complement by immune

complexes is dependent on N-glycans in IgG antibodies. *Arthritis Rheum* (2008) 58:3081–9. doi:10.1002/art.23865
165. Kaneko Y, Nimmerjahn F, Ravetch JV. Anti-inflammatory activity of immunoglobulin G resulting from Fc sialylation. *Science* (2006) 313:670–3. doi:10.1126/science.1129594
166. Karsten CM, Pandey MK, Figge J, Kilchenstein R, Taylor PR, Rosas M, et al. Anti-inflammatory activity of IgG1 mediated by Fc galactosylation and association of FcgammaRIIB and dectin-1. *Nat Med* (2012) 18:1401–6. doi:10.1038/nm.2862
167. Parekh RB, Dwek RA, Sutton BJ, Fernandes DL, Leung A, Stanworth D, et al. Association of rheumatoid arthritis and primary osteoarthritis with changes in the glycosylation pattern of total serum IgG. *Nature* (1985) 316:452–7. doi:10.1038/316452a0
168. Ercan A, Cui J, Chatterton DE, Deane KD, Hazen MM, Brintnell W, et al. Aberrant IgG galactosylation precedes disease onset, correlates with disease activity, and is prevalent in autoantibodies in rheumatoid arthritis. *Arthritis Rheum* (2010) 62:2239–48. doi:10.1002/art.27533
169. Rombouts Y, Ewing E, van de Stadt LA, Selman MH, Trouw LA, Deelder AM, et al. Anti-citrullinated protein antibodies acquire a pro-inflammatory Fc glycosylation phenotype prior to the onset of rheumatoid arthritis. *Ann Rheum Dis* (2015) 74:234–41. doi:10.1136/annrheumdis-2013-203565
170. Alavi A, Arden N, Spector TD, Axford JS. Immunoglobulin G glycosylation and clinical outcome in rheumatoid arthritis during pregnancy. *J Rheumatol* (2000) 27:1379–85.
171. Rook GA, Steele J, Brealey R, Whyte A, Isenberg D, Sumar N, et al. Changes in IgG glycoform levels are associated with remission of arthritis during pregnancy. *J Autoimmun* (1991) 4:779–94. doi:10.1016/0896-8411(91)90173-A
172. van de Geijn FE, Wuhrer M, Selman MH, Willemsen SP, de Man YA, Deelder AM, et al. Immunoglobulin G galactosylation and sialylation are associated with pregnancy-induced improvement of rheumatoid arthritis and the postpartum flare: results from a large prospective cohort study. *Arthritis Res Ther* (2009) 11:R193. doi:10.1186/ar2892
173. Rademacher TW, Williams P, Dwek RA. Agalactosyl glycoforms of IgG autoantibodies are pathogenic. *Proc Natl Acad Sci U S A* (1994) 91:6123–7. doi:10.1073/pnas.91.13.6123
174. van de Bovenkamp FS, Hafkenscheid L, Rispens T, Rombouts Y. The emerging importance of IgG Fab glycosylation in immunity. *J Immunol* (2016) 196:1435–41. doi:10.4049/jimmunol.1502136
175. Kempers AC, Hafkenscheid L, Scherer HU, Toes REM. Variable domain glycosylation of ACPA-IgG: a missing link in the maturation of the ACPA response? *Clin Immunol* (2018) 186:34–7. doi:10.1016/j.clim.2017.09.001
176. Hafkenscheid L, Bondt A, Scherer HU, Huizinga TW, Wuhrer M, Toes RE, et al. Structural analysis of variable domain glycosylation of anti-citrullinated protein antibodies in rheumatoid arthritis reveals the presence of highly sialylated glycans. *Mol Cell Proteomics* (2017) 16:278–87. doi:10.1074/mcp.M116.062919
177. Lundstrom SL, Fernandes-Cerqueira C, Ytterberg AJ, Ossipova E, Hensvold AH, Jakobsson PJ, et al. IgG antibodies to cyclic citrullinated peptides exhibit profiles specific in terms of IgG subclasses, Fc-glycans and a fab-peptide sequence. *PLoS One* (2014) 9:e113924. doi:10.1371/journal.pone.0113924
178. Scherer HU, van der Woude D, Ioan-Facsinay A, el-Bannoudi H, Trouw LA, Wang J, et al. Glycan profiling of anti-citrullinated protein antibodies isolated from human serum and synovial fluid. *Arthritis Rheum* (2010) 62:1620–9. doi:10.1002/art.27414
179. Trouw LA, Haisma EM, Levarht EW, van der Woude D, Ioan-Facsinay A, Daha MR, et al. Anti-cyclic citrullinated peptide antibodies from rheumatoid arthritis patients activate complement via both the classical and alternative pathways. *Arthritis Rheum* (2009) 60:1923–31. doi:10.1002/art.24622
180. van Venrooij WJ, van Beers JJ, Pruijn GJ. Anti-CCP antibodies: the past, the present and the future. *Nat Rev Rheumatol* (2011) 7:391–8. doi:10.1038/nrrheum.2011.76
181. Witalison EE, Thompson PR, Hofseth LJ. Protein arginine deiminases and associated citrullination: physiological functions and diseases associated with dysregulation. *Curr Drug Targets* (2015) 16:700–10. doi:10.2174/1389450116666150202160954
182. Knuckley B, Causey CP, Jones JE, Bhatia M, Dreyton CJ, Osborne TC, et al. Substrate specificity and kinetic studies of PADs 1, 3, and 4 identify potent and selective inhibitors of protein arginine deiminase 3. *Biochemistry* (2010) 49:4852–63. doi:10.1021/bi100363t
183. Willis VC, Banda NK, Cordova KN, Chandra PE, Robinson WH, Cooper DC, et al. Protein arginine deiminase 4 inhibition is sufficient for the amelioration of collagen-induced arthritis. *Clin Exp Immunol* (2017) 188:263–74. doi:10.1111/cei.12932
184. Vossenaar ER, Smeets TJ, Kraan MC, Raats JM, van Venrooij WJ, Tak PP. The presence of citrullinated proteins is not specific for rheumatoid synovial tissue. *Arthritis Rheum* (2004) 50:3485–94. doi:10.1002/art.20584
185. Kastbom A, Strandberg G, Lindroos A, Skogh T. Anti-CCP antibody test predicts the disease course during 3 years in early rheumatoid arthritis (the Swedish TIRA project). *Ann Rheum Dis* (2004) 63:1085–9. doi:10.1136/ard.2003.016808
186. Schellekens GA, de Jong BA, van den Hoogen FH, van de Putte LB, van Venrooij WJ. Citrulline is an essential constituent of antigenic determinants recognized by rheumatoid arthritis-specific autoantibodies. *J Clin Invest* (1998) 101:273–81. doi:10.1172/JCI1316
187. Lee DM, Schur PH. Clinical utility of the anti-CCP assay in patients with rheumatic diseases. *Ann Rheum Dis* (2003) 62:870–4. doi:10.1136/ard.62.9.870
188. Pinheiro GC, Scheinberg MA, Aparecida da Silva M, Maciel S. Anti-cyclic citrullinated peptide antibodies in advanced rheumatoid arthritis. *Ann Intern Med* (2003) 139:234–5. doi:10.7326/0003-4819-139-3-200308050-00021
189. Rantapaa-Dahlqvist S, de Jong BA, Berglin E, Hallmans G, Wadell G, Stenlund H, et al. Antibodies against cyclic citrullinated peptide and IgA rheumatoid factor predict the development of rheumatoid arthritis. *Arthritis Rheum* (2003) 48:2741–9. doi:10.1002/art.11223
190. Suzuki K, Sawada T, Murakami A, Matsui T, Tohma S, Nakazono K, et al. High diagnostic performance of ELISA detection of antibodies to citrullinated antigens in rheumatoid arthritis. *Scand J Rheumatol* (2003) 32:197–204. doi:10.1080/03009740310003677
191. van Venrooij WJ, Hazes JM, Visser H. Anticitrullinated protein/peptide antibody and its role in the diagnosis and prognosis of early rheumatoid arthritis. *Neth J Med* (2002) 60:383–8.
192. Vasishta A. Diagnosing early-onset rheumatoid arthritis: the role of anti-CCP antibodies. *Am Clin Lab* (2002) 21:34–6.
193. Sokolove J, Zhao X, Chandra PE, Robinson WH. Immune complexes containing citrullinated fibrinogen costimulate macrophages via toll-like receptor 4 and Fcgamma receptor. *Arthritis Rheum* (2011) 63:53–62. doi:10.1002/art.30081
194. Anquetil F, Clavel C, Offer G, Serre G, Sebbag M. IgM and IgA rheumatoid factors purified from rheumatoid arthritis sera boost the Fc receptor- and complement-dependent effector functions of the disease-specific anti-citrullinated protein autoantibodies. *J Immunol* (2015) 194:3664–74. doi:10.4049/jimmunol.1402334
195. Ohmura K, Terao C, Maruya E, Katayama M, Matoba K, Shimada K, et al. Anti-citrullinated peptide antibody-negative RA is a genetically distinct subset: a definitive study using only bone-erosive ACPA-negative rheumatoid arthritis. *Rheumatology* (2010) 49:2298–304. doi:10.1093/rheumatology/keq273
196. Shi J, Knevel R, Suwannalai P, van der Linden MP, Janssen GM, van Veelen PA, et al. Autoantibodies recognizing carbamylated proteins are present in sera of patients with rheumatoid arthritis and predict joint damage. *Proc Natl Acad Sci U S A* (2011) 108:17372–7. doi:10.1073/pnas.1114465108
197. Stoop JN, Liu BS, Shi J, Jansen DT, Hegen M, Huizinga TW, et al. Antibodies specific for carbamylated proteins precede the onset of clinical symptoms in mice with collagen induced arthritis. *PLoS One* (2014) 9:e102163. doi:10.1371/journal.pone.0102163
198. Dekkers JS, Verheul MK, Stoop JN, Liu B, Ioan-Facsinay A, van Veelen PA, et al. Breach of autoreactive B cell tolerance by post-translationally modified proteins. *Ann Rheum Dis* (2017) 76:1449–57. doi:10.1136/annrheumdis-2016-210772
199. Nakabo S, Hashimoto M, Ito S, Furu M, Ito H, Fujii T, et al. Carbamylated albumin is one of the target antigens of anti-carbamylated protein antibodies. *Rheumatology* (2017) 56:1217–26. doi:10.1093/rheumatology/kex088
200. Verheul MK, Vierboom MPM, t Hart BA, Toes REM, Trouw LA. Anti-carbamylated protein antibodies precede disease onset in monkeys with collagen-induced arthritis. *Arthritis Res Ther* (2017) 19:246. doi:10.1186/s13075-017-1455-1
201. Verheul MK, Yee A, Seaman A, Janssen GM, van Veelen PA, Drijfhout JW, et al. Identification of carbamylated alpha 1 anti-trypsin (A1AT) as an

antigenic target of anti-CarP antibodies in patients with rheumatoid arthritis. *J Autoimmun* (2017) 80:77–84. doi:10.1016/j.jaut.2017.02.008
202. Wooley PH, Seibold JR, Whalen JD, Chapdelaine JM. Pristane-induced arthritis. The immunologic and genetic features of an experimental murine model of autoimmune disease. *Arthritis Rheum* (1989) 32:1022–30. doi:10.1002/anr.1780320812
203. Keystone EC, Schorlemmer HU, Pope C, Allison AC. Zymosan-induced arthritis: a model of chronic proliferative arthritis following activation of the alternative pathway of complement. *Arthritis Rheum* (1977) 20:1396–401. doi:10.1002/art.1780200714
204. Finnegan A, Mikecz K, Tao P, Glant TT. Proteoglycan (aggrecan)-induced arthritis in BALB/c mice is a Th1-type disease regulated by Th2 cytokines. *J Immunol* (1999) 163:5383–90.
205. Koga T, Kakimoto K, Hirofuji T, Kotani S, Ohkuni H, Watanabe K, et al. Acute joint inflammation in mice after systemic injection of the cell wall, its peptidoglycan, and chemically defined peptidoglycan subunits from various bacteria. *Infect Immun* (1985) 50:27–34.
206. Sakaguchi S, Takahashi T, Hata H, Nomura T, Sakaguchi N. SKG mice, a new genetic model of rheumatoid arthritis. *Arthritis Res Ther* (2003) 5(Suppl 3):10. doi:10.1186/ar811
207. Brackertz D, Mitchell GF, Mackay IR. Antigen-induced arthritis in mice. I. Induction of arthritis in various strains of mice. *Arthritis Rheum* (1977) 20:841–50. doi:10.1002/art.1780200314
208. Courtenay JS, Dallman MJ, Dayan AD, Martin A, Mosedale B. Immunisation against heterologous type II collagen induces arthritis in mice. *Nature* (1980) 283:666–8. doi:10.1038/283666a0
209. Terato K, Harper DS, Griffiths MM, Hasty DL, Ye XJ, Cremer MA, et al. Collagen-induced arthritis in mice: synergistic effect of *E. coli* lipopolysaccharide bypasses epitope specificity in the induction of arthritis with monoclonal antibodies to type II collagen. *Autoimmunity* (1995) 22:137–47. doi:10.3109/08916939508995311
210. Kouskoff V, Korganow AS, Duchatelle V, Degott C, Benoist C, Mathis D. Organ-specific disease provoked by systemic autoimmunity. *Cell* (1996) 87:811–22. doi:10.1016/S0092-8674(00)81989-3
211. Kouskoff V, Korganow AS, Duchatelle V, Degott C, Benoist C, Mathis D. A new mouse model of rheumatoid arthritis: organ-specific disease provoked by systemic autoimmunity. *Ryumachi* (1997) 37:147.
212. Butler DM, Malfait AM, Mason LJ, Warden PJ, Kollias G, Maini RN, et al. DBA/1 mice expressing the human TNF-alpha transgene develop a severe, erosive arthritis: characterization of the cytokine cascade and cellular composition. *J Immunol* (1997) 159:2867–76.
213. Horai R, Saijo S, Tanioka H, Nakae S, Sudo K, Okahara A, et al. Development of chronic inflammatory arthropathy resembling rheumatoid arthritis in interleukin 1 receptor antagonist-deficient mice. *J Exp Med* (2000) 191:313–20. doi:10.1084/jem.191.2.313
214. Trentham DE, Townes AS, Kang AH. Autoimmunity to type II collagen an experimental model of arthritis. *J Exp Med* (1977) 146:857–68. doi:10.1084/jem.146.3.857
215. Cathcart ES, Hayes KC, Gonnerman WA, Lazzari AA, Franzblau C. Experimental arthritis in a nonhuman primate. I. Induction by bovine type II collagen. *Lab Invest* (1986) 54:26–31.
216. Yoo TJ, Kim SY, Stuart JM, Floyd RA, Olson GA, Cremer MA, et al. Induction of arthritis in monkeys by immunization with type II collagen. *J Exp Med* (1988) 168:777–82. doi:10.1084/jem.168.2.777
217. Andriopoulos NA, Mestecky J, Miller EJ, Bennett JC. Antibodies to human native and denatured collagens in synovial fluids of patients with rheumatoid arthritis. *Clin Immunol Immunopathol* (1976) 6:209–12. doi:10.1016/0090-1229(76)90112-4
218. Tanaka S, Toki T, Akimoto T, Morishita K. Lipopolysaccharide accelerates collagen-induced arthritis in association with rapid and continuous production of inflammatory mediators and anti-type II collagen antibody. *Microbiol Immunol* (2013) 57:445–54. doi:10.1111/1348-0421.12052
219. Banda NK, Kraus D, Vondracek A, Huynh LH, Bendele A, Holers VM, et al. Mechanisms of effects of complement inhibition in murine collagen-induced arthritis. *Arthritis Rheum* (2002) 46:3065–75. doi:10.1002/art.10591
220. Ioan-Facsinay A, el-Bannoudi H, Scherer HU, van der Woude D, Menard HA, Lora M, et al. Anti-cyclic citrullinated peptide antibodies are a collection of anti-citrullinated protein antibodies and contain overlapping and non-overlapping reactivities. *Ann Rheum Dis* (2011) 70:188–93. doi:10.1136/ard.2010.131102
221. Mullazehi M, Wick MC, Klareskog L, van Vollenhoven R, Ronnelid J. Anti-type II collagen antibodies are associated with early radiographic destruction in rheumatoid arthritis. *Arthritis Res Ther* (2012) 14:R100. doi:10.1186/ar3825
222. Andersson EC, Hansen BE, Jacobsen H, Madsen LS, Andersen CB, Engberg J, et al. Definition of MHC and T cell receptor contacts in the HLA-DR4 restricted immunodominant epitope in type II collagen and characterization of collagen-induced arthritis in HLA-DR4 and human CD4 transgenic mice. *Proc Natl Acad Sci U S A* (1998) 95:7574–9. doi:10.1073/pnas.95.13.7574
223. Brunsberg U, Gustafsson K, Jansson L, Michaelsson E, Ahrlund-Richter L, Pettersson S, et al. Expression of a transgenic class II Ab gene confers susceptibility to collagen-induced arthritis. *Eur J Immunol* (1994) 24:1698–702. doi:10.1002/eji.1830240736
224. Hietala MA, Jonsson MI, Tarkowski A, Kleinau S, Pekna M. Complement deficiency ameliorates collagen-induced arthritis in mice. *J Immunol* (2002) 169:454–9. doi:10.4049/jimmunol.169.1.454
225. Watson WC, Townes AS. Genetic susceptibility to murine collagen II autoimmune arthritis. Proposed relationship to the IgG2 autoantibody subclass response, complement C5, major histocompatibility complex (MHC) and non-MHC loci. *J Exp Med* (1985) 162:1878–91. doi:10.1084/jem.162.6.1878
226. Luross JA, Williams NA. The genetic and immunopathological processes underlying collagen-induced arthritis. *Immunology* (2001) 103:407–16. doi:10.1046/j.1365-2567.2001.01267.x
227. Holmdahl R, Jansson L, Gullberg D, Rubin K, Forsberg PO, Klareskog L. Incidence of arthritis and autoreactivity of anti-collagen antibodies after immunization of DBA/1 mice with heterologous and autologous collagen II. *Clin Exp Immunol* (1985) 62:639–46.
228. Wooley PH, Luthra HS, Lafuse WP, Huse A, Stuart JM, David CS. Type II collagen-induced arthritis in mice. III. Suppression of arthritis by using monoclonal and polyclonal anti-Ia antisera. *J Immunol* (1985) 134:2366–74.
229. Seki N, Sudo Y, Yoshioka T, Sugihara S, Fujitsu T, Sakuma S, et al. Type II collagen-induced murine arthritis. I. Induction and perpetuation of arthritis require synergy between humoral and cell-mediated immunity. *J Immunol* (1988) 140:1477–84.
230. Morgan K, Clague RB, Shaw MJ, Firth SA, Twose TM, Holt PJ. Native type II collagen – induced arthritis in the rat: the effect of complement depletion by cobra venom factor. *Arthritis Rheum* (1981) 24:1356–62. doi:10.1002/art.1780241104
231. Stuart JM, Dixon FJ. Serum transfer of collagen-induced arthritis in mice. *J Exp Med* (1983) 158:378–92. doi:10.1084/jem.158.2.378
232. Kerwar SS, Englert ME, McReynolds RA, Landes MJ, Lloyd JM, Oronsky AL, et al. Type II collagen-induced arthritis. Studies with purified anticollagen immunoglobulin. *Arthritis Rheum* (1983) 26:1120–31. doi:10.1002/art.1780260910
233. Goodfellow RM, Williams AS, Levin JL, Williams BD, Morgan BP. Soluble complement receptor one (sCR1) inhibits the development and progression of rat collagen-induced arthritis. *Clin Exp Immunol* (2000) 119:210–6. doi:10.1046/j.1365-2249.2000.01129.x
234. Dreja H, Annenkov A, Chernajovsky Y. Soluble complement receptor 1 (CD35) delivered by retrovirally infected syngeneic cells or by naked DNA injection prevents the progression of collagen-induced arthritis. *Arthritis Rheum* (2000) 43:1698–709. doi:10.1002/1529-0131(200008)43:8<1698::AID-ANR5>3.0.CO;2-8
235. Holers M, Banda N, Mehta G, Fridkis-Hareli M, Or E, Storek M, et al. The human complement receptor type 2 (CR2)/CR1 fusion protein TT32, a targeted inhibitor of the classical and alternative pathway C3 convertases, prevents arthritis in active immunization and passive transfer models and acts by CR2-dependent targeting of CR1 regulatory activity. *Immunobiology* (2012) 217:1210. doi:10.1016/j.imbio.2012.08.232
236. Weisman HF, Bartow T, Leppo MK, Marsh HC Jr, Carson GR, Concino MF, et al. Soluble human complement receptor type 1: in vivo inhibitor of complement suppressing post-ischemic myocardial inflammation and necrosis. *Science* (1990) 249:146–51. doi:10.1126/science.2371562
237. Makrides SC, Scesney SM, Ford PJ, Evans KS, Carson GR, Marsh HC Jr. Cell surface expression of the C3b/C4b receptor (CR1) protects Chinese hamster ovary cells from lysis by human complement. *J Biol Chem* (1992) 267:24754–61.

238. Kang HJ, Bao L, Xu Y, Quigg RJ, Giclas PC, Holers VM. Increased serum C3 levels in Crry transgenic mice partially abrogates its complement inhibitory effects. *Clin Exp Immunol* (2004) 136:194–9. doi:10.1111/j.1365-2249.2004.02450.x
239. Banda NK, Kraus DM, Muggli M, Bendele A, Holers VM, Arend WP. Prevention of collagen-induced arthritis in mice transgenic for the complement inhibitor complement receptor 1-related gene/protein y. *J Immunol* (2003) 171:2109–15. doi:10.4049/jimmunol.171.4.2109
240. Mizuno M, Nishikawa K, Spiller OB, Morgan BP, Okada N, Okada H, et al. Membrane complement regulators protect against the development of type II collagen-induced arthritis in rats. *Arthritis Rheum* (2001) 44:2425–34. doi:10.1002/1529-0131(200110)44:10<2425::AID-ART407>3.0.CO;2-4
241. Wang Y, Rollins SA, Madri JA, Matis LA. Anti-C5 monoclonal antibody therapy prevents collagen-induced arthritis and ameliorates established disease. *Proc Natl Acad Sci U S A* (1995) 92:8955–9. doi:10.1073/pnas.92.19.8955
242. Wang Y, Kristan J, Hao L, Lenkoski CS, Shen Y, Matis LA. A role for complement in antibody-mediated inflammation: C5-deficient DBA/1 mice are resistant to collagen-induced arthritis. *J Immunol* (2000) 164:4340–7. doi:10.4049/jimmunol.164.8.4340
243. Andersson M, Goldschmidt TJ, Michaelsson E, Larsson A, Holmdahl R. T-cell receptor V beta haplotype and complement component C5 play no significant role for the resistance to collagen-induced arthritis in the SWR mouse. *Immunology* (1991) 73:191–6.
244. Banerjee S, Anderson GD, Luthra HS, David CS. Influence of complement C5 and V beta T cell receptor mutations on susceptibility to collagen-induced arthritis in mice. *J Immunol* (1989) 142:2237–43.
245. Spinella DG, Jeffers JR, Reife RA, Stuart JM. The role of C5 and T-cell receptor Vb genes in susceptibility to collagen-induced arthritis. *Immunogenetics* (1991) 34:23–7. doi:10.1007/BF00212308
246. Woodruff TM, Nandakumar KS, Tedesco F. Inhibiting the C5-C5a receptor axis. *Mol Immunol* (2011) 48:1631–42. doi:10.1016/j.molimm.2011.04.014
247. Andersson C, Wenander CS, Usher PA, Hebsgaard JB, Sondergaard BC, Rono B, et al. Rapid-onset clinical and mechanistic effects of anti-C5aR treatment in the mouse collagen-induced arthritis model. *Clin Exp Immunol* (2014) 177:219–33. doi:10.1111/cei.12338
248. Nandakumar KS, Jansson A, Xu B, Rydell N, Ahooghalandari P, Hellman L, et al. A recombinant vaccine effectively induces c5a-specific neutralizing antibodies and prevents arthritis. *PLoS One* (2010) 5:e13511. doi:10.1371/journal.pone.0013511
249. Williams AS, Mizuno M, Richards PJ, Holt DS, Morgan BP. Deletion of the gene encoding CD59a in mice increases disease severity in a murine model of rheumatoid arthritis. *Arthritis Rheum* (2004) 50:3035–44. doi:10.1002/art.20478
250. Terato K, Hasty KA, Reife RA, Cremer MA, Kang AH, Stuart JM. Induction of arthritis with monoclonal antibodies to collagen. *J Immunol* (1992) 148:2103–8.
251. Nandakumar KS, Holmdahl R. Efficient promotion of collagen antibody induced arthritis (CAIA) using four monoclonal antibodies specific for the major epitopes recognized in both collagen induced arthritis and rheumatoid arthritis. *J Immunol Methods* (2005) 304:126–36. doi:10.1016/j.jim.2005.06.017
252. Nandakumar KS, Holmdahl R. Collagen antibody induced arthritis. *Methods Mol Med* (2007) 136:215–23. doi:10.1007/978-1-59745-402-5_16
253. Ge C, Tong D, Liang B, Lonnblom E, Schneider N, Hagert C, et al. Anti-citrullinated protein antibodies cause arthritis by cross-reactivity to joint cartilage. *JCI Insight* (2017) 2:1–19. doi:10.1172/jci.insight.93688
254. Vossenaar ER, Nijenhuis S, Helsen MM, van der Heijden A, Senshu T, van den Berg WB, et al. Citrullination of synovial proteins in murine models of rheumatoid arthritis. *Arthritis Rheum* (2003) 48:2489–500. doi:10.1002/art.11229
255. Klareskog L, Amara K, Malmstrom V. Adaptive immunity in rheumatoid arthritis: anticitrulline and other antibodies in the pathogenesis of rheumatoid arthritis. *Curr Opin Rheumatol* (2014) 26:72–9. doi:10.1097/BOR.0000000000000016
256. Burkhardt H, Sehnert B, Bockermann R, Engstrom A, Kalden JR, Holmdahl R. Humoral immune response to citrullinated collagen type II determinants in early rheumatoid arthritis. *Eur J Immunol* (2005) 35:1643–52. doi:10.1002/eji.200526000
257. Uysal H, Bockermann R, Nandakumar KS, Sehnert B, Bajtner E, Engstrom A, et al. Structure and pathogenicity of antibodies specific for citrullinated collagen type II in experimental arthritis. *J Exp Med* (2009) 206:449–62. doi:10.1084/jem.20081862
258. Kuhn KA, Kulik L, Tomooka B, Braschler KJ, Arend WP, Robinson WH, et al. Antibodies against citrullinated proteins enhance tissue injury in experimental autoimmune arthritis. *J Clin Invest* (2006) 116:961–73. doi:10.1172/JCI25422
259. Turunen S, Koivula MK, Risteli L, Risteli J. Anticitrulline antibodies can be caused by homocitrulline-containing proteins in rabbits. *Arthritis Rheum* (2010) 62:3345–52. doi:10.1002/art.27644
260. Aggarwal A, Bhardwaj A, Alam S, Misra R. Evidence for activation of the alternate complement pathway in patients with juvenile rheumatoid arthritis. *Rheumatology* (2000) 39:189–92. doi:10.1093/rheumatology/39.2.189
261. Jarvis JN, Iobidze M, Taylor H, DeJonge J, Chang S. A comparison of immunoglobulin G-containing high-molecular-weight complexes isolated from children with juvenile rheumatoid arthritis and congenital human immunodeficiency virus infection. *Pediatr Res* (1993) 34:781–4. doi:10.1203/00006450-199312000-00017
262. Schaapherder AF, Gooszen HG, te Bulte MT, Daha MR. Human complement activation via the alternative pathway on porcine endothelium initiated by IgA antibodies. *Transplantation* (1995) 60:287–91. doi:10.1097/00007890-199508000-00014
263. Banda NK, Thurman JM, Kraus D, Wood A, Carroll MC, Arend WP, et al. Alternative complement pathway activation is essential for inflammation and joint destruction in the passive transfer model of collagen-induced arthritis. *J Immunol* (2006) 177:1904–12. doi:10.4049/jimmunol.177.3.1904
264. Banda NK, Levitt B, Wood AK, Takahashi K, Stahl GL, Holers VM, et al. Complement activation pathways in murine immune complex-induced arthritis and in C3a and C5a generation in vitro. *Clin Exp Immunol* (2010) 159:100–8. doi:10.1111/j.1365-2249.2009.04035.x
265. Takahashi M, Ishida Y, Iwaki D, Kanno K, Suzuki T, Endo Y, et al. Essential role of mannose-binding lectin-associated serine protease-1 in activation of the complement factor D. *J Exp Med* (2010) 207:29–37. doi:10.1084/jem.20090633
266. Takahashi M, Iwaki D, Kanno K, Ishida Y, Xiong J, Matsushita M, et al. Mannose-binding lectin (MBL)-associated serine protease (MASP)-1 contributes to activation of the lectin complement pathway. *J Immunol* (2008) 180:6132–8. doi:10.4049/jimmunol.180.9.6132
267. Takahashi M, Sekine H, Endo Y, Fujita T. Comment on "Mannan-binding lectin-associated serine protease (MASP)-1 is crucial for lectin pathway activation in human serum, whereas neither MASP-1 nor MASP-3 is required for alternative pathway function". *J Immunol* (2013) 190:2477. doi:10.4049/jimmunol.1390003
268. Banda NK, Takahashi M, Levitt B, Glogowska M, Nicholas J, Takahashi K, et al. Essential role of complement mannose-binding lectin-associated serine proteases-1/3 in the murine collagen antibody-induced model of inflammatory arthritis. *J Immunol* (2010) 185:5598–606. doi:10.4049/jimmunol.1001564
269. Arend WP, Mehta G, Antonioli AH, Takahashi M, Takahashi K, Stahl GL, et al. Roles of adipocytes and fibroblasts in activation of the alternative pathway of complement in inflammatory arthritis in mice. *J Immunol* (2013) 190:6423–33. doi:10.4049/jimmunol.1300580
270. Banda NK, Acharya S, Scheinman RI, Mehta G, Coulombe M, Takahashi M, et al. Mannan-binding lectin-associated serine protease 1/3 cleavage of pro-factor D into factor D in vivo and attenuation of collagen antibody-induced arthritis through their targeted inhibition by RNA interference-mediated gene silencing. *J Immunol* (2016) 197:3680–94. doi:10.4049/jimmunol.1600719
271. Banda NK, Desai D, Casterano A, Scheinman RI, Acharya S, Sekine H, et al. siRNA-mediated targeting of hepatocyte mannan-binding lectin-associated serine protease-3 for the treatment of murine collagen-antibody-inducsed arthritis (CAIA), a model for human rheumatoid arthritis. *Mol Immunol* (2017) 89:161. doi:10.1016/j.molimm.2017.06.129
272. Dobo J, Harmat V, Beinrohr L, Sebestyen E, Zavodszky P, Gal P. MASP-1, a promiscuous complement protease: structure of its catalytic region reveals the basis of its broad specificity. *J Immunol* (2009) 183:1207–14. doi:10.4049/jimmunol.0901141

273. Ruseva MM, Takahashi M, Fujita T, Pickering MC. C3 dysregulation due to factor H deficiency is mannan-binding lectin-associated serine proteases (MASP)-1 and MASP-3 independent in vivo. *Clin Exp Immunol* (2014) 176:84–92. doi:10.1111/cei.12244
274. Banda NK, Hyatt S, Antonioli AH, White JT, Glogowska M, Takahashi K, et al. Role of C3a receptors, C5a receptors, and complement protein C6 deficiency in collagen antibody-induced arthritis in mice. *J Immunol* (2012) 188:1469–78. doi:10.4049/jimmunol.1102310
275. Vergunst CE, Gerlag DM, Dinant H, Schulz L, Vinkenoog M, Smeets TJ, et al. Blocking the receptor for C5a in patients with rheumatoid arthritis does not reduce synovial inflammation. *Rheumatology* (2007) 46:1773–8. doi:10.1093/rheumatology/kem222
276. Hornum L, Hansen AJ, Tornehave D, Fjording MS, Colmenero P, Watjen IF, et al. C5a and C5aR are elevated in joints of rheumatoid and psoriatic arthritis patients, and C5aR blockade attenuates leukocyte migration to synovial fluid. *PLoS One* (2017) 12:e0189017. doi:10.1371/journal.pone.0189017
277. Borodovsky A, Yucius K, Sprague A, Banda NK, Holers VM, Vaishnaw A, et al. Aln-CC5, an investigational RNAi therapeutic targeting C5 for complement inhibition. *Blood* (2014) 124:1606.
278. Mehta G, Ferreira VP, Skerka C, Zipfel PF, Banda NK. New insights into disease-specific absence of complement factor H related protein C in mouse models of spontaneous autoimmune diseases. *Mol Immunol* (2014) 62:235–48. doi:10.1016/j.molimm.2014.06.028
279. Syed SN, Rau E, Ziegelmann M, Sogkas G, Brune B, Schmidt RE. C5aR activation in the absence of C5a: a new disease mechanism of autoimmune hemolytic anemia in mice. *Eur J Immunol* (2017) 48:696–704. doi:10.1002/eji.201747238
280. Friese MA, Hellwage J, Jokiranta TS, Meri S, Muller-Quernheim HJ, Peter HH, et al. Different regulation of factor H and FHL-1/reconectin by inflammatory mediators and expression of the two proteins in rheumatoid arthritis (RA). *Clin Exp Immunol* (2000) 121:406–15. doi:10.1046/j.1365-2249.2000.01285.x
281. Hellwage J, Eberle F, Babuke T, Seeberger H, Richter H, Kunert A, et al. Two factor H-related proteins from the mouse: expression analysis and functional characterization. *Immunogenetics* (2006) 58:883–93. doi:10.1007/s00251-006-0153-y
282. Vik DP, Munoz-Canoves P, Kozono H, Martin LG, Tack BF, Chaplin DD. Identification and sequence analysis of four complement factor H-related transcripts in mouse liver. *J Biol Chem* (1990) 265:3193–201.
283. Cserhalmi M, Csincsi AI, Mezei Z, Kopp A, Hebecker M, Uzonyi B, et al. The murine factor H-related protein FHR-B promotes complement activation. *Front Immunol* (2017) 8:1145. doi:10.3389/fimmu.2017.01145
284. Antonioli AH, White J, Crawford F, Renner B, Marchbank KJ, Hannan JP, et al. Modulation of the alternative pathway of complement by murine factor H-related proteins. *J Immunol* (2018) 200:316–26. doi:10.4049/jimmunol.1602017
285. Vetto AA, Mannik M, Zatarain-Rios E, Wener MH. Immune deposits in articular cartilage of patients with rheumatoid arthritis have a granular pattern not seen in osteoarthritis. *Rheumatol Int* (1990) 10:13–9. doi:10.1007/BF02274776
286. Matsumoto I, Staub A, Benoist C, Mathis D. Arthritis provoked by linked T and B cell recognition of a glycolytic enzyme. *Science* (1999) 286:1732–5. doi:10.1126/science.286.5445.1732
287. Ji H, Gauguier D, Ohmura K, Gonzalez A, Duchatelle V, Danoy P, et al. Genetic influences on the end-stage effector phase of arthritis. *J Exp Med* (2001) 194:321–30. doi:10.1084/jem.194.3.321
288. Nandakumar KS, Holmdahl R. Antibody-induced arthritis: disease mechanisms and genes involved at the effector phase of arthritis. *Arthritis Res Ther* (2006) 8:223. doi:10.1186/ar2089
289. Yang D, Dong J, Ge H, Zhu X, Sun G, Ouyang W, et al. The diagnostic significance of glucose-6-phosphate isomerase (G6PI) antigen and anti-G6PI antibody in rheumatoid arthritis patients. *Adv Biosci Biotechnol* (2013) 4:818–22. doi:10.4236/abb.2013.48108
290. Schaller M, Burton DR, Ditzel HJ. Autoantibodies to GPI in rheumatoid arthritis: linkage between an animal model and human disease. *Nat Immunol* (2001) 2:746–53. doi:10.1038/90696
291. Xu W, Seiter K, Feldman E, Ahmed T, Chiao JW. The differentiation and maturation mediator for human myeloid leukemia cells shares homology with neuroleukin or phosphoglucose isomerase. *Blood* (1996) 87:4502–6.
292. Fan LY, Zong M, Wang Q, Yang L, Sun LS, Ye Q, et al. Diagnostic value of glucose-6-phosphate isomerase in rheumatoid arthritis. *Clin Chim Acta* (2010) 411:2049–53. doi:10.1016/j.cca.2010.08.043
293. Herve CA, Wait R, Venables PJ. Glucose-6-phosphate isomerase is not a specific autoantigen in rheumatoid arthritis. *Rheumatology* (2003) 42:986–8. doi:10.1093/rheumatology/keg271
294. Kassahn D, Kolb C, Solomon S, Bochtler P, Illges H. Few human autoimmune sera detect GPI. *Nat Immunol* (2002) 3:411–412; author reply 412–413. doi:10.1038/ni0502-411b
295. Foulquier C, Sebbag M, Clavel C, Chapuy-Regaud S, Al Badine R, Mechin MC, et al. Peptidyl arginine deiminase type 2 (PAD-2) and PAD-4 but not PAD-1, PAD-3, and PAD-6 are expressed in rheumatoid arthritis synovium in close association with tissue inflammation. *Arthritis Rheum* (2007) 56:3541–53. doi:10.1002/art.22983
296. Auger I, Charpin C, Balandraud N, Martin M, Roudier J. Autoantibodies to PAD4 and BRAF in rheumatoid arthritis. *Autoimmun Rev* (2012) 11:801–3. doi:10.1016/j.autrev.2012.02.009
297. Ji H, Ohmura K, Mahmood U, Lee DM, Hofhuis FM, Boackle SA, et al. Arthritis critically dependent on innate immune system players. *Immunity* (2002) 16:157–68. doi:10.1016/S1074-7613(02)00275-3
298. Okroj M, Heinegard D, Holmdahl R, Blom AM. Rheumatoid arthritis and the complement system. *Ann Med* (2007) 39:517–30. doi:10.1080/07853890701477546
299. Solomon S, Kolb C, Mohanty S, Jeisy-Walder E, Preyer R, Schollhorn V, et al. Transmission of antibody-induced arthritis is independent of complement component 4 (C4) and the complement receptors 1 and 2 (CD21/35). *Eur J Immunol* (2002) 32:644–51. doi:10.1002/1521-4141(200203)32:3<644::AID-IMMU644>3.0.CO;2-5
300. Kimura Y, Zhou L, Miwa T, Song WC. Genetic and therapeutic targeting of properdin in mice prevents complement-mediated tissue injury. *J Clin Invest* (2010) 120:3545–54. doi:10.1172/JCI41782

5

Complementing Cancer Metastasis

Dawn M. Kochanek[†], *Shanawaz M. Ghouse*[†], *Magdalena M. Karbowniczek** *and Maciej M. Markiewski**

Department of Immunotherapeutics and Biotechnology, School of Pharmacy, Texas Tech University Health Sciences Center, Abilene, TX, United States

Correspondence:
Magdalena M. Karbowniczek
magdalena.karbowniczek@ttuhsc.edu;
Maciej M. Markiewski
maciej.markiewski@ttuhsc.edu

[†]*These authors have contributed equally to this work.*

Complement is an effector of innate immunity and a bridge connecting innate immunity and subsequent adaptive immune responses. It is essential for protection against infections and for orchestrating inflammatory responses. Recent studies have also demonstrated contribution of the complement system to several homeostatic processes that are traditionally not considered to be involved in immunity. Thus, complement regulates homeostasis and immunity. However, dysregulation of this system contributes to several pathologies including inflammatory and autoimmune diseases. Unexpectedly, studies of the last decade have also revealed that complement promotes cancer progression. Since the initial discovery of tumor promoting role of complement, numerous preclinical and clinical studies demonstrated contribution of several complement components to regulation of tumor growth through their direct interactions with the corresponding receptors on tumor cells or through suppression of antitumor immunity. Most of this work, however, focused on a role of complement in regulating growth of primary tumors. Only recently, a few studies showed that complement promotes cancer metastasis through its contribution to epithelial-to-mesenchymal transition and the premetastatic niche. This latter work has shown that complement activation and generation of complement effectors including C5a occur in organs that are target for metastasis prior to arrival of the very first tumor cells. C5a through its interactions with C5a receptor 1 inhibits antitumor immunity by activating and recruiting immunosuppressive cells from the bone marrow to the premetastatic niche and by regulating function and self-renewal of pulmonary tissue-resident alveolar macrophages. These new advancements provide additional evidence for multifaceted functions of complement in cancer.

Keywords: complement system proteins, cancer, metastasis, alveolar macrophages, myeloid-derived suppressor cells, epithelial–mesenchymal transition

INTRODUCTION

In both mouse models of cancer and patients, the expression of several complement genes is increased, resulting in higher than normal concentrations of complement proteins in plasma or other body fluids (1, 2, 3). In addition, complement activation is thought to occur in cancers because activated complement fragments are deposited within tumors (4, 5). This deposition of complement cleavage products and complement protein complexes including the C5b-9 terminal complement complex was observed in breast cancer (6) and in papillary thyroid carcinoma (7, 8). Complement activation through the lectin pathway was shown in colorectal carcinoma (9, 10). Complement fragments were detected in ascites from ovarian carcinoma patients (11). Complement activation in cancer patients is also supported by detection of C5a circulating in plasma of non-small cell lung carcinoma patients (2). The early studies reporting upregulation and activation of the complement pathway led to a notion that complement, similar to lysing bacteria, may contribute to lysis of tumor cells and, consequently, participates in tumor immune surveillance. However, this is disputable because of the resistance of cancer cells to complement-mediated lysis, which, however, become obvious mainly in the context of use of monoclonal antibodies for cancer immunotherapy (12, 13). This resistance results from high expression of membrane complement regulatory proteins (CRPs) on tumor cells (14) and secretion of soluble complement regulators from these cells (15), especially in solid tumors (13, 16). In contrast, in hematologic malignancies, complement mediated killing can be relevant, at least in the therapeutic context. For example, rituximab, a chimeric CD20 monoclonal antibody used to treat B cell lymphomas utilizes complement-mediated cytotoxicity (CDC) to kill tumor cells. There is growing interest in targeting complement regulators to improve efficacy of monoclonal antibody therapy in cancer (13, 17). Another approach to improve complement-mediated killing of tumor cells is the use of the "hexabody" platform. This technology stems from a seminal discovery that IgGs form hexamers after binding to antigen on the activating surface. This process is mediated by noncovalent interactions between Fc fragments of IgGs (18). Engineering Fc segments can be utilized to enhance formation of hexamers and, consequently, improvement of CDC toward tumor cells (19). Additional example of antitumor complement functions is participation of the complement anaphylatoxins C3a and C5a in enhancing antitumor immunity after radiotherapy. Interestingly, dexamethasone, a drug often administrated during radiotherapy limited complement activation and, consequently, inhibited antitumor immunity (20).

In contrast to these beneficial outcomes of complement activity, it is conceivable that without the discussed here therapeutic interventions, complement enhances tumor growth through its proinflammatory properties (4, 5). This possibility is consistent with a well-established tumor promoting role of chronic inflammation (21). Indeed, the first work to demonstrate tumor promoting properties of complement showed that several complement deficiencies were associated with reduced tumor growth through mechanisms linked to improvement of antitumor immunity (22). Several follow-up studies demonstrated immunoregulatory properties of various complement proteins (23). In addition, complement enhances tumor growth through direct regulation of tumor cell proliferation and invasiveness through C3a and C5a receptors expressed on carcinoma cells (24). Interestingly, the receptors for anaphylatoxins are also expressed in several leukemia and lymphoma cell lines and the blasts from chronic myeloid leukemia and acute myeloid leukemia patients. These cells responded robustly to C3a and C5a stimulation *in vitro* through chemotaxis and this process is negatively regulated by heme oxygenase 1 (HO-1) (25). These findings indicate that trafficking and spread of tumor cells in hematologic malignancies is perhaps, at least partially, controlled by complement system, therefore, inhibiting complement or upregulating HO-1 offer a new therapeutic opportunity for hematologic malignancies.

Together, studies of the last decade provide compelling evidence for a pivotal role of the complement system in tumor growth and targeting complement for anticancer therapy. Interestingly, recent developments point to regulation of cancer metastasis by complement, which appears, in some studies, to be independent from complement functions in primary tumors. This work links complement to a phase of metastatic process that only recently has been proved experimentally and is termed the premetastatic niche (26). We focus our discussion here on these new advancements on complement in metastasis. We also discuss contributions of complement to epithelial-to-mesenchymal transition (EMT), which initiates metastasis in primary tumors.

COMPLEX COMPLEMENT

The complement system is an assembly of more than 50 proteins that work together to provide immunity from infections, regulate several homeostatic processes, and trigger responses to tissue damage or injury (23). Although the textbook definition places complement in the center of innate immunity, recent developments demonstrated that this versatile system functions beyond limits of the immune system, regulating, for example, synaptic pruning (27), tissue regeneration/repair (28, 29), and bone homeostasis (30). In addition to its key function in innate immunity, complement regulates adaptive immunity. The receptors for the complement activation fragments are expressed in B and T cells and their signaling is pivotal for maintaining efficient protection against infection (31, 32). The stimulation of the complement receptor 2 (CR2) through antigen coated with C3d reduces the threshold for B cell activation rendering costimulation for best antibody production (33, 34). The studies on a role of complement in regulating T cell responses has led to surprising discovery that complement proteins in the cytoplasm regulate several intracellular process, mainly of a metabolic nature, essential for T cell homeostasis. The intracellular complement, termed "complosome," interacts with other intracellular innate sensor systems to control processes that are fundamental for adaptive immune responses such as metabolic reprograming necessary for generation of effector T cells (35).

The complement system also includes soluble fluid-phase or membrane-bound proteins, cofactors, regulators, and receptors (36). Upon stimulation by either pathogen or danger-associated molecular patterns, or antibodies, a cascade of events occurs that leads to activation of complement through different complement pathways. The alternative pathway is initiated by bacterial surfaces or unconstrained fluid phase hydrolysis of the complement C3 thioester (37). The lectin pathway is triggered through binding of mannose binding lectin or the ficolins (termed ficolin-1, ficolin-2, ficolin-3) to particular carbohydrates or N-acteyl residues (38, 39). The classical pathway starts when C1q binds to at least two IgG molecules (or one IgM) in a complex with antigen (40). In addition, complement fragments can be cleaved and thus activated through proteolytic enzymes that are not traditionally linked to the complement system. We grouped these additional ways of complement activation under the "umbrella" of the "fourth extrinsic pathway" (41). All three traditional complement activation pathways lead to cleavage of a complement fragment C3, which results in generation of C3a anaphylatoxin (10 kDa) and a large component—C3b. The C3b is deposited on the bacterial or other activating surfaces (42, 43). Following cleavage of C3 by an enzymatic complex—C3 convertase, C5 is cleaved by C5 convertase and similar to C3 cleavage, small C5a and large C5b fragments are generated. C3b and C4b opsonize pathogens, e.g., flag them for phagocytosis by myeloid professional phagocytes that express receptors for C3 cleavage fragments. The large C5 cleavage product, C5b, binds to an activating surface and supports subsequent binding of C6, C7, C8, and finally C9 [membrane attack complex (MAC)]. The multiple C9 fragments polymerize and form a pore in the cell membrane resulting in cell lysis or cell activation in certain circumstances (44). The complement anaphylatoxins C3a, C4a, and C5a are potent mediators that orchestrate events of inflammation (41, 45).

Excessive complement activation can be deleterious; therefore, this process is tightly controlled by CRPs (46). There are both soluble and membrane bound CRPs that can be grouped into several functional categories: (i) CRPs with decay-acceleration activity that increases the rate of C3 convertase breakdown and (ii) with cofactor activity resulting in the cleavage of C3b and C4b, thus, stopping C3 convertase formation (47). Three additional important CRPs are factor H, C1 inhibitor (C1NH), and CD59. Factor H acts in the alternative pathway as a C3 convertase decay accelerator and as a cofactor for factor I-mediated cleavage of C3b. CD59 is the only CRP, which acts to prevent assembly of the MAC. C1NH acts in both the classical and lectin pathways by inactivating C1r, C1s, and mannose-binding lectin serine proteases (47, 48, 49).

COMPLEMENT AND CANCER

In 2008, complement C3, C4, and C5a receptor 1-deficient mice were shown to have slower tumor growth in a model of human papilloma virus-induced cancer (22). This paper was the first study to contradict a well-accepted, at that time, notion of complement participation in immune surveillance. Tumor promoting functions of complement, at least in this model, were linked to C5a/C5a receptor 1 (C5aR1)-mediated activation and recruitment of myeloid-derived suppressor cells (MDSC) to tumors and inhibition of antitumor immunity. At the time of this publication, concerns were raised that the observed phenotypes may be restricted to a single tumor model (4, 5, 50). However, multiple preclinical and clinical studies in the last decade supported tumor-promoting properties of different complement components (16, 49). For example, studies by Corrales and colleagues demonstrated that C5a regulates MDSC in a lung cancer model (2). The blockade of C5aR1 led to a reduction in expression of genes that suppress antitumor immunity including *Arg1, Il-6, Il-10, Ctla4, Lag3, and Cd234 (PDL1)* (2). Recently, it has been shown that C3aR and C5aR1 signaling have an important impact on the IL-10-mediated cytotoxic properties of $CD8^+$ T cells infiltrating tumors in models of melanoma and breast cancer (E0771) (51). In this manuscript, tumor infiltrating $CD8^+$ T cells were shown to produce C3, which in autocrine manner inhibited the expression of IL-10. This cytokine appears to be essential for the cytotoxic properties of these cells. Mechanistically, IL-10 was associated with C3aR and C5aR1 signaling in $CD8^+$ T cells. Complement's role in recruiting tumor-associated macrophages (TAMs) and controlling their proangiogenic characteristics was proposed in a work, exploring antitumor functions of pentraxin 3 (52).

In addition to research demonstrating contributions of complement to inhibition of antitumor immunity, several studies showed other mechanisms behind tumor promoting functions of complement. In ovarian carcinoma models, tumor cells were demonstrated to produce complement components. C3a and C5a generated through activation of complement fragments produced in tumor cells regulated proliferation and invasiveness of tumor cells in autocrine fashion (24). C1q deposited in several human malignancies and mouse tumors seems to accelerate tumor growth through its proangiogenic properties and direct regulation of tumor cell motility and proliferation (53). Of value, Ajona et. al recently demonstrated improved efficacy of programmed cell-death 1 (PD-1) blockade in the presence of complement inhibition in reducing progression of tumors in a model of lung cancer (54). These new findings divulge a feasible path for targeting the complement system with the use of immunotherapeutic agents along with T cell check inhibitors. The detailed and comprehensive descriptions of a role in regulating tumor growth can be found in recent reviews (16, 23, 49). Here, we focus the discussion on the role of complement in regulating metastasis, a role that seems to involve different mechanisms.

METASTASIS A HALLMARK OF MALIGNANCY

Cancer metastasis is a process of relocation of tumor cells from a primary to a distant (disconnected from primary tumor) site, through lymph or blood. In fact, a metastatic potential determines the malignant character of primary growth (55). Cancer metastasis are responsible for approximately 90 percent of cancer-associated deaths, however, paradoxically, mechanisms regulating metastasis remain the most obscure aspect of cancer biology (56). The metastatic spread of cancer is a multistep and complex chain of alterations in tumor and host cells, and tumor stroma, known as the invasion-metastasis cascade (56, 57). This cascade involves processes in primary tumor sites, circulation, and metastasis-targeted organs. Some of the first steps in the metastatic cascade involve acquisition of the ability to migrate and invade and degrade the tumor stroma by tumor cells. This goal is achieved through triggering in tumor cells several cellular programs that are collectively termed EMT, which is also an essential process during embryogenesis and wound healing (58). The EMT occurs perhaps in several malignancies; however, the current understanding of these cellular adaptations stems from studies in the models of epithelial-origin neoplasms carcinomas (59).

Complement has been linked to EMT in two recent studies (**Figure 1**) (60, 61). In the first study, increased expression of C5aR1 was found in hepatocellular carcinoma and hepatocellular carcinoma-derived cell lines and positively correlated with stage and invasion of liver capsule by tumor cells. The stimulation of C5aR1 *via* C5a induced EMT, as demonstrated by downregulation of E-cadherin and Claudin-1 expression, and upregulation

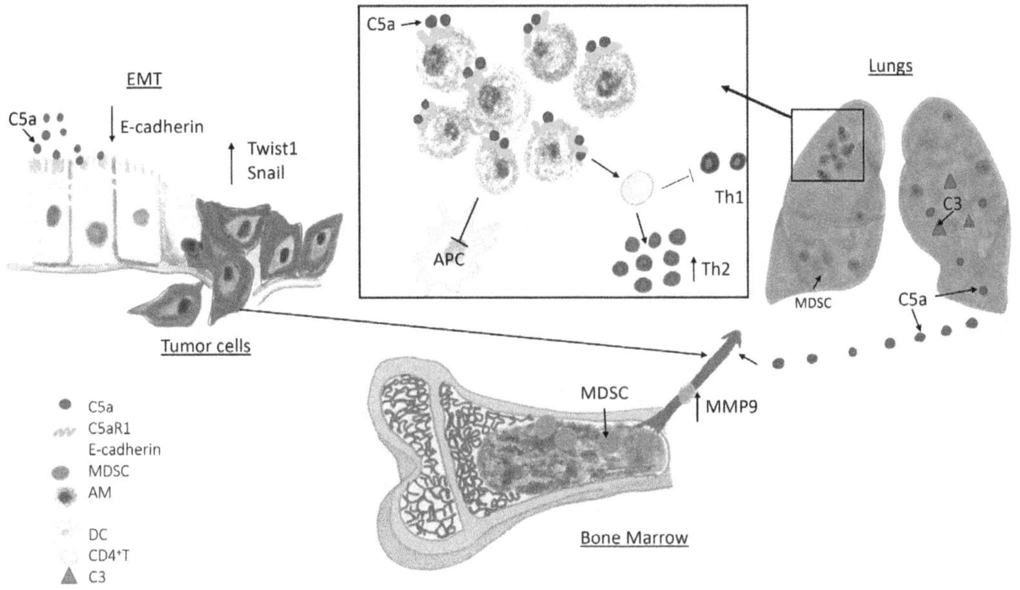

FIGURE 1 | Overview of a role of complement in cancer metastasis. The C5a/C5aR1 axis contributes to the initial step of the invasion-metastasis cascade epithelial-to-mesenchymal transition, which is essential for tumor cell motility, invasion of extracellular matrix blood vessels. C5aR1 signaling contributes to the formation of the premetastatic niche by recruiting immunosuppressive myeloid-derived suppressor cell from bone marrow to the lungs and by regulating self-renewal of alveolar macrophages that impair antitumor immunity *via* reducing antigen-presenting capacity of dendritic cells (APC) and polarizing T cell response toward Th2 phenotype.

of Snail. Mechanistically, C5aR1-mediated EMT was linked to ERK1/2 signaling (61). In another study, C3 expressed in ovarian carcinoma-derived cells reduced expression of E-cadherin through C3a and Krüppel-like factor 5. Interestingly, C3 expression in tumor cells is transcriptionally regulated by twist basic helix–loop–helix transcription factor 1 (TWIST1), which binds to the *C3* promoter and enhances its expression. TWIST1 and C3 colocalized at the invasive tumor edges, and in the neural crest and limb buds of mouse embryos. Therefore, this work identified TWIST1 as a transcription factor that regulates *C3* expression during pathologic and physiologic EMT (60). The phenotypes associated with EMT program resemble phenotypes of cancer stem cells (CSCs) that are essential for metastatic spread. The recent work showed that $CD10^+$ cancer-associated fibroblasts that express a second C5a receptor (C5L2) provide a survival niche for CSCs through C5L2-mediated NF-kβ activation (62). Through EMT, tumor cells reduce their attachment to neighboring tumor cells and surrounding stromal elements, increase motility, and acquire the ability to invade stroma, blood, or lymphatic vessels, thereby gaining access to the vasculature.

The invasion of blood or lymphatic vessels enables tumor cells to intravasate and enter the circulation. The histopathological identification of vasculature invasion is itself a poor prognostic factor and often correlates with advanced metastatic disease (63). The lymph node metastases are a critical factor in cancer staging and are independent prognostic factors in several malignancies (64). However, mortality in cancer patients results from hematogenous spread to the vital organs including lungs, liver, and ultimately brain. Although initially lymph node metastases were thought to precede the subsequent hematogenous spread of cancer, evidence that draining lymph nodes are just temporary "parking" sites for cancer cells, before their departure to blood, is rather limited. It seems that lymph nodes represent a final destination for some cancer cells while other tumor cells, for unclear reasons, spread through the blood vessels (59). Upon successful intravasation, tumor cells move with the bloodstream to distant sites. However, only a small fraction of tumor cells that enter circulation safely reach their destination in the capillary beds of lungs and liver or cross the blood–brain barrier. This low efficacy of metastatic spread in blood results from hemodynamic stress and elimination of circulating tumor cells by the innate immunity, mainly natural killer (NK) cells (65). In contrast to NK cells, interactions with platelets (66) and neutrophils (67, 68) appear to facilitate metastasis.

After reaching their final destination, tumor cells are trapped in the capillary beds of the vital organs because their size is usually larger than the diameter of a single capillary. The halting of tumor cells in narrow capillaries facilitates their interaction with endothelium that is required for adhesion to endothelial cells and subsequent crossing of this endothelial barrier by extravasating tumor cells (transendothelial migration). Several substances secreted by tumor and host cells in the capillary beds enhance adhesiveness of tumor and endothelial cells and increase vascular permeability (69, 70), thereby, facilitating tumor cell extravasation. In the liver and kidneys, the fenestrated endothelium seems to facilitate seeding of these organs by metastasizing tumor cells. Perhaps the mechanisms contributing to extravasation of tumor cells in different organs vary, depending on the location and intrinsic properties of metastasizing cells.

After successful seeding of distant sites, tumor cells usually persist in an indolent state as single disseminated tumor cells or subclinical microscopic metastases, sometimes for years. The reasons for tumor cells to remain in a dormant state are unclear; however, poor adaptation of tumor cells to new microenvironment of metastasis-targeted organs seems to play a significant role (59). In addition, transition to rapidly growing and clinically overt metastasis, known as metastatic colonization, requires robust angiogenesis and immune evasion that may not be evident during a dormant phase of metastatic progression (71). For breast, prostate, and kidney cancers, a dormant phase may last even for decades after initial therapy and eradication of a primary tumor (59). Therefore, dormant tumor cells need to find a microenvironment-niche that allows them to slowly self-renew, provides needed nutrients, and protects from anticancer drugs and elimination by the immune system (72). For example, prostate carcinoma cells often metastasize to bones where they compete for residence in the endosteal niche with hematopoietic stem cells (73). In multiple organs including lungs, bones, and brain, tumor cells reside in close proximity to blood vessels in a region known as the perivascular niche (72, 74).

Interestingly, as much as EMT is necessary to trigger the invasion-metastasis cascade in primary sites, the reversal of this process, called mesenchymal-to-epithelial transition (MET), contributes to metastatic colonization, which is a final stage of metastatic disease. In metastatic tumors, MET appears to be critical in restoring a complex and heterogonous structure resembling primary tumors (75). Metastatic colonization leads to development of clinically overt and rapidly growing metastatic lesions, which are the ultimate reason for cancer-associated mortality. The transition from dormant to rapidly growing metastases requires acquisition of specific cellular programs by tumor cells, such as, discussed already MET, but also complex and well-orchestrated changes in the microenvironment of metastasis-targeted organs that include angiogenesis (72, 76), inflammation (77), remodeling of extracellular matrix (78, 79, 80), and evasion of antitumor immunity (81).

THE PREMETASTATIC NICHE

Surprisingly, in several mouse models of cancer, changes that appear to be essential for metastatic colonization, e.g., a final stage of the invasion-metastatic cascade, including vascular alterations, remodeling of extracellular matrix, inflammation, and immunosuppression are observed in certain organs that seem to be marked for metastasis even before the arrival of the tumor cells. These alterations, collectively known as the premetastatic niche, are thought to facilitate seeding of these organs by disseminated tumor cells and their survival after they arrive to distant sites. The establishment of the premetastatic niche is triggered by the primary tumors (82) because efficiency of seeding of metastasis-targeted organs by intravenously (i.v.) injected tumor cells is greatly enhanced by the presence of these tumors (3). Tumor-free mice i.v. injected with murine cancer cells developed significantly less lung metastases-derived from these i.v. injected cells than breast tumor-bearing mice i.v. injected with the same amounts of cells, indicating that the presence of primary breast malignancy facilitated seeding of the lungs by circulating (i.v. injected) tumor cells (3). It also appears that different types of cancer selectively prepare the premetastatic niche in different organs. This reflects the tendency of some malignancies to metastasize preferentially to specific locations. This specificity, known also as organotropism, was initially noted by Stephan Paget in 1889 (82), however, mechanisms regulating organotropism remain unclear until now. These mechanisms perhaps involve complex interactions between tumor cells and metastasis targeted organs that were proposed by Paget in his "seeds (tumor cells) and soil (microenvironment of premetastatic sites) theory." However, until seminal studies of the last decade (83, 84), which indeed established the field of premetastatic niche, the experimental proof for Paget's theory was missing. It is increasingly accepted that the premetastatic niche is created by tumor-secreted factors and tumor-shed extracellular vesicles, mainly exosomes. These factors seem to collectively control the stepwise development of premetastatic niche that begins with vascular alterations and progresses through activation of resident cells, extracellular matrix remodeling, and recruitment of bone marrow-derived cells (85).

Secreted Factors

The evidence that tumor-secreted factors contribute to the premetastatic niche and organotropism, was, perhaps, first provided by experiments showing that melanoma-conditioned medium injected into mice, directed the metastasis of Lewis lung carcinoma cells (which normally metastasize only to the lungs) to sites typical for experimental melanoma metastasis (84). Among several identified factors secreted by tumors, vascular endothelial growth factor A (VEGFA), placental growth factor (84), transforming growth factor β (TGF-β), and tumor necrosis factor (TNF) were first demonstrated to prepare "soil" for tumor cells (26, 83).

Exosomes

Exosomes, small extracellular vesicles formed on the cell surface through a budding mechanism, contain diverse cargo that facilitates cell-to-cell communication and homeostatic cell regulation (86). However, in patients and mouse models, formation of exosomes by tumor cells is increased compared to normal cells (87). Tumor-derived exosomes were isolated from plasma of cancer patients and mice with experimental tumors and found to carry tumor-derived cargo that promotes disease progression (87). This exosomal cargo, which includes tumor-derived miRNA and proteins, reprograms the target cells toward a pro-metastatic and pro-inflammatory phenotype, resulting in their contribution to the formation of the premetastatic niche. For example, melanoma B16-derived exosomes increase the expression of the receptor tyrosine kinase and MET in bone marrow progenitors, causing their exit from bone marrow and migration to the lungs, where they contributed to the premetastatic niche. Importantly, MET expression is also elevated in circulating $CD45^{-}C\text{-}KIT^{low/+}TIE2^{+}$ bone marrow progenitors from patients with metastatic melanoma (87). B16-derived exosomes increase vascular permeability and enhance expression of TNF, S100A8, and S100A9, contributing to recruitment of bone marrow cells to the lung premetastatic niche. Of note, the source of S100 proteins was not identified in this study (87).

Abundant Complement

In contrast to tumor-derived secreted factors and exosomes, complement proteins are present in abundance in plasma and body fluids (41, 88) and, therefore, are readily available to participate in the premetastatic niche in patients or mice even with very small tumors. Increased concentration of complement components in plasma and other bodily fluids has been observed in both cancer patients and mouse models of cancer (1, 2, 3) suggesting upregulation of the complement pathway. These higher amounts of complement proteins may be linked to enhanced expression and production of complement by the liver, however, local increases in expression of complement genes in tumors and organs targeted by metastasis contribute to augmented levels of complement fragments because endothelial and immune cells synthesize complement fragments (89, 90) and these cells are an integral component of the tumor microenvironment (81, 91) and the premetastatic niche (26). Thus, they are possible sites of origin for several complement proteins in tumors and metastatic sites. For example, in a mouse model of breast cancer with spontaneous metastatic spread mimicking human malignancy, increased concentrations of C3 were found in plasma and bronchoalveolar lavage indicating increased production of complement proteins (3). These higher levels of complement fragments correlated with increases in expression of C3 and C5 genes in the lungs (3, 92). Cytotoxic CD8$^+$ T cells were found to synthesize C3 in mouse models of melanoma and breast cancer (51). Importantly, tumor cells also produce complement proteins. Mouse ovarian carcinoma tumor cells and human ovarian carcinoma cell lines were demonstrated to produce C3 (24). In a squamous cell carcinoma model, expression of C3, factor B, and factor I were also demonstrated (93, 94). Boire and colleagues recently demonstrated that C3 produced and secreted from tumor cells has prosurvival functions and facilitates leptomeningeal metastasis (95).

Complement proteins are secreted from cells in their inactive forms, as zymogens. To exert their functions, these fragments are activated through a series of proteolytic cleavages that form a complement cascade, which ends with generation of complement effectors (41). Therefore, if complement plays a role in regulating metastatic progression, complement activation in metastasis-targeted organs or tumors is anticipated. This activation can be revealed by detecting deposited complement fragments in tissue or secreted effectors such as complement anaphylatoxins, C3a, C4a, and C5a. The cleavage fragments of C3 were found to be deposited in the lungs prior to metastasis, indicating complement activation and participation of the complement system in the lung premetastatic (3). These data were obtained through a use of a syngeneic mouse model of metastatic breast cancer (4T1), in which tumor cells are injected into the mammary fat pad, and breast tumors formed there subsequently metastasize to distant sites, similar to human malignancy (96). The deposition of C3 cleavage fragments in the lungs correlated with increasing levels of C5a in plasma over time (**Figure 1**) (3).

Vasculature

Increased vascular permeability is one of the earliest changes observed in the premetastatic niche and is associated with increased metastatic burden (97, 98). The factors secreted from primary tumors, including epithelial growth factor receptor ligand epiregulin, metalloproteinases MMP1, and MMP2, are known to impact vascular permeability in primary tumors and distant sites, helping tumor cells to intravasate in a primary and then extravasate in a distant site, respectively (99). In a melanoma model, tumor cells secrete factors upregulating angiopoietin 2, MMP3, and MMP10 that synergistically destabilize vasculature in the premetastatic organs (97). Factors affecting vascular permeability can also be secreted from different cell populations recruited to the premetastatic niche. For example, myeloid cells were shown to produce MMP9 (100) and VEGFA (101). Endothelial cells, which are often targets for vasoactive substances, can themselves participate in vascular alterations in the premetastatic niche. VEGFA-dependent upregulation of E-selectin on the luminal surface of endothelium facilities adhesion of tumor cells to endothelium and subsequent extravasation (102).

The complement effectors, especially C5a, are powerful inflammatory mediators that are actively engaged in bringing leukocytes to sites of inflammation. C5a can achieve this goal, acting as a potent chemoattractant that causes cytoskeleton changes in leukocytes that are responsible for cell movement (103). However, it also enhances (directly and indirectly) vascular permeability, further adding to accumulation of leukocytes in inflammatory foci (103). The complement C3 cleavage fragments were found to be deposited in the premetastatic lungs as early as 4 days after injecting tumor cells into the mammary fat pad in a model of breast cancer (before any tumor cells are present in the lungs). Since C3 is a central component of complement cascade, on which all complement activation pathways converge, deposition of C3 cleavage fragments indicates complement activation and subsequent generation of C5a (88), which indeed was present in sera of these mice (3). It is, therefore, conceivable that complement contributes directly to increased vascular permeability in the premetastatic niche similar to its participation in inflammatory vascular alterations; however, a direct experimental evidence for these C5a functions in the premetastatic niche has yet to be provided. The indirect impact of complement on vascular changes can be attributed to recruitment of MDSC (3) because these cells can produce and release several vasoactive factors including MMP9, which is intimately involved in regulating vascular integrity in the premetastatic niche (83, 84). Genetic ablation of *Mmp9* was shown to normalize the aberrant vasculature in the premetastatic lungs and reduce metastatic burden (100). The seminal recent work has also demonstrated that cancer-cell-derived C3/C3a through C3aR in the choroid plexus disrupts the blood–cerebrospinal fluid barrier. The increased permeability of this barrier facilities the entry of plasma proteins that are essential for tumor growth into the cerebrospinal fluid, thereby, facilitating leptomeningeal metastasis (95).

Resident Cells

Resident cells in metastasis-targeted organs are naturally suited to participate in the premetastatic niche because they are present before the arrival of tumor cells. Tumors can reach and potentially hijack these cells through several mechanisms including secreted tumor-derived factors, exosomes, and recruitment of bone marrow-derived cells that subsequently interact with resident components of the premetastatic niche. Recent work also demonstrated that complement activation regulates resident cells in the lungs (**Figure 1**) (92). As discussed already, endothelial cells are targets for several vasoactive substances whether derived from tumors, recruited cells, or generated locally. Fibroblasts contribute to remodeling of extracellular matrix through deposition of new extracellular matrix components or by secreting enzymes that affect preexisting components of the matrix (104). S100A4 expressing pulmonary fibroblasts incorporate exosomal cargo derived from breast cancer cells and through this mechanism upregulates S100 proteins (82). Exosomal cargo from pancreatic carcinoma induces similar changes in the liver-resident macrophages, Kupffer cells (105). S100 proteins were linked to recruitment of myeloid-origin cells to the premetastatic niche (106). Similar to Kupffer cells in the liver, another population of tissue-resident macrophages, pulmonary alveolar macrophages, were recently demonstrated to contribute to the premetastatic niche (92).

These recent developments on participation of tissue-resident macrophages to metastasis are of particular interest because roles of these cells in cancer remain unclear, in contrast to very well-studied TAMs or inflammatory monocytes/macrophages recruited to the lungs with metastases by CCL2 (101). Several early studies yielded conflicting results on how liver Kupffer cells and lung alveolar macrophages contribute to cancer progression (107). A role of these cells in cancer requires revision because recently published linage-tracing data demonstrated that these cells have a different origin and biology than inflammatory macrophages (108). Unlike inflammatory macrophages and TAMs that are recruited from bone marrow to sites of inflammation or tumors, respectively, tissue-resident macrophages migrate to different organs during embryogenesis prior to hematopoiesis, and self-renew thereafter (109). Pulmonary alveolar macrophages are the resident macrophages of the lungs, and while they have well-known immunoregulatory and homeostatic roles in healthy lungs (110), they appear to be well-suited to partake in preconditioning the lungs for metastasis through their immunoregulatory properties. In support of this notion, alveolar macrophages were found to accumulate in premetastatic lungs and this accumulation was the result of cell proliferation rather than recruitment from bone marrow (92). The mechanisms controlling proliferation of these cells were linked to C5aR1 signaling because tumor-bearing C5aR1-deficient mice presented with a lower total number of these cells in the lungs compared to tumor-bearing wild-type controls and this reduced cell number associated with reduced Ki-67 expression. Immunoregulatory functions of these cells appeared to be related to skewing effector $CD4^+$ T cells responses toward Th2 phenotype, which plays limited role in antitumor immunity in contrast to Th1 responses (92). In addition, alveolar macrophages in tumor-bearing hosts reduced number and antigen-presenting capacity of lung dendritic cells through regulation of TGF-β1 in lung infiltrating leukocytes (**Figure 1**). The depletion of alveolar macrophages reversed immunosuppression and reduced lung metastatic burden (92).

Extracellular Matrix Remodeling

The continuous remodeling of extracellular matrix by tumor-derived secreted factors, resident fibroblasts, and recruited bone marrow-derived cells is an integral part of the premetastatic niche (111). This remodeling is achieved through deposition of new extracellular matrix components or modification of existing components. For example, deposition of fibronectin produced by activated fibroblast provides a docking site for bone marrow-derived cells that express fibronectin receptor VLA-4 (84). These stromal fibroblasts, stimulated with tumor-derived TGF-β, produce periostin in a mouse model of breast cancer (78). Periostin directly interacts with type I collagen, fibronectin, and Notch1 through its amino-terminal EMI domain and interacts with tenascin-C and BMP-1 through its fas I domains. These periostin interactions with mainly extracellular matrix molecules occur at first intracellularly. In addition, periostin serves as a ligand for integrins such as αvβ3 and αvβ5 and promotes cell motility by acting outside the cell (112). Periostin was demonstrated to facilitate melanoma metastasis to wounds (113) and to regulate immunosuppressive functions of MDSC during early stages of breast cancer metastasis (114). MDSC (mainly monocytic-MDSC), which accumulated in the premetastatic lung of MMTV-PyMT spontaneous breast tumor-bearing mice, secrete versican, an extracellular matrix proteoglycan. Versican contributed to MET and the formation of macrometastasis in the lungs (115). Enzymatic modulation of extracellular matrix proteins also occurs in the premetastatic niche and is mediated mainly by metalloproteinases produced by cells that are recruited to the premetastatic niche. In addition, the members of the LOX family crosslink collagen type I and IV and this crosslinking facilitates adhesion of bone marrow-derived cells to the extracellular matrix of the premetastatic niche. These cells produce more metalloproteinases contributing to further remodeling of extracellular matrix.

Although complement was not directly linked to extracellular-matrix remodeling in the premetastatic niche, studies in different model systems demonstrated that fibronectin can interact with several complement components including C1q (116) and C3 cleavage fragments (117). C3 cleavage fragments can also bind to different components of extracellular matrix including collagen (118). Interestingly, binding of C1q to fibronectin was not associated with complement activation but was connected to enhancement of phagocytosis of C1q coated particles through fibronectin. Therefore, functional significance of complement interactions with extracellular matrix proteins in the premetastatic niche remain to be elucidated. However, it is reasonable to theorize that complement C3 cleavage fragments, bound to extracellular matrix proteins, interact with its receptors broadly expressed on myeloid-origin cells that are recruited to the premetastatic niche. The receptors for C3 degradation products include CR1, which binds C3b and iC3b, CR2 (CD21), which binds the degradation products of C3b (iC3b, C3dg, C3d), CR3 (CD11b/CD18 or Mac-1), which binds iC3b, and CR4 (CD11c/CD18), which binds iC3b, however, through a different domain than CR3 (119). C5a leads to upregulation of CR3 on MDSC, which may facilitate adhesion of these cells to endothelium and recruitment to tumors (22); however, it may also contribute to adhesion of MDSC to extracellular matrix in the premetastatic niches.

Recruited Cells

The identification of bone-marrow derived cells in the premetastatic niche and discovery of their roles in facilitating seeding of these niches by tumor cells, provided perhaps the first experimental evidence confirming the "seed and soil" theory (83, 84). A seminal work by Hiratsuka and colleagues defined Mac1 (CR3) positive macrophages as a source of MMP9 in the lungs in addition to endothelial cells. These macrophages were recruited to the lungs because resident alveolar macrophages do not express CD11b (https://www.immgen.org/). The study by Kaplan and colleagues demonstrated recruitment of VEGFR1 and VLA-4 expressing hematopoietic progenitors to the premetastatic lungs and their participation in the premetastatic niche (84). These studies opened an avenue for further investigations into discovery of other recruited components of the premetastatic niche. Less than a decade later, MDSC, which were long recognized as modulators of the primary tumor microenvironment (120), were identified as contributors to the premetastatic niche (100, 115). However, these studies reported on metastasis promoting properties of MDSC linked to increased vascular permeability (100) and remodeling of extracellular matrix (115) rather than to their well-established immunoregulatory roles.

The C5aR1/C5a signaling axis recruits MDSC to primary tumors (2, 22), therefore, it was explored whether similar mechanisms operate in the premetastatic niche. Utilizing a syngeneic mouse model of metastatic breast cancer, it has been demonstrated that C5aR1 knockout or wild-type mice administrated with a specific C5aR1 inhibitor (PMX-53) had decreased lung and liver metastatic burden compared to control mice. Interestingly, C5aR1 appear to regulate only metastasis in this model because lack of C5aR1in mice did not affect primary breast tumors. The differences in lung metastasis were associated with differences in a degree of infiltration of the lungs and livers by MDSC. The lung infiltrating MDSC were found mainly in interavleolar septa and due to intensity of this infiltration, the morphological picture resembled interstitial pneumonia. Therefore, the term the premetastatic pneumonia has been proposed to emphasize intensity of MDSC infiltration and specific localization of these cells in the lungs (3). These MDSC were recruited to the premetastatic sites through C5a since C5aR1 was expressed in blood MDSC and complement activation, leading to C5a generation, was observed in the premetastatic niche (**Figure 1**). To further investigate the role of C3 cleavage fragments and MDSC, tumor-draining lymph nodes from breast cancer patients were examined; they observed that C3 fragments' deposition and local C3 production were both intensified in lymph nodes with metastases (3). The decreased metastasis in mice lacking C5aR1 resulted from improved antitumor immunity due to escalated infiltration of the lungs by $CD8^+$ and $CD4^+$ T cells. In addition, the increases in these T cell subsets were found in peripheral blood and C5aR1-deficiency favored Th1 response. Also observed was a decrease in Tregs in both the blood and the lungs in C5aR1-knockout mice. The T cell subsets including $CD4^+$ and $CD8^+$ T cells isolated from the lungs of C5aR1 knockout mice produced increased amounts of IFN-γ. The elimination of cytotoxic $CD8^+$ T cells by neutralizing antibody erased the inhibitory effect of C5aR1-deficiency on metastasis, supporting notion that this effect was caused by stimulating antitumor immunity. Importantly, these data also indicate immunoregulatory functions of MDSC in the premetastatic niche (3).

CONCLUDING REMARKS

The evidence supporting contributions of complement to cancer metastasis is scarce and limited to a few recent papers. However, it appears that complement affects key steps in the invasion-metastasis cascade including EMT and the premetastatic niche (**Figure 1**). Given ubiquitous presence of complement in body fluids and tissues, the potential contributions of complement to regulating metastasis are significant. Our recent work demonstrated that C5aR1 regulates resident (alveolar macrophages) (92) and recruited (MDSC) (3) cells in the premetastatic niche. The significance of this regulation was underscored by complete protection from lung metastasis in mice depleted of alveolar macrophages and treated with C5aR1 inhibitor (92). Thus, despite an early phase of studies on complement participation in metastasis, several complement fragments appear to be promising targets for therapies seeking to stop cancer metastasis.

AUTHOR CONTRIBUTIONS

All authors listed have made a substantial, direct, and intellectual contribution to the work, and approved it for publication.

FUNDING

This work was supported by the National Institute of Health (R01CA190209 to MM), the Cancer Prevention and Research Institute of Texas (RP120168 to MK), the U.S. Department of Defense (TS140010 to MK), Laura W. Bush Institute for Women's Health (seed grants to MM and MK). We thank the Development Corporation of Abilene for continued financial support.

REFERENCES

1. Gminski J, Mykala-Ciesla J, Machalski M, Drozdz M, Najda J. Immunoglobulins and complement components levels in patients with lung cancer. *Rom J Intern Med* (1992) 30(1):39–44.
2. Corrales L, Ajona D, Rafail S, Lasarte JJ, Riezu-Boj JI, Lambris JD, et al. Anaphylatoxin C5a creates a favorable microenvironment for lung cancer progression. *J Immunol* (2012) 189(9):4674–83. doi:10.4049/jimmunol.1201654
3. Vadrevu SK, Chintala NK, Sharma SK, Sharma P, Cleveland C, Riediger L, et al. Complement c5a receptor facilitates cancer metastasis by altering T-cell responses in the metastatic niche. *Cancer Res* (2014) 74(13):3454–65. doi:10.1158/0008-5472.CAN-14-0157
4. Markiewski MM, Lambris JD. Is complement good or bad for cancer patients? A new perspective on an old dilemma. *Trends Immunol* (2009) 30(6):286–92. doi:10.1016/j.it.2009.04.002
5. Markiewski MM, Lambris JD. Unwelcome complement. *Cancer Res* (2009) 69(16):6367–70. doi:10.1158/0008-5472.CAN-09-1918
6. Niculescu F, Rus HG, Retegan M, Vlaicu R. Persistent complement activation on tumor cells in breast cancer. *Am J Pathol* (1992) 140(5):1039–43.
7. Yamakawa M, Yamada K, Tsuge T, Ohrui H, Ogata T, Dobashi M, et al. Protection of thyroid cancer cells by complement-regulatory factors. *Cancer*

(1994) 73(11):2808–17. doi:10.1002/1097-0142(19940601)73:11<2808::AID-CNCR2820731125>3.0.CO;2-P

8. Lucas SD, Karlsson-Parra A, Nilsson B, Grimelius L, Akerstrom G, Rastad J, et al. Tumor-specific deposition of immunoglobulin G and complement in papillary thyroid carcinoma. *Hum Pathol* (1996) 27(12):1329–35. doi:10.1016/S0046-8177(96)90346-9
9. Baatrup G, Qvist N, Junker A, Larsen KE, Zimmermann-Nielsen C. Activity and activation of the complement system in patients being operated on for cancer of the colon. *Eur J Surg* (1994) 160(9):503–10.
10. Ytting H, Jensenius JC I, Christensen J, Thiel S, Nielsen HJ. Increased activity of the mannan-binding lectin complement activation pathway in patients with colorectal cancer. *Scand J Gastroenterol* (2004) 39(7):674–9. doi:10.1080/00365520410005603
11. Bjorge L, Hakulinen J, Vintermyr OK, Jarva H, Jensen TS, Iversen OE, et al. Ascitic complement system in ovarian cancer. *Br J Cancer* (2005) 92(5):895–905. doi:10.1038/sj.bjc.6602334
12. Fishelson Z, Donin N, Zell S, Schultz S, Kirschfink M. Obstacles to cancer immunotherapy: expression of membrane complement regulatory proteins (mCRPs) in tumors. *Mol Immunol* (2003) 40(2–4):109–23. doi:10.1016/S0161-5890(03)00112-3
13. Taylor RP, Lindorfer MA. Cytotoxic mechanisms of immunotherapy: harnessing complement in the action of anti-tumor monoclonal antibodies. *Semin Immunol* (2016) 28(3):309–16. doi:10.1016/j.smim.2016.03.003
14. Donin N, Jurianz K, Ziporen L, Schultz S, Kirschfink M, Fishelson Z. Complement resistance of human carcinoma cells depends on membrane regulatory proteins, protein kinases and sialic acid. *Clin Exp Immunol* (2003) 131(2):254–63. doi:10.1046/j.1365-2249.2003.02066.x
15. Jurianz K, Ziegler S, Donin N, Reiter Y, Fishelson Z, Kirschfink M. K562 erythroleukemic cells are equipped with multiple mechanisms of resistance to lysis by complement. *Int J Cancer* (2001) 93(6):848–54. doi:10.1002/ijc.1406
16. Reis ES, Mastellos DC, Ricklin D, Mantovani A, Lambris JD. Complement in cancer: untangling an intricate relationship. *Nat Rev Immunol* (2017) 18(1):5–18. doi:10.1038/nri.2017.97
17. Gelderman KA, Lam S, Gorter A. Inhibiting complement regulators in cancer immunotherapy with bispecific mAbs. *Expert Opin Biol Ther* (2005) 5(12):1593–601. doi:10.1517/14712598.5.12.1593
18. Diebolder CA, Beurskens FJ, de Jong RN, Koning RI, Strumane K, Lindorfer MA, et al. Complement is activated by IgG hexamers assembled at the cell surface. *Science* (2014) 343(6176):1260–3. doi:10.1126/science.1248943
19. Cook EM, Lindorfer MA, van der Horst H, Oostindie S, Beurskens FJ, Schuurman J, et al. Antibodies that efficiently form hexamers upon antigen binding can induce complement-dependent cytotoxicity under complement-limiting conditions. *J Immunol* (2016) 197(5):1762–75. doi:10.4049/jimmunol.1600648
20. Surace L, Lysenko V, Fontana AO, Cecconi V, Janssen H, Bicvic A, et al. Complement is a central mediator of radiotherapy-induced tumor-specific immunity and clinical response. *Immunity* (2015) 42(4):767–77. doi:10.1016/j.immuni.2015.03.009
21. Balkwill F, Mantovani A. Inflammation and cancer: back to Virchow? *Lancet* (2001) 357(9255):539–45. doi:10.1016/S0140-6736(00)04046-0
22. Markiewski MM, DeAngelis RA, Benencia F, Ricklin-Lichtsteiner SK, Koutoulaki A, Gerard C, et al. Modulation of the antitumor immune response by complement. *Nat Immunol* (2008) 9(11):1225–35. doi:10.1038/ni.1655
23. Kolev M, Markiewski MM. Targeting complement-mediated immunoregulation for cancer immunotherapy. *Semin Immunol* (2018) 37:85–97. doi:10.1016/j.smim.2018.02.003
24. Cho MS, Vasquez HG, Rupaimoole R, Pradeep S, Wu S, Zand B, et al. Autocrine effects of tumor-derived complement. *Cell Rep* (2014) 6(6):1085–95. doi:10.1016/j.celrep.2014.02.014
25. Abdelbaset-Ismail A, Borkowska-Rzeszotek S, Kubis E, Bujko K, Brzezniakiewicz-Janus K, Bolkun L, et al. Activation of the complement cascade enhances motility of leukemic cells by downregulating expression of HO-1. *Leukemia* (2017) 31(2):446–58. doi:10.1038/leu.2016.198
26. Sceneay J, Smyth MJ, Moller A. The pre-metastatic niche: finding common ground. *Cancer Metastasis Rev* (2013) 32(3–4):449–64. doi:10.1007/s10555-013-9420-1
27. Stevens B, Allen NJ, Vazquez LE, Howell GR, Christopherson KS, Nouri N, et al. The classical complement cascade mediates CNS synapse elimination. *Cell* (2007) 131(6):1164–78. doi:10.1016/j.cell.2007.10.036
28. Strey CW, Markiewski M, Mastellos D, Tudoran R, Spruce LA, Greenbaum LE, et al. The proinflammatory mediators C3a and C5a are essential for liver regeneration. *J Exp Med* (2003) 198(6):913–23. doi:10.1084/jem.20030374
29. Markiewski MM, DeAngelis RA, Lambris JD. Liver inflammation and regeneration: two distinct biological phenomena or parallel pathophysiologic processes? *Mol Immunol* (2006) 43(1–2):45–56. doi:10.1016/j.molimm.2005.06.019
30. Modinger Y, Loffler B, Huber-Lang M, Ignatius A. Complement involvement in bone homeostasis and bone disorders. *Semin Immunol* (2018) 37:53–65. doi:10.1016/j.smim.2018.01.001
31. Kemper C, Atkinson JP. T-cell regulation: with complements from innate immunity. *Nat Rev Immunol* (2007) 7(1):9–18. doi:10.1038/nri1994
32. Laumonnier Y, Karsten CM, Köhl J. Novel insights into the expression pattern of anaphylatoxin receptors in mice and men. *Mol Immunol* (2017) 89:44–58. doi:10.1016/j.molimm.2017.05.019
33. Dempsey PW, Allison ME, Akkaraju S, Goodnow CC, Fearon DT. C3d of complement as a molecular adjuvant: bridging innate and acquired immunity. *Science* (1996) 271(5247):348–50. doi:10.1126/science.271.5247.348
34. Carroll MC, Isenman DE. Regulation of humoral immunity by complement. *Immunity* (2012) 37(2):199–207. doi:10.1016/j.immuni.2012.08.002
35. West EE, Kolev M, Kemper C. Complement and the regulation of T cell responses. *Annu Rev Immunol* (2018) 36:309–38. doi:10.1146/annurev-immunol-042617-053245
36. Ricklin D, Lambris JD. Complement in immune and inflammatory disorders: pathophysiological mechanisms. *J Immunol* (2013) 190(8):3831–8. doi:10.4049/jimmunol.1203487
37. Rodríguez de Córdoba S, Harris CL, Morgan BP, Llorca O. Lessons from functional and structural analyses of disease-associated genetic variants in the complement alternative pathway. *Biochim Biophys Acta* (2011) 1812(1):12–22. doi:10.1016/j.bbadis.2010.09.002
38. Bajic G, Degn SE, Thiel S, Andersen GR. Complement activation, regulation, and molecular basis for complement-related diseases. *EMBO J* (2015) 34(22):2735–57. doi:10.15252/embj.201591881
39. Hein E, Garred P. The lectin pathway of complement and biocompatibility. *Adv Exp Med Biol* (2015) 865:77–92. doi:10.1007/978-3-319-18603-0_5
40. Merle NS, Church SE, Fremeaux-Bacchi V, Roumenina LT. Complement system part I – molecular mechanisms of activation and regulation. *Front Immunol* (2015) 6:262. doi:10.3389/fimmu.2015.00262
41. Markiewski MM, Lambris JD. The role of complement in inflammatory diseases from behind the scenes into the spotlight. *Am J Pathol* (2007) 171(3):715–27. doi:10.2353/ajpath.2007.070166
42. Elvington M, Liszewski MK, Atkinson JP. Evolution of the complement system: from defense of the single cell to guardian of the intravascular space. *Immunol Rev* (2016) 274(1):9–15. doi:10.1111/imr.12474
43. Lukacsi S, Nagy-Balo Z, Erdei A, Sandor N, Bajtay Z. The role of CR3 (CD11b/CD18) and CR4 (CD11c/CD18) in complement-mediated phagocytosis and podosome formation by human phagocytes. *Immunol Lett* (2017) 189:64–72. doi:10.1016/j.imlet.2017.05.014
44. Towner LD, Wheat RA, Hughes TR, Morgan BP. Complement membrane attack and tumorigenesis: a systems biology approach. *J Biol Chem* (2016) 291(29):14927–38. doi:10.1074/jbc.M115.708446
45. Wang H, Ricklin D, Lambris JD. Complement-activation fragment C4a mediates effector functions by binding as untethered agonist to protease-activated receptors 1 and 4. *Proc Natl Acad Sci U S A* (2017) 114(41):10948–53. doi:10.1073/pnas.1707364114
46. Holers VM. Complement and its receptors: new insights into human disease. *Annu Rev Immunol* (2014) 32:433–59. doi:10.1146/annurev-immunol-032713-120154
47. Nesargikar PN, Spiller B, Chavez R. The complement system: history, pathways, cascade and inhibitors. *Eur J Microbiol Immunol (Bp)* (2012) 2(2):103–11. doi:10.1556/EuJMI.2.2012.2.2
48. Ferreira VP, Pangburn MK, Cortes C. Complement control protein factor H: the good, the bad, and the inadequate. *Mol Immunol* (2010) 47(13):2187–97. doi:10.1016/j.molimm.2010.05.007
49. Afshar-Kharghan V. The role of the complement system in cancer. *J Clin Invest* (2017) 127(3):780–9. doi:10.1172/JCI90962

50. Loveland BE, Cebon J. Cancer exploiting complement: a clue or an exception? *Nat Immunol* (2008) 9(11):1205–6. doi:10.1038/ni1108-1205
51. Wang Y, Sun SN, Liu Q, Yu YY, Guo J, Wang K, et al. Autocrine complement inhibits IL10-dependent T-cell-mediated antitumor immunity to promote tumor progression. *Cancer Discov* (2016) 6(9):1022–35. doi:10.1158/2159-8290.CD-15-1412
52. Bonavita E, Gentile S, Rubino M, Maina V, Papait R, Kunderfranco P, et al. PTX3 is an extrinsic oncosuppressor regulating complement-dependent inflammation in cancer. *Cell* (2015) 160(4):700–14. doi:10.1016/j.cell.2015.01.004
53. Bulla R, Tripodo C, Rami D, Ling GS, Agostinis C, Guarnotta C, et al. C1q acts in the tumour microenvironment as a cancer-promoting factor independently of complement activation. *Nat Commun* (2016) 7:10346. doi:10.1038/ncomms10346
54. Ajona D, Ortiz-Espinosa S, Moreno H, Lozano T, Pajares MJ, Agorreta J, et al. A combined PD-1/C5a blockade synergistically protects against lung cancer growth and metastasis. *Cancer Discov* (2017) 7(7):694–703. doi:10.1158/2159-8290.CD-16-1184
55. Chambers AF, Groom AC, MacDonald IC. Dissemination and growth of cancer cells in metastatic sites. *Nat Rev Cancer* (2002) 2(8):563–72. doi:10.1038/nrc865
56. Gupta GP, Massague J. Cancer metastasis: building a framework. *Cell* (2006) 127(4):679–95. doi:10.1016/j.cell.2006.11.001
57. Talmadge JE, Fidler IJ. AACR centennial series: the biology of cancer metastasis: historical perspective. *Cancer Res* (2010) 70(14):5649–69. doi:10.1158/0008-5472.CAN-10-1040
58. Nieto MA, Huang RY, Jackson RA, Thiery JP. Emt: 2016. *Cell* (2016) 166(1):21–45. doi:10.1016/j.cell.2016.06.028
59. Lambert AW, Pattabiraman DR, Weinberg RA. Emerging biological principles of metastasis. *Cell* (2017) 168(4):670–91. doi:10.1016/j.cell.2016.11.037
60. Cho MS, Rupaimoole R, Choi HJ, Noh K, Chen J, Hu Q, et al. Complement component 3 is regulated by TWIST1 and mediates epithelial-mesenchymal transition. *J Immunol* (2016) 196(3):1412–8. doi:10.4049/jimmunol.1501886
61. Hu WH, Hu Z, Shen X, Dong LY, Zhou WZ, Yu XX. C5a receptor enhances hepatocellular carcinoma cell invasiveness via activating ERK1/2-mediated epithelial-mesenchymal transition. *Exp Mol Pathol* (2016) 100(1):101–8. doi:10.1016/j.yexmp.2015.10.001
62. Su S, Chen J, Yao H, Liu J, Yu S, Lao L, et al. CD10(+)GPR77(+) cancer-associated fibroblasts promote cancer formation and chemoresistance by sustaining cancer stemness. *Cell* (2018) 172(4):841–56.e16. doi:10.1016/j.cell.2018.01.009
63. Gujam FJ, Going JJ, Edwards J, Mohammed ZM, McMillan DC. The role of lymphatic and blood vessel invasion in predicting survival and methods of detection in patients with primary operable breast cancer. *Crit Rev Oncol Hematol* (2014) 89(2):231–41. doi:10.1016/j.critrevonc.2013.08.014
64. de Boer M, van Dijck JA, Bult P, Borm GF, Tjan-Heijnen VC. Breast cancer prognosis and occult lymph node metastases, isolated tumor cells, and micrometastases. *J Natl Cancer Inst* (2010) 102(6):410–25. doi:10.1093/jnci/djq008
65. Headley MB, Bins A, Nip A, Roberts EW, Looney MR, Gerard A, et al. Visualization of immediate immune responses to pioneer metastatic cells in the lung. *Nature* (2016) 531(7595):513–7. doi:10.1038/nature16985
66. Gasic GJ, Gasic TB, Stewart CC. Antimetastatic effects associated with platelet reduction. *Proc Natl Acad Sci U S A* (1968) 61(1):46–52. doi:10.1073/pnas.61.1.46
67. Spicer JD, McDonald B, Cools-Lartigue JJ, Chow SC, Giannias B, Kubes P, et al. Neutrophils promote liver metastasis via Mac-1-mediated interactions with circulating tumor cells. *Cancer Res* (2012) 72(16):3919–27. doi:10.1158/0008-5472.CAN-11-2393
68. Cools-Lartigue J, Spicer J, McDonald B, Gowing S, Chow S, Giannias B, et al. Neutrophil extracellular traps sequester circulating tumor cells and promote metastasis. *J Clin Invest* (2013) 123(8):3446–58. doi:10.1172/JCI67484
69. Padua D, Zhang XH, Wang Q, Nadal C, Gerald WL, Gomis RR, et al. TGFbeta primes breast tumors for lung metastasis seeding through angiopoietin-like 4. *Cell* (2008) 133(1):66–77. doi:10.1016/j.cell.2008.01.046
70. Reymond N, d'Agua BB, Ridley AJ. Crossing the endothelial barrier during metastasis. *Nat Rev Cancer* (2013) 13(12):858–70. doi:10.1038/nrc3628
71. Aguirre Ghiso JA, Kovalski K, Ossowski L. Tumor dormancy induced by downregulation of urokinase receptor in human carcinoma involves integrin and MAPK signaling. *J Cell Biol* (1999) 147(1):89–104. doi:10.1083/jcb.147.1.89
72. Ghajar CM, Peinado H, Mori H, Matei IR, Evason KJ, Brazier H, et al. The perivascular niche regulates breast tumour dormancy. *Nat Cell Biol* (2013) 15(7):807–17. doi:10.1038/ncb2767
73. Shiozawa Y, Pedersen EA, Havens AM, Jung Y, Mishra A, Joseph J, et al. Human prostate cancer metastases target the hematopoietic stem cell niche to establish footholds in mouse bone marrow. *J Clin Invest* (2011) 121(4):1298–312. doi:10.1172/JCI43414
74. Ghajar CM. Metastasis prevention by targeting the dormant niche. *Nat Rev Cancer* (2015) 15(4):238–47. doi:10.1038/nrc3910
75. Brabletz T. To differentiate or not – routes towards metastasis. *Nat Rev Cancer* (2012) 12(6):425–36. doi:10.1038/nrc3265
76. Kienast Y, von Baumgarten L, Fuhrmann M, Klinkert WE, Goldbrunner R, Herms J, et al. Real-time imaging reveals the single steps of brain metastasis formation. *Nat Med* (2010) 16(1):116–22. doi:10.1038/nm.2072
77. De Cock JM, Shibue T, Dongre A, Keckesova Z, Reinhardt F, Weinberg RA. Inflammation triggers Zeb1-dependent escape from tumor latency. *Cancer Res* (2016) 76(23):6778–84. doi:10.1158/0008-5472.CAN-16-0608
78. Malanchi I, Santamaria-Martinez A, Susanto E, Peng H, Lehr HA, Delaloye JF, et al. Interactions between cancer stem cells and their niche govern metastatic colonization. *Nature* (2011) 481(7379):85–9. doi:10.1038/nature10694
79. Oskarsson T, Acharyya S, Zhang XH, Vanharanta S, Tavazoie SF, Morris PG, et al. Breast cancer cells produce tenascin C as a metastatic niche component to colonize the lungs. *Nat Med* (2011) 17(7):867–74. doi:10.1038/nm.2379
80. Cox TR, Erler JT. Molecular pathways: connecting fibrosis and solid tumor metastasis. *Clin Cancer Res* (2014) 20(14):3637–43. doi:10.1158/1078-0432.CCR-13-1059
81. Quail DF, Joyce JA. Microenvironmental regulation of tumor progression and metastasis. *Nat Med* (2013) 19(11):1423–37. doi:10.1038/nm.3394
82. Peinado H, Zhang H, Matei IR, Costa-Silva B, Hoshino A, Rodrigues G, et al. Pre-metastatic niches: organ-specific homes for metastases. *Nat Rev Cancer* (2017) 17(5):302–17. doi:10.1038/nrc.2017.6
83. Hiratsuka S, Nakamura K, Iwai S, Murakami M, Itoh T, Kijima H, et al. MMP9 induction by vascular endothelial growth factor receptor-1 is involved in lung-specific metastasis. *Cancer Cell* (2002) 2(4):289–300. doi:10.1016/S1535-6108(02)00153-8
84. Kaplan RN, Riba RD, Zacharoulis S, Bramley AH, Vincent L, Costa C, et al. VEGFR1-positive haematopoietic bone marrow progenitors initiate the pre-metastatic niche. *Nature* (2005) 438(7069):820–7. doi:10.1038/nature04186
85. Psaila B, Lyden D. The metastatic niche: adapting the foreign soil. *Nat Rev Cancer* (2009) 9(4):285–93. doi:10.1038/nrc2621
86. Raposo G, Stoorvogel W. Extracellular vesicles: exosomes, microvesicles, and friends. *J Cell Biol* (2013) 200(4):373–83. doi:10.1083/jcb.201211138
87. Peinado H, Aleckovic M, Lavotshkin S, Matei I, Costa-Silva B, Moreno-Bueno G, et al. Melanoma exosomes educate bone marrow progenitor cells toward a pro-metastatic phenotype through MET. *Nat Med* (2012) 18(6):883–91. doi:10.1038/nm.2753
88. Walport MJ. Complement. First of two parts. *N Engl J Med* (2001) 344(14):1058–66. doi:10.1056/NEJM200104053441406
89. Morgan B, Gasque P. Extrahepatic complement biosynthesis: where, when and why? *Clin Exp Immunol* (1997) 107(1):1–7. doi:10.1046/j.1365-2249.1997.d01-890.x
90. Lubbers R, van Essen MF, van Kooten C, Trouw LA. Production of complement components by cells of the immune system. *Clin Exp Immunol* (2017) 188(2):183–94. doi:10.1111/cei.12952
91. Gajewski TF, Schreiber H, Fu YX. Innate and adaptive immune cells in the tumor microenvironment. *Nat Immunol* (2013) 14(10):1014–22. doi:10.1038/ni.2703
92. Sharma SK, Chintala NK, Vadrevu SK, Patel J, Karbowniczek M, Markiewski MM. Pulmonary alveolar macrophages contribute to the pre-metastatic niche by suppressing antitumor T cell responses in the lungs. *J Immunol* (2015) 194(11):5529–38. doi:10.4049/jimmunol.1403215
93. Riihilä P, Nissinen L, Farshchian M, Kivisaari A, Ala-Aho R, Kallajoki M, et al. Complement factor I promotes progression of cutaneous squamous

cell carcinoma. *J Invest Dermatol* (2015) 135(2):579–88. doi:10.1038/jid.2014.376
94. Riihilä P, Nissinen L, Farshchian M, Kallajoki M, Kivisaari A, Meri S, et al. Complement component C3 and complement factor B promote growth of cutaneous squamous cell carcinoma. *Am J Pathol* (2017) 187(5):1186–97. doi:10.1016/j.ajpath.2017.01.006
95. Boire A, Zou Y, Shieh J, Macalinao DG, Pentsova E, Massagué J. Complement component 3 adapts the cerebrospinal fluid for leptomeningeal metastasis. *Cell* (2017) 168(6):1101–13.e13. doi:10.1016/j.cell.2017.02.025
96. Pulaski BA, Ostrand-Rosenberg S. Mouse 4T1 breast tumor model. *Curr Protoc Immunol* (2001) Chapter 20:Unit 20.2. doi:10.1002/0471142735.im2002s39
97. Huang Y, Song N, Ding Y, Yuan S, Li X, Cai H, et al. Pulmonary vascular destabilization in the premetastatic phase facilitates lung metastasis. *Cancer Res* (2009) 69(19):7529–37. doi:10.1158/0008-5472.CAN-08-4382
98. Hiratsuka S, Ishibashi S, Tomita T, Watanabe A, Akashi-Takamura S, Murakami M, et al. Primary tumours modulate innate immune signalling to create pre-metastatic vascular hyperpermeability foci. *Nat Commun* (2013) 4:1853. doi:10.1038/ncomms2856
99. Gupta GP, Nguyen DX, Chiang AC, Bos PD, Kim JY, Nadal C, et al. Mediators of vascular remodelling co-opted for sequential steps in lung metastasis. *Nature* (2007) 446(7137):765–70. doi:10.1038/nature05760
100. Yan HH, Pickup M, Pang Y, Gorska AE, Li Z, Chytil A, et al. Gr-1+CD11b+ myeloid cells tip the balance of immune protection to tumor promotion in the premetastatic lung. *Cancer Res* (2010) 70(15):6139–49. doi:10.1158/0008-5472.CAN-10-0706
101. Qian BZ, Li J, Zhang H, Kitamura T, Zhang J, Campion LR, et al. CCL2 recruits inflammatory monocytes to facilitate breast-tumour metastasis. *Nature* (2011) 475(7355):222–5. doi:10.1038/nature10138
102. Hiratsuka S, Goel S, Kamoun WS, Maru Y, Fukumura D, Duda DG, et al. Endothelial focal adhesion kinase mediates cancer cell homing to discrete regions of the lungs via E-selectin up-regulation. *Proc Natl Acad Sci U S A* (2011) 108(9):3725–30. doi:10.1073/pnas.1100446108
103. Guo RF, Ward PA. Role of C5a in inflammatory responses. *Annu Rev Immunol* (2005) 23:821–52. doi:10.1146/annurev.immunol.23.021704.115835
104. Cox TR, Bird D, Baker AM, Barker HE, Ho MW, Lang G, et al. LOX-mediated collagen crosslinking is responsible for fibrosis-enhanced metastasis. *Cancer Res* (2013) 73(6):1721–32. doi:10.1158/0008-5472.CAN-12-2233
105. Costa-Silva B, Aiello NM, Ocean AJ, Singh S, Zhang H, Thakur BK, et al. Pancreatic cancer exosomes initiate pre-metastatic niche formation in the liver. *Nat Cell Biol* (2015) 17(6):816–26. doi:10.1038/ncb3169
106. Hiratsuka S, Watanabe A, Sakurai Y, Akashi-Takamura S, Ishibashi S, Miyake K, et al. The S100A8-serum amyloid A3-TLR4 paracrine cascade establishes a pre-metastatic phase. *Nat Cell Biol* (2008) 10(11):1349–55. doi:10.1038/ncb1794
107. Qian BZ, Pollard JW. Macrophage diversity enhances tumor progression and metastasis. *Cell* (2010) 141(1):39–51. doi:10.1016/j.cell.2010.03.014
108. Davies LC, Rosas M, Jenkins SJ, Liao CT, Scurr MJ, Brombacher F, et al. Distinct bone marrow-derived and tissue-resident macrophage lineages proliferate at key stages during inflammation. *Nat Commun* (2013) 4:1886. doi:10.1038/ncomms2877
109. Davies LC, Jenkins SJ, Allen JE, Taylor PR. Tissue-resident macrophages. *Nat Immunol* (2013) 14(10):986–95. doi:10.1038/ni.2705
110. Holt PG, Strickland DH, Wikstrom ME, Jahnsen FL. Regulation of immunological homeostasis in the respiratory tract. *Nat Rev Immunol* (2008) 8(2):142–52. doi:10.1038/nri2236
111. Sleeman JP. The metastatic niche and stromal progression. *Cancer Metastasis Rev* (2012) 31(3–4):429–40. doi:10.1007/s10555-012-9373-9
112. Kudo A. Periostin in fibrillogenesis for tissue regeneration: periostin actions inside and outside the cell. *Cell Mol Life Sci* (2011) 68(19):3201–7. doi:10.1007/s00018-011-0784-5
113. Fukuda K, Sugihara E, Ohta S, Izuhara K, Funakoshi T, Amagai M, et al. Periostin is a key niche component for wound metastasis of melanoma. *PLoS One* (2015) 10(6):e0129704. doi:10.1371/journal.pone.0129704
114. Wang Z, Xiong S, Mao Y, Chen M, Ma X, Zhou X, et al. Periostin promotes immunosuppressive premetastatic niche formation to facilitate breast tumour metastasis. *J Pathol* (2016) 239(4):484–95. doi:10.1002/path.4747
115. Gao D, Joshi N, Choi H, Ryu S, Hahn M, Catena R, et al. Myeloid progenitor cells in the premetastatic lung promote metastases by inducing mesenchymal to epithelial transition. *Cancer Res* (2012) 72(6):1384–94. doi:10.1158/0008-5472.CAN-11-2905
116. Bing DH, Almeda S, Isliker H, Lahav J, Hynes RO. Fibronectin binds to the C1q component of complement. *Proc Natl Acad Sci U S A* (1982) 79(13):4198–201. doi:10.1073/pnas.79.13.4198
117. Hautanen A, Keski-Oja J. Interaction of fibronectin with complement component C3. *Scand J Immunol* (1983) 17(3):225–30. doi:10.1111/j.1365-3083.1983.tb00785.x
118. Shields KJ, Stolz D, Watkins SC, Ahearn JM. Complement proteins C3 and C4 bind to collagen and elastin in the vascular wall: a potential role in vascular stiffness and atherosclerosis. *Clin Transl Sci* (2011) 4(3):146–52. doi:10.1111/j.1752-8062.2011.00304.x
119. Bajic G, Yatime L, Sim RB, Vorup-Jensen T, Andersen GR. Structural insight on the recognition of surface-bound opsonins by the integrin I domain of complement receptor 3. *Proc Natl Acad Sci U S A* (2013) 110(41):16426–31. doi:10.1073/pnas.1311261110
120. Talmadge JE, Gabrilovich DI. History of myeloid-derived suppressor cells. *Nat Rev Cancer* (2013) 13(10):739–52. doi:10.1038/nrc3581

6

The Complement System in Dialysis: A Forgotten Story?

Felix Poppelaars[1], Bernardo Faria[1,2,3], Mariana Gaya da Costa[1], Casper F. M. Franssen[1], Willem J. van Son[1], Stefan P. Berger[1], Mohamed R. Daha[1,4] and Marc A. Seelen[1]*

[1] Department of Internal Medicine, Division of Nephrology, University Medical Center Groningen, Groningen, Netherlands, [2] Nephrology and Infectious Diseases Research and Development Group, University of Porto, Porto, Portugal, [3] Department of Nephrology, Hopsital Braga, Braga, Portugal, [4] Department of Nephrology, Leiden University Medical Centre, Leiden, Netherlands

***Correspondence:**
Felix Poppelaars
f.poppelaars@umcg.nl

Significant advances have lead to a greater understanding of the role of the complement system within nephrology. The success of the first clinically approved complement inhibitor has created renewed appreciation of complement-targeting therapeutics. Several clinical trials are currently underway to evaluate the therapeutic potential of complement inhibition in renal diseases and kidney transplantation. Although, complement has been known to be activated during dialysis for over four decades, this area of research has been neglected in recent years. Despite significant progress in biocompatibility of hemodialysis (HD) membranes and peritoneal dialysis (PD) fluids, complement activation remains an undesired effect and relevant issue. Short-term effects of complement activation include promoting inflammation and coagulation. In addition, long-term complications of dialysis, such as infection, fibrosis and cardiovascular events, are linked to the complement system. These results suggest that interventions targeting the complement system in dialysis could improve biocompatibility, dialysis efficacy, and long-term outcome. Combined with the clinical availability to safely target complement in patients, the question is not if we should inhibit complement in dialysis, but when and how. The purpose of this review is to summarize previous findings and provide a comprehensive overview of the role of the complement system in both HD and PD.

Keywords: complement, kidney, dialysis, hemodialysis, peritoneal dialysis

INTRODUCTION

An estimated 2.6 million people are treated for end-stage kidney disease (ESKD) worldwide (1). The majority of ESKD patients are dialysis-dependent. The choice between peritoneal dialysis (PD) and hemodialysis (HD) involves various determinants. Nonetheless, there is no major difference in

Abbreviations: AP, alternative pathway; C1-INH, C1 esterase inhibitor; C3aR, C3a-receptor; C5aR, C5a-receptor; C5aRA, C5a-receptor antagonist; CARPA, complement activation-related pseudo allergy; MCP, membrane cofactor protein; CD55, decay accelerating factor; CD59, membrane attack complex-inhibitory protein; CP, classical pathway; CR1, complement receptor 1; CR3, complement receptor 3; CRP, C-reactive protein; CV-event, cardiovascular event; DAF, decay accelerating factor; ESKD, end-stage kidney disease; HD, hemodialysis; IgG, immunoglobulin G; IgM, immunoglobulin M; IL, interleukin; LDL, low-density lipoprotein; LP, lectin pathway; MAC, membrane attack complex; MBL, mannose-binding lectin; MCP-1, monocyte chemoattractant protein-1; PD, peritoneal dialysis; sC5b-9, soluble C5b-9; sCR1, soluble complement receptor 1; TGF-β, tumor growth factor beta; TNF-α, tumor necrosis factor alfa.

mortality between HD and PD patients (2). Although considerable progress has been made in survival rates of dialysis patients, cardiovascular morbidity and mortality remain extremely high (3). Both traditional risk factors (such as hypertension, dyslipidemia, and diabetes), as well as non-traditional risk factors (such as oxidative stress, endothelial dysfunction and chronic inflammation), contribute to the high cardiovascular risk (4). In order to lower the high morbidity and mortality rates in dialysis patients, the chronic inflammation seen in these patients must be tackled. The systemic inflammation in dialysis patients can be attributed to the (remaining) uremia, the underlying renal disease, comorbidities, and dialysis-related factors (5). The latter represents an issue that has been present in dialysis throughout history, and still remains unresolved, namely bioincompatibility.

BIOCOMPATIBILITY

The term "biocompatible" refers to the "capacity of a material/solutions to exist in contact with the human body without causing a (inappropriate) host response" (6). The biocompatibility of the materials used in dialysis remains an important clinical challenge. In HD, the membrane provokes an inflammatory response, as it is the site where blood has direct contact with a foreign surface (7). Additionally, PD fluids containing high glucose levels, hyperosmolarity and acidic pH are considered biologically "unfriendly" and this lack of compatibility causes peritoneal membrane damage (8). Improving biocompatibility in HD and PD is a critical factor to ensure dialysis adequacy and enable long-term treatment (7–9). The challenge of biocompatibility is not confined to dialysis but equally important for other medical devices in contact with either tissue or blood (10). The incompatibility reaction is complex and poorly understood; however, platelets, leukocytes, the complement, and the coagulation system have been shown to be involved (11, 12). In general, incompatibility will lead to inflammation, thrombosis, and fibrosis (11–13). These events will negatively impact the clinical performance and lead to adverse events. The complement system is an important mediator of incompatibility because it can discriminate between self and non-self (14). In accordance, complement has been shown to be activated during cardiopulmonary bypass (15), low-density lipoprotein (LDL) apheresis (16), plasmapheresis (17), and immunoadsorption (18). Additionally, the complement system is also involved in biomaterial-induced complications of medical devices that are not in direct contact with the circulation, such as surgical meshes and prostheses (19, 20). Yet, it should be emphasized that the trigger by which complement is activated is different and depends on the properties of the biomaterial used (20). Proposed mechanisms of indirect complement activation include: (1) immunoglobulin G binding to the biomaterial initiating the classical pathway (CP); (2) lectin pathway (LP) activation by carbohydrate structures or acetylated compounds; or (3) activation of the alternative pathway (AP) by altered surfaces, e.g., plasma protein-coated biomaterials. In addition, complement initiators can also directly bind to the biomaterial, leading to complement activation (20). Irrespective of the pathway, complement activation always leads to the cleavage of C3, forming C3a and C3b (**Figure 1**). Increased levels of C3b result in the generation of the C5-convertase, cleaving C5 in C5a, a powerful anaphylatoxin and chemoattractant, and C5b. Next, C5b binds to the surface and interacts with C6–C9, forming the membrane attack complex (MAC/C5b-9) (14).

HEMODIALYSIS

Hemodialysis is a general term including several techniques such as low or high-flux HD (diffusion-based dialysis) and online haemodiafiltration (combined convective and diffusive therapy). Overall, HD remains the most-used form of renal replacement in adult ESKD patients (1). The dialysis membrane can be divided into two main groups, cellulose-based and synthetic membranes (7, 21). In the past, HD membranes were based on cuprophane (a copper-substituted cellulose) because these were inexpensive and thin-walled. The disadvantage of cellulose-based membranes was the immunoreactivity due to the many free hydroxyl-groups. Subsequently, modified cellulosic membranes were developed to improve biocompatibility by replacing the free hydroxyl-groups with different substitutions (especially acetate). The following step was the development of "synthetic" membranes, such as polyacrylonitrile, acrylonitrile-sodium methallyl sulfonate, polysulfone, polycarbonate, polyamide, and polymethylmethacrylate membranes. Nowadays, synthetic membranes are the most commonly used in clinical practice (21). The benefits of these membranes are the varying pore size and reduced immunoreactivity. The complement system is critical in the bioincompatibility of extracorporeal circulation procedures, because complement is abundantly present in blood. Moreover, innate immune activation during HD is a neglected but potentially vital mechanism that contributes to the high morbidity and mortality in these patients (4).

Complement Activation in HD

In the 1970s, HD was already known to affect the complement system (22). Several studies have since then looked at complement activation during HD, the complement pathway responsible and additional mechanisms contributing to complement activation. In the past, an important adverse event in dialysis was the "first-use syndrome," named after the fact that these reactions were most severe with new dialyzers. This incompatibility reaction was the result of complement activation by the membrane and closely resembles the pseudo-anaphylactic clinical picture that is nowadays known as complement activation-related pseudoallergy (CARPA) (23, 24). Furthermore, these early studies provided important information on the kinetics of complement activation. During HD, C3 activation, resulting in the generation of C3a, peaks during the first 10–15 min, whereas terminal pathway activation, resulting in C5a and C5b-9 formation occurs at a later stage of dialysis (25). Over the past decades, membranes have been developed with improved biocompatibility. Nonetheless, even with modern "biocompatible" HD membranes significant complement activation still occurs (23, 26, 27). During a single HD session soluble C5b-9 (sC5b-9) levels and C3d/C3-ratios in the plasma increase up to 70% (23, 26). Yet, this is most likely an underestimation of the amount of complement activation, since these values represent fluid phase activation. Complement activation takes place in the plasma (the fluid phase), but also on

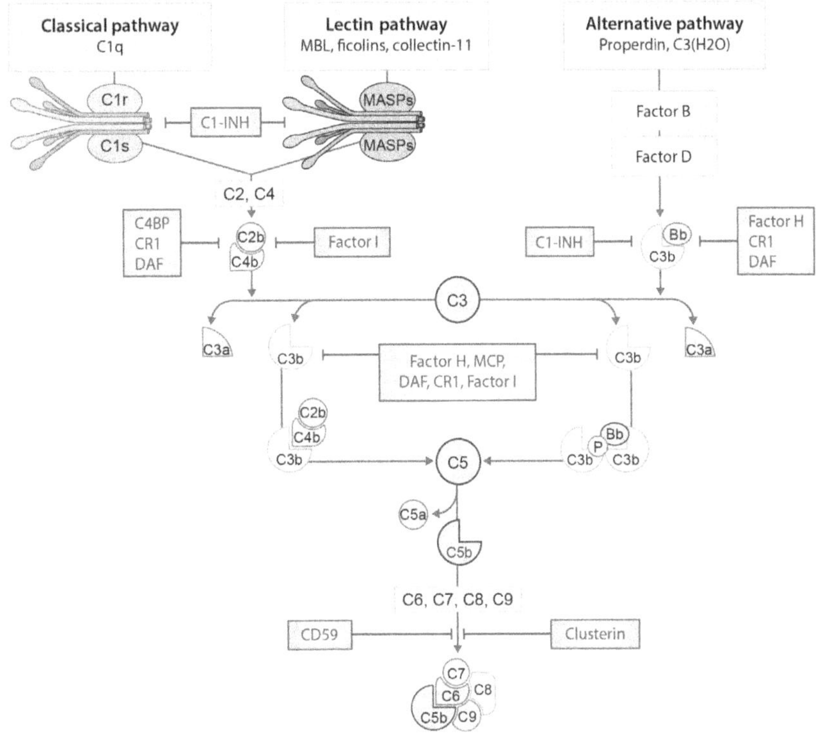

FIGURE 1 | The complement system. A schematic view of activation of the complement system and its regulation. The classical pathway (CP) is initiated by C1q binding to immune complexes or other molecules (e.g., CRP), thereby activating C1r and C1s resulting in the cleavage of C2 and C4 thereby forming the C3-convertase (C4b2b). The lectin pathway (LP) is initiated by mannose-binding lectin (MBL), ficolins, or collectin-11 binding to carbohydrates or other molecules (e.g., IgA), thereby activating MASP-1 and MASP-2, forming the same C3-convertase as the CP. Subsequently, the C3-convertase cleavages C3 into C3a and C3b. Activation of the alternative pathway (AP) occurs *via* properdin binding to certain cell surfaces (e.g., LPS) or by spontaneous hydrolysis of C3 into C3(H_2O). Next, binding of factor B creates the AP C3-convertase (C3bBb). Increased levels of C3b results in the formation of the C5-convertases, which cleaves C5 in C5a, a powerful anaphylatoxin, and C5b. Next, C5b binds to the surface and interactions with C6–C9, generating the membrane attack complexes (MAC/C5b-9). Several complement regulators (either soluble and membrane-bound) prevent or restrain complement activation. C1 esterase inhibitor (C1-INH) inhibits the activation of early pathway activation of all three pathways, while C4b-binding protein (C4BP) controls activation at the C4 level of the CP and LP. Factor I and factor H regulate the C3 and C5-convertase. Furthermore, the membrane-bound inhibitors include complement receptor 1 (CR1), membrane cofactor protein (MCP) that acts as an co-factors for factor I and decay accelerating factor (DAF) which accelerates the decay of C3-convertases. The membrane-bound regulator Clusterin and CD59 prevents the generation of the C5b-9.

surfaces (the solid phase) (14). Fittingly, in addition to fluid phase activation, complement depositions have also been shown on the surface of the HD membranes (28).

Different studies have tried to dissect the pathway responsible for complement activation in HD. Early evidence emerged from a study by Cheung et al., demonstrating AP activation by cellulose membranes (29). Initially, the involvement of the CP or LP was excluded, since it was reported that plasma C4d concentrations remained unaffected during HD (30). However, others were able to show C4 activation by cellulose membranes (31, 32). The increase in C4d levels correlated with the rise in C3d levels, implying that the CP or LP is (at least partly) responsible for the complement activation seen in HD (32). More recently, a role for the LP was demonstrated in complement activation by polysulfone membranes (33, 34). An elegant study by Mares et al., using mass spectrometry, showed a 26-fold change in eluate-to-plasma ratio for ficolin-2 (previously called L-ficolin), suggesting preferential adsorption by the membrane (33). A follow-up study using proteomics analysis of dialyzer eluates revealed that C3c, ficolin-2, mannose-binding lectin (MBL) and properdin were most enriched (28). In addition, plasma ficolin-2 levels decreased by 41% during one HD session, corresponding with the excessive adsorption to the membrane. The decrease in plasma ficolin-2 levels was associated with C5a production and leukopenia during HD (28). The adsorption of properdin to the dialyzer, confirms earlier studies regarding AP activation by HD (28, 29). To summarize, the principal mechanism of complement activation in HD is the binding of MBL and ficolin-2 to the membrane, resulting in LP activation; while, simultaneously, properdin and/or C3b bind to the membrane resulting in AP activation (**Figure 2**). The latter is supported by the evidence that in C4-deficient patients, systemic complement activation and C3b deposition on the HD membrane are reduced during dialysis but not abolished (31). These results show the importance of the LP, while demonstrating the crucial contribution of the AP.

A second mechanism that could modulate complement activation during HD is the loss of complement inhibitors *via* absorption to the membrane. In HD, polysulfone membranes

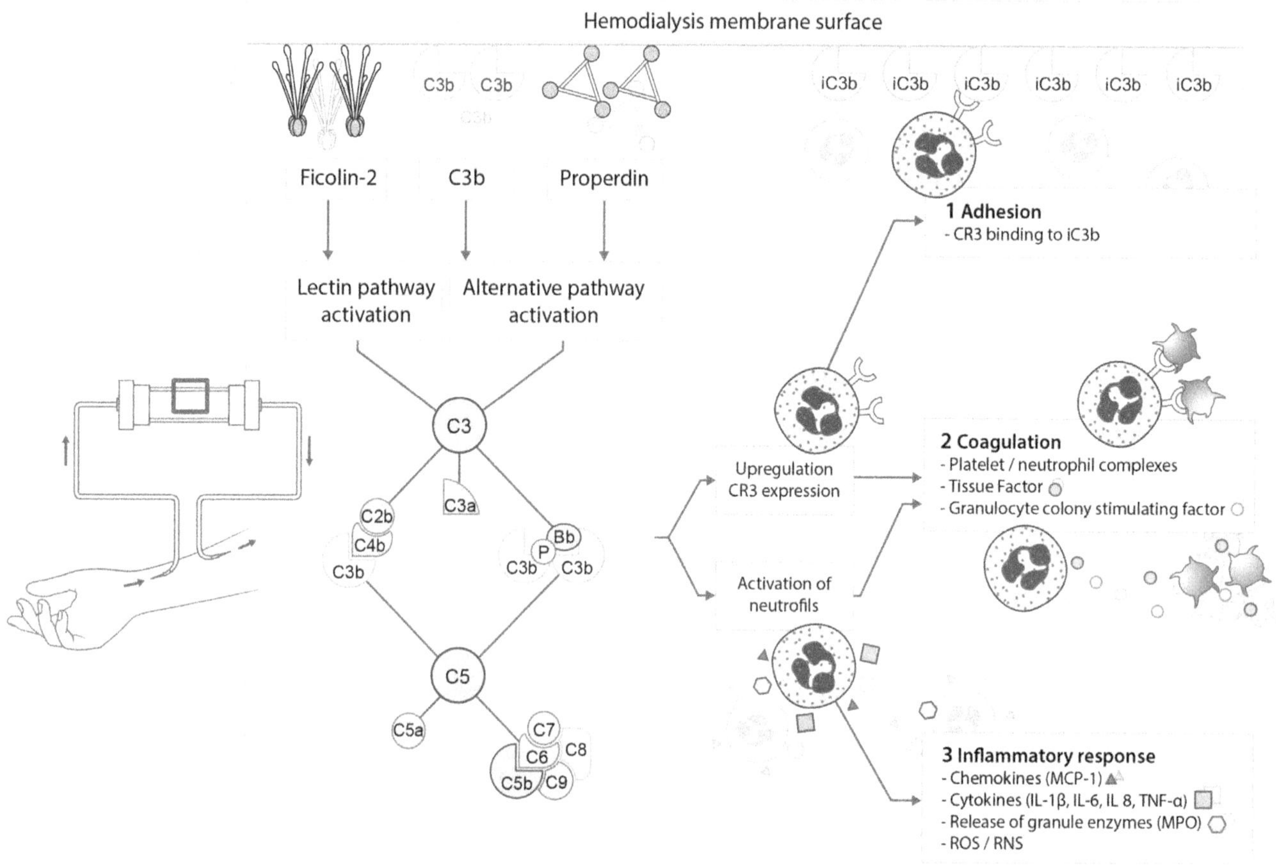

FIGURE 2 | Proposed model for complement activation in hemodialysis (HD). The principal mechanism leading to complement activation in HD is the binding of ficolin-2 to the membrane, resulting in lectin pathway activation. Simultaneously, properdin and/or C3b bind to the membrane resulting in alternative pathway activation. Complement activation will result in the formation of anaphylatoxins (C3a, C5a), opsonins (C3b, iC3b), and the membrane attack complex (C5b-9). First, complement activation leads to the upregulation of complement receptor 3 (CR3) allowing leukocytes to bind C3 fragments deposited on the membrane, leading to leukopenia. Second, CR3 on neutrophils is also important for the formation of platelet-neutrophil complexes, which contributes to thrombotic processes. Furthermore, C5a generation during HD leads to the expression of tissue factor and granulocyte colony-stimulating factor in neutrophils, shifting HD patients to a procoagulant state. Third, complement activation also promotes recruitment and activation of leukocytes resulting in the oxidative burst and the release of pro-inflammatory cytokines and chemokine's. More specifically, the activation of neutrophils by C5a leads to the release of granule enzymes, e.g., myeloperoxidase (MPO).

were shown to absorb factor H and clusterin (28, 33). Factor H is an important inhibitor of C3, while clusterin prevent terminal pathway activation thereby stopping the formation of C5a and C5b-9 (**Figure 1**) (14). The loss of these inhibitors would cause dysregulation of the AP, leading to further complement activation in the fluid phase (i.e., in the circulation) in HD patients.

Effector Functions and Clinical Implications of Complement Activation

Complement activation will lead to the generation of effector molecules, which can result in a variety of biological responses (14). In HD, the most important effector functions of complement activation are the induction of inflammation, promoting coagulation and impaired host defense due to accelerated consumption of complement proteins (20, 35, 36).

The generation of C3a and C5a during HD promotes recruitment and activation of leukocytes (37, 38). Leukocyte activation results in the oxidative burst and the release of pro-inflammatory cytokines and chemokine's, such as interleukin (IL)-1β, IL-6, IL-8, tumor necrosis factor-α, monocyte chemoattractant protein-1, and interferon-γ. More specifically, the activation of PMNs by C5a leads to the release of granule enzymes such as myeloperoxidase and elastase (39–41). Furthermore, complement activation in HD patients results in the upregulation of adhesion molecules on leukocytes, especially complement receptor 3 (CR3). The C5a-activated leukocytes will then bind C3 fragments (iC3b) deposited on the membrane *via* CR3, leading to leukopenia (20, 28, 39). Likewise, CR3 on PMNs is also important for the formation of platelet–PMN complexes, which can contribute to both inflammatory and thrombotic processes (42). The crosstalk between activation of the complement and coagulation system has correspondingly been described in HD. It has been demonstrated that C5a generation during HD leads to the expression of tissue factor and granulocyte colony-stimulating factor in PMNs, shifting HD patients to a procoagulative state (35). In conformity, plasma C3 levels have been shown to positively correlated with a denser clot structure in HD patients (43). On the other hand, the coagulation system has also been shown to impact complement activation (44).

Inflammation and coagulation are principally involved in the pathogenesis of cardiovascular disease. Accordingly, complement has been associated to the susceptibility to cardiovascular disease in HD patients (26, 27, 45–47). Plasma C3 levels, prior to a HD session, were found to be higher in patients who develop a cardiovascular event (CV-event) than HD patients who remained event-free. Moreover, an association was found between C3 levels and the development of CV-events (27). A similar trend of higher C3 levels in HD patients who develop a CV-event was seen in our study (26). A possible explanation would be that higher C3 levels prior to HD might reflect the potential for HD-evoked complement activation. Additionally, another association was found for baseline sC5b-9 levels with the occurrence of CV-events as well as mortality. This association was complex and showed an U-shaped relationship, indicating that both high and low sC5b-9 levels led to a higher risk, whereas HD patients with mid-range values were protected (27). Furthermore, a common factor H gene polymorphism was found to be an independent predictor of cardiovascular disease in HD patients (47). Homozygous HD patients for the Y402H polymorphism had an odds ratio of 7.28 for the development of CV-events compared to controls. This polymorphism affects the binding sites for heparin and C-reactive protein (CRP) and it has, therefore, been hypothesized that the reduced binding of factor H to the patient's endothelial cells would increase their risk of a CV-event. Alternatively, the link between the factor H polymorphism and the cardiovascular risk in HD patients could be mediated through CRP, since factor H binds CRP and thereby undermines its pro-inflammatory activity (48, 49). The Y402H polymorphism of factor H results in inadequate binding to CRP and thus leaves the pro-inflammatory activity of CRP unchecked. Furthermore, several studies have demonstrated that CRP levels in HD patients are associated to cardiovascular mortality (50–52). *Buraczynska* et al. revealed that in HD patients the complement receptor 1 (CR1) gene polymorphism C5507G is independently associated with the susceptibility for cardiovascular disease (46). Whether this effect is mediated *via* the complement inhibitory capacity of CR1 or *via* the recently discovered function of CR1 in the binding and clearance of native LDL remains to be elucidated (53). Another study showed that low serum C1q-adiponectin/C1q ratios were linked to cardiovascular disease in HD patients (45). The mechanism behind this connection is not understood but it has been demonstrated that adiponectin protects against activation of C1q-induced inflammation (54). Thus, in HD patients increased complement activation, as well as increased complement activity and the loss of complement inhibitors have all been linked to a higher risk of cardiovascular disease (**Table 1**). Recently, our group showed that low MBL levels are also associated with the occurrence of cardiovascular disease in HD patients (26). The higher risk in these patients was attributed to CV-events linked to atherosclerosis. In support of this, low MBL levels have been linked to enhanced arterial stiffness in HD patients (55). Accordingly, Satomura et al. demonstrated that low MBL levels were an independent predictor of all-cause mortality in HD patients (56). We, therefore, postulate that in HD patients, low MBL levels promote cardiovascular disease by enhancing atherosclerosis due to the inadequate removal of atherogenic particles.

In HD patients, little is known about the changes in complement components overtime. The plasma levels of C3 have been shown to decrease after 12 months compared to baseline (27). In this study, the C3 levels also negatively correlated with the dialysis vintage. In addition, the ability to activate complement has also been shown to be decreased in HD patients compared to healthy controls (23). In theory, these acquired deficiencies of complement proteins could explain the higher infection and sepsis risk seen in HD patients. Conversely, there was no association between low MBL levels and the risk of infection in HD patients (57). However, the authors concluded that this might be due to a compensation mechanism of higher ficolin-2 and MASP-2 levels in MBL-deficient individuals. Furthermore, another study found that long-term HD patients have decreased levels of clusterin, factor B and factor H compared to short-term HD patients (58). Thus far, no study has analyzed the link between HD-acquired complement deficiencies and infection risk. The clinical consequences of the HD-induced ficolin-2 reduction would be the most interesting to examine (28, 33). It is highly likely that this reduction would have a tremendous impact on HD patients' health and outcome. A genetic deficiency in ficolin-2 has not been reported to date, highlighting the essential function of this component within host defense. In conformity, ficolin-2 has been shown to be involved in the elimination of numerous pathogens (59).

Therapeutic Options

Several types of interventions have been proposed or tested in HD patients to decrease inflammation or target cardiovascular risk factors with mixed success. Hence, the clinical need for better therapeutic options that limit the inflammation and decrease cardiovascular risk in HD patients is on-going. The complement system is considered to be a promising target during HD to limit the inflammation and decrease cardiovascular risk (60). Therapies modulating HD-induced complement activation have focused on three treatment strategies: (1) reduction in the complement activating-capacity of the HD membrane; (2) the use of non-specific complement inhibitors (e.g., anticoagulants with a complement inhibitory property); and (3) specific complement-directed therapies.

Prevention is better than cure; therefore, creating a truly biocompatible membrane would, therefore, be ideal to prevent complement activation during HD. Much progress has been made with the development of more biologically compatible membranes by surface modifications and reducing protein retention. Today, the most common HD membranes contain sulfonyl-groups (7). To further improve biocompatibility, it is vital to understand the structures that initiate complement activation as it has the potential to develop HD membranes with enhanced biocompatibility. In modern HD membranes, ficolin-2 seems to

TABLE 1 | The association between complement proteins and morbidity and mortality in HD patients.

Study	Complement protein	Outcome	Association[a]	Possible mechanism
Poppelaars et al. (26, 67)	MBL levels	CV-events	Low MBL levels OR = 3.98 (1.88–8.24)	Low MBL levels promote atherosclerosis due to the inadequate removal of atherogenic particles
Satomura et al. (56)	MBL levels	All-cause mortality	Low MBL levels OR = 7.63 (2.24–25.96)	Low MBL levels promote atherosclerosis due to the inadequate removal of atherogenic particles
Kishida et al. (45)	C1q-adiponectin levels	CV-events	Low C1q-adiponectin levels	Adiponectin protects against activation of C1q-induced inflammation
Lines et al. (27)	C3 levels	CV-events	Higher C3 levels (per 0.1 mg/ml) HR = 1.20 (1.01–1.42)	Increased complement activity
Lines et al. (27)	sC5b-9 levels	CV-events	Low and high sC5b-9 levels U-shaped relationship	(1) Increased complement activation. (2) Complement depletion by local complement activation on the HD membrane
		All-cause mortality	Low and high sC5b-9 levels U-shaped relationship	
Buraczynska et al. (47)	Factor H gene polymorphism (Y402H)	CV-events	The CC genotype OR = 7.28 (5.32–9.95)	(1) The loss of complement inhibition, leading to complement activation. (2) Reduced binding of factor H to endothelial cells.
Buraczynska et al. (46)	CR1 gene polymorphism (C5507G)	CV-events	The GG genotype OR = 3.44 (2.23–5.3)	(1) The loss of complement inhibition, leading to complement activation. (2) Reduced binding and clearance of native low-density lipoprotein by CR1.

[a]*Data are presented as hazard or OR plus 95% confidence interval.*
OR, odds ratio; HR, hazard ratio; HD, hemodialysis; MBL, mannose-binding lectin; CR1, complement receptor 1; CV-event, cardiovascular event; sC5b-9, soluble C5b-9.

be an important mediator in HD-induced complement activation (28, 33). Ficolin-2 is unfortunately a highly promiscuous molecule with numerous binding partners, several of which are acetylated compounds (59).

Anticoagulants have been used extensively to render biomaterial-blood incompatibility, through inhibition of the coagulation, contact and complement system. The effect of citrate anticoagulation on complement activation has widely been studied in HD. Citrate has calcium-chelating properties and thereby reduces complement activation (61, 62). During the initial phase of HD with cellulose membranes, citrate anticoagulation reduced C3a levels by almost 50% compared to heparin (63). However, no complement inhibition was seen by citrate anticoagulation during HD in other studies with cellulose or synthetic membranes (64–66). Heparinoids are also known to prevent complement activation, although this inhibition is strictly concentration dependent (67). Although heparin has been tested extensively in HD, sadly none of these studies determined the effect on complement activation.

In the past decade, numerous complement inhibitors have been developed; two are currently used in the clinics and others are now undergoing clinical trials. Purified C1 esterase inhibitor (C1-INH) is a protease that is clinically used to treat hereditary angioedema. Eculizumab, a C5 antibody is used for the treatment of paroxysmal nocturnal hemoglobinuria and atypical hemolytic uremic syndrome (14, 68). In HD, specific complement-directed therapies have predominantly been evaluated in experimental settings, still valuable information has been uncovered and shown that the use of complement inhibitors are a promising tool to reduce the inflammatory response and subsequent consequences in these patients (60). The potential of complement inhibition in HD is further underlined by the successful use of complement inhibitors for biomaterial-induced complement activation in cardiopulmonary bypass systems (19). In patients undergoing cardiopulmonary bypass surgery, treatment with soluble CR1 (sCR1/TP30), an inhibitor of C3, lead to a decrease in mortality and morbidity as well as a reduced need for intra-aortic balloon pump support (69). Consequently, soluble complement inhibitors may be equally effective in HD, since there is the recurrent need of complement inhibition for short periods. Specifically, the short half-life of sCR1 matches the need for restricted complement inhibition in HD, which is only needed during dialysis, after which complement activity should be reestablished between sessions. This approach would also prevent complications of long-term immunosuppression. In a pre-clinical monkey model of HD, another C3-inhibitor (compstatin) was used to attenuate HD-induced complement activation (70). Despite the use of HD membranes with high biocompatibility and standard heparin treatment in their study, severe complement activation still occurred in monkeys. In this study, animals received a bolus injection prior to the HD and a continuous infusion of compstatin during the 4 h HD procedure. Treatment completely blocked complement activation and C3 activation products stayed at basal levels throughout the HD session. Strikingly, a second treatment regimen with only a bolus injection of compstatin at the start of the session was also sufficient to abolished complement activation throughout the procedure. Furthermore, complement inhibition lead to the increase of IL-10, an anti-inflammatory cytokine. Unfortunately, the effect of complement inhibition on other inflammatory markers could not be assessed, since one HD session was insufficient to induce substantial levels of pro-inflammatory cytokines. Next to inhibition of the central component C3, blockage of early complement components may be equally successful. C1-INH forms a therapeutic option, since HD leads to LP activation and C1-INH could attenuate this (67). Additionally, C1-INH also affects the coagulation and contact system, which could add to the success of this therapeutic approach. Given the strong involvement of complement activation effector molecules in HD, more specifically C5a, another attractive option would be the inhibition of C5 or C5a-receptor antagonists (C5aRA) (35). This could be either done by the anti-C5 antibody or by C5aRA. Eculizmab blocks the generation of C5a and C5b-9 and could thus be more effective than C5aRA. However, the long half-life and the high costs form important disadvantages. In contrast, C5aRA tends to be more cost-effective (71). These drugs could significantly reduce activation of leukocytes and thereby inflammation in HD. Currently, the most likely candidate to be used in HD is PMX-53, a C5aRA, since this compound is currently tested in different clinical trials (72). Another promising approach is coating biomaterials with complement inhibitors (20). One of these molecules, the 5C6 peptide is a molecule that has strong binding affinity toward factor H without modifying its inhibitory activity. More importantly, polystyrene surfaces coated with 5C6 were shown to bind factor H and thereby prevent complement activation when exposed to human plasma, thus enhancing biocompatibility (73). However, it is unknown whether the reduction of systemic factor H levels by 5C6 during HD could have undesirable consequences, such as seen in factor H-deficient individuals. Finally, the cost of the different complement inhibitors should be taken into account, considering the high frequency of treatments required in HD patients.

PERITONEAL DIALYSIS

Peritoneal dialysis is the most common used dialysis technique at home and is equally effective as HD for the treatment of CKD (74). Nevertheless, the advantages of PD include; better preservation of residual renal function, lower infectious risk and higher satisfaction rates. Despite the good results seen with PD, this dialysis technique remains underused (1). In PD, unlike in HD, no synthetic membrane is used. In contrast, the peritoneum in the abdominal cavity of the patients acts as a semi-permeable membrane allowing diffusion between the dialysis fluid and the circulation. The osmotic gradient during PD is based on high glucose levels in the dialysate. However, glucose acts as a double edge sword, since it serves as an osmotic agent but it is also responsible for the incompatibility reaction. The peritoneal membrane is made up of an inner mesothelial layer and these cells are, therefore, directly in contact with the dialysis fluid. Long-term exposure to dialysate leads to tissue remodeling of this layer resulting in peritoneal fibrosis (75). This progressive fibrosis forms a major limitation for chronic PD treatment. Another common complication in PD is peritonitis (76). Patients who develop peritonitis can have irreversible peritoneum damage, PD failure and significant morbidity or even mortality. For this reason, avoiding PD failure due to peritonitis or fibrosis remains a challenge for nephrologists (77).

Complement Activation in PD

The link between the complement system and PD seems less obvious, because there is no direct contact with blood. However, mesothelial cells produce and secrete different complement factors, including C4, C3, and C5 till C9 (78, 79). In accordance, different studies have found the presence of complement in the peritoneal dialysate. Additionally, the amount of C3 in the PD fluid does not depend on the serum concentration, suggesting that the C3 originates from local production (80). The study by Oliveira et al. found strong protein abundance of Factor D in six adult PD patients (81), whereas a similar approach in 76 PD patients by Wen et al. found significant protein expression of C4 and C3 only (82). Altogether, proteomic analyses of the dialysate of healthy PD patients has revealed the presence of C4, C3, Factor B, Factor D, Factor H, Factor I, and C9 (81–85). Proteomic profiling in the peritoneal fluid of children identified a total number of 189 proteins, of which 18 complement components (84). The discrepancies between the various proteomic studies could be explained by differences in the underlying cause of renal failure, since diabetic patients on PD have been shown to have lower levels of C4 in the dialysate compared to controls (83). Obviously, other patient's characteristics such as ethnicity and differences in the accuracy and sensitive of the analysis have to be taken into account as well. Complement production by mesothelial cells has been shown to be increased in uremic patients and it can be further stimulated upon exposure to PD solutions containing glucose (78, 79). Next to complement production; mesothelial cells also express important complement regulators; e.g., MCP, DAF, and CD59 (79, 80).

Systemically, PD patients have lower MBL levels compared to HD patients and healthy controls, even after adjusting for the effect of mutations (86). This could indicate loss of systemic MBL *via* the peritoneal route, independent of the reduced renal function. However, MBL has so far not been assessed in peritoneal dialysates. Furthermore, serum levels of C1q, C4, C3d, factor D, and properdin were shown to be higher in pediatric PD patients compared to healthy controls, however, not in comparison to patients with ESKD (87). Overall, the higher plasma levels of the complement components are likely caused by increased synthesis by the liver due to the pro-inflammatory state in ESKD patients. Moreover, the increased levels of C3d in PD patients are believed to be the consequence of reduced elimination of factor D by the kidney, creating enhanced AP activation. However, while systemic complement activation (the fluid phase) is similar between PD patients and patients with ESKD, higher intravascular complement depositions (solid phase) have been shown in children with PD compared to non-PD children with ESKD. Omental and parietal arterioles from PD patients demonstrated a higher presence of C1q, C3d, and C5b-9 (88).

Evidence has also been provided for complement activation in the peritoneal cavity in PD patients (80, 89). Previously, it was demonstrated that the dialysate/serum ratios of factor D and C3d were elevated in PD, whereas the dialysate/serum ratios of C3, C4, and properdin were decreased (89). The high dialysate levels of C3d demonstrate local complement activation, while the comparatively low dialysate/serum ratios of complement components are likely caused by intraperitoneal complement consumption. In accordance, the presence of sC5b-9 in the peritoneal dialysate has also been shown. In the dialysate of PD patients, sC5b-9 levels up to 200 pg/μg of total protein level have been reported (80). Considering the high molecular weight of sC5b-9 (>1,000 kDa), it is very likely that the sC5b-9 in the dialysate is produced in the peritoneal cavity and does not originate from the circulation.

One of the proposed mechanisms of complement activation in PD patients is that PD therapy modifies the expression of complement regulators on the peritoneal mesothelium, leading to local complement activation (**Figure 3**). In accordance, CD55 expression is lower on mesothelial cells from PD patients than non-CKD patients and the reduced expression of CD55 is accompanied by higher peritoneal levels of sC5b-9 (80). Likewise, complement regulators were also shown to be downregulated in arterioles of PD patients. Furthermore, the C5b-9 deposition seen in the arterioles of PD patients correlated with the level of dialytic glucose exposure (88). However, this is probably not the only mechanism responsible for complement activation in PD patients. Hypothetically, cellular debris as a result of direct peritoneal damage by bioincompatible PD fluids as well as antibodies against microorganisms could contribute to local complement activation during PD. Unfortunately, most of the reviewed studies are relatively old and there is, therefore, a need for novel studies to assess the effect of newer PD solutions on complement production and activation.

Effector Functions and Clinical Implications of Complement Activation

During PD, complement activation occurs locally within the peritoneal cavity and leads to the generation of opsonins, anaphylatoxins, and the MAC. The effects of complement activation during PD include the induction of tissue injury, inflammation, coagulation, and fibrosis. However, complement activation in PD patients has also been linked to long-term effects such as cardiovascular risk (88). In different experimental models, complement

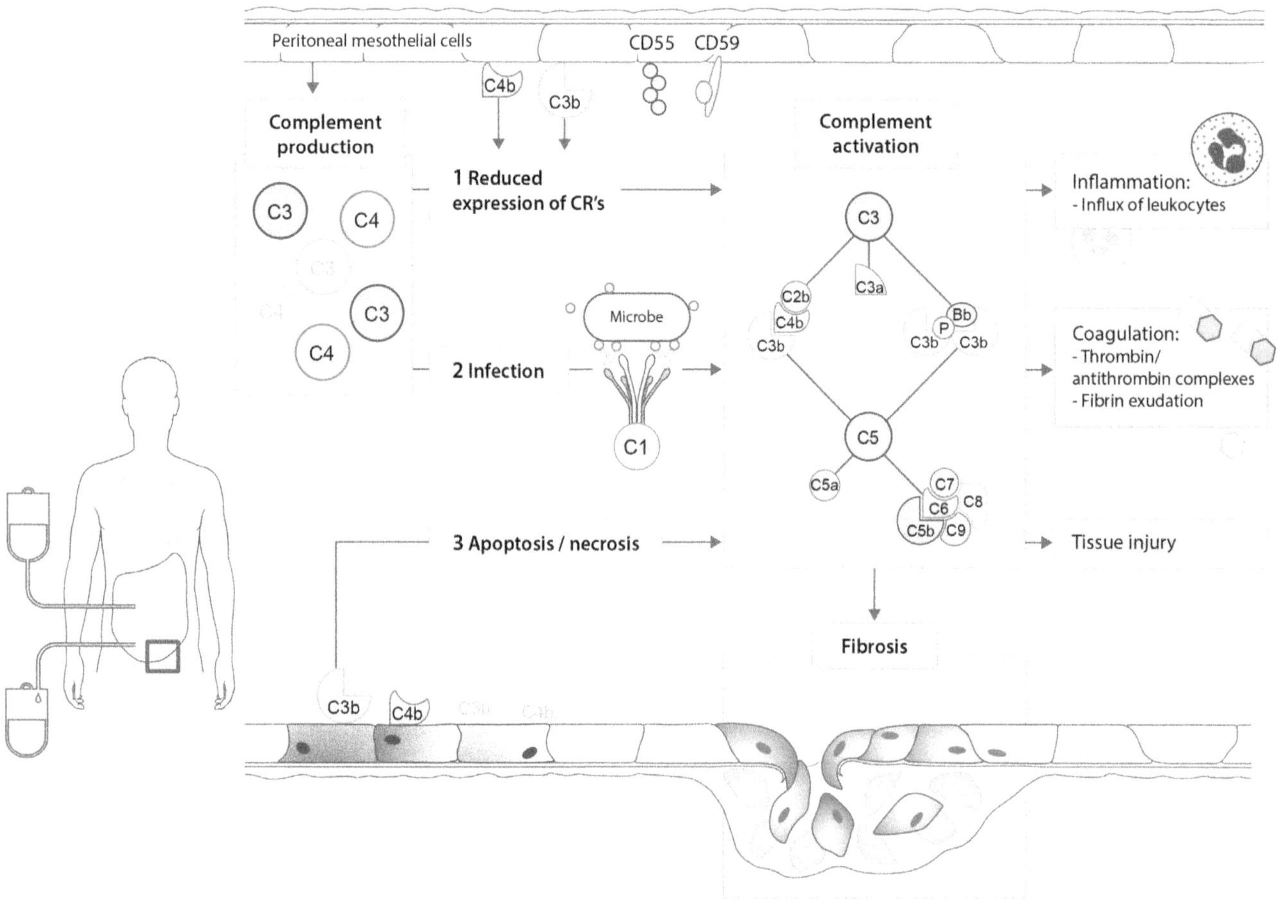

FIGURE 3 | Proposed model for complement activation in peritoneal dialysis (PD). In PD patients, mesothelial cells produce and secrete different complement factors. One of the proposed mechanisms of complement activation in PD patients is that PD therapy decreases the expression of complement regulators such as CD55 and CD59 on the peritoneal mesothelium, leading to local complement activation. In addition, cellular debris as a result of direct peritoneal damage by bioincompatible PD fluids as well as antibodies against microorganisms could contribute to local complement activation during PD. Complement activation will result in the formation of anaphylatoxins (C3a, C5a), opsonins (C3b, iC3b), and the membrane attack complex (C5b-9). First, complement activation leads to the influx of leukocytes, predominantly neutrophils. Second, complement activation increased the production of thrombin anti-thrombin complexes and fibrin exudation on the surface of the injured peritoneum. Altogether, these events indicate the activation of the coagulation system. Third, complement activation during PD leads to direct damage of the peritoneum. Moreover, recent evidence suggests that complement activation promotes the progression to fibrosis after tissue injury. In PD, complement activation could stimulate mesothelial cells to undergo epithelial-to-mesenchymal transition, resulting in the accumulation of myofibroblasts and consequently peritoneal fibrosis.

activation during PD leads to direct damage of the peritoneum. The complement-induced peritoneal damage seems to be mediated *via* activation of the terminal pathway, specifically C5a and C5b-9 (90–92). Additionally, complement activation leads to inflammation. In a rat model of peritoneal fluid infusion, the numbers of neutrophils increased significantly overtime, and this process was largely dependent on C5 activation. In conformity, intraperitoneal injections with C3a and C5a in mice lead to the influx of leukocytes, predominantly neutrophils (93). The effect of C5a is mediated *via* C5aR1, while the effect of C3a is presumably mediated *via* the C3a-receptor. The crosstalk between activation of the complement and coagulation system has also been described in PD. Thrombin anti-thrombin complexes increased significantly in experimental models of PD and this process was partly dependent on C5 activation (92). Mizuno et al. showed that intraperitoneal complement activation leads to fibrin exudation on the surface of the injured peritoneum (94). Altogether these findings indicate that activation of the coagulation system by the PD therapy is at least (partly) complement dependent. The fibrin exudate can also be a sign of PD-associated fibrosis.

The link between fibrosis and complement is relatively new; nevertheless, recent evidence suggests that complement activation promotes the progression to fibrosis after tissue injury (95). In PD, high peritoneal transport is associated with progression of peritoneal fibrosis (96). Proteomics analysis of PD fluid showed enhanced expression of C3 in patients with high transporter status, while expression of C4 is lower in low transporters (82, 97). Furthermore, in PD mesothelial cells undergo epithelial-to-mesenchymal transition, resulting in the accumulation of myofibroblasts and consequently peritoneal fibrosis (98). In other disease models, complement has been shown to induce epithelial-to-mesenchymal transition (99). This effect is mediated *via* the C5aR1, since in rodent models of infection-induced peritoneal fibrosis $C5aR1^{-/-}$ mice were protected against fibrosis (100). The C5aR1 is also involved in the production of profibrotic and inflammatory mediators by peritoneal leukocytes (100). In addition, Bartosova et al. reported that in the peritoneal arterioles of PD patient's, high abundance of complement deposition was found to correlate with TGF-b signaling (88). More specifically, C1q and C5b-9 deposition were associated with an increased phosphorylation of SMAD2/3, and enhanced vasculopathy. Interestingly, the TGF-b–SMAD pathway has also been recently linked to cardiovascular disease (101). Encapsulating peritoneal sclerosis is another long-term complication of PD, which is the result of abnormal thickening and fibrosis of the peritoneum, leading to a fibrous cocoon thereby encapsulating the intestines causing obstruction (102). The exact cause of this rare complication is unknown, but it is linked to the bioincompatibility of the glucose-based PD solutions (103). The bioincompatibility of these solutions presumably promotes the expression TGF-b, thereby stimulating the transition of mesothelial cells to myofibroblasts. Recently, a prospective proteomics study identified complement components as a possible biomarker of encapsulating peritoneal sclerosis (85). Factors B and factor I were elevated in the PD fluid of patients up to 5 years prior to developing encapsulating peritoneal sclerosis. In patients with stable membrane function, factor I was present in the PD fluid in lower amounts and decreased overtime, while factor B was barely detectable in the PD fluid of controls. However, whether the elevated levels of these complement factors are merely an acute phase response or involved in the pathogenesis remains to be investigated. Yet, based on the current literature, complement activation is likely to play a role in the mechanisms of peritoneal fibrosis. Nevertheless, additional studies are needed to further elucidate the specific role of the complement system in this process.

Peritonitis is another common complication with significant morbidity and mortality. Complement has been proposed to be involved in the risk of PD patients for peritonitis. First, a variation in the FCN2 gene was shown to be more prevalent in PD patients with a history of peritonitis (104). In addition, local activation will lead to a further decline of already low levels of complement components in PD fluid and may thereby additionally impair host defense. Complement activation products have also been suggested as a biomarker during peritonitis. Mizuno et al. showed that C4, C3, and sC5b-9 levels in the peritoneal fluid are significantly higher in PD patients with poor prognosis after peritonitis (105). Complement markers in peritoneal fluid have, therefore, the potential to serve as a biomarker for the prediction of the prognosis of PD-related peritonitis. Finally, the risk of peritonitis could form a major Achilles heel for complement inhibition in PD.

Therapeutic Options

Treatment aimed at attenuating or blocking complement activation in PD has mostly focused on the terminal pathway. The advantage of this approach is the elimination effector functions of C5a and/or C5b-9, while proximal complement functions stay intact. *In vitro*, inhibition of the C5aR1 on peritoneal leukocytes, isolated from PD fluid, reduced bacteria-induced profibrotic (TGF-β) and inflammatory (IL-6 and IL-8) mediator production (100). In addition, the systemic administration of a C5aR1 antagonist in a rat model of PD prevented influx of inflammatory cells and reduced tissue damage of the peritoneal cavity (91). Furthermore, blockage of C5 in PD improved ultrafiltration and additionally reduced activation of the blood clotting system (92). Other studies have confirmed these results; showing that C5 blockade significantly increased the ultrafiltration volume *via* reduced peritoneal glucose transport, most likely by preventing C5a-induced vasodilatation (106). In contrast, C3 inhibition through complement depletion by cobra venom factor, also led to diminished chemoattractant release, neutrophil recruitment and enhanced ultrafiltration (106). Anticoagulants have also been tested for the treatment of the inflammatory reaction to PD fluids (106, 107). The addition of low-molecular-weight heparin to the PD fluid not only prevented thrombin formation but also inhibited the complement activation, neutrophil recruitment, and improved ultrafiltration (107). In brief, results about complement inhibition in PD look promising, but many hurdles remain to be solved.

CONCLUSION

In conclusion, biocompatibility remains an important clinical challenge within dialysis. Due to bioincompatibility, complement is systemically activated during HD, while PD leads to local complement activation. Moreover, important effector functions of complement activation include promoting inflammation and coagulation. In addition, long-term complications of dialysis, such as infection, fibrosis, and cardiovascular events, are linked to the complement system. These results indicate the possibility for complement interventions in dialysis to improve biocompatibility, dialysis efficacy, and long-term outcome.

AUTHOR CONTRIBUTIONS

FP and MG performed the literature search. MD, SB, and MS helped with the interpretation of the literature. BF and CF provided the review with clinical information and the clinical relevance. FP, BF, and MG wrote the review. WS, CF, SB, MD, and MS critically reviewed the manuscript prior to submission.

REFERENCES

1. Robinson BM, Akizawa T, Jager KJ, Kerr PG, Saran R, Pisoni RL. Factors affecting outcomes in patients reaching end-stage kidney disease worldwide: differences in access to renal replacement therapy, modality use, and haemodialysis practices. *Lancet* (2016) 388:294–306. doi:10.1016/S0140-6736(16)30448-2
2. Yeates K, Zhu N, Vonesh E, Trpeski L, Blake P, Fenton S. Hemodialysis and peritoneal dialysis are associated with similar outcomes for end-stage renal disease treatment in Canada. *Nephrol Dial Transplant* (2012) 27:3568–75. doi:10.1093/ndt/gfr674
3. Weiner DE, Tighiouart H, Amin MG, Stark PC, MacLeod B, Griffith JL, et al. Chronic kidney disease as a risk factor for cardiovascular disease and all-cause mortality: a pooled analysis of community-based studies. *J Am Soc Nephrol* (2004) 15:1307–15. doi:10.1097/01.ASN.0000123691.46138.E2
4. Ekdahl KN, Soveri I, Hilborn J, Fellström B, Nilsson B. Cardiovascular disease in haemodialysis: role of the intravascular innate immune system. *Nat Rev Nephrol* (2017) 13:285–96. doi:10.1038/nrneph.2017.17
5. Jofré R, Rodriguez-Benitez P, Ló Pez-Gó Mez JM, Pérez-Garcia R. Inflammatory syndrome in patients on hemodialysis. *J Am Soc Nephrol* (2006) 17:274–80. doi:10.1681/ASN.2006080926
6. Williams DF. On the mechanisms of biocompatibility. *Biomaterials* (2008) 29:2941–53. doi:10.1016/j.biomaterials.2008.04.023
7. Kokubo K, Kurihara Y, Kobayashi K, Tsukao H, Kobayashi H. Evaluation of the biocompatibility of dialysis membranes. *Blood Purif* (2015) 40:293–7. doi:10.1159/000441576
8. Cho Y, Johnson DW, Craig JC, Strippoli GF, Badve SV, Wiggins KJ. Biocompatible dialysis fluids for peritoneal dialysis. In: Cho Y, editor. *Cochrane Database of Systematic Reviews*. UK: John Wiley & Sons, Ltd. (2014) CD007554 p.
9. Chaudhary K, Khanna R. Biocompatible peritoneal dialysis solutions: do we have one? *Clin J Am Soc Nephrol* (2010) 5:723–32. doi:10.2215/CJN.05720809
10. Helmus MN, Gibbons DF, Cebon D. Biocompatibility: meeting a key functional requirement of next-generation medical devices. *Toxicol Pathol* (2008) 36:70–80. doi:10.1177/0192623307310949
11. Christo SN, Diener KR, Bachhuka A, Vasilev K, Hayball JD. Innate immunity and biomaterials at the Nexus: friends or foes. *Biomed Res Int* (2015) 2015:342304. doi:10.1155/2015/342304
12. Gorbet MB, Sefton MV. Biomaterial-associated thrombosis: roles of coagulation factors, complement, platelets and leukocytes. *Biomaterials* (2004) 25:5681–703. doi:10.1016/j.biomaterials.2004.01.023
13. Love RJ, Jones KS. Biomaterials, fibrosis, and the use of drug delivery systems in future antifibrotic strategies. *Crit Rev Biomed Eng* (2009) 37:259–81. doi:10.1615/CritRevBiomedEng.v37.i3.20
14. Ricklin D, Hajishengallis G, Yang K, Lambris JD. Complement: a key system for immune surveillance and homeostasis. *Nat Immunol* (2010) 11:785–97. doi:10.1038/ni.1923
15. Hein E, Munthe-Fog L, Thiara AS, Fiane AE, Mollnes TE, Garred P. Heparin-coated cardiopulmonary bypass circuits selectively deplete the pattern recognition molecule ficolin-2 of the lectin complement pathway *in vivo*. *Clin Exp Immunol* (2015) 179:294–9. doi:10.1111/cei.12446
16. Lappegård KT, Enebakk T, Thunhaug H, Ludviksen JK, Mollnes TE, Hovland A. LDL apheresis activates the complement system and the cytokine network, whereas PCSK9 inhibition with evolocumab induces no inflammatory response. *J Clin Lipidol* (2016) 10:1481–7. doi:10.1016/j.jacl.2016.09.001
17. Burnouf T, Eber M, Kientz D, Cazenave J-P, Burkhardt T. Assessment of complement activation during membrane-based plasmapheresis procedures. *J Clin Apher* (2004) 19:142–7. doi:10.1002/jca.20019
18. Eskandary F, Wahrmann M, Biesenbach P, Sandurkov C, Konig F, Schwaiger E, et al. ABO antibody and complement depletion by immunoadsorption combined with membrane filtration – a randomized, controlled, cross-over trial. *Nephrol Dial Transplant* (2014) 29:706–14. doi:10.1093/ndt/gft502
19. Kourtzelis I, Rafail S, DeAngelis RA, Foukas PG, Ricklin D, Lambris JD. Inhibition of biomaterial-induced complement activation attenuates the inflammatory host response to implantation. *FASEB J* (2013) 27:2768–76. doi:10.1096/fj.12-225888
20. Nilsson B, Ekdahl KN, Mollnes TE, Lambris JD. The role of complement in biomaterial-induced inflammation. *Mol Immunol* (2007) 44:82–94. doi:10.1016/j.molimm.2006.06.020
21. Kerr PG, Huang L. Review: membranes for haemodialysis. *Nephrology (Carlton)* (2010) 15:381–5. doi:10.1111/j.1440-1797.2010.01331.x
22. Craddock PR, Fehr J, Brigham KL, Kronenberg RS, Jacob HS. Complement and leukocyte-mediated pulmonary dysfunction in hemodialysis. *N Engl J Med* (1977) 296:769–74. doi:10.1056/NEJM197704072961401
23. Hempel JC, Poppelaars F, Gaya Da Costa M, Franssen CF, de Vlaam TP, Daha MR, et al. Distinct in vitro complement activation by various intravenous iron preparations. *Am J Nephrol* (2017) 45:49–59. doi:10.1159/000451060
24. Szebeni J. Complement activation-related pseudoallergy: a stress reaction in blood triggered by nanomedicines and biologicals. *Mol Immunol* (2014) 61:163–73. doi:10.1016/j.molimm.2014.06.038
25. Chenoweth DE, Cheung AK, Henderson LW. Anaphylatoxin formation during hemodialysis: effects of different dialyzer membranes. *Kidney Int* (1983) 24:764–9. doi:10.1038/ki.1983.225
26. Poppelaars F, Gaya da Costa M, Berger SP, Assa S, Meter-Arkema AH, Daha MR, et al. Strong predictive value of mannose-binding lectin levels for cardiovascular risk of hemodialysis patients. *J Transl Med* (2016) 14:236. doi:10.1186/s12967-016-0995-5
27. Lines SW, Richardson VR, Thomas B, Dunn EJ, Wright MJ, Carter AM. Complement and cardiovascular disease – the missing link in haemodialysis patients. *Nephron* (2015) 132:5–14. doi:10.1159/000442426
28. Mares J, Richtrova P, Hricinova A, Tuma Z, Moravec J, Lysak D, et al. Proteomic profiling of blood-dialyzer interactome reveals involvement of lectin complement pathway in hemodialysis-induced inflammatory response. *Proteomics Clin Appl* (2010) 4:829–38. doi:10.1002/prca.201000031
29. Cheung AK, Parker CJ, Wilcox L, Janatova J. Activation of the alternative pathway of complement by cellulosic hemodialysis membranes. *Kidney Int* (1989) 36:257–65. doi:10.1038/ki.1989.188
30. Hauser AC, Derfler K, Stockenhuber F, Janata O, Balcke P. Generation of the membrane attack complex during haemodialysis: impact of classical and alternative pathway components. *Clin Sci (Lond)* (1990) 79:471–6. doi:10.1042/cs0790471
31. Lhotta K, Würzner R, Kronenberg F, Oppermann M, König P. Rapid activation of the complement system by cuprophane depends on complement component C4. *Kidney Int* (1998) 53:1044–51. doi:10.1111/j.1523-1755.1998.00836.x
32. Innes A, Farrell AM, Burden RP, Morgan AG, Powell RJ. Complement activation by cellulosic dialysis membranes. *J Clin Pathol* (1994) 47:155–8. doi:10.1136/jcp.47.2.155
33. Mares J, Thongboonkerd V, Tuma Z, Moravec J, Matejovic M. Specific adsorption of some complement activation proteins to polysulfone dialysis membranes during hemodialysis. *Kidney Int* (2009) 76:404–13. doi:10.1038/ki.2009.138
34. Inoshita H, Ohsawa I, Onda K, Tamano M, Horikoshi S, Ohi H, et al. An analysis of functional activity via the three complement pathways during hemodialysis sessions: a new insight into the association between the lectin pathway and C5 activation. *Clin Kidney J* (2012) 5:401–4. doi:10.1093/ckj/sfs089

35. Kourtzelis I, Markiewski MM, Doumas M, Rafail S, Kambas K, Mitroulis I, et al. Complement anaphylatoxin C5a contributes to hemodialysis-associated thrombosis. *Blood* (2010) 116:631–9. doi:10.1182/blood-2010-01-264051
36. Sharif MR, Chitsazian Z, Moosavian M, Raygan F, Nikoueinejad H, Sharif AR, et al. Immune disorders in hemodialysis patients. *Iran J Kidney Dis* (2015) 9:84–96.
37. Johnson RJ, Burhop KE, Van Epps DE. Infusion of ovine C5a into sheep mimics the inflammatory response of hemodialysis. *J Lab Clin Med* (1996) 127:456–69. doi:10.1016/S0022-2143(96)90063-3
38. Rousseau Y, Carreno MP, Poignet JL, Kazatchkine MD, Haeffner-Cavaillon N. Dissociation between complement activation, integrin expression and neutropenia during hemodialysis. *Biomaterials* (1999) 20:1959–67. doi:10.1016/S0142-9612(99)00101-5
39. Bergseth G, Lambris JD, Mollnes TE, Lappegård KT. Artificial surface-induced inflammation relies on complement factor 5: proof from a deficient person. *Ann Thorac Surg* (2011) 91:527–33. doi:10.1016/j.athoracsur.2010.10.084
40. Lin YF, Chang DM, Shaio MF, Lu KC, Chyr SH, Li BL, et al. Cytokine production during hemodialysis: effects of dialytic membrane and complement activation. *Am J Nephrol* (1996) 16:293–9. doi:10.1159/000169012
41. Lappegard KT, Christiansen D, Pharo A, Thorgersen EB, Hellerud BC, Lindstad J, et al. Human genetic deficiencies reveal the roles of complement in the inflammatory network: lessons from nature. *Proc Natl Acad Sci U S A* (2009) 106:15861–6. doi:10.1073/pnas.0903613106
42. Hamad OA, Mitroulis I, Fromell K, Kozarcanin H, Chavakis T, Ricklin D, et al. Contact activation of C3 enables tethering between activated platelets and polymorphonuclear leukocytes via CD11b/CD18. *Thromb Haemost* (2015) 114:1207–17. doi:10.1160/TH15-02-0162
43. Schuett K, Savvaidis A, Maxeiner S, Lysaja K, Jankowski V, Schirmer SH, et al. Clot structure: a potent mortality risk factor in patients on hemodialysis. *J Am Soc Nephrol* (2017) 28(5):1622–30. doi:10.1681/ASN.2016030336
44. Wiegner R, Chakraborty S, Huber-Lang M. Complement-coagulation cross-talk on cellular and artificial surfaces. *Immunobiology* (2016) 221:1073–9. doi:10.1016/j.imbio.2016.06.005
45. Kishida K, Kishida N, Arima M, Nakatsuji H, Kobayashi H, Funahashi T, et al. Serum C1q-binding adiponectin in maintenance hemodialysis patients. *BMC Nephrol* (2013) 14:50. doi:10.1186/1471-2369-14-50
46. Buraczynska M, Ksiazek P, Wacinski P, Zukowski P, Dragan M, Bednarek-Skublewska A. Complement receptor 1 gene polymorphism and cardiovascular disease in dialyzed end-stage renal disease patients. *Hum Immunol* (2010) 71:878–82. doi:10.1016/j.humimm.2010.06.001
47. Buraczynska M, Ksiazek P, Zukowski P, Benedyk-Lorens E, Orlowska-Kowalik G. Complement factor H gene polymorphism and risk of cardiovascular disease in end-stage renal disease patients. *Clin Immunol* (2009) 132:285–90. doi:10.1016/j.clim.2009.04.005
48. Okemefuna AI, Nan R, Miller A, Gor J, Perkins SJ. Complement factor H binds at two independent sites to C-reactive protein in acute phase concentrations. *J Biol Chem* (2010) 285:1053–65. doi:10.1074/jbc.M109.044529
49. Molins B, Fuentes-Prior P, Adán A, Antón R, Arostegui JI, Yagüe J, et al. Complement factor H binding of monomeric C-reactive protein downregulates proinflammatory activity and is impaired with at risk polymorphic CFH variants. *Sci Rep* (2016) 6:22889. doi:10.1038/srep22889
50. Zimmermann J, Herrlinger S, Pruy A, Metzger T, Wanner C. Inflammation enhances cardiovascular risk and mortality in hemodialysis patients. *Kidney Int* (1999) 55:648–58. doi:10.1046/j.1523-1755.1999.00273.x
51. Yeun JY, Levine RA, Mantadilok V, Kaysen GA. C-reactive protein predicts all-cause and cardiovascular mortality in hemodialysis patients. *Am J Kidney Dis* (2000) 35:469–76. doi:10.1016/S0272-6386(00)70200-9
52. Wanner C, Zimmermann J, Schwedler S, Metzger T. Inflammation and cardiovascular risk in dialysis patients. *Kidney Int* (2002) 61:S99–102. doi:10.1046/j.1523-1755.61.s80.18.x
53. Klop B, van der Pol P, van Bruggen R, Wang Y, de Vries MA, van Santen S, et al. Differential complement activation pathways promote C3b deposition on native and acetylated LDL thereby inducing lipoprotein binding to the complement receptor 1. *J Biol Chem* (2014) 289:35421–30. doi:10.1074/jbc.M114.573840
54. Ebina K, Oshima K, Matsuda M, Fukuhara A, Maeda K, Kihara S, et al. Adenovirus-mediated gene transfer of adiponectin reduces the severity of collagen-induced arthritis in mice. *Biochem Biophys Res Commun* (2009) 378:186–91. doi:10.1016/j.bbrc.2008.11.005
55. Hornum M, Bay JT, Clausen P, Melchior Hansen J, Mathiesen ER, Feldt-Rasmussen B, et al. High levels of mannose-binding lectin are associated with lower pulse wave velocity in uraemic patients. *BMC Nephrol* (2014) 15:162. doi:10.1186/1471-2369-15-162
56. Satomura A, Endo M, Fujita T, Ohi H, Ohsawa I, Fuke Y, et al. Serum mannose-binding lectin levels in maintenance hemodialysis patients: impact on all-cause mortality. *Nephron Clin Pract* (2006) 102:c93–9. doi:10.1159/000089666
57. Ishii M, Ohsawa I, Inoshita H, Kusaba G, Onda K, Wakabayashi M, et al. Serum concentration of complement components of the lectin pathway in maintenance hemodialysis patients, and relatively higher levels of L-Ficolin and MASP-2 in Mannose-binding lectin deficiency. *Ther Apher Dial* (2011) 15:441–7. doi:10.1111/j.1744-9987.2011.00936.x
58. Lin Y-P, Yang C-Y, Liao C-C, Yu W-C, Chi C-W, Lin C-H. Plasma protein characteristics of long-term hemodialysis survivors. *PLoS One* (2012) 7:e40232. doi:10.1371/journal.pone.0040232
59. Hein E, Garred P. The lectin pathway of complement and biocompatibility. In: Lambris J, Ekdahl K, Ricklin D, Nilsson B, editors. *Immune Responses to Biosurfaces. Advances in Experimental Medicine and Biology*. Vol. 865. Cham: Springer (2015).
60. DeAngelis RA, Reis ES, Ricklin D, Lambris JD. Targeted complement inhibition as a promising strategy for preventing inflammatory complications in hemodialysis. *Immunobiology* (2012) 217:1097–105. doi:10.1016/j.imbio.2012.07.012
61. Seelen MA, Roos A, Wieslander J, Mollnes TE, Sjöholm AG, Wurzner R, et al. Functional analysis of the classical, alternative, and MBL pathways of the complement system: standardization and validation of a simple ELISA. *J Immunol Methods* (2005) 296:187–98. doi:10.1016/j.jim.2004.11.016
62. Huang S, Sandholm K, Jonsson N, Nilsson A, Wieslander A, Grundström G, et al. Low concentrations of citrate reduce complement and granulocyte activation in vitro in human blood. *Clin Kidney J* (2015) 8:31–7. doi:10.1093/ckj/sfu127
63. Böhler J, Schollmeyer P, Dressel B, Dobos G, Hörl WH. Reduction of granulocyte activation during hemodialysis with regional citrate anticoagulation: dissociation of complement activation and neutropenia from neutrophil degranulation. *J Am Soc Nephrol* (1996) 7:234–41.
64. Gabutti L, Ferrari N, Mombelli G, Keller F, Marone C. The favorable effect of regional citrate anticoagulation on interleukin-1beta release is dissociated from both coagulation and complement activation. *J Nephrol* (2004) 17:819–25.
65. Opatrný K, Richtrová P, Polanská K, Wirth J, Šefrna F, Brandl M, et al. Citrate anticoagulation control by ionized calcium levels does not prevent hemostasis and complement activation during hemodialysis. *Artif Organs* (2007) 31:200–7. doi:10.1111/j.1525-1594.2007.00365.x
66. Dhondt A, Vanholder R, Tielemans C, Glorieux G, Waterloos MA, De Smet R, et al. Effect of regional citrate anticoagulation on leukopenia, complement activation, and expression of leukocyte surface molecules during hemodialysis with unmodified cellulose membranes. *Nephron* (2000) 85:334–42. doi:10.1159/000045683
67. Poppelaars F, Damman J, de Vrij EL, Burgerhof JGM, Saye J, Daha MR, et al. New insight into the effects of heparinoids on complement inhibition by C1-inhibitor. *Clin Exp Immunol* (2016) 184:378–88. doi:10.1111/cei.12777
68. Ricklin D, Lambris JD. Progress and trends in complement therapeutics. *Adv Exp Med Biol* (2013) 735:1–22. doi:10.1007/978-1-4614-4118-2_1
69. Lazar HL, Bokesch PM, van Lenta F, Fitzgerald C, Emmett C, Marsh HC, et al. Soluble human complement receptor 1 limits ischemic damage in cardiac surgery patients at high risk requiring cardiopulmonary bypass. *Circulation* (2004) 110:II-274–279. doi:10.1161/01.CIR.0000138315.99788.eb
70. Reis ES, DeAngelis RA, Chen H, Resuello RRG, Ricklin D, Lambris JD. Therapeutic C3 inhibitor Cp40 abrogates complement activation induced by modern hemodialysis filters. *Immunobiology* (2015) 220:476–82. doi:10.1016/j.imbio.2014.10.026
71. Qu H, Ricklin D, Lambris JD. Recent developments in low molecular weight complement inhibitors. *Mol Immunol* (2009) 47:185–95. doi:10.1016/j.molimm.2009.08.032
72. Köhl J. Drug evaluation: the C5a receptor antagonist PMX-53. *Curr Opin Mol Ther* (2006) 8:529–38.

73. Wu Y-Q, Qu H, Sfyroera G, Tzekou A, Kay BK, Nilsson B, et al. Protection of nonself surfaces from complement attack by factor H-binding peptides: implications for therapeutic medicine. *J Immunol* (2011) 186:4269–77. doi:10.4049/jimmunol.1003802
74. Li PK, Chow KM. Peritoneal dialysis–first policy made successful: perspectives and actions. *Am J Kidney Dis* (2013) 62:993–1005. doi:10.1053/j.ajkd.2013.03.038
75. Shi J, Yu M, Sheng M. Angiogenesis and inflammation in peritoneal dialysis: the role of adipocytes. *Kidney Blood Press Res* (2017) 42:209–19. doi:10.1159/000476017
76. Akoh JA. Peritoneal dialysis associated infections: an update on diagnosis and management. *World J Nephrol* (2012) 1:106–22. doi:10.5527/wjn.v1.i4.106
77. Zhou Q, Bajo M-A, del Peso G, Yu X, Selgas R. Preventing peritoneal membrane fibrosis in peritoneal dialysis patients. *Kidney Int* (2016) 90:515–24. doi:10.1016/j.kint.2016.03.040
78. Tang S, Leung JCK, Chan LYY, Tsang AWL, Chen CXR, Zhou W, et al. Regulation of complement C3 and C4 synthesis in human peritoneal mesothelial cells by peritoneal dialysis fluid. *Clin Exp Immunol* (2004) 136:85–94. doi:10.1111/j.1365-2249.2004.02407.x
79. Barbano G, Cappa F, Prigione I, Tedesco F, Pausa M, Gugliemino R, et al. Peritoneal mesothelial cells produce complement factors and express CD59 that inhibits C5b-9-mediated cell lysis. *Adv Perit Dial* (1999) 15:253–7.
80. Sei Y, Mizuno M, Suzuki Y, Imai M, Higashide K, Harris CL, et al. Expression of membrane complement regulators, CD46, CD55 and CD59, in mesothelial cells of patients on peritoneal dialysis therapy. *Mol Immunol* (2015) 65:302–9. doi:10.1016/j.molimm.2015.02.005
81. Oliveira E, Araújo JE, Gómez-Meire S, Lodeiro C, Perez-Melon C, Iglesias-Lamas E, et al. Proteomics analysis of the peritoneal dialysate effluent reveals the presence of calcium-regulation proteins and acute inflammatory response. *Clin Proteomics* (2014) 11:17. doi:10.1186/1559-0275-11-17
82. Wen Q, Zhang L, Mao H-P, Tang X-Q, Rong R, Fan J-J, et al. Proteomic analysis in peritoneal dialysis patients with different peritoneal transport characteristics. *Biochem Biophys Res Commun* (2013) 438:473–8. doi:10.1016/j.bbrc.2013.07.116
83. Wang HY, Tian YF, Chien CC, Kan WC, Liao PC, Wu HY, et al. Differential proteomic characterization between normal peritoneal fluid and diabetic peritoneal dialysate. *Nephrol Dial Transplant* (2010) 25:1955–63. doi:10.1093/ndt/gfp696
84. Raaijmakers R, Pluk W, Schroder CH, Gloerich J, Cornelissen EAM, Wessels HJCT, et al. Proteomic profiling and identification in peritoneal fluid of children treated by peritoneal dialysis. *Nephrol Dial Transplant* (2008) 23:2402–5. doi:10.1093/ndt/gfn212
85. Zavvos V, Buxton AT, Evans C, Lambie M, Davies SJ, Topley N, et al. A prospective, proteomics study identified potential biomarkers of encapsulating peritoneal sclerosis in peritoneal effluent. *Kidney Int* (2017) 92:988–1002. doi:10.1016/j.kint.2017.03.030
86. Lam MF, Leung JCK, Tang CCS, Lo WK, Tse KC, Yip TP, et al. Mannose binding lectin level and polymorphism in patients on long-term peritoneal dialysis. *Nephrol Dial Transplant* (2005) 20:2489–96. doi:10.1093/ndt/gfi089
87. Reddingius RE, Schröder CH, Daha MR, Monnens LA. The serum complement system in children on continuous ambulatory peritoneal dialysis. *Perit Dial Int* (1993) 13:214–8.
88. Bartosova M, Schaefer B, Bermejo JL, Tarantino S, Lasitschka F, Macher-Goeppinger S, et al. Complement activation in peritoneal dialysis-induced arteriolopathy. *J Am Soc Nephrol* (2018) 29(1):268–82. doi:10.1681/ASN.2017040436
89. Reddingius RE, Schröder CH, Daha MR, Willems HL, Koster AM, Monnens LA. Complement in serum and dialysate in children on continuous ambulatory peritoneal dialysis. *Perit Dial Int* (1995) 15:49–53.
90. Mizuno T, Mizuno M, Morgan BP, Noda Y, Yamada K, Okada N, et al. Specific collaboration between rat membrane complement regulators Crry and CD59 protects peritoneum from damage by autologous complement activation. *Nephrol Dial Transplant* (2011) 26:1821–30. doi:10.1093/ndt/gfq683
91. Mizuno T, Mizuno M, Imai M, Suzuki Y, Kushida M, Noda Y, et al. Anti-C5a complementary peptide ameliorates acute peritoneal injury induced by neutralization of Crry and CD59. *Am J Physiol Renal Physiol* (2013) 305:F1603–16. doi:10.1152/ajprenal.00681.2012
92. Bazargani F, Rother RP, Braide M. The roles of complement factor C5a and CINC-1 in glucose transport, ultrafiltration, and neutrophil recruitment during peritoneal dialysis. *Perit Dial Int* (2006) 26:688–96.
93. Poppelaars F, van Werkhoven MB, Kotimaa J, Veldhuis ZJ, Ausema A, Broeren SGM, et al. Critical role for complement receptor C5aR2 in the pathogenesis of renal ischemia-reperfusion injury. *FASEB J* (2017) 31(7):3193–204. doi:10.1096/fj.201601218R
94. Mizuno M, Ito Y, Mizuno T, Harris CL, Suzuki Y, Okada N, et al. Membrane complement regulators protect against fibrin exudation increases in a severe peritoneal inflammation model in rats. *Am J Physiol Renal Physiol* (2012) 302:F1245–51. doi:10.1152/ajprenal.00652.2011
95. Danobeitia JS, Djamali A, Fernandez LA. The role of complement in the pathogenesis of renal ischemia-reperfusion injury and fibrosis. *Fibrogenesis Tissue Repair* (2014) 7:16. doi:10.1186/1755-1536-7-16
96. Rumpsfeld M, McDonald SP, Johnson DW. Higher peritoneal transport status is associated with higher mortality and technique failure in the Australian and New Zealand peritoneal dialysis patient populations. *J Am Soc Nephrol* (2006) 17:271–8. doi:10.1681/ASN.2005050566
97. Sritippayawan S, Chiangjong W, Semangoen T, Aiyasanon N, Jaetanawanitch P, Sinchaikul S, et al. Proteomic analysis of peritoneal dialysate fluid in patients with different types of peritoneal membranes. *J Proteome Res* (2007) 6:4356–62. doi:10.1021/pr0702969
98. Yáñez-Mó M, Lara-Pezzi E, Selgas R, Ramírez-Huesca M, Domínguez-Jiménez C, Jiménez-Heffernan JA, et al. Peritoneal dialysis and epithelial-to-mesenchymal transition of mesothelial cells. *N Engl J Med* (2003) 348:403–13. doi:10.1056/NEJMoa020809
99. Tang Z, Lu B, Hatch E, Sacks SH, Sheerin NS. C3a mediates epithelial-to-mesenchymal transition in proteinuric nephropathy. *J Am Soc Nephrol* (2009) 20:593–603. doi:10.1681/ASN.2008040434
100. Raby A-C, Colmont CS, Kift-Morgan A, Köhl J, Eberl M, Fraser D, et al. Toll-like receptors 2 and 4 are potential therapeutic targets in peritoneal dialysis-associated fibrosis. *J Am Soc Nephrol* (2017) 28:461–78. doi:10.1681/ASN.2015080923
101. Zeng L, Dang TA, Schunkert H. Genetics links between transforming growth factor β pathway and coronary disease. *Atherosclerosis* (2016) 253:237–46. doi:10.1016/j.atherosclerosis.2016.08.029
102. Moinuddin Z, Summers A, Van Dellen D, Augustine T, Herrick SE. Encapsulating peritoneal sclerosis-a rare but devastating peritoneal disease. *Front Physiol* (2014) 5:470. doi:10.3389/fphys.2014.00470
103. Cnossen TT, Konings CJAM, Kooman JP, Lindholm B. Peritoneal sclerosis—aetiology, diagnosis, treatment and prevention. *Nephrol Dial Transplant* (2006) 21:ii38–41. doi:10.1093/ndt/gfl189
104. Meijvis SCA, Herpers BL, Endeman H, de Jong B, van Hannen E, van Velzen-Blad H, et al. Mannose-binding lectin (MBL2) and ficolin-2 (FCN2) polymorphisms in patients on peritoneal dialysis with staphylococcal peritonitis. *Nephrol Dial Transplant* (2011) 26:1042–5. doi:10.1093/ndt/gfq474
105. Mizuno M, Suzuki Y, Higashide K, Sei Y, Iguchi D, Sakata F, et al. High levels of soluble C5b-9 complex in dialysis fluid may predict poor prognosis in peritonitis in peritoneal dialysis patients. *PLoS One* (2017) 12:e0169111. doi:10.1371/journal.pone.0169111
106. Bazargani F. Acute inflammation in peritoneal dialysis: experimental studies in rats. Characterization of regulatory mechanisms. *Swed Dent J Suppl* (2005):1–57.
107. Bazargani F, Albrektsson A, Yahyapour N, Braide M. Low molecular weight heparin improves peritoneal ultrafiltration and blocks complement and coagulation. *Perit Dial Int* (2005) 25:394–404.

7

Complement Factor H-Related Protein 4A is the Dominant Circulating Splice Variant of *CFHR4*

Richard B. Pouw[1,2], Mieke C. Brouwer[1], Anna E. van Beek[1,2], Mihály Józsi[3], Diana Wouters[1†] and Taco W. Kuijpers[2,4†]*

[1] *Department of Immunopathology, Sanquin Research and Landsteiner Laboratory of the Academic Medical Center, University of Amsterdam, Amsterdam, Netherlands,* [2] *Department of Pediatric Hematology, Immunology and Infectious Diseases, Emma Children's hospital, Academic Medical Center, Amsterdam, Netherlands,* [3] *MTA-ELTE "Lendület" Complement Research Group, Department of Immunology, ELTE Eötvös Loránd University, Budapest, Hungary,* [4] *Department of Blood Cell Research, Sanquin Research and Landsteiner Laboratory of the Academic Medical Center, University of Amsterdam, Amsterdam, Netherlands*

***Correspondence:**
Richard B. Pouw
r.pouw@sanquin.nl

†These authors have contributed equally to this work.

Recent research has elucidated circulating levels of almost all factor H-related (FHR) proteins. Some of these proteins are hypothesized to act as antagonists of the important complement regulator factor H (FH), fine-tuning complement regulation on human surfaces. For the *CFHR4* splice variants FHR-4A and FHR-4B, the individual circulating levels are unknown, with only total levels being described. Specific reagents for FHR-4A or FHR-4B are lacking due to the fact that the unique domains in FHR-4A show high sequence similarity with FHR-4B, making it challenging to distinguish them. We developed an assay that specifically measures FHR-4A using novel, well-characterized monoclonal antibodies (mAbs) that target unique domains in FHR-4A only. Using various FHR-4A/FHR-4B-specific mAbs, no FHR-4B was identified in any of the serum samples tested. The results demonstrate that FHR-4A is the dominant splice variant of *CFHR4* in the circulation, while casting doubt on the presence of FHR-4B. FHR-4A levels (avg. 2.55 ± 1.46 μg/mL) were within the range of most of the previously reported levels for all other FHRs. FHR-4A was found to be highly variable among the population, suggesting a strong genetic regulation. These results shed light on the physiological relevance of the previously proposed role of FHR-4A and FHR-4B as antagonists of FH in the circulation.

Keywords: factor H-related-4A, factor H-related-4B, factor H, factor H-related proteins, CFHR4 gene, the complement system

INTRODUCTION

The complement system is an evolutionarily ancient protein cascade which, through a series of events, recognizes, attacks, and kills foreign cells like bacteria, but can also target host cells [reviewed by Ricklin et al. (1)]. In order to prevent damage of healthy host cells, humans possess several complement regulators. Some are membrane bound and expressed on the cell surface; however, one of the most important regulators, complement factor H (FH) circulates freely in plasma. FH is a 155 kDa glycoprotein that circulates in blood with a reported average concentration ranging from 233 up to 400 μg/mL or 1.5–2.6 μM (2–6). FH is a crucial regulator of the alternative activation pathway of the complement system, orchestrating complement activation toward foreign cells by specifically binding to and inhibiting complement on human cells. FH belongs to the FH protein family, which consists of eight proteins derived from six genes, encoded in tandem in the *CFH* locus. The *CFH* gene itself encodes two proteins, FH and its splice-variant FH-like 1 (FHL-1). Next to FH and FHL-1, six factor H-related (FHR) proteins are found in plasma. Like FH and FHL-1, the FHRs are completely comprised of domains called short consensus repeat (SCR) domains. FHR-1, FHR-2, FHR-3, and FHR-5 are encoded separately by corresponding genes (*CFHR1, CFHR2, CFHR3,* and *CFHR5*), while FHR-4A and FHR-4B are splice variants encoded by *CFHR4* (7, 8). FHR-4A is the largest FHR (86 kDa) and comprises nine SCR domains, while FHR-4B has been predicted to consist of five SCR domains (43 kDa) (7, 8). The five SCR domains of FHR-4B are completely identical to SCR 1 and SCRs 6–9 of FHR-4A (**Figure 1B**). The unique four SCR domains between SCRs 1 and 6 of FHR-4A appear to have arisen from an internal duplication in *CFHR4* and are highly similar to the other SCR domains in FHR-4A and, therefore, also to FHR-4B (8). SCR 1 is highly similar to SCR 5 (85%), 2–6 (90%), 3–7 (93%), and SCR 4 to SCR 8 (87%) in FHR-4A. This makes it challenging to specifically distinguish FHR-4A from FHR-4B in immunoassays.

It is still unclear what the role of FHR-4A and FHR-4B is within the complement system. Increasing evidence indicates that FHRs act as antagonists of FH, competing with FH for the binding to complement C3b and human cell surfaces [reviewed by Józsi et al. (9)]. FHR-4A and -4B seem to lack physiologically relevant complement inhibitory activities on their own. FHR-4A has been reported to enhance the co-factor activity of FH at supraphysiological concentrations (10, 11). Furthermore, binding of

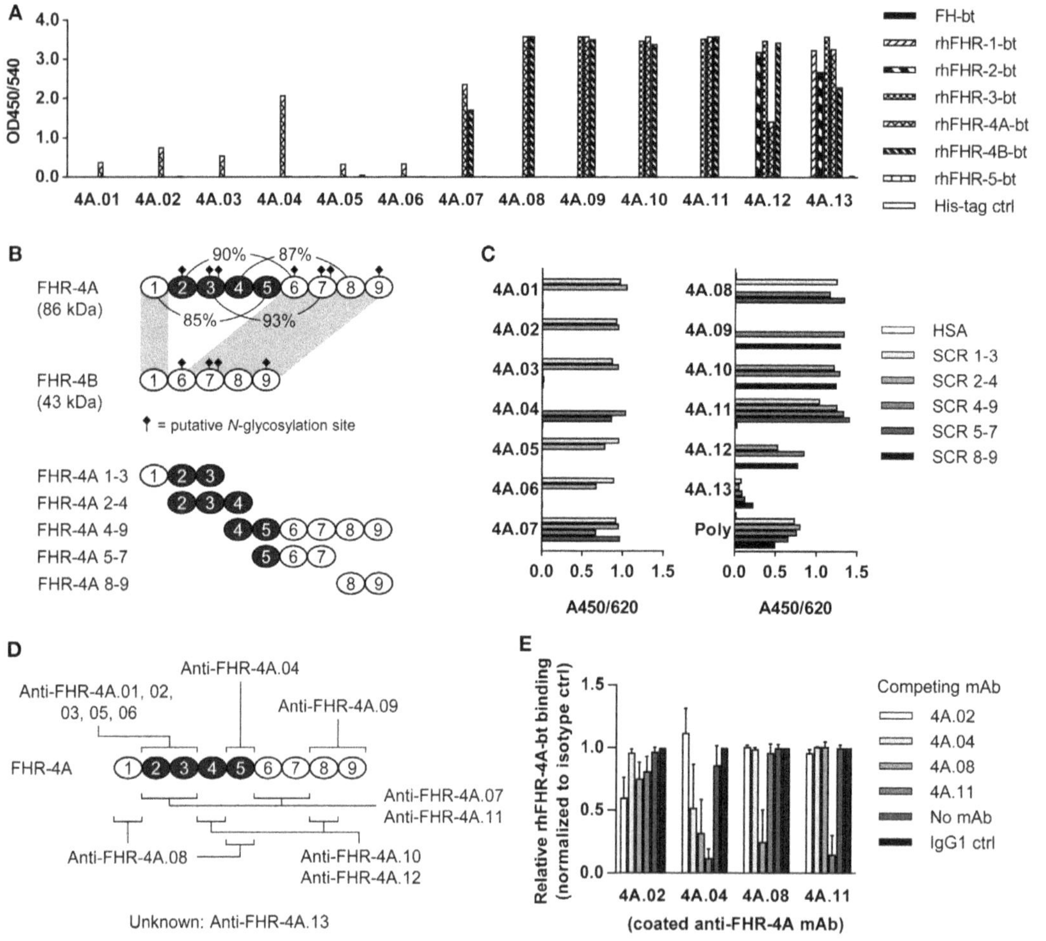

FIGURE 1 | Characterization of anti-FHR-4A monoclonal antibodies (mAbs). **(A)** Cross-reactivity of the anti-FHR-4A mAbs to biotinylated rhFHR proteins and biotinylated plasma-derived FH was determined by ELISA. **(B)** Schematic representation of FHR-4A, FHR-4B, and the recombinant fragments of FHR-4A used for epitope mapping, with the duplicated SCR domains in FHR-4A depicted in black. Corresponding percentage of sequence identity between the domains in FHR-4A is indicated. Domains 1 and 6–9 of FHR-4A are completely identical to the domains of FHR-4B (indicated by gray shading). **(C)** Epitope mapping of anti-FHR-4A antibodies using the fragments of rhFHR-4A as depicted in **(B)**, determined by ELISA. As a control, polyclonal anti-FHR-3 (poly), which cross-reacts with all FHR proteins was used. **(D)** Schematic representation of the epitope location of each of the anti-FHR-4A mAbs. Single epitope mAbs are listed above FHR-4A, mAbs with multiple epitopes below. Note that most cross-reactive mAbs have two epitopes in FHR-4A, due to the high sequence similarity of the SCR domains. **(E)** Competition ELISA with monospecific mAbs (anti-FHR-4A.02 and 4A.04) and cross-reactive mAbs (anti-FHR-4A.08 and 4A.11). Binding of biotinylated rhFHR-4A is expressed as relative to the binding of biotinylated rhFHR-4A without any competing mAb. Bars represent mean of independent replicates with error bars indicating SD. All graphs are representative of multiple independent experiments.

FHR-4A and FHR-4B instead of FH allows complement activation to occur on the surface (11) and FHR-4A and FHR-4B might act as a competitor of FH. This form of regulation might serve to fine-tune complement inhibition by FH on surfaces where balanced complement activation is required for clearance, such as on necrotic and apoptotic cells. This hypothesis would also explain associations between genetic variation in *CFHR* genes and various diseases. For instance, the lack of *CFHR3* and *CFHR1* due to copy number variation (CNV) has been reported to be protective against age-related macular degeneration (12, 13). However, no such link with disease has yet been found for *CFHR4*. Like other FHRs, FHR-4A and FHR-4B bind to C3b and C-reactive protein, allowing complement activation to occur (11, 14, 15). Furthermore, FHR-4A has been reported to recruit CRP to necrotic cells *in vitro*, allowing more complement activation to occur, and is found to be accumulated in necrotic tissue (14). However, in contrast to all other members of the FH protein family, FHR-4A and FHR-4B seem to lack any affinity toward heparin (16, 17).

Highly relevant for the proposed antagonistic properties of FHR proteins is their physiological concentration, especially in relation to FH. Recently, we have reported normal protein concentrations for all FHRs in >100 healthy individuals, except for FHR-4A and FHR-4B. FHR-1/1 homodimers, FHR-2/2 homodimers, and FHR-1/2 heterodimers circulate at average concentrations of 14.6 (±3.0), 0.7 (±0.4), and 5.8 (±2.4) µg/mL, respectively, in healthy donors with two *CFHR1* copies, whereas FHR-5/5 homodimers circulate at 1.7 (±0.4) µg/mL in healthy donors (18). Of note, the FHR-1 total levels have recently also been reported to be 122 (±26) µg/mL, without distinguishing between homo- or heterodimers, nor fully describing the calibration used (19). However, a third, independent, group recently reported combined, total FHR-1, FHR-2, and FHR-5 levels, measured in an immunoassay, to be 10.7 (±5.4) µg/mL, thus supporting the lower levels for FHR-1 and FHR-2 (20). FHR-3 circulates at average concentrations of 0.7–1.1 µg/mL (6, 21). For FHR-4A and FHR-4B, only total FHR-4 levels ranging from 6.5 to 53.9 µg/mL with an average concentration of 25.4 µg/mL have been described, measured in only 11 healthy individuals (11). These levels were determined without distinguishing between FHR-4A and FHR-4B. Therefore, in order to specifically measure FHR-4A and FHR-4B, as well as establishing normal levels in a larger cohort of healthy individuals, we have developed specific reagents for FHR-4A and FHR-4B. Monoclonal antibodies (mAbs) were used to specifically detect FHR-4A, but we were unable to detect any freely circulating FHR-4B in human serum, despite the use of various cross-reactive mAbs. Finally, we demonstrate that FHR-4A levels vary greatly among healthy individuals.

MATERIALS AND METHODS

Samples

Healthy donor serum samples were collected as part of a previous study from anonymous, healthy volunteers with informed, written consent in accordance with Dutch regulations and this study was approved by the Sanquin Ethical Advisory Board in accordance with the Declaration of Helsinki (6). Normal human serum (NHS) pool comprises serum from 400 healthy donors. FHR-3-deficient serum pool comprises serum of four healthy donors previously genotyped by multiplex ligation-dependent probe amplification to carry no *CFHR3* gene copies (6). Samples of patients with confirmed bacterial infections were collected as part of the EUCLIDS project (van Beek et al., manuscript in preparation). CRP levels were determined in these samples as part of routine testing.

Proteins and Reagents

Rat anti-mouse kappa (RM-19) mAb was from Sanquin Reagents (Sanquin, Amsterdam, the Netherlands). High-performance ELISA buffer (HPE) was provided by Sanquin. Proteins were biotinylated according to the manufacturer's instructions using EZ-Link Sulfo-NHS-LC-Biotin, No-Weigh Format (Thermo Scientific, Waltham, MA, USA), when indicated. Polyclonal anti-FHR-3 antibodies and mAb clone anti-FHR-3.3 were obtained and characterized as part of a previous study (6). Recombinant human (rh) FHR proteins, containing a C-terminal 6×-histidine tag, were produced and purified as previously described (6). In short, proteins were expressed by transient transfection of pcDNA3.1 expression vectors in HEK293F cells, after which proteins were purified from the supernatant by Ni^{2+} affinity chromatography using HisTrap™ High Performance 1 mL columns (GE Healthcare Life Sciences, Freiburg, Germany). rhFHRs were filtered and concentrated using Amicon® Ultra Centrifugal Filter Devices (Merck Millipore, Darmstadt, Germany) according to the manufacturer's instructions using appropriate molecular weight cut-offs. For rhFHR-4A, a 100 kDa cut-off Amicon® Filter was used to further purify rhFHR-4A from any high molecular weight aggregates observed after Ni^{2+} affinity chromatography purification (Figures S1A,B in Supplemental Material).

Immunization, mAb Generation, and Characterization

Anti-FHR-4A mAbs were generated, screened, and purified as previously described, using rhFHR-4A as immunogen (6). Isotypes of mAbs were determined by ELISA or with the use of the Mouse mAb Isotyping Kit (Hycult Biotech, Uden, the Netherlands) according to the manufacturer's instructions. Cross-reactivity against other FH protein family members was determined as previously described (6).

Epitope Mapping

The epitope location of each of the anti-FHR-4A mAbs was determined using rhFHR-4A, rhFHR-4B, and rhFHR-4A fragments consisting of SCR domains 1–3, 2–4, 4–9, 5–7, or 8–9 as previously described (15). Proteins and fragments were coated (4 µg/mL in PBS) onto Nunc Maxisorp 96-well microtiter plates (Invitrogen, Life Technologies, Carlsbad, CA, USA) by overnight (O/N) incubation at 4°C. Plates were washed three times with PBS + 0.02% (w/v) Tween-20 (PT) and blocked with 4% (w/v) BSA in PBS by incubation for 1 h. After another wash with PT, wells were incubated with the anti-FHR-4A mAbs diluted in PT for 1 h. Unbound anti-FHR-4A mAbs were washed away by washing the wells five times with PT, followed by incubating with 0.05% (v/v) HRP-conjugated rabbit anti-mouse IgG (Dako Agilent, Santa Clara, CA, USA) for 1 h and subsequently washing the plates five times. The ELISA was developed using 3,5,3′,5′-tetramethylbenzidine (TMB) solution and the reaction was stopped using 50 μL 2 M H_2SO_4. As a positive control, FHR-4A fragments were detected using polyclonal rabbit anti-FHR-4A, followed by HRP-conjugated goat anti-rabbit IgG (Dako Agilent). All ELISA steps were performed with a final volume of 50 μL per well and incubated at room temperature while shaking unless stated otherwise. Absorption was measured at 450 nm and corrected for background absorbance at 620 nm.

Competition ELISA

To determine whether the mAbs competed for the binding of rhFHR-4A, Nunc Maxisorp 96-well microtiter plates (Invitrogen) were coated with 100 μL of 2 μg/mL anti-FHR-4A mAbs, in PBS, by incubating O/N at room temperature. Next, the plates were washed with PT. Biotinylated rhFHR-4A (0.1 μg/mL, in HPE) was incubated with 10 μg/mL of each mAb for 20 min, followed by incubation on the washed plate for 1 h. Next, unbound biotinylated rhFHR-4A was washed away and the wells were incubated with 0.01% (v/v) strep-poly-HRP (Sanquin), diluted in HPE, for 20 min. After washing, the assay was developed by addition of 100 μL of 100 μg/mL TMB in 0.11 M sodium acetate containing 0.003% (v/v) H_2O_2, pH 5.5. Substrate conversion was stopped after approximately 10 min by addition of 100 μL 2 M H_2SO_4. Absorbance was measured at 450 nm and corrected for the absorbance at 540 nm with a Synergy 2 Multi-Mode plate reader (BioTek Instruments, Winooski, VT, USA). All ELISA steps were performed with a volume of 100 μL per well and incubated at room temperature while shaking unless stated otherwise.

Sucrose Gradient

Sucrose gradients were described previously (18). In short, NHS or FHR-3-deficient serum (150 μL of 50%, v/v, pooled serum, diluted in PBS) were loaded on 5–32.9% (w/v) sucrose (Merck 1.07654) gradients. Gradients were centrifuged for 20 h at 160,000 × *g* after which they were fractionated in 24 fractions of 500 μL. Proteins were immunoprecipitated and visualized on Western Blots as described below.

Immunoprecipitation (IP)

Factor H-related-4A and FHR-4B were immunoprecipitated from human healthy donor serum or sucrose gradient fractions using indicated mAbs. IP was performed by incubating 200 μL serum or 250 μL sucrose gradient fraction with 500 μL of 5 mg/mL CNBr-activated sepharose (GE Healthcare, Little Chalfont, UK) to which RM-19 was coupled (25 mg mAb per 1 g sepharose), and 50 μL of 100 μg/mL mAb, diluted in PBS supplemented with 0.1% Tween-20, 0.1% BSA, and 10 mM EDTA. Following overnight incubation at 4°C, while rotating, the sepharose was washed three times with 1 mL PT and two times with 1 mL PBS. Precipitated proteins were eluted by addition of 50 μL 1× NuPAGE Sample buffer solution (Invitrogen) and incubation at 70°C for 10 min. After spinning down the sepharose, SDS-PAGE under non-reducing conditions was performed using a Novex NuPAGE 10 or 4–12% Bis–Tris gel followed by Western Blot onto a nitrocellulose membrane (Novex iBlot Gel Transfer kit, Invitrogen). Membranes were blocked with 1% (v/v) Western Blocking Reagent (WBR) (Roche, Basel, Switzerland) in PBS for 30 min and incubated with 1 μg/mL biotinylated polyclonal rabbit anti-FHR-3 in PBS + 0.5% (v/v) WBR, O/N. After washing three times with PT, membranes were incubated with 0.1% (v/v) Strep-HRP in PBS + 0.5% (v/v) WBR. After 1 h, the membranes were washed three times with PT followed by two washes with PBS. Western Blots were developed with the Pierce ECL 2 Western Blotting substrate kit (Thermo Scientific) according to the manufacturer's instructions and analyzed using the ChemiDoc™ MP System (BioRad, Hercules, CA, USA).

FHR-4A ELISA

To measure FHR-4A in serum, RM-19 was coated (3 μg/mL in PBS) onto Nunc Maxisorp 96-well microtiter plates (Invitrogen) by O/N incubation at room temperature. After coating, plates were washed five times with PT, followed by incubation with 1 μg/mL anti-FHR-4A.04 in HPE, for 1 h. After washing, samples, diluted in HPE, were added and incubated for 1 h. Following washing with PT, 0.5 μg/mL biotinylated polyclonal anti-FHR-3 (in HPE) was incubated on the plate for 1 h. Next, unbound conjugate was washed away and the wells were incubated with 0.01% (v/v) strep-poly-HRP (Sanquin), diluted in HPE, for 20 min. After washing, the assay was developed as described above using TMB and measuring absorbance at 450 nm and correcting for the absorbance at 540 nm. All ELISA steps were performed with a volume of 100 μL per well and incubated at room temperature while shaking unless stated otherwise. For the calibration of the FHR-4A ELISA, highly pure rhFHR-4A was used (Figure S1B in Supplemental Material) of which the concentration was determined by measuring the absorbance at 280 nm and using an absorbance coefficient of 2.134 (0.1% w/v solution).

Statistical Analysis

Analysis and statistical tests were performed using GraphPad Prism, version 7.03 (GraphPad Software, La Jolla, CA, USA).

RESULTS

Characterization of mAbs Against FHR-4A

We characterized 13 mouse mAbs raised against rhFHR-4A. All mAbs were first tested for cross-reactivity against all other members of the FH protein family (**Figure 1A**). The mAbs were named in order of increasing cross-reactivity: anti-FHR-4A.01 to 4A.06 being mono-specific for rhFHR-4A, anti-FHR-4A.07, and 4A.08 recognizing both rhFHR-4A and -4B, anti-FHR-4A.09 to 4A.11 recognizing rhFHR-3, 4A, and -4B, anti-FHR-4A.12 binding rhFHR-2, -3, -4A, and -4B, whereas anti-FHR-4A.13 recognizes all rhFHRs except rhFHR-5. None of the anti-FHR-4 mAbs showed cross-reactivity with either FHR-5 or FH.

With the use of recombinant fragments comprising different FHR-4A domains (**Figure 1B**), the epitope location of almost all anti-FHR-4A mAbs were mapped. As expected, all FHR-4A-specific mAbs (anti-FHR-4A.01 to 4A.06) bound to an epitope located in domains 2–5, which are unique for rhFHR-4A and not present in rhFHR-4B (**Figures 1C,D**). Of these FHR-4A specific mAbs, only anti-FHR-4A.04 recognized an epitope located in domain 5, whereas all other mAbs bound to an epitope in domain 2 or 3. Anti-FHR-4A.01, 4A.02, 4A.03, 4A.05, and 4A.06, competed with each other for the binding of rhFHR-4A, indicating identical or partially overlapping epitopes (data not shown).

Of the mAbs that cross-reacted with rhFHR-4B and other FHR protein family members, most appeared to bind to either of two epitopes in rhFHR-4A, reflecting the high degree of similarity between these SCR domains 2–5 in FHR-4A and the domains 1, 6, 7, and 8 in FHR-4A and FHR-4B.

Only anti-FHR-4A.09 appeared to have one epitope in domain 8 or 9, recognizing both rhFHR-4A and rhFHR-4B, while also cross-reacting with FHR-3.

The cross-reactive mAbs anti-FHR-4A.08 and anti-FHR-4A.11 were able to block binding of rhFHR-4A to the monospecific FHR-4A mAbs; however, in the reverse setting, this cross-blocking was not achieved (**Figure 1E**). This is in line with the presence of two epitopes for anti-FHR-4A.08 and 4A.11 in rhFHR-4A. It indicates that one of the two epitopes for anti-FHR-4A.08 and anti-FHR-4A.11 is partially overlapping or sterically hindering the binding site of the monospecific mAbs. The epitope location of anti-FHR-4A.13 could not be mapped due to a very low and ambiguous binding signal when the fragments were used. However, binding of rhFHR-4A to anti-FHR-4A.13 could be blocked with anti-FHR-4A.09, suggesting an epitope location in either domain 8 or 9 for anti-FHR-4A.13. An overview of the mAbs characteristics, the mapped epitope location, and the cross-reactivity is given in **Table 1**.

Only FHR-4A Is Detected in NHS

Next, we tested whether the anti-FHR-4A mAbs capture FHR-4A and FHR-4B from NHS. To this end, an IP followed by Western Blot was performed, which was developed with cross-reactive biotinylated polyclonal anti-FHR-3. Of the specific anti-FHR-4A mAbs, only anti-FHR-4A.04 seemed to efficiently capture FHR-4A from NHS, resulting in a clear protein band corresponding to the molecular weight of FHR-4A (86 kDa) (**Figure 2A**). Only a very faint FHR-4A band was visible in the precipitates of anti-FHR-4A.01, 4A.02, 4A.03, 4A.05, and 4A.06. In addition, both anti-FHR-4A.07 and anti-FHR-4A.13 were neither able to efficiently immunoprecipitate FHR-4A from serum nor any of the other FHR proteins with which these mAbs cross-react. A band corresponding to FHR-4B (43 kDa) in the IP with

TABLE 1 | Anti-factor H-related (FHR)-4A monoclonal antibodies characterized in this study.

Designation	Mouse isotype	Epitope location (domain) 1st	Epitope location (domain) 2nd	Cross-reactivity	Competes with
Anti-FHR-4A.01	IgG1, Kappa	2–3	–	None	4A.02, 4A.03, 4A.05, 4A.06
Anti-FHR-4A.02	IgG1, Kappa	2–3	–	None	4A.01, 4A.03, 4A.05, 4A.06
Anti-FHR-4A.03	IgG1, Kappa	2–3	-	None	4A.01, 4A.02, 4A.05, 4A.06
Anti-FHR-4A.04	IgG1, Kappa	5	–	None	None
Anti-FHR-4A.05	IgG2b, Kappa	2–3	–	None	4A.01, 4A.02, 4A.03, 4A.06
Anti-FHR-4A.06	IgG1, Kappa	2–3	–	None	4A.01, 4A.02, 4A.03, 4A.05
Anti-FHR-4A.07	IgG1, Kappa	2–3	6–7	rhFHR-4B	None
Anti-FHR-4A.08	IgG1, Kappa	1	5	rhFHR-4B	4A.01, 4A.02, 4A.03, 4A.05, 4A.06
Anti-FHR-4A.09	IgG1, Kappa	8–9	–	rhFHR-3, -4B	None
Anti-FHR-4A.10	IgG1, Kappa	4	8	rhFHR-3, -4B	None
Anti-FHR-4A.11	IgG1, Kappa	2–3	6–7	rhFHR-3, -4B	4A.01, 4A.02, 4A.03, 4A.05, 4A.06
Anti-FHR-4A.12	IgG1, Kappa	4	8	rhFHR-2, -3, -4B	None
Anti-FHR-4A.13	IgG1, Kappa	Unknown	Unknown	rhFHR-1, -2, -3, -4B	4A.09

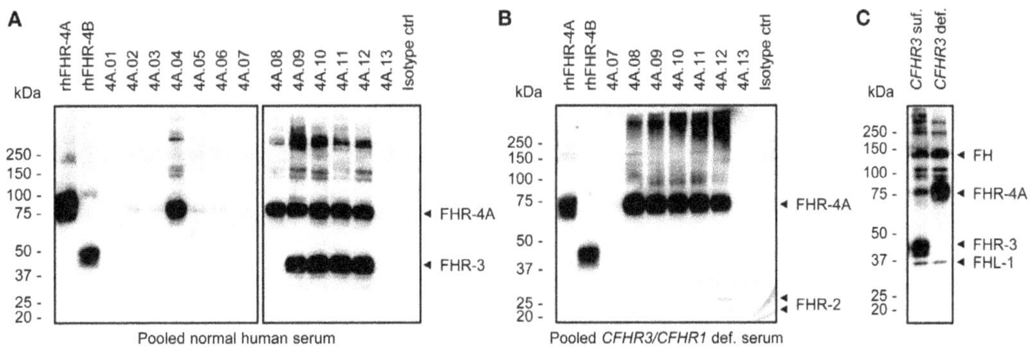

FIGURE 2 | Immunoprecipitation (IP) of plasma-derived factor H-related (FHR) proteins by the anti-FHR-4A monoclonal antibodies (mAbs). **(A)** Western blot following IP from pooled normal human serum using the indicated mAbs. For comparison, 100 ng rhFHR-4A and rhFHR-4B were loaded on the left side of the gel. Precipitated proteins are indicated with arrowheads on the right side of the blot. **(B)** As in **(A)**, but with pooled serum of healthy donors who are deficient for *CFHR3* and *CFHR1* and using only the cross-reactive anti-FHR-4A mAbs for IP. **(C)** IP using polyclonal anti-FHR-3 and serum of two healthy donors with either two *CFHR3* (*CFHR3* suf.) or no *CFHR3* (*CFHR3* def.) gene copies. All Western blots were stained with cross-reactive biotinylated polyclonal anti-FHR-3. Precipitated proteins are indicated with arrowheads on the right side of each blot. Results are representative of multiple independent experiments.

anti-FHR-4A.08 also appeared to be missing, while the mAb was found to be cross-reactive with rhFHR-4B in the ELISA. A protein band corresponding to FHR-4B could not be distinguished in the IP of anti-FHR-4A.09 to anti-FHR-4A.12, as these mAbs also precipitated FHR-3 (43–50 kDa), which migrates at the same expected molecular weight and is also recognized by the polyclonal antibody. Therefore, to better visualize the IP of FHR-4B, an IP from a FHR-3-deficient serum pool was performed, using the cross-reactive mAbs. However, also in these conditions, no band corresponding to FHR-4B was detected in the IP of anti-FHR-4A.08 to anti-FHR-4A.12, which was unexpected given the cross-reactivity we observed with rhFHR-4B in ELISA (**Figure 2B**). On the other hand, anti-FHR-4A.12 did immunoprecipitate FHR-2 from NHS, confirming the cross-reactivity results obtained with rhFHR-2. As a control, the IP was repeated with the cross-reactive polyclonal anti-FHR-3 using serum of two healthy donors, one with two *CFHR3* gene copies, and one with no *CFHR3* gene copies. This resulted in the precipitation of FH, FHL-1, FHR-3, and FHR-4A (**Figure 2C**). However, also with this set-up, no FHR-4B was detected.

Serum fractionated by sucrose gradients was previously used to investigate the molecular size of FHR proteins in their native state (18). Using a recently characterized anti-FHR-3 mAb that cross-reacts with FH, rhFHR-4A, rhFHR-4B, and FHL-1 (clone anti-FHR-3.3) (6), we investigated the circulating molecular size of FHR-4A relative to FH and FHR-3, by IP of these proteins from sucrose gradient fractions. As expected, FH was precipitated from the fractions also containing IgG, while FHR-3 was mainly present in the fractions containing albumin, corresponding with their respective molecular weights (155 and 50 kDa) (**Figure 3A**). FHR-4A was found in the fractions corresponding with its molecular weight (86 kDa), between the main fractions containing FH and FHR-3. Again, no bands corresponding with FHR-4B were found in the sucrose gradient fractions of neither the FHR-3 sufficient nor the FHR-3-deficient serum pool (**Figure 3B**).

FHR-4A Levels Vary Greatly Between Individuals

As we could not detect FHR-4B in human serum, we next focused on specifically measuring FHR-4A by ELISA. FHR-4A was measured using the monospecific mAb anti-FHR-4A.04, captured on immobilized RM-19, and using biotinylated polyclonal anti-FHR-3 antibody as a conjugate. The specificity

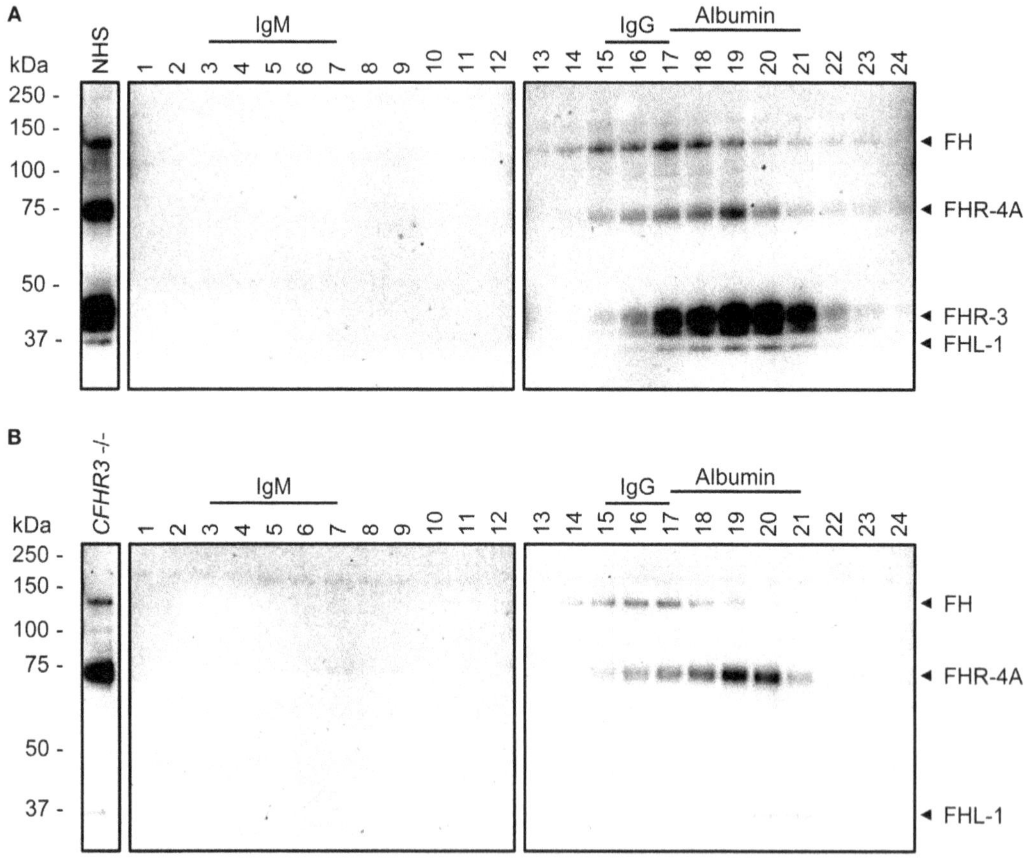

FIGURE 3 | Sucrose gradients of normal human serum (NHS) and *CFHR3*-deficient serum. Western Blots of immunoprecipitation (IP) of fractions (1–24) from a sucrose gradient with **(A)** NHS or **(B)** a serum pool deficient for FHR-3 (*CFHR3*$^{-/-}$). IP was performed using anti-FHR-3.3, Western Blots were stained with biotinylated polyclonal anti-FHR-3 antibody. Fractions containing IgM (970 kDa, fractions 3–7), IgG (150 kDa, fractions 15–17), or albumin (66 kDa, fractions 17–21) are indicated above the blots and used as size reference. Identified proteins are indicated with arrowheads on the right side.

of the FHR-4A ELISA was confirmed using rhFHR proteins and plasma purified FH, giving a clear signal for rhFHR-4A (**Figure 4A**). Both rhFHR-3 and rhFHR-4B were detected at the highest concentrations we tested, but the FHR-4A ELISA was found to be 843-fold and 1,490-fold more sensitive for rhFHR-4A compared to rhFHR-4B or rhFHR-3, respectively. Next, using purified rhFHR-4A, we calibrated a NHS pool to contain 2.33 µg/mL FHR-4A, which was subsequently used as a calibration curve in the FHR-4A ELISA (**Figure 4B**). FHR-4A levels in serum and plasma did not differ (**Figure 4C**, $P > 0.05$), nor were the levels affected by repeated freeze/thaw cycles (**Figure 4D**). Next, we measured the levels of FHR-4A in serum from 129 healthy donors. The average concentration of FHR-4A was found to be close to the concentration found in the NHS pool, being 2.55 µg/mL or 29.65 nM. Moreover, FHR-4A levels were found to be highly variable with a SD of 1.46 µg/mL and ranging from 0.26 up to 6.20 µg/mL (**Figure 4E**). We subsequently investigated whether FHR-4A behaves as an acute phase protein. To this end, we measured FHR-4A levels in 78 patients during an acute bacterial infection. No correlation was found for FHR-4A with CRP levels ($r = 0.024$, $P = 0.834$, **Figure 4F**). Of note, no total deficiency for FHR-4A was found in any healthy donor or patient measured during this study.

DISCUSSION

The FHR proteins are hypothesized to act as antagonists of complement regulator FH, competing for binding to ligands and allowing, instead of inhibiting, complement activation on surfaces (9). Several reports have shown that recombinant FHR-4A and -4B indeed bind to known FH ligands and allow complement activation to occur *in vitro* (11, 14, 15). To date, normal levels of FHR-1, FHR-2, FHR-3, and FHR-5 have been reported and were found to be circulating at much lower concentration as compared to FH (6, 18, 21, 22). In this report, we describe the circulating levels of FHR-4A in healthy individuals, using novel, well-characterized anti-FHR-4A mAbs. FHR-4B is apparently absent in blood, implying that FHR-4A is the dominant splice variant of *CFHR4*.

We obtained thirteen mAbs that were raised against rhFHR-4A, of which, six were found to be monospecific for FHR-4A. Their epitopes were mapped to be located within the four SCR domains unique for FHR-4A (and absent in FHR-4B). Of the seven cross-reactive mAbs that could also recognize the rhFHR-4B protein, six mAbs were found to bind to two epitopes within rhFHR-4A, corresponding to SCR domains that share high sequence similarity within rhFHR-4A because of the known internal gene duplication. The presence of two epitopes for

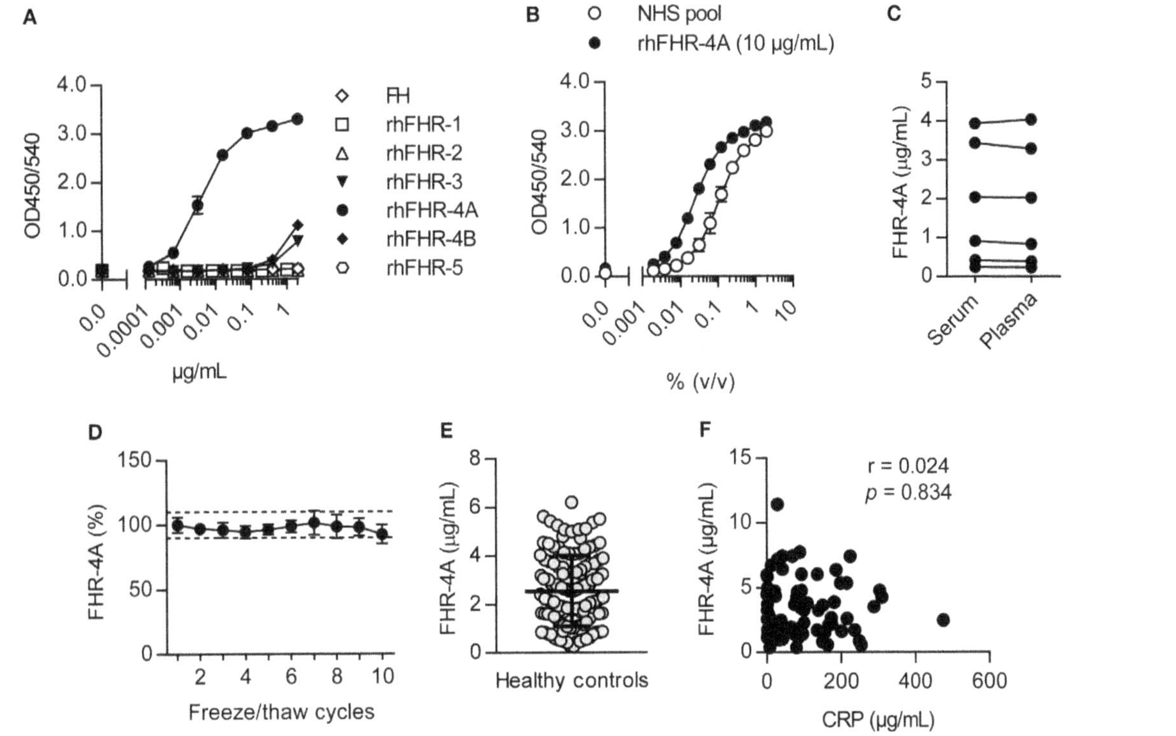

FIGURE 4 | Development of the factor H-related (FHR)-4A specific ELISA. **(A)** Representative result on the reactivity of the FHR-4A ELISA against rhFHR proteins and plasma-derived FH. Anti-FHR-4A.04 was used as monospecific catching mAb, and binding of antigen was detected using cross-reactive polyclonal anti-FHR-3. **(B)** Calibration of pooled normal human serum using rhFHR-4A (10 µg/mL) in the FHR-4A ELISA. **(C)** Comparison of FHR-4A levels in seven paired serum and EDTA plasma samples using the FHR-4A ELISA. Each point represents the mean of three independent measurements per sample. **(D)** Effect of multiple freeze/thaw cycles. Each point represents the mean of three independent measurements per sample with error bars indicating SD. Dashed lines indicate 90–110% range. **(E)** Concentration of FHR-4A in 129 healthy donor sera, measured by ELISA. Each point represents the mean of three independent measurements per serum sample. Line indicates mean with SD. **(F)** Scatter plot of FHR-4A levels versus CRP levels determined in 78 patients with acute bacterial infection. Correlation was assessed using Spearman's correlation test.

these mAbs in rhFHR-4A was further supported by competition experiments. The rhFHR-4A-specific mAbs (one epitope) were not able to prevent binding of rhFHR-4A to cross-reactive mAbs (two epitopes), whereas the cross-reactive mAbs blocked binding to the specific mAbs, indicating that one of the two epitopes of the cross-reactive mAbs is overlapping with the epitope of the specific anti-FHR-4A mAbs.

Seven mAbs (anti-FHR-4A.01, -4A.02, -4A.03, -4A.05, -4A.06, -4A.07, and -4A.13) seemed unable or very inefficient in immunoprecipitating FHR-4A from NHS. The lack thereof is indicative for a much lower binding affinity for plasma-derived FHR-4A compared to rhFHR-4A. Strikingly, the epitopes of anti-FHR-4A.01, -4A.02, -4A.03, -4A.05, -4A.06, and -4A.07 are all located in SCR domains of FHR-4A that contain (multiple) putative *N*-linked glycosylation sites. While rhFHR-4A is produced by HEK293F cells and thus possesses glycans from human origin, it is possible that differences in the exact glycan composition from those found *in vivo* are involved in the apparent lack of binding affinity toward serum-derived FHR-4A. This might also be the case for anti-FHR-4A.13, for which we could not precisely map the epitope location.

We were unable to identify a band corresponding to FHR-4B in the IP by five different cross-reactive mAbs against rhFHR-4A and rhFHR-4B. These mAbs were able to precipitate FHR-4A from serum. Because anti-FHR-4A.08, -4A.10, -4A.11, and -4A.12 all recognized two epitopes in rhFHR-4A, it is possible that the lack of FHR-4B detection following IP was caused by a difference in binding avidity, favoring FHR-4A over FHR-4B. However, anti-FHR-4A.09, which also did not precipitate FHR-4B from human serum, only recognized one epitope in domain 8/9 or 4/5 of FHR-4A and FHR-4B, respectively. Thus far, only one report has suggested the presence of FHR-4B in human serum, being distinguished from FHR-3 by Western blotting following 2D electrophoresis separation (23). These blots were stained using cross-reactive polyclonal antibodies, making it unclear whether it is truly FHR-4B that was originally detected or not. Even if present, the levels of freely circulating FHR-4B must be extremely low compared to FHR-4A, since it was undetectable in any of our assays. Our current results are supported by previous reports, in which Western Blot analysis of human plasma also seems to indicate that FHR-4A is the dominant splice variant (8, 24). Hence, we developed an ELISA capable of specifically measuring FHR-4A and determined the normal average concentration of FHR-4A at 2.55 μg/mL (i.e., 29.65 nM). This is a 67.5-fold molar difference compared to the ~2 μM concentration of FH in human serum. The FHR-4A levels reported here are in line with previous reported levels determined by mass spectrometry (25) but stand in great contrast with the FHR-4 concentration of 25.4 μg/mL, as determined previously by an immunoassay (11). As discussed above, it seems unlikely that FHR-4B, which in theory was also measured in the previous report, can account for this difference. Both ELISAs catch FHR-4A with a monoclonal antibody while detecting it with a polyclonal antibody. Hence, it is more likely that there is a difference in the Sf9-derived rhFHR-4A previously used (14) and the HEK293F-derived rhFHR-4A used here for the calibration of the assays. Considering the recently reported normal values for all other FHR proteins (6, 18, 21, 22), ranging from 0.7 to 12 μg/mL (with FHR-1 being the most abundant FHR protein), it seems the values that we report for FHR-4A are likely to be correct.

We found considerable variation in FHR-4A concentration among healthy individuals, which is in line with previous observations by others (8, 17). This high degree of variation is also found in FHR-3 (6). However, the variation in FHR-3 levels can, to a major extent, be explained by the *CFHR3/CFHR1* deletion, which is relatively common with an allele frequency of about 20% in the Western population (12, 13, 26–30). The second known deletion in the *CFH-CFHR* locus, encompassing *CFHR1* and *CFHR4*, is far less common with an allele frequency of about 0.9% in the Western population (31). Thus, it is unlikely that CNV of *CFHR4* explains the variation seen in FHR-4A levels, suggesting that other as yet unknown genetic variations determine the concentrations of FHR-4A, which is independent of inflammation since FHR-4A did not behave as an early acute phase protein. Studies investigating the genetic variation(s) resulting in altered FHR-4A expression are currently ongoing.

In summary, we characterized novel anti-FHR-4A mAbs, which were employed to develop a highly specific FHR-4A ELISA. FHR-4A was found to be the dominant splice variant of *CFHR4* and circulates in healthy individuals at an average concentration of 2.55 (±1.46) μg/mL. Similar to the other FHR proteins, the circulating levels of FHR-4A are much lower as compared to FH (~0.03 versus ~2 μM, respectively).

AUTHOR CONTRIBUTIONS

RP, DW, and TK designed the study. RP, MJ, DW, and TK designed experiments. RP, MB, and AvB performed experiments. All authors analyzed and discussed data. RP, DW, and TK wrote the first draft of the manuscript. All authors revised the data and contributed to the final version of the manuscript.

ACKNOWLEDGMENTS

The authors would like to express thanks to the blood donors and patients for their contribution. Research leading to these results has received funding from the European Union's seventh Framework program under EC-GA no. 279185 (EUCLIDS; www.euclids-project.eu).

REFERENCES

1. Ricklin D, Reis ES, Lambris JD. Complement in disease: a defence system turning offensive. *Nat Rev Nephrol* (2016) 12:383–401. doi:10.1038/nrneph.2016.70
2. Esparza-Gordillo J, Soria JM, Buil A, Almasy L, Blangero J, Fontcuberta J, et al. Genetic and environmental factors influencing the human factor H plasma levels. *Immunogenetics* (2004) 56:77–82. doi:10.1007/s00251-004-0660-7
3. Hakobyan S, Tortajada A, Harris CL, Rodríguez de Córdoba S, Morgan BP. Variant-specific quantification of factor H in plasma identifies null alleles associated with atypical hemolytic uremic syndrome. *Kidney Int* (2010) 78:782–8. doi:10.1038/ki.2010.275
4. Ansari M, Mckeigue PM, Skerka C, Hayward C, Rudan I, Vitart V, et al. Genetic influences on plasma CFH and CFHR1 concentrations and their role in susceptibility to age-related macular degeneration. *Hum Mol Genet* (2013) 22:4857–69. doi:10.1093/hmg/ddt336
5. Sofat R, Mangione PP, Gallimore JR, Hakobyan S, Hughes TR, Shah T, et al. Distribution and determinants of circulating complement factor H concentration determined by a high-throughput immunonephelometric assay. *J Immunol Methods* (2013) 390:63–73. doi:10.1016/j.jim.2013.01.009
6. Pouw RB, Brouwer MC, Geissler J, van Herpen LV, Zeerleder SS, Wuillemin WA, et al. Complement factor H-related protein 3 serum levels are low compared to factor H and mainly determined by gene copy number variation in CFHR3. *PLoS One* (2016) 11:e0152164. doi:10.1371/journal.pone.0152164
7. Skerka C, Hellwage J, Weber W, Tilkorn A, Buck F, Marti T, et al. The human factor H-related protein 4 (FHR-4). *J Biol Chem* (1997) 272:5627–34. doi:10.1074/jbc.272.9.5627
8. Józsi M, Richter H, Löschmann I, Skerka C, Buck F, Beisiegel U, et al. FHR-4A: a new factor H-related protein is encoded by the human FHR-4 gene. *Eur J Hum Genet* (2005) 13:321–9. doi:10.1038/sj.ejhg.5201324
9. Józsi M, Tortajada A, Uzonyi B, Goicoechea de Jorge E, Rodríguez de Córdoba S. Factor H-related proteins determine complement-activating surfaces. *Trends Immunol* (2015) 36:374–84. doi:10.1016/j.it.2015.04.008
10. Hellwage J, Jokiranta TS, Koistinen V, Vaarala O, Meri S, Zipfel PF. Functional properties of complement factor H-related proteins FHR-3 and FHR-4: binding to the C3d region of C3b and differential regulation by heparin. *FEBS Lett* (1999) 462:345–52. doi:10.1016/S0014-5793(99)01554-9
11. Hebecker M, Józsi M. Factor H-related protein 4 activates complement by serving as a platform for the assembly of alternative pathway C3 convertase via its interaction with C3b protein. *J Biol Chem* (2012) 287:19528–36. doi:10.1074/jbc.M112.364471
12. Schmid-Kubista KE, Tosakulwong N, Wu Y, Ryu E, Hecker LA, Baratz KH, et al. Contribution of copy number variation in the regulation of complement activation locus to development of age-related macular degeneration. *Investig Ophthalmol Vis Sci* (2009) 50:5070–9. doi:10.1167/iovs.09-3975
13. Sawitzke J, Im KM, Kostiha B, Dean M, Gold B. Association assessment of copy number polymorphism and risk of age-related macular degeneration. *Ophthalmology* (2011) 118:2442–6. doi:10.1016/j.ophtha.2011.05.027
14. Mihlan M, Hebecker M, Dahse H-M, Hälbich S, Huber-Lang M, Dahse R, et al. Human complement factor H-related protein 4 binds and recruits native pentameric C-reactive protein to necrotic cells. *Mol Immunol* (2009) 46:335–44. doi:10.1016/j.molimm.2008.10.029
15. Hebecker M, Okemefuna AI, Perkins SJ, Mihlan M, Huber-Lang M, Józsi M. Molecular basis of C-reactive protein binding and modulation of complement activation by factor H-related protein 4. *Mol Immunol* (2010) 47:1347–55. doi:10.1016/j.molimm.2009.12.005
16. Hellwage J, Skerka C, Zipfel PF. Biochemical and functional characterization of the factor-H-related protein 4 (FHR-4). *Immunopharmacology* (1997) 38:149–57. doi:10.1016/S0162-3109(97)00075-1
17. Närkiö-Mäkelä M, Hellwage J, Tahkokallio O, Meri S. Complement-regulator factor H and related proteins in otitis media with effusion. *Clin Immunol* (2001) 100:118–26. doi:10.1006/clim.2001.5043
18. van Beek AE, Pouw RB, Brouwer MC, van Mierlo G, Ooijevaar-de Heer P, de Boer M, et al. FHR-1 and FHR-2 form homo- and heterodimers, while FHR-5 circulates only as homodimer in human plasma. *Front Immunol* (2017) 8:1328. doi:10.3389/fimmu.2017.01328
19. Tortajada A, Gutiérrez E, Goicoechea de Jorge E, Anter J, Segarra A, Espinosa M, et al. Elevated factor H-related protein 1 and factor H pathogenic variants decrease complement regulation in IgA nephropathy. *Kidney Int* (2017) 92(4):953–63. doi:10.1016/j.kint.2017.03.041
20. Kopczynska M, Zelek W, Touchard S, Gaughran F, Di Forti M, Mondelli V, et al. Complement system biomarkers in first episode psychosis. *Schizophr Res* (2017). doi:10.1016/j.schres.2017.12.012
21. Schäfer N, Grosche A, Reinders J, Hauck S, Pouw RB, Kuijpers TW, et al. Complement regulator FHR-3 is elevated either locally or systemically in a selection of autoimmune diseases. *Front Immunol* (2016) 7:542. doi:10.3389/fimmu.2016.00542
22. McRae JL, Duthy TG, Griggs KM, Ormsby RJ, Cowan PJ, Cromer BA, et al. Human factor H-related protein 5 has cofactor activity, inhibits C3 convertase activity, binds heparin and C-reactive protein, and associates with lipoprotein. *J Immunol* (2005) 174:6250–6. doi:10.4049/jimmunol.174.10.6250
23. Abarrategui-Garrido C, Martínez-Barricarte R, López-Trascasa M, Rodríguez de Córdoba S, Sánchez-Corral P. Characterization of complement factor H-related (CFHR) proteins in plasma reveals novel genetic variations of CFHR1 associated with atypical hemolytic uremic syndrome. *Blood* (2009) 114:4261–71. doi:10.1182/blood-2009-05-223834
24. Skerka C, Chen Q, Frémeaux-Bacchi V, Roumenina LT. Complement factor H related proteins (CFHRs). *Mol Immunol* (2013) 56:170–80. doi:10.1016/j.molimm.2013.06.001
25. Zhang P, Zhu M, Geng-Spyropoulos M, Shardell M, Gonzalez-Freire M, Gudnason V, et al. A novel, multiplexed targeted mass spectrometry assay for quantification of complement factor H (CFH) variants and CFH-related proteins 1-5 in human plasma. *Proteomics* (2017) 17:1–29. doi:10.1002/pmic.201600237.This
26. Hageman GS, Hancox LS, Taiber AJ, Gehrs KM, Anderson DH, Johnson LV, et al. Extended haplotypes in the complement factor H (CFH) and CFH-related (CFHR) family of genes protect against age-related macular degeneration: characterization, ethnic distribution and evolutionary implications. *Ann Med* (2006) 38:592–604. doi:10.1080/07853890601097030
27. Zipfel PF, Edey M, Heinen S, Józsi M, Richter H, Misselwitz J, et al. Deletion of complement factor H-related genes CFHR1 and CFHR3 is associated with atypical hemolytic uremic syndrome. *PLoS Genet* (2007) 3:e41. doi:10.1371/journal.pgen.0030041
28. Sivakumaran TA, Igo RP, Kidd JM, Itsara A, Kopplin LJ, Chen W, et al. A 32 kb critical region excluding Y402H in CFH mediates risk for age-related macular degeneration. *PLoS One* (2011) 6:e25598. doi:10.1371/journal.pone.0025598
29. Zhao J, Wu H, Khosravi M, Cui H, Qian X, Kelly JA, et al. Association of genetic variants in complement factor H and factor H-related genes with systemic lupus erythematosus susceptibility. *PLoS Genet* (2011) 7:e1003079. doi:10.1371/journal.pgen.1002079
30. Holmes LV, Strain L, Staniforth SJ, Moore I, Marchbank KJ, Kavanagh D, et al. Determining the population frequency of the CFHR3/CFHR1 deletion at 1q32. *PLoS One* (2013) 8:e60352. doi:10.1371/journal.pone.0060352
31. Moore I, Strain L, Pappworth I, Kavanagh D, Barlow PN, Herbert AP, et al. Association of factor H autoantibodies with deletions of CFHR1, CFHR3, CFHR4, and with mutations in CFH, CFI, CD46, and C3 in patients with atypical hemolytic uremic syndrome. *Blood* (2010) 115:379–87. doi:10.1182/blood-2009-05-221549

8

Both Monoclonal and Polyclonal Immunoglobulin Contingents Mediate Complement Activation in Monoclonal Gammopathy Associated-C3 Glomerulopathy

Sophie Chauvet[1,2,3*], *Lubka T. Roumenina*[2,3,4], *Pierre Aucouturier*[5,6], *Maria-Chiara Marinozzi*[2,5], *Marie-Agnès Dragon-Durey*[2,3,7], *Alexandre Karras*[1], *Yahsou Delmas*[8], *Moglie Le Quintrec*[9], *Dominique Guerrot*[10], *Noémie Jourde-Chiche*[11], *David Ribes*[12], *Pierre Ronco*[4,13,14], *Frank Bridoux*[15,16] and *Véronique Fremeaux-Bacchi*[2,3,5]

[1] Assistance Publique-Hôpitaux de Paris, Hôpital Européen Georges Pompidou, Department of Nephrology, Paris, France, [2] INSERM UMRS1138, Centre de Recherche des Cordeliers, Team "Complément et Maladies", Paris, France, [3] Université Paris Descartes Sorbonne Paris-Cité, Paris, France, [4] Sorbonne Université, Paris, France, [5] Assistance Publique-Hôpitaux de Paris, Hôpital Saint Antoine, Department of Immunology, Paris, France, [6] INSERM UMRS 938, Sorbonne Universités, UPMC Univ Paris 06, Hôpital Saint-Antoine, Paris, France, [7] Assistance Publique-Hôpitaux de Paris, Hôpital Européen Georges Pompidou, Department of Immunology, Paris, France, [8] Department of Nephrology, Centre Hospitalier Universitaire de Bordeaux, Bordeaux, France, [9] Department of Nephrology, Hôpital de Foch, Suresnes, France, [10] Department of Nephrology, Centre Hospitalier Universitaire de Rouen, Rouen, France, [11] Aix-Marseille Univ, UMRS 1076 Vascular Research Center of Marseille, Department of Nephrology, AP-HM, Marseille, France, [12] Department of Nephrology, Centre Hospitalier Universitaire de Toulouse, Toulouse, France, [13] Assistance Publique-Hôpitaux de Paris, Hôpital Tenon, Department of Nephrology, Paris, France, [14] INSERM UMRS1155, Hôpital Tenon, Paris, France, [15] Department of Nephrology, INSERM CIC 1402, Centre Hospitalier Universitaire de Poitiers, Poitiers, France, [16] Centre National de Référence Maladies Rares: Amylose al et Autres Maladies à Dépôts d'Immunoglobulines Monoclonales, Université de Poitiers, Poitiers, France

***Correspondence:**
Sophie Chauvet
sophiechauvet@ymail.com

C3 glomerulopathy (C3G) results from acquired or genetic abnormalities in the complement alternative pathway (AP). C3G with monoclonal immunoglobulin (MIg-C3G) was recently included in the spectrum of "monoclonal gammopathy of renal significance." However, mechanisms of complement dysregulation in MIg-C3G are not described and the pathogenic effect of the monoclonal immunoglobulin is not understood. The purpose of this study was to investigate the mechanisms of complement dysregulation in a cohort of 41 patients with MIg-C3G. Low C3 level and elevated sC5b-9, both biomarkers of C3 and C5 convertase activation, were present in 44 and 78% of patients, respectively. Rare pathogenic variants were identified in 2/28 (7%) tested patients suggesting that the disease is acquired in a large majority of patients. Anti-complement auto-antibodies were found in 20/41 (49%) patients, including anti-FH (17%), anti-CR1 (27%), anti-FI (5%) auto-antibodies, and C3 Nephritic Factor (7%) and were polyclonal in 77% of patients. Using cofactor assay, the regulation of the AP was altered in presence of purified IgG from 3/9 and 4/7 patients with anti-FH or anti-CR1 antibodies respectively. By using fluid and solid phase AP activation, we showed that total purified IgG of 22/34 (65%) MIg-C3G patients were able to enhance C3 convertase activity. In five documented cases, we showed that the C3 convertase enhancement was mostly due to the monoclonal immunoglobulin, thus paving the way for a new mechanism of complement dysregulation in C3G. All together the results highlight the contribution of both polyclonal and monoclonal Ig in MIg-C3G. They provide direct insights to treatment approaches and opened up a potential way to a personalized therapeutic strategy based on chemotherapy adapted to the B cell clone or immunosuppressive therapy.

Keywords: complement, alternative pathway activation, C3 glomerulopathies, monoclonal gammopathy, autoantibodies

INTRODUCTION

C3 glomerulopathy (C3G) is a heterogeneous group of rare glomerular diseases, characterized by predominant C3 deposition in glomeruli (1–3) and resulting from dysregulation of the complement alternative pathway (AP) (4–6). In physiological conditions, the complement AP is continuously activated at a low level and is amplified on activating surfaces, such as bacteria or dying cells (7). To avoid undesirable auto-amplification, the AP is tightly regulated in the fluid-phase and on cell surfaces by the plasma regulatory proteins factor H (FH), factor I (FI), membrane cofactor protein (MCP, CD46), complement receptor 1 (CR1, CD35), and decay accelerating factor (DAF, CD55) (8). Together, these regulators act by preventing the formation of and by dissociating the AP C3 convertase (FH, CR1, and DAF) and by serving as cofactors for FI-mediated inactivation of C3b to iC3b (FH, MCP, and CR1). Properdin is the only positive regulator of the AP, stabilizing the AP C3/C5 convertase (8, 9). Many of these factors are involved in complement dysregulation in C3G. Rare pathogenic variants in AP genes are identified in ~25% of C3G patients (5, 6, 10). In most cases, complement dysregulation is acquired, induced by the presence of Nephritic Factors (C3NeF and C5NeF), i.e., autoantibodies targeting the AP C3/C5 convertase (6, 10) or anti-FH antibodies (11, 12). Recently, C3G has been proposed to be included in the spectrum of monoclonal gammopathy of renal significance (MGRS) because of the high prevalence of monoclonal immunoglobulins (MIg) in C3G patients aged over 50, without criteria for multiple myeloma, that reached 30–71% in two small series, and 65% in the French C3G cohorts (13–16). Although this association and the favorable effect of clone-targeted therapy on renal outcomes (16) suggests a role of MIg in the occurrence of the renal disease, the exact pathophysiological link between MIg and AP dysregulation remains to be elucidated.

The aim of the current work was to determine the mechanism of acquired complement AP dysregulation in patients with MIg-C3G in order to clarify the causal relationship between the MIg and the occurrence of C3G.

METHODS

Study Population

Between 2000 and June 2014, 201 plasma samples from patients aged over 18 were received at the Laboratory of Immunology (European Hospital Georges Pompidou) for complement exploration in the context of C3G. The diagnosis of C3G was assessed by immunofluorescence according to consensus recommendations, with bright diffuse predominant C3 glomerular staining (≥2+), of at least two orders of magnitude greater than any other immune reactant (i.e., Ig). Patients with trace or weak amounts of IgM staining on glomerular sclerotic lesions were included, but those with weak staining for IgG, IgA or Ig light chains were excluded (2). The diagnosis of DDD was confirmed by demonstration of diffuse, highly electron-dense osmiophilic deposits within the lamina densa by EM. By contrast, the diagnosis of C3GN was established in patients showing deposits of lesser density without the characteristic distribution and "sausage shape" appearance of DDD (1). All patients with positive hepatitis B or C serology, antinuclear antigen autoantibodies, anti- double-stranded DNA antibodies, or cryoglobulinemia are excluded from the French C3G registry.

Search for monoclonal gammopathy was performed by immunofixation in all patients aged over 40. Of the 201 adult patients in the French registry of C3G, 60 patients (G1-G60) had a detectable MIg. Among them, 50 were included in a retrospective clinical study regarding the effect of chemotherapy on renal outcomes (16). In the current study, 41/60 MIg-C3G patients with available blood samples were included (**Supplemental Figure 1**). Two of 28 patients screened for genetic abnormalities carried a rare variant of undetermined significance (p.Asp130Asn in CFH and p.Glu548Gln in CFI), as previously described (16). As 96% of MIg-C3G patients displayed a C3GN pattern on kidney biopsy, 107 adult patients with C3GN without MIg extracted from the French cohort of C3G, and 8 patients with MIg without kidney disease, were used as control population. The local ethics committee approved the study and the study was approved by the Commission Nationale de L'informatique et des Libertés (CCP number 192 12 23) and all legal representative of children gave written informed consent for genetic analysis.

Assays for Complement Component and for C3 and C5 Nephritic Factors

EDTA plasma samples were obtained from all patients. Plasma protein concentrations of C3, C4 were measured by nephelometry (Dade Behring, Deerfield, IL, USA). Soluble C5b-9 level determination was done using the MicroVue sC5b-9 Plus EIA Assay (Quidel, San Diego, CA), according to manufacturer instructions. Normal values were established from plasma samples from 100 healthy donors. C3NeF and C5NeF activities were determined by assessing the ability of purified plasma IgG to stabilize the membrane-bound C3bBb and C3bBbP convertases (6).

ELISA Detection for anti-FH, anti-FI, anti-CR1, anti-C3b and anti-FB Antibodies

ELISA plates were coated with 10 to 15μg/ml of FH (11), FI, FB, C3b (17) (all from Complement Technologies, Tylor, Texas), CR1 (RandD System) in PBS for 1 h, followed by blocking of the plates with PBS-0.4% Tween 20. Plasma was diluted 1/200 in PBS-0.1% Tween 20 and applied for 1 h. Bound IgG or IgA was revealed by anti-human IgG antibody conjugated with HRP (Southern Biotech) or anti-human IgA antibody conjugated with HRP (Sigma) diluted in PBS-0.1% Tween 20, followed by TMB substrate system.

Study of IgG Binding to CR1 by Surface Plasmon Resonance (SPR)

The interaction of patient IgG with CR1 was analyzed in real time using a ProteOn XPR36 SPR equipment (BioRad, Marne-la-coquette, France). CR1 (RandD System) was covalently immobilized to a GLC sensor chip (BioRad) following the manufacturer's procedure. Protein G purified IgG from the patients or healthy donors (at 100 μg/ml) were injected for 300 s in PBS 0.005% Tween 20 containing running buffer. The dissociation was followed for 300 s. The signal from the interspots, reflecting the background binding was subtracted, as recommended by the manufacturer.

Study of C3b Interaction With CR1 in Presence of Patients IgG by Surface Plasmon Resonance

IgG from patients with anti-CR1 antibodies were tested for their capacity to alter the C3b binding to CR1 using SPR. CR1 was coupled to individual flow channels of GLC biosensor chip using standard amine-coupling, according to the manufacturer's instruction. Total purified IgG were flowed at a concentration 100 mg/ml followed by injection of C3b (Complement Technologies) at concentrations starting from 1 μg/ml. Five concentrations and a running buffer were injected at 30 μl/min in HEPES buffer (10 mM Hepes, 25 mM NaCl, Tween 0.005%, pH 7.4) for 300 s across the immobilized ligand. Data were analyzed using ProteOn Manager software and the data from the blank channel were subtracted. Kinetic parameters were calculated by fitting the obtained sensorgrams into a two-state interaction model.

Determination of Light Chain and Heavy Chain Isotype Specificity of Anti-complement Protein Antibodies

The light chain (LC) isotype of antibodies was determined by ELISA. After plasma incubation and washing, isotype-specific goat antibodies directed against kappa and lambda LC (Southern Biotech), diluted in PBS-0.1% Tween 20 were incubated 1 h. Bound Ig was revealed by a Rabbit anti goat IgG Ab (Santa Cruz) diluted in PBS-0.1% Tween 20, followed by TMB substrate system. The ratios of the optical densities obtained with the anti-k and anti-l Abs (k/l) were calculated for all samples. A k/l ratio < 0.1 or >3 indicated the predominance of anti-complement autoantibody of lambda or kappa LC specificity respectively, as previously described. A ratio between 0.1 and 3 indicated both kappa and lambda reactivity (11). The heavy chain (HC) IgG subtypes of anti FH and anti CR1 IgG Ab were determined by an anti-FH or anti-CR1 ELISA. After plasma incubation and washing, isotype-specific mouse antibodies directed against IgG1, IgG2, IgG3, and IgG4 (NL16 for IgG1, GOM2 for IgG2, ZG4 for IgG3, and RJ4 or IgG4) (Unipath, Bedford, UK), diluted PBS-0.1% Tween 20 were incubated 1 h. Bound IgG was revealed by a rabbit anti mouse IgG Ab (Jackson ImmunoResearch) diluted in PBS-0.1% Tween 20, followed by TMB substrate system.

Determination of LC and HC Isotype Specificity of Monoclonal Immunoglobulin

The analysis of serum MIg of 29/41 patients was performed by a western blotting. Serum dilutions were adjusted to normalized gamma globulin levels. Proteins were separated by high-resolution thin layer agarose electrophoresis and transferred on nitrocellulose sheets. After saturation with skimmed milk, the blots were probed with polyclonal antibodies specific for a, g, m, k or l Ig chains or with monoclonal antibodies specific for IgG subclasses with NL16 for IgG1, GOM2 for IgG2, ZG4 for IgG3, and RJ4 or IgG4 (Unipath, Bedford, UK), followed by peroxydase coupled rabbit anti mouse IgG antibodies (Jackson ImmunoResearch). The signal was developed by chemo luminescence using ECL kit (Perkin Elmer) and MyECL Imager (Thermo Scientific).

IgG Purification

Total IgG Purification

IgG were purified from plasma of MIg-C3G patients or from plasma of control patients (healthy donors, patients with positive C3NeF and patients with MIg but without kidney disease) by using Protein G beads (GE Healthcare), as recommended by the manufacturer. The concentration of the IgG was determined by a Nanodrop spectrophotometer.

Purification of Monoclonal And Polyclonal Igs by Chromatography

Monoclonal and polyclonal Ig fractions of 5 patients (with monoclonal IgG) were purified using ion exchange column chromatography. Each plasma sample was dialyzed against 10 mM Tris (pH8). Prepaked diethyl-aminoethyl (DEAE) trisacryl column (Life Science) was equilibrated with 10 mM Tris (pH8). The dialyzed samples were loaded onto the column followed by elution with a 0–0.2 M NaCl gradient in 10 mM Tris buffer (pH8). Serial 1 ml fractions were collected and assayed for protein concentration (280 nm OD). The fractions were tested by agarose electrophoresis and immunofixation to determine which fractions contained polyclonal or MIg.

Cofactor Assays

C3 protein (20 μg/ml; Calbiochem) was incubated at 37°C for 0, 1, 5, or 10 min with FI (10 μg/ml; Complement Technologies) and FH (20 μg/ml; Complement Technologies, Tylor, Texas), or soluble CR1 (10 μg/ml; RandD Systems) in 10 mM Tris,

150 mM NaCl, pH 7.4 in presence of 100 μg/ml of total purified IgG. Samples were boiled and the cleavage of the C3 was probed by a Western blot, using SNAP system (Millipore). After blocking with Tris 10 mM, NaCl 150 mM, 0.1% Tween, 1% BSA, the blots were probed with a 1:5,000 dilution of goat anti-human C3 IgG (Calbiochem) followed by HRP-conjugated rabbit anti-goat IgG (Santa Cruz). The signal was developed by chemiluminescence using ECL kit (Perkin Elmer) and MyECL Imager (Thermo Scientific). Cleavage efficiency was evaluated by the appearance of the α43 band and the disappearance of the α-chain at 10 min and quantitated by densitometry of the scanned images. The ratio between α43 and the β bands (representing the % of C3b cleaved) was plotted vs. the time of incubation.

TABLE 1 | Comparison of immunological findings in 41 MIg-C3G patients and 107 C3GN adults patients without MIg.

	MIg-C3G $N = 41$	Adults C3GN $N = 107$	*p*-value
IMMUNOLOGICAL FINDINGS			
C3 (mg/L)	703 (78-1220)	781 (67-1760)	0.86
Low C3 level, n(%)	18 (44%)	56 (40%)	0.71
C4 (mg/L)	250 (104-575)*	252 (94-751)*	1
sC5b-9 (ng/mL)	848 (164-2880)	478 (94-2582)	0.005
Elevated sC5b9 (upper 420ng/mL)	29/37 (78%)	47/76 (62%)	0.09
Elevated sC5b-9 (upper twice the normal)	15/37 (41%)	13/76 (17%)	0.01
C3NeF, n(%)	3 (7%)	44/98 (45%)	0.0001
C5NeF, n(%)	0/12 (0%)	11/21(52%)	0.002
Anti-FH Abs, n(%)	9 (17%)	10/91 (11%)	0.09
Anti-FI Abs, n(%)	2 (5%)	NA	-
Anti-CR1 Abs, n(%)	11 (27%)	3/84 (4%)	0.0001
GENETIC ANALYSIS			
Pathogenic variants	2/28(7%)	27/99 (27%)**	0.02

** C4 level was normal in all patients*
***99 on 107 C3GN patients without monoclonal gammopathy were screened for genetics abnormalities of complement proteins. Results are described in Servais et al. (4) and Marinozzi et al. (6).*

C3 Convertase Formation in Normal Human Serum in Presence of Patients' IgG

Purified total IgG from patients or healthy donors were incubated for 30 min at 37°C with normal human serum diluted 1:3 in presence of EGTA-Mg to block the classical pathway (10 mM $MgCl_2$,10 mM EGTA, 40 mM NaCl Hepes buffer). The generation of C3a was quantified by the Micro Vue C3a Kit (Quidel) according to the manufacturer's instructions. IgG from 8 patients with MIg without kidney disease were used as controls.

Fluid Phase C3 Convertase Activation in Presence of Patients' IgG

Total purified IgG (100 μg/ml) were incubated for 45 min at 37°C with C3 (25 μg/ml), FB (0 to 50 ng), FD (0.05 μg/ml) (all from Complement Technologies, Tylor, Texas) in Hepes, 40 mM NaCl supplemented with 10 mM $MgCl_2$. The reaction was stopped by adding DTT-containing sample buffer. The cleavage of C3 was probed by a Western blot, using SNAP system (Millipore). After blocking with Tris 10 mM, NaCl 150 mM, 0.1% Tween, 1% BSA, blots were probed with a 1:5,000 dilution of goat anti-human C3 IgG (Calbiochem) followed by HRP-conjugated rabbit anti-goat IgG (Santa Cruz). The signal was developed by chemiluminescence using ECL kit (Perkin Elmer) and MyECL Imager (Thermo Scientific). Percentage of C3 cleavage revealing convertase formation was characterized by the appearance of α'-band and quantitated by densitometry of the scanned images. The ratio between α' and the β bands was calculated at 50 ng of FB. The same experiment was reproduced with monoclonal and polyclonal Ig fractions of 5 patients and with IgG of 3

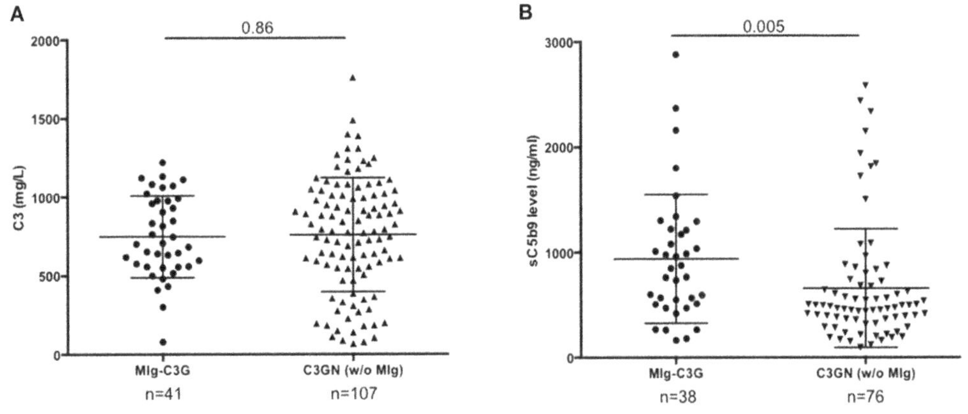

FIGURE 1 | C3 and s C5b9 levels in C3G patients. **(A)** Plasma levels of C3 and **(B)** sC5b-9 of 41 patients with MIg-C3G (including 39 with C3GN and 2 with DDD pattern) and adult C3GN patients without MIg (n = 107). For measurement of sC5b9, 76/107 C3GN patients were tested. Fifty healthy controls were used to calculate the normal range of sC5b-9 (below 460 ng/ml). The mean ± standard deviation of each group is indicated.

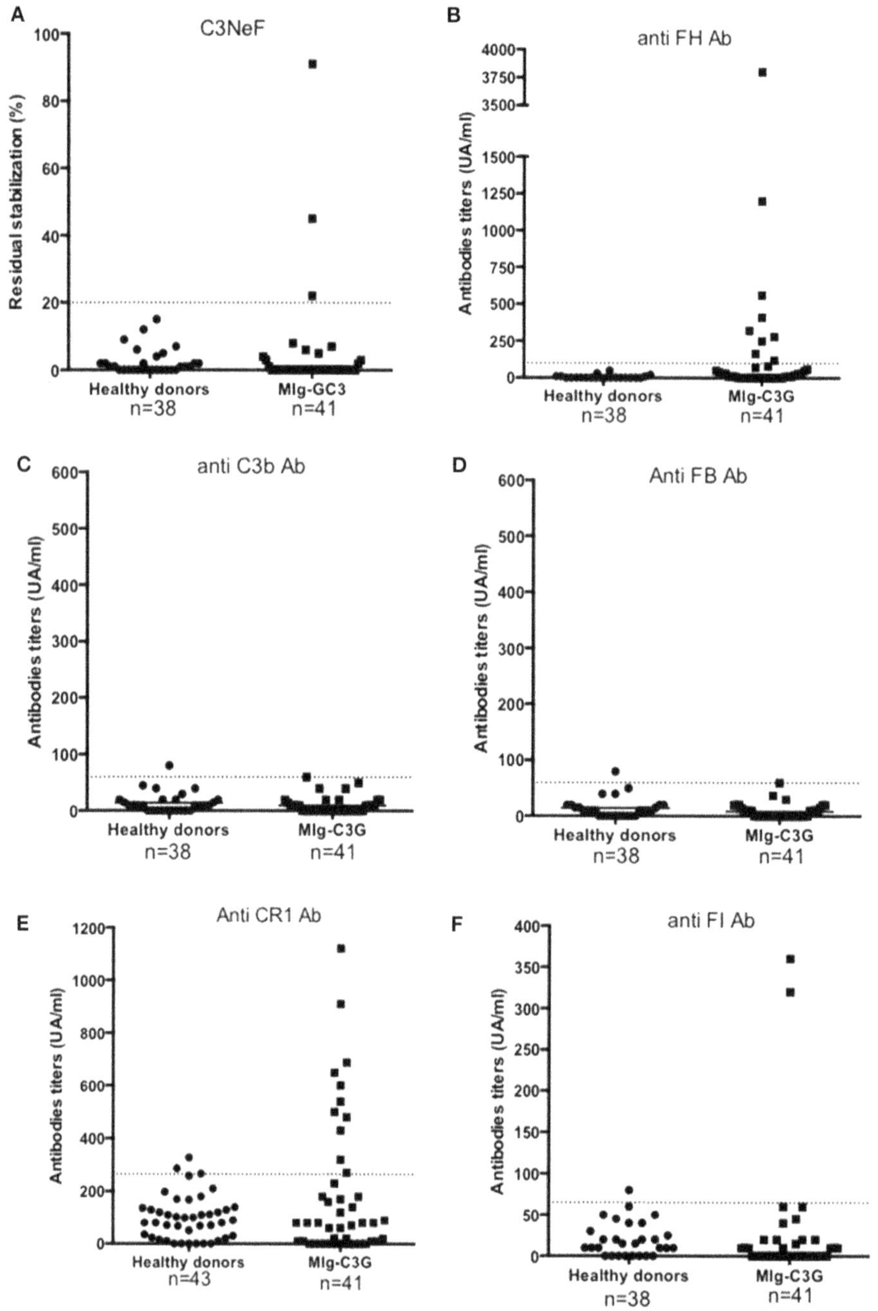

FIGURE 2 | Detection of auto-antibodies against complement proteins. **(A–F)** Reactivity of Ig in plasma samples against FH, C3b, FB, CR1, FI, and C3 convertase (C3NeF assay). Samples from 41 MIg-C3G patients and 38 healthy individuals were tested. Results of C3NeF and other antibodies are expressed as percentage of residual stabilization, and in arbitrary units (UA), respectively. For anti-FH, anti-C3b and anti-FB antibodies, we used positive controls as previously described (one patient positive for anti-FH auto-antibodies in the setting of atypical HUS and one patient positive for both anti-C3b and anti-FB auto-antibodies) (11, 17). For the other ELISA assays, results were considered as positive when the OD was upper the mean +2SD (of the OD obtained with IgG from healthy donors). The patient's sample with the higher OD value was then used to determine the UA.

MIg-C3GN patients after chemotherapy adapted to the B cell clone. IgG from 8 patients with MIg without kidney disease were used as controls. The same experiment was reproduced with monoclonal and polyclonal fractions of 5 MIg-C3G patients IgG.

C3 Convertase Activation on Immobilized Patient IgG

Coating of ELISA plate was performed at 20μg/ml of purified IgG in PBS for 1 h followed by a blocking of the plates by PBS-0.4% Tween 20. After washing, C3 convertase was formed

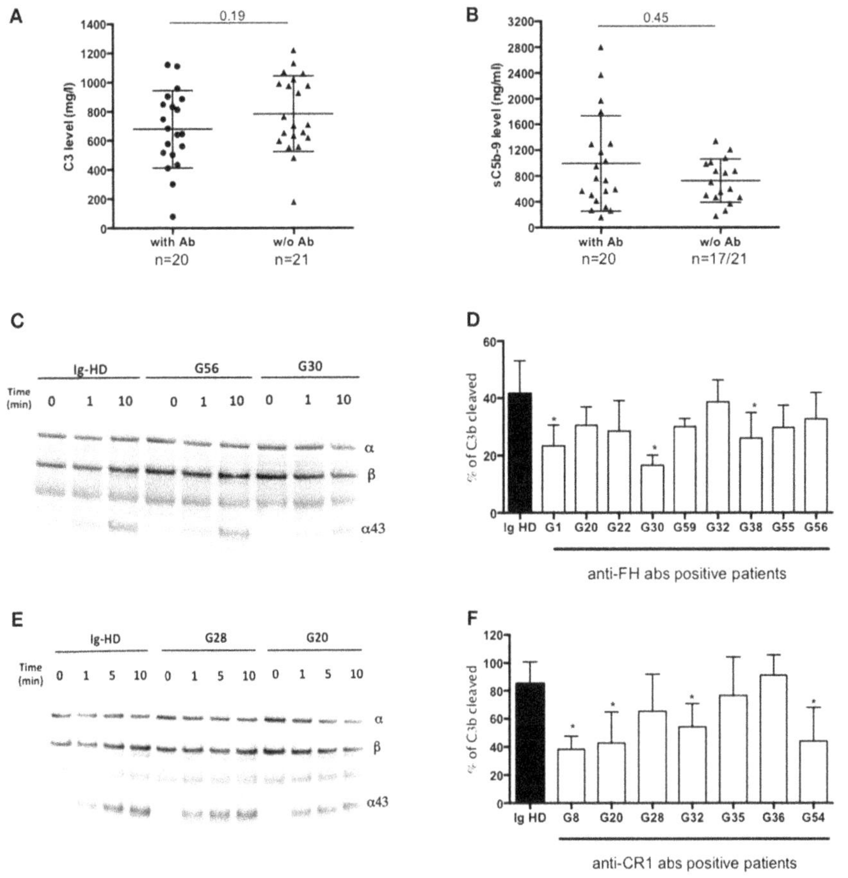

FIGURE 3 | Functional consequences of anti-complement antibodies. **(A)** Plasma levels of C3 and **(B)** sC5b-9 of 22 MIg-C3G patients with anti-complement protein antibodies and 19 MIg-C3G without antibodies. **(C-D)** Analysis of Factor I-dependant cofactor activity of FH in presence of IgG from patients positive for anti-FH antibodies and **(E-F)** of CR1 in presence of IgG from patients positive for anti-CR1 antibodies. Cleavage of C3b to iC3b was indicated by the generation of α43 fragment and decrease of the α-chain. The percentage of C3b cleaved was determined by the ratio α43/β chain ($n = 3$ experiments). $^*p < 0.05$.

by adding C3 (25 μg/ml), FB (0–50 ng), FD (0.05 μg/ml) (all from Complement Technologies, Tylor, Texas) diluted in Hepes, 40 mM NaCl supplemented with 10 mM $MgCl_2$. The cleavage of C3 was probed by a Western blot and quantified as described above.

Statistical Analyses

Data are expressed as median (with range) for continuous variables and percentage for categorical variables. Statistical analyses were performed using the Mann-Whitney and Kruskal-Wallis tests, as appropriate, for comparison of continuous variables. Chi-square or Fisher's exact tests were used for comparison of categorical variables. *P*-values below 0.05 were considered significant. Results were analyzed using the Graph Pad Prism software.

RESULTS

MIg-C3G Is Associated With Biomarkers of C3/C5 Convertase Activation

Forty-one patients from the French registry of C3G met inclusion criteria (**Supplemental Figure 1**). Baseline clinical data and complement biomarkers are detailed in **Supplemental Table 1** and **Table 1**. At diagnosis, 18/41 (44%) MIg-C3G patients had a low C3 level and a normal C4 (**Table 1**). Median C3 level of MIg-C3G patients and C3GN patients without MIg were similar ($p = 0.86$) (**Figure 1A**). Soluble C5b-9 was increased in 29/37 (78%) MIg-C3G patients and in 47/76 (62%) C3GN patients without MIg ($p = 0.09$) (**Table 1**). Median sC5b-9 level was significantly higher in MIg-C3G patients compared to patients without MIg ($p = 0.005$) (**Figure 1B**).

Detection of Anti-complement Protein Auto-antibodies in MIg-C3G

Samples were screened for C3 NeF/C5 NeF and auto-antibodies targeting 5 proteins of the AP (**Figures 2A-F**). Anti-FH auto-antibodies, C3NeF and anti-FI auto-antibodies were detected in 17% (9/41), 7% (3/41), and 5% (2/41) of MIg-C3G patients, respectively. None had anti-C3b, anti-FB antibodies or C5NeF. Eleven patients were positive for anti-CR1 auto-antibodies (11/41, 27%) (**Figure 2E** and **Supplemental Figure 2A**). The characteristics of the binding of anti-CR1 positive IgG to CR1 by Surface Plasmon Resonance (SPR) are provided (**Supplemental Figures 2B-C**). Overall, anti-complement

TABLE 2 | Heavy and light chain characterization of anti-complement protein Ab and monoclonal immunoglobulin.

Patient	MIg	Anti-complement protein Ab			Similar HC and LC specificity between Ab and MIg
		Spécificity	HC	LC	
G30	IgG1λ	Anti FH	γ3	κ and λ	No
G22	IgG4k	Anti FH	γ2	κ and λ	No
G38	IgG2k	Anti FH	γ2	κ	Yes
G55	IgAk	Anti FH	α	κ	Yes
G8	IgG4l	Anti CR1	γ1	κ and λ	No
G13	IgG1k	Anti CR1	γ1	κ and λ	No
G15	IgG1λ	Anti CR1	γ1, γ4	κ and λ	No
G35	IgG3k	Anti CR1	γ1	κ and λ	No
G28	IgG2k	Anti CR1	γ1	κ and λ	No
G54	LCk	Anti CR1	γ1	κ and λ	No
G40	IgAk	Anti FI	α	κ	Yes
G20	IgG2λ	Anti FH/CR1	Anti-FH γ1 and Anti-CR1	κ and λ	No
G32	IgG4l	anti FH/anti CR1	Anti-FH γ2 and Anti-CR1 γ1	κ and λ	No

Abbreviations: Ab, antibody, HC: heavy chain, LC: light chain, MIg: monoclonal immunoglobulin

auto-antibodies were detected in 20/41 (49%) MIg-C3G patients, including 4 patients with combined anti-FH and anti-CR1 antibodies and 1 with anti-FI and anti-FH antibodies.

C3 and sC5b9 levels were similar in patients with or without antibodies (**Figures 3A,B**). Compared to C3GN patients without MIg, MIg-C3G patients had significantly lower frequency of C3NeF [3/41(7%) vs. 44/98(45%); $p = 0.0001$] and C5NeF ($p = 0.002$), higher frequency of anti-CR1 auto-antibodies [11/41(27%) vs. 3/84(4%); $p = 0.0001$] and similar frequency of anti-FH auto-antibodies (**Table 1**).

Functional studies were carried out in patients with anti-FH, anti-CR1 and anti-FI antibodies. We studied the impact of anti-FH antibodies on AP regulation by studying the capacity of FI to cleave C3b in iC3b in presence of FH. We performed a fluid phase cofactor assay in presence of total IgG purified from patients with anti-FH antibodies or healthy donors (HD). The C3b cleavage was revealed by Western Blot and ratio α43-chain on β-chain of C3b, determined by densitometry, was used to determine the % of C3b cleavage. C3b cleavage was significantly decreased in 3/9 patients with anti-FH antibodies (**Figures 3C,D**).

We next studied the functional properties of anti-CR1 antibodies. The presence of anti-CR1 antibodies resulted in decreased capacity (from 12 to 25%) of C3b to bind CR1, as demonstrated by SPR-based technology (**Supplemental Figures 2D–F**). Moreover, by Western blot, significant reduced CR1 cofactor activity for FI was obtained in presence of IgG purified from 4/7 anti-CR1 positive patients (**Figures 3E,F**). In 2 patients with anti-FI antibodies, C3b cleavage by FI in presence of FH was not decreased (data not shown).

Study of Light and Heavy Chain Isotype Specificity of Anti-complement Protein Antibodies

MIg heavy chain (HC) and light chain (LC) isotype specificities were determined by immunoblot in 29 patients (**Supplemental Table 2**).

Using ELISA, we determined heavy chain (HC) and light chain (LC) isotype specificity of anti-complement antibodies in 13 positive patients. In 3 cases, anti-FI IgA, anti-FH IgG or anti-FH IgA antibodies displayed similar HC and LC restriction as the MIg. In 10/13 (77%) positive patients, the MIg HC (all of IgG isotype) and/or LC did not match those of the respective auto-antibodies (**Table 2**).

Patients' Ig Induce Fluid-Phase and Solid-Phase AP Convertase Activation

To test the capacity of total purified IgG (containing the MIg) of MIg-C3G patients to activate complement AP, we measured C3a release in normal human serum (NHS) by ELISA after incubation with patients' IgG or IgG from healthy donors (**Supplemental Figure 3**). For 10/32 patients' IgG, C3a level was above the mean+2SD cut-off obtained with IgG from healthy donors (**Supplemental Figure 3A**). C3a release was similar in MIg-C3G patients with or without anti-complement protein auto-antibodies (**Supplemental Figure 3B**).

To demonstrate that IgG of MIg-C3G patients directly enhance the C3 cleavage into C3b without the influence of auto-antibodies, purified C3, FB, FD were incubated with total IgG from controls (Healthy-donors (HD) and patients with MIg without kidney disease) and MIg-C3G patients and tested in solution or on IgG-coated plate in presence of EGTA-Mg^{2+}. The % of C3 cleavage into C3b was determined by Western blot, by measuring the ratio between α′chain and βchain of C3b, determined by densitometry. Mean % of C3 cleavage was 38% in the presence of IgG from HDs in solution (mean + 2DS of the ratio = 56%) and 39% on HD-IgG-coated plate (mean + 2DS of the ratio = 59%). Cleavage of C3 was increased (higher than mean+2SD) in presence of 12/34 MIg-C3G patients' IgG in solution (**Figures 4A,B**) and on 13/34 IgG-coated plates (**Figures 4C,D**). Total IgG purified from 3 patients increased C3b formation both in solution and on coated IgG. Patients' IgG that activated the C3 convertase in solution or on coated phase were named "C3-activating IgG." Altogether 22/34 tested patients' IgG displayed capacity to cleave C3. In both experimental conditions, C3b formation was significantly higher compared to that obtained in presence of total IgG from patients with MIg but without kidney disease (**Figures 4B,D**). C3 cleavage was similar in MIg-C3G patients with or without anti-complement protein antibodies (**Supplemental Figures 3C,D**).

C3 levels were significantly lower in patients positive for C3-activating IgG than in those negative ($P = 0.03$) (**Figure 4E**), whereas there was no difference for sC5b9 in plasma ($p = 0.94$) (**Figure 4F**). Plasma sC5b9 levels were upper than twice the normal value in 12/22 (57%) patients with C3-activating IgG and in 3/14 (21%) patients without this capacity ($p = 0.04$).

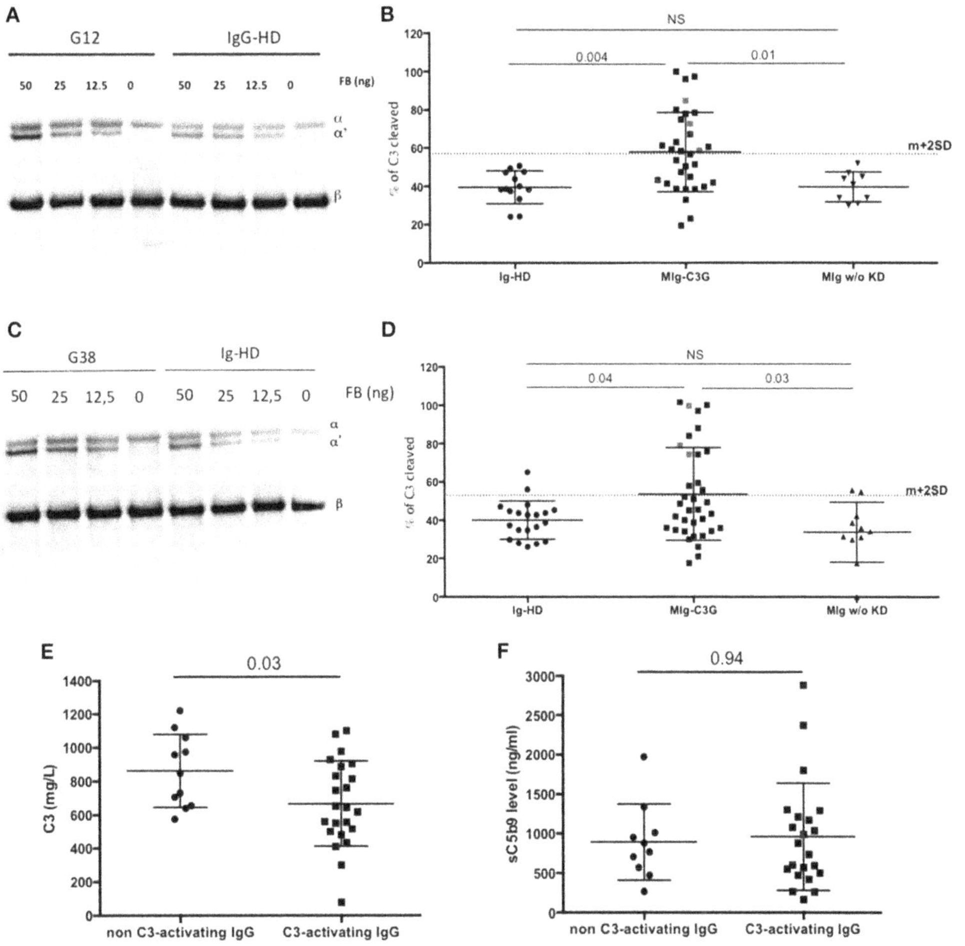

FIGURE 4 | AP convertase activation in presence of patients' total purified IgG. **(A)** MIg-C3G patients' IgG were tested for their capacity to enhance fluid phase AP C3 convertase formation. Cleavage of C3 to C3b by fluid phase C3 convertase was measured by the generation of the α' chain. Result of patient G12 is provided compared to Healthy donor (HD) **(B)** C3 convertase activity was significantly increased in presence of MIg-C3G patients' IgG compared to Ig from HD or Ig from patients with MIg without kidney disease (MIg w/o KD). In presence of Ig from 12/34 patients, % of C3 cleavage was significantly increased [above the cut-off (mean+2SD)]. **(C)** MIg-C3G patients' IgG coated on well plates were tested for their capacity to enhance AP C3 convertase formation. Cleavage of C3–C3b by fluid phase C3 convertase was measured by the generation of the α' chain. Result of patient G38 is provided compared to HD **(D)** C3 convertase activity was significantly increased in presence of MIg-C3G patients' IgG compared to Ig from healthy donors or Ig from patients with MIg without kidney disease (MIg w/o KD). IgG from patients able to enhance C3 convertase in fluid phase or on well plate were named "C3-activating" Ig **(E)** C3 level of patients with "C3-activating" IgG was significantly increased compared to patients without "C3-activating" IgG. **(F)** sC5b9 level of patients with "C3-activating" IgG was similar to patients without "C3-activating" IgG.

Monoclonal Ig Are Able to Enhance Fluid Phase C3 Convertase Overactivation

To identify the components involved in the AP activation, the MIg was separated from polyclonal Ig by chromatography in 2 patients with C3-activating IgG (G12, G20) and 3 patients without C3 activating IgG in fluid phase (G38, G40, G24). In samples from patients G12 and G20, C3b formation was increased in presence of the MIg compared to the polyclonal Ig (**Figures 5A,B**).

We also investigated whether the capacity of total IgG to activate the AP disappeared after complete hematological response (as assessed by negative serum immunofixation) following chemotherapy. Blood samples from 3 patients (G5, G37, G53) in whom total IgG were responsible for C3 cleavage in solution were available. In all three cases, C3 cleavage was significantly reduced in presence of total IgG purified from blood after treatment compared to that obtained with IgG from the same patients at diagnosis (**Figures 5C–E**).

DISCUSSION

We described for the first time the mechanisms of complement alternative pathway dysregulation in a peculiar group of patients with C3G associated with monoclonal immunoglobulin (MIg-C3G). We found anti complement antibodies in more than 50% of patients but with different target compare to C3G patients without monoclonal gammopathy suggesting that the two diseases are distinct. Moreover, our results

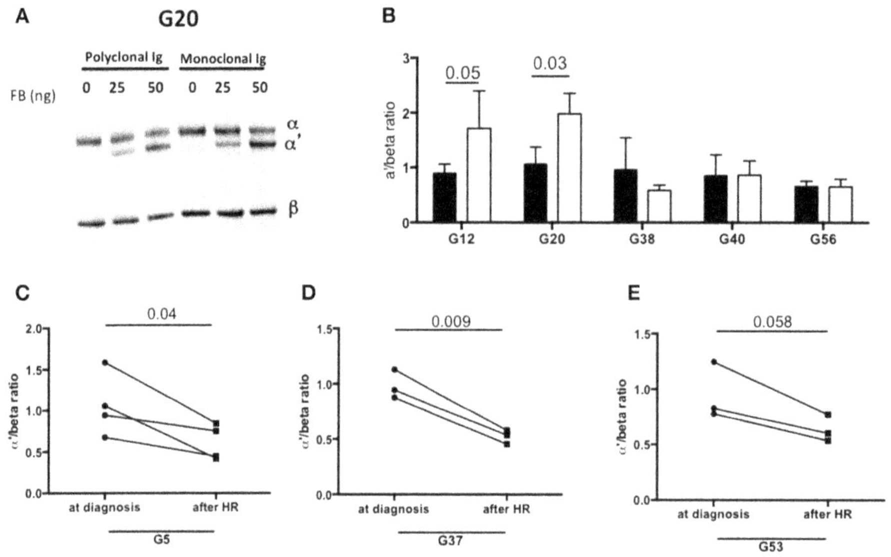

FIGURE 5 | Monoclonal Ig promotes fluid phase C3 convertase activation. **(A)** Polyclonal and monoclonal Ig fractions of 5 MIg-C3G patients were tested for their capacity to enhance fluid phase AP C3 convertase. Cleavage of C3 to C3b by C3 convertase was indicated by generation of the α' chain. **(B)** In 2 out 5 patients (G12, G20), C3 cleavage was increased in presence of the monoclonal Ig fraction (white bars) compared to polyclonal fraction (black bars) ($n = 3$ experiments). In the samples with C3-activating IgG on coated plate, negative for the tests in solution (G38 and G40) and "non C3-activating IgG (G56), C3 convertase activity was similar in presence of the monoclonal and polyclonal Ig fractions. **(C–E)** C3 cleavage by a fluid phase C3 convertase was decreased in 3 patients with "fluid phase activator " Ig (G5, G37, G53) in presence of Ig purified from plasma collected after hematological response (HR) compared to Ig purified from plasma collected at diagnosis of C3G ($n = 3$ experiments).

highlight a contribution of both monoclonal and polyclonal Ig in the inappropriate activation of complement AP in MIg-C3G patients, paving the way to new therapeutic strategies.

In the French cohort of adult C3G without detectable MIg, impaired complement control is driven by C3NeF and by genetic variation in complement genes in 45 and 27%, respectively. Genetic abnormalities were identified in only 7% of tested MIg-C3G patients, suggesting that genetic factors do not play a major role in MIg-C3G. This result is in agreement with those of a recent study in which none of 21 tested patients had any genetic abnormalities (18). Exhaustive screening identified auto-antibodies targeting complement proteins in about 50% of MIg-C3G patients. However, the targets of anti-complement auto-antibodies were different between C3G patients with and without MIg. Indeed, C3NeF was found in only 7% of MIg-C3G patients. This is in agreement with previous small cohort studies, which identified C3NeF in 0/6 and 2/9 MIg-C3G patients (14, 15). The presence of C5NeF stabilizing the C5 convertase has been recently described in 56% of patients with C3GN (6). Interestingly, despite elevated sC5b-9 level in 80% of MIg-C3G cases, C5NeF was negative in all tested patients. The frequency of anti-FH auto-antibodies was low and similar to C3G patients without MIg (11, 12). In contrast, we found that 27% of MIg-C3G patients had anti-CR1 auto-antibodies, undetectable in C3G patients without MIg. Interestingly, CR1 which is expressed by podocytes, emerges as a novel disease-relevant target in C3G (19) and auto-antibodies targeting CR1 have been found in patients with multiple myeloma (20). We further explored functional consequences of these antibodies. Cofactor activity of both CR1 and FH was decreased in 4/7 and 3/9 patients positive for anti-FH or anti-CR1 antibodies, respectively, whereas it was normal in two patients with anti-FI antibodies suggesting that these antibodies have limited functional consequences on AP regulation. C3 and sC5B9 levels were similar in patients with or without anti-complement protein antibodies, confirming the weak contribution of these antibodies in AP dysregulation in MIg-C3G.

The initial assumption was that autoantibodies targeting complement proteins were monoclonal. Indeed, in 1999, Jokiranta et al. demonstrated that a dimeric monoclonal lambda LC, identified in a patient with glomerulonephritis and predominant C3 deposits, was able to bind FH as an auto-antibody, resulting in uncontrolled AP activation *in vitro* (21). In the current study, we showed a concordance in the heavy and light chain isotypes of MIg and anti-complement protein auto-antibodies in only 3/13 patients. Therefore, our results suggest that in most cases anti-complement protein reactivity is not borne by the MIg. This result is in agreement with other kidney diseases mediated by auto-antibodies, where the implication of monoclonal autoantibodies remains exceptional (22, 23).

Further, we tested a new hypothesis according to which the MIg could serve directly as a complement-activating surface. We designed an experiment to study C3 cleavage without interference with the regulatory proteins and thus without the contribution of anti-complement protein antibodies. In 22/34 (65%) of cases, patients' IgG enhanced C3 cleavage, and therefore they could be considered as C3-activating IgG. Interestingly, C3 level was significantly lower in patients with C3-activating IgG than in those without. Moreover, the percentage of patients with sC5b9 levels higher than twice the normal value was significantly increased in patients with C3-activating IgG compared to those patients without C3-activating IgG. Interestingly, the capacity of patients' IgG to enhance C3 cleavage was not increase in patients with MIg but without kidney disease and the link between an ongoing complement activation in MIg-C3G patients and the MIg remains speculative. The direct role of the MIg in AP activation was strongly suggested in 5 patients. Indeed, in 3 of them, we demonstrated the disappearance of the capacity of total IgG to activate the C3 convertase once the MIg had become undetectable after chemotherapy. In 2 patients, we showed the increased capacity of the MIg to enhance fluid phase C3 convertase activity compared to the polyclonal IgG from the same patients. It is well established that MIg have peculiar physicochemical properties due to different profiles of glycosylation or mutations/deletions of the variable or constant domain (24). These peculiarities are likely to account for the variable capacity of these MIg to enhance C3 convertase *in vitro*. It is tempting to speculate that the nascent C3b, generated by slow fluid phase activation of C3, binds to MIg and forms a starting point for the subsequent assembly of C3 convertase.

In a recent clinical study, we demonstrated that achievement of rapid and deep hematological response with clone-targeted chemotherapy significantly improved renal survival in MIg-C3G patients and that C3 levels in patients with hematological response were significantly higher compared with pretreatment C3 levels (16). The present provides more support for a link between the monoclonal Ig and renal disease. Therefore targeting the responsible clone should be a therapeutic goal to preserve or improve renal function in these patients.

Our study has some limitations. It is a retrospective study with a relatively low number of patients. Most patients had low amounts of MIg making the MIg purification process difficult or even impossible. These limitations did not allow us to investigate the direct contribution of MIg in AP dysregulation in all patients, and further studies are needed to depict the full pathophysiological spectrum of MIg in C3GP.

In conclusion, our study highlight different complement AP activation mechanisms in C3G associated with MIg compared to C3G without MIg. We demonstrated that IgG isolated from MIg-C3G patients directly activate the AP in 65% of cases and our findings provide further evidence that monoclonal gammopathy is a cause of the disease, particularly in patients with very high levels of sC5b9 at diagnosis. Our results highlight the need to consider chemotherapy targeting the B cell clone in the treatment strategy of MIg-C3G patients.

AUTHOR CONTRIBUTIONS

The study was conceived and designed by SC and VF-B. SC conducted the experiments and analysis; SC and VF-B were involved in the writing of the manuscript. VF-B and LR reviewed the data analysis; SC, VF-B, FB, and all other authors contributed to the conduct of the study, recruited patients, and were involved in the review of results and final approval of the manuscript.

DISCLOSURE

VF-B received fees for participation in advisory boards, experts meetings and/or teaching courses from Alexion Pharmaceutical. YD received honoraria from Alexion Pharmaceutical for teaching symposia.

FUNDING

This work was supported by the EU FP7 grant 2012-305608 (EURenOmics) (to VF-B), the KIDNEEDS research grant 2015 (to VF-B), the ANR research grant (ANR-16-CE18-0015-01, CompC3) (to VF-B), the Fondation du rein (FRM, Prix 2012 FDR) (to VF -B), the Association pour l'Information et la Recherche dans les maladies Rénales génétiques (AIRG France), the Fondation Pour La Recherche Medicale (FDM 20130727355) (to SC) and the Fondation Française pour la Recherche contre le Myélome et les Gammapathies monoclonales (SC, VF-B).

ACKNOWLEDGMENTS

We gratefully acknowledge Morgane Mignotet for technical support and all colleagues who participated in this study: Dr Rémi Boudet (department of Nephrology, Brives), Pr Eric Daugas (department of Nephrology, Bichat, APHP), Pr Fadi Fakhouri (department of Nephrology, Nantes), Dr Florence Gallen Labbe (department of Nephrology, Valence), Dr Pierre Gobert (department of Nephrology, Avignon), Pr Marc Hazzan (department of Nephrology, Lille), Dr Lucile Mercadal (department of Nephrology, Pitié Salpétrière, APHP), Dr Mathilde Nouvier (department of Nephrology, Lyon), Dr Nicolas Martin Silva (department of Medicine, Caen), Dr Merabet (department of Hematology, Versailles), Dr Eric Renaudineau (department of Nephrology, Saint Malo), Dr Jean Baptiste Philit (department of Nephrology, Chambery), Dr Damien Sarret (department of Nephrology, Val de Grâce, Paris), Dr Aude Servais (department of Nephrology, Necker, APHP), Dr Lili Taghipour (department of Nephrology, Armentières), Dr Aurélien Tiple (department of Nephrology, Clermont-Ferrand), Pr Guy Touchard and Jean-Michel Goujon (department of Pathology, Poitiers).

REFERENCES

1. Fakhouri F, Frémeaux-Bacchi V, Noël L-H, Cook HT, Pickering MC. C3 glomerulopathy: a new classification. *Nat Rev Nephrol.* (2010) 6:494–9. doi: 10.1038/nrneph.2010.85
2. Pickering MC, D'Agati VD, Nester CM, Smith RJ, Haas M, Appel GB, et al. C3 glomerulopathy: a new classification. *Kidney Int.* (2013) 84:1079–89. doi: 10.1038/ki.2013.377
3. Hou J, Markowitz GS, Bomback AS, Appel GB, Herlitz LC, Barry Stokes M, et al. Toward a working definition of C3 glomerulopathy by immunofluorescence. *Kidney Int.* (2014) 85:450–6. doi: 10.1038/ki.2013.340
4. Servais A, Noël L-H, Roumenina LT, Le Quintrec M, Ngo S, Dragon-Durey M-A, et al. Acquired and genetic complement abnormalities play a critical role in dense deposit disease and other C3 glomerulopathies. *Kidney Int.* (2012) 82:454–64. doi: 10.1038/ki.2012.63
5. Sethi S, Fervenza FC, Zhang Y, Nasr SH, Leung N, Vrana J, et al. Proliferative glomerulonephritis secondary to dysfunction of the alternative pathway of complement. *Clin J Am Soc Nephrol.* (2011) 6:1009–17. doi: 10.2215/CJN.07110810
6. Marinozzi M-C, Chauvet S, Le Quintrec M, Mignotet M, Petitprez F, Legendre C, et al. C5 nephritic factors drive the biological phenotype of C3 glomerulopathies. *Kidney Int.* (2017) 92:1232–41. doi: 10.1016/j.kint.2017.04.017
7. Merle NS, Noe R, Halbwachs-Mecarelli L, Fremeaux-Bacchi V, Roumenina LT. Complement system part II: role in immunity. *Front Immunol.* (2015) 6:257. doi: 10.3389/fimmu.2015.00257
8. Merle NS, Church SE, Fremeaux-Bacchi V, Roumenina LT. Complement system part I - molecular mechanisms of activation and regulation. *Front Immunol.* (2015) 6:262. doi: 10.3389/fimmu.2015.00262
9. Pedersen DV, Roumenina L, Jensen RK, Gadeberg TA, Marinozzi C, Picard C, et al. Functional and structural insight into properdin control of complement alternative pathway amplification. *EMBO J.* (2017) 36:1084–99. doi: 10.15252/embj.201696173
10. Iatropoulos P, Noris M, Mele C, Piras R, Valoti E, Bresin E, et al. Complement gene variants determine the risk of immunoglobulin-associated MPGN and C3 glomerulopathy and predict long-term renal outcome. *Mol Immunol.* (2016) 71:131–42. doi: 10.1016/j.molimm.2016.01.010
11. Blanc C, Togarsimalemath SK, Chauvet S, Le Quintrec M, Moulin B, Buchler M, et al. Anti-factor H autoantibodies in C3 glomerulopathies and in atypical hemolytic uremic syndrome: one target, two diseases. *J Immunol.* (2015) 194:5129–38. doi: 10.4049/jimmunol.1402770
12. Goodship THJ, Pappworth IY, Toth T, Denton M, Houlberg K, McCormick F, et al. Factor H autoantibodies in membranoproliferative glomerulonephritis. *Mol Immunol.* (2012) 52:200–6. doi: 10.1016/j.molimm.2012.05.009
13. Sethi S, Zand L, Leung N, Smith RJH, Jevremonic D, Herrmann SS, et al. Membranoproliferative glomerulonephritis secondary to monoclonal gammopathy. *Clin J Am Soc Nephrol.* (2010) 5:770–82. doi: 10.2215/CJN.06760909
14. Zand L, Kattah A, Fervenza FC, Smith RJH, Nasr SH, Zhang Y, et al. C3 glomerulonephritis associated with monoclonal gammopathy: a case series. *Am J Kidney Dis Off J Natl Kidney Found.* (2013) 62:506–14. doi: 10.1053/j.ajkd.2013.02.370
15. Bridoux F, Desport E, Frémeaux-Bacchi V, Chong CF, Gombert J-M, Lacombe C, et al. Glomerulonephritis with isolated C3 deposits and monoclonal gammopathy: a fortuitous association? *Clin J Am Soc Nephrol.* (2011) 6:2165–74.
16. Chauvet S, Frémeaux-Bacchi V, Petitprez F, Karras A, Daniel L, Burtey S, et al. Treatment of B-cell disorder improves renal outcome of patients with monoclonal gammopathy-associated C3 glomerulopathy. *Blood* (2017) 129:1437–47. doi: 10.2215/CJN.06180710
17. Marinozzi MC, Roumenina LT, Chauvet S, Hertig A, Bertrand D, Olagne J, et al. Anti-factor B and Anti-C3b autoantibodies in C3 glomerulopathy and Ig-associated membranoproliferative GN. *J Am Soc Nephrol.* (2017) 28:1603–13. doi: 10.1681/ASN.2016030343
18. Ravindran A, Fervenza FC, Smith RJH, Sethi S. C3 glomerulopathy associated with monoclonal Ig is a distinct subtype. *Kidney Int.* (2018) 94:178–86. doi: 10.1016/j.kint.2018.01.037
19. Chauvet S, Roumenina LT, Bruneau S, Marinozzi MC, Rybkine T, Schramm EC, et al. A familial C3GN secondary to defective C3 regulation by complement receptor 1 and factor H. *J Am Soc Nephrol.* (2015) 27:1665–77. doi: 10.1681/ASN.2015040348
20. Sadallah S, Hess C, Trendelenburg M, Vedeler C, Lopez-Trascasa M, Schifferli JA. Autoantibodies against complement receptor 1 (CD35) in SLE, liver cirrhosis and HIV-infected patients. *Clin Exp Immunol.* (2003) 131:174–81. doi: 10.1046/j.1365-2249.2003.02045.x
21. Jokiranta TS, Solomon A, Pangburn MK, Zipfel PF, Meri S. Nephritogenic lambda light chain dimer: a unique human miniautoantibody against complement factor H. *J Immunol.* (1999) 163:4590–6.
22. Debiec H, Hanoy M, Francois A, Guerrot D, Ferlicot S, Johanet C, et al. Recurrent membranous nephropathy in an allograft caused by IgG3κ targeting the PLA2 receptor. *J Am Soc Nephrol.* (2012) 23:1949–54. doi: 10.1681/ASN.2012060577
23. Rigothier C, Delmas Y, Roumenina LT, Contin-Bordes C, Lepreux S, Bridoux F, et al. Distal angiopathy and atypical hemolytic uremic syndrome: clinical and functional properties of an anti-factor H IgAλ antibody. *Am J Kidney Dis Off J Natl Kidney Found.* (2015) 66:331–6. doi: 10.1053/j.ajkd.2015.03.039
24. Cogné M, Silvain C, Khamlichi AA, Preud'homme JL. Structurally abnormal immunoglobulins in human immunoproliferative disorders. *Blood* (1992) 79:2181–95.

9

Interpretation of Serological Complement Biomarkers in Disease

Kristina N. Ekdahl[1,2]*, *Barbro Persson*[1], *Camilla Mohlin*[2], *Kerstin Sandholm*[2], *Lillemor Skattum*[3] *and Bo Nilsson*[1]

[1] *Rudbeck Laboratory C5:3, Department of Immunology, Genetics and Pathology, Uppsala University, Uppsala, Sweden,* [2] *Centre of Biomaterials Chemistry, Linnaeus University, Kalmar, Sweden,* [3] *Section of Microbiology, Immunology and Glycobiology, Department of Laboratory Medicine, Clinical Immunology and Transfusion Medicine, Lund University, Lund, Sweden*

Correspondence:
Kristina N. Ekdahl
Kristina.Nilsson_Ekdahl@igp.uu.se

Complement system aberrations have been identified as pathophysiological mechanisms in a number of diseases and pathological conditions either directly or indirectly. Examples of such conditions include infections, inflammation, autoimmune disease, as well as allogeneic and xenogenic transplantation. Both prospective and retrospective studies have demonstrated significant complement-related differences between patient groups and controls. However, due to the low degree of specificity and sensitivity of some of the assays used, it is not always possible to make predictions regarding the complement status of individual patients. Today, there are three main indications for determination of a patient's complement status: (1) complement deficiencies (acquired or inherited); (2) disorders with aberrant complement activation; and (3) C1 inhibitor deficiencies (acquired or inherited). An additional indication is to monitor patients on complement-regulating drugs, an indication which may be expected to increase in the near future since there is now a number of such drugs either under development, already in clinical trials or in clinical use. Available techniques to study complement include quantification of: (1) individual components; (2) activation products, (3) function, and (4) autoantibodies to complement proteins. In this review, we summarize the appropriate indications, techniques, and interpretations of basic serological complement analyses, exemplified by a number of clinical disorders.

Keywords: complement, deficiency, activation products, functional test, complement regulatory drugs

THE COMPLEMENT SYSTEM

Activation of Complement

The complement system comprises approximately 50 proteins that are found in the fluid phase of the blood or bound to cells where they function as receptors or regulators of complement activation (**Figure 1A**). The system is organized in three activation pathways: the lectin pathway (LP), the classical pathway (CP), and the alternative pathway (AP), each with different recognition molecules. Complement activation leads to the formation of two proteolytic enzyme complexes, convertases which have C3, the central and most abundant complement component as their common substrate.

The LP is activated when one of several recognition molecules, mannan-binding lectin (MBL), collectins, or ficolins bind to carbohydrates, e.g., on a pathogen surface, and often on polymers. The CP is activated when C1q binds to IgM or IgG, which may be in the form of immune complexes or bound in an altered conformation to artificial surfaces, such as in medical devices. In addition, the CP can also become activated by pentraxins, e.g., C-reactive protein (CRP), and a variety of negatively charged molecules that includes DNA, LPS and heparin. This activation leads to activation of fluid phase proteolytic enzymes: mannan associated serine proteases (MASP)−1 and MASP-2 within the LP and C1r and C1s within the CP. These proteases mediate formation of the CP/LP C3 convertase C4bC2a.

Activation of the AP is accomplished by conformationally altered C3, either as a result of tick-over to C3b or C3(H_2O) or by its binding to surfaces, but AP activation can also be facilitated through the binding of properdin to damage-associated molecular patterns (DAMPs) on pathogens (1).

Through these processes of activation, the formation of the AP C3 convertase, C3bBbP, is induced. The labile C3 convertases cleave C3 into the anaphylatoxin C3a and the larger C3b fragment. In the presence of an acceptor surface, e.g., a pathogen or antigen-antibody complex, C3b can form a covalent bond to amino acid or sugar residues. Then C3b can be cleaved in three steps by the plasma protease factor I, in cooperation with one of several co-factors. The two first cleavages generate iC3b, which promotes phagocytosis via interaction with different complement receptors (CR)-1 (CD35), CR3 (CD11b/CD18), CR4 (CD11c/CD18), and/or CRIg (complement receptor of the immunoglobulin family). The third factor I mediated cleavage separates the molecule into the target bound C3d,g fragment which is a ligand for CR2 (CD21), and C3c which is released from the activating surface. The same digestion also takes place in the fluid phase indicating that complement activation *in vivo* or *in vitro* can be monitored by measuring C3d,g, iC3b or C3a.

In addition to being a trigger of complement activation the AP also provides a potent amplification loop. Since each deposited C3b residue (regardless of the nature of the initial activation trigger) is the potential nucleus of a novel C3bBb C3 convertase, it has the potential capacity to activate numerous other C3 molecules. Deposition of additional C3b molecules to or in the vicinity of either of the C3 convertases alters their enzymatic specificity from C3 to C5. Cleavage of C5 yields the anaphylatoxin C5a and initiates the generation of the terminal pathway (TP) where the end product is the terminal complement complex, C5b-9, which may remain in the plasma as soluble C5b-9 (sC5b-9) or be inserted in the cell membrane as membrane attack complex (MAC). MAC may induce cell lysis (primarily in non-nucleated cells) and gram-negative bacteria or inflammation and upregulation of tissue factor, e.g., on endothelial cells, at sub-lytic concentrations (2, 3).

The anaphylatoxins C3a and C5a bind to their receptors C3aR and C5aRs, expressed on phagocytes: polymorphonuclear cells (PMNs), and monocytes, thereby attracting and activating them, thus further fuelling the inflammation.

Regulation of Complement

A number of regulators protect surfaces of autologous cells against complement attack. These regulators include (but are not restricted to) cell-bound molecules, such as CR1, decay acceleration factor (DAF; CD55), and membrane cofactor protein (MCP; CD46), all of which inactivate the C3 convertases in different ways. Additional regulators, C4b-binding protein (C4BP, which regulates the CP/LP convertase) and factor H (the main regulator of the AP), found in the plasma are recruited via glycoseaminoglycans and/or deposited C3 fragments to the cell surface, thus providing further down-regulation of complement.

Regulation at the level of the TP is accomplished by cell bound CD59, and clusterin and vitronectin in the fluid phase, which all inhibit MAC formation and its insertion into the membrane of autologous cells. Furthermore, C1 inhibitor (C1-INH) inhibits the proteases generated within the CP and LP; C1r/C1s and MASP-1/MASP-2, respectively, (**Figure 1A**). However, C1-INH is not specific for complement system-associated serine proteases but also inhibits proteases generated by the activation of the contact system like Factor (F)XIIa, FXIa, and kallikrein.

Pathology of Complement

The pathogenesis of many inflammatory diseases includes different complement deficiencies as well as excessive complement activation. Complement is engaged in a number of diseases exemplified in **Figure 2**. The pathologic effect may be caused either by an increased and persistent activation or an altered expression or function of various complement inhibitors resulting in defective control. Systemic lupus erythematosus (SLE), myasthenia gravis and other autoimmune disorders are examples of the former, where the presence of soluble or solid-phase antibody-antigen complexes induce excessive complement activation. C3 glomerulopathy (C3G), paroxysmal nocturnal haemoglobinuria (PNH), and atypical haemolytic uremic syndrome (aHUS), are diseases which are associated with insufficient complement inhibition/regulation, e.g., as discussed in (4, 5) and quoted in the references.

In many cases the complement activation is a part of reactions resulting from activation of all cascade systems of blood, and under conditions such as ischemia/reperfusion injury (IRI), there is a combination of excessive activation and insufficient control. IRI can occur under many pathological conditions but also during medical treatments. Cardiac infarction and stroke are associated with ischemia followed by reperfusion of an organ or blood vessel. Ischemia which is often complicated with IRI can also occur after transplantation (both allogeneic and xenogeneic) as well as during cardiovascular surgery facilitated by cardiopulmonary bypass. In IRI, excessive complement activation in combination with insufficient complement regulation play important roles and the resulting damage appears to be associated with all three pathways of complement. This complement activation leads to an inflammatory response which consists of generation of anaphylatoxins and other mediators which collectively induce activation of endothelial cells and phagocytes resulting in recrutiment and extravasation of PMNs, as described in (6) and cited references.

Despite the clear involvement of complement in a large number of conditions, there are only a limited number of diseases where serological complement biomarkers have been established as differential markers of disease. In the majority of other conditions, the biomarkers are able to distinguish between patients and normal individuals at group level. However, these markers can often be used to follow individual patients if the baseline values are known or can be anticipated e.g. as in trauma and shock (7), sepsis (8), in neurological diseases such

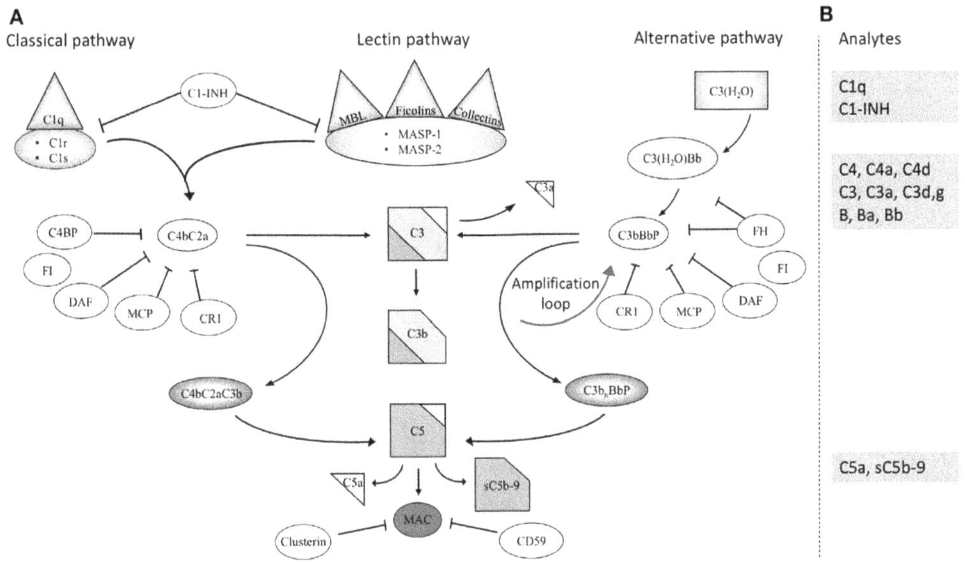

FIGURE 1 | Overview of the complement system. **(A)** Activation and regulation of the complement system. The complement system can be activated by three different pathways: the classical (CP), lectin (LP), and alternative pathways (AP). Recognition molecules within the three pathways bind to structures present on pathogens, and then activate the serine proteases C1r and C1s of the CP and MASP-1, MASP-2 of the LP, respectively. These proteases initiate the assembly of the CP/LP C3 convertase (C4bC2a) while formation of the AP C3 convertase (C3bBbP) is initiated either by hydrolysis of C3 to $C3(H_2O)$ or by other mechanisms. The convertases cleave C3 to the opsonin C3b and the anaphylatoxin C3a. Subsequent action of the C5 convertases generates the anaphylatoxin C5a and initiates the assembly of the C5b-9 complex. Complement activation is under strict control of a number of membrane-bound and fluid phase inhibitors, the majority of which control the activity of the convertases. These include (but are not restricted to) C4b-binding protein (C4BP), decay acceleration factor (DAF), membrane cofactor protein (MCP), and complement receptor 1 (CR1), factor H (FH), and factor I (FI). In addition, formation of the C5b-9 complex is under control of CD59 and clusterin, while the CP and LP serine proteases are inhibited by C1- inhibitor (C1-INH). Color coding: recognition molecules: gray triangles; initiators serine proteases and $C3(H_2O)$: orange symbols; convertases: green ovals; inhibitors: bright yellow ovals; anaphylatoxins: dim yellow triangles. **(B)** Selected analytes commonly used clinically to assess complement function and activation. C1q, C1-INH, C4, C3 factor B (B) and their activation fragments, as well as C5a and sC5b-9.

as myasthenia gravis (9), in ophthalmic diseases such as age-related macular degeneration, (AMD) (10), bullous pemphigoid (11), antineutrophil cytoplasmic antibody (ANCA)-associated vasculitis (12) etc. They can also be used for research purposes.

This review will describe the indications and specific methods that are used to determine the complement status of a patient and how the results of these assays are interpreted.

ANALYTICAL METHODS

Activation *in vivo* vs. Activation *in vitro*

Complement system activation via different pathways in blood plasma is a feature of a large number of diseases. For example, in immune complex diseases, the CP and the TP components are mainly activated while in renal diseases the AP and the TP components are predominantly engaged. When a component is activated *in vivo* either by proteolytic cleavage and/or by induced conformational changes triggered by protein-protein interactions, the component is taken up by receptors of e.g., leukocytes and Kupffer cells. This results in consumption of complement components. If a whole pathway (CP+TP or AP+TP) is activated, all components are consumed and the function is reduced along this pathway and systemic activation products will be moderately increased. Poor function via either the LP/CP or the AP will also affect the other pathway if the activation is strong enough since the components of the common TP will be consumed. If on the other hand the pathway (CP+TP, LP+TP or AP+TP) is activated *in vitro* all components are inactivated along this path and the function of this activation pathway is also reduced, but unlike the *in vivo* situation the activated proteins remain in the sample and are not consumed and the activation products will stay at high levels in the tube. If EDTA-plasma is prepared, any further activation of complement is stopped, since EDTA chelates Ca^{2+} and Mg^{2+} and thereby blocks the function of the C1 complex and the two C3 convertases, respectively. If, by contrast, serum is prepared, further activation of the sample *in vitro* is possible and it can be used for functional testing, e.g., using haemolytic assays (**Figure 3**) (13).

Preanalytical Factors

With this in mind, EDTA-plasma is suitable for analyses of individual components and for activation products, while serum is used for analysis of complement function. Serum can be replaced by plasma anticoagulated with the specific thrombin inhibitor lepirudin (i.e., recombinant hirudin) or any other thrombin or FXa inhibitor, which does not affect complement function (14). In order to maintain the function of the complement components and avoid further activation of individual components the samples must be kept cold until they

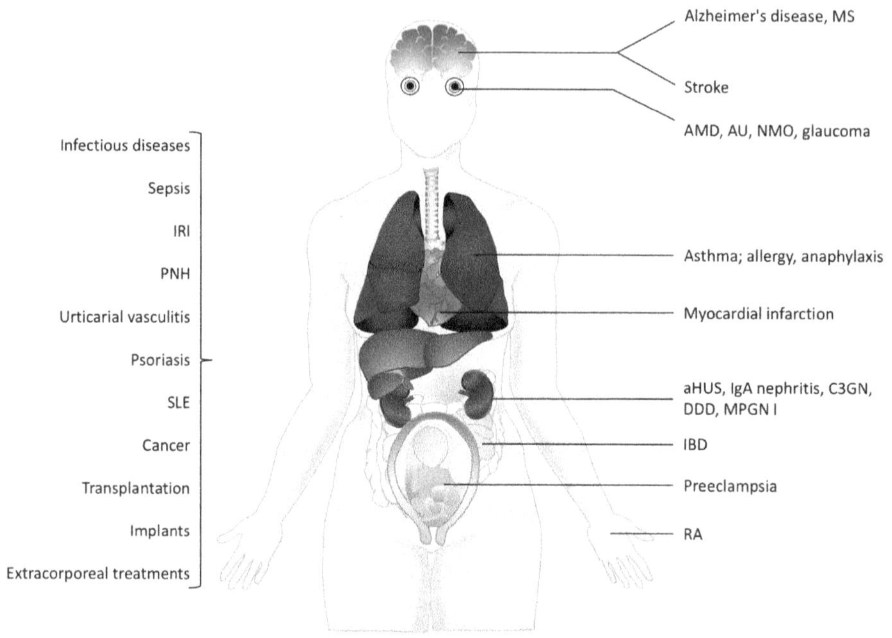

FIGURE 2 | Examples of pathological conditions involving the complement system. The pathogenesis of many inflammatory diseases includes excessive or uncontrolled complement activation. Some of these pathological conditions are organ-specific while others are systemic. In addition, different treatment modalities such as transplantation, implants or extracorporeal treatments also trigger complement activation. See the text for details. IRI, ischemia reperfusion injury, PNH, paroxysmal nocturnal hemoglobinuria; SLE, systemic lupus erythematosus; MS, multiple sclerosis, AMD, age-related macular degeneration; AU, autoimmune uveitis; NMO, neuromyelitis optica; aHUS, atypical haemolytic uremic syndrome; C3GN, C3 glomerulonephritis; DDD, dense deposit disease; MPGN, membranoproliferative glomerulonephritis; IBD, irritable bowel disease; RA, rheumatoid arthritis.

are frozen at −80°C, which should be done preferably within 120 but no longer than 240 min. It is important not to freeze the samples at −20°C, not even temporarily, since this creates a slow freezing rate and further activation/inactivation of individual components. During transportation dry ice must be used and the samples should be transferred directly from the to 80°C freezer to the dry ice (13).

Analysis of Complement in Plasma/Serum

Quantification of Individual Complement Components

Different types of immunoassays, most commonly immunoprecipitation assays, are used to determine the concentration of individual complement components. Previously, rocket immuno electrophoresis (RIE), radial immunoprecipitation or enzyme immune assays (EIAs) were most common, but have today to a great extent been replaced by nephelometry and turbidimetry. These techniques utilize polyclonal antibodies against the analyte, e.g., C1-INH, C4, C3, or factor B or activation fragments of these proteins (**Figure 1B**). These antibodies are added in excess to the sample and bind to their target, forming antigen-antibody complexes. Detection is performed by passing a light beam though the sample and which will be dispersed or absorbed by the formed immune complexes.

All techniques which use polyclonal antibodies for detection are relatively robust regarding the effect of preanalytical factors such as proteolytic cleavage or denaturation of the target protein induced during suboptimal sample handling. However, it is important to be aware that when polyclonal antibodies which are raised against C3c are being used, these assays will detect all forms of C3 which contain the C3c moiety, i.e, intact, non-activated C3 and its activated proteolytic fragments C3b, iC3b, and C3c. In analogy, anti-C4c antibodies will detect the corresponding forms of C4. Consequently, this type of assay is useful to determine the *in vivo* concentration of the protein (i.e., to monitor consumption or deficiency) but gives no information of the activation state or conformation of the protein.

More recently, multiplex assays for complement components have been developed and are now commercially available. The advantage of such assays is that they enable the simultaneous determination of several components, thereby saving both time and sample volume. So far, the analytes in the available kits are restricted to components with fairly high plasma concentrations, and to our knowledge, no LP-specific panels are yet on the market.

Quantification of Activation Products

The sequential proteolytic cleavage which occurs during complement activation generates activation products with different properties than those of the non-activated zymogen molecules (**Figure 1B**). In general, two principles are used in assays designed to determine the degree of complement activation: one is to use monoclonal antibodies (mAbs) which detect amino acid sequences

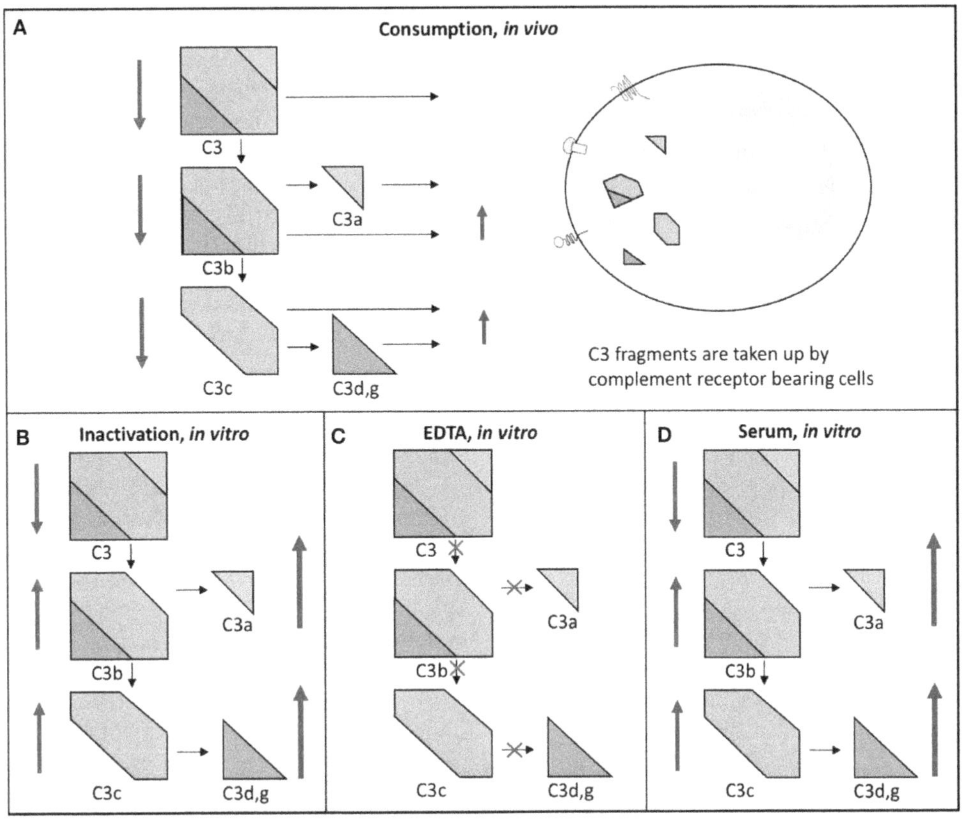

FIGURE 3 | Activation and consumption of complement *in vivo* and *in vitro*. Activation of C3 yields the activation products C3a, C3b/iC3b, C3d,g, and C3c (indicated by arrows). *In vivo*, a portion of the C3 fragments get eliminated by complement receptor-bearing cells **(A)**. The complement system can also be activated *in vitro* in serum **(D)** or in maltreated samples **(B)**, but in these cases the activation products remain in the fluid phase. In order to avoid complement activation *in vitro*, blood can be drawn in the presence of EDTA which inhibits all further activation is **(C)**. In each panel, the degree of C3 cleavage is indicated by the length of the arrows.

that are inaccessible in the native zymogen molecule but become exposed when the protein is activated (i.e., neo-epitopes). Most commercially available assays for C3a, C3b/iC3b/C3c, C4a, C4b, C4d, Ba, Bb, C5a, and sC5b-9 are based on neo-epitope mAbs. The other option is to use polyclonal antibodies but this often requires fractionation of zymogen molecules and activation products according to size. One example is C3d,g which is detected by EIA or nephelometry/turbidimetry, but since the polyclonal antibodies (in this case raised against C3d,g) also recognize intact C3, C3b, and iC3b in addition to C3d,g, these larger molecules must be removed by precipitation before analysis (15).

In vivo there is a continuous physiological turnover of C3 which leads to generation of activation fragments including C3a and C3d,g. Consequently, in order to monitor ongoing complement activation it is mandatory to determine a ratio of C3a or C3d,g level to the total level of C3 (C3a or C3d,g/C3), e.g., during an exacerbation in SLE (15). Furthermore, in obese individuals, the levels of a number of complement components, including C3, are greatly increased, resulting in corresponding higher levels of C3a; this problem further underscores the importance of calculating a ratio as a measure of relative activation (16).

Formation of the lytic C5b-9 (MAC) complex is the last step of the complement cascade which causes cell damage or lysis as a result of its insertion into the cell membrane, or endothelial cell activation at sub-lytic concentrations (2, 3). Complement activation of the TP can be monitored by quantification of sC5b-9 in the fluid phase, with an EIA which uses a mAb specific for a neo-epitope in C9 for capture. The epitope for this mAb is exposed in conformationally changed complex-bound C9 but not in intact C9. After capture, the sC5b-9 complexes can be detected by using polyclonal antibodies against another protein present in the same macromolecular complex, e.g., C5 or C6 (17).

Most, if not all, complement activation markers can rapidly be produced by complement activation *in vitro*. Consequently, it is of utmost importance that samples intended for detection of complement activation are collected and handled properly. In particular, there is a great risk that C3a will be generated *in vitro* if samples are improperly handled (14). It should also be taken into account that different C3 activation products vary greatly with regard to their *in vivo* half-life: approximately 0.5 h for C3a (18) and 4 h for C3d,g (19). Since C3d,g is a more robust marker, it is more suitable for diagnostic use while the generation of C3a is the more common analysis in experimental settings (20).

Quantification of Complement Function

In order to maintain full function in an individual complement activation pathway it is necessary for each of the participating proteins to be active, i.e., a deficiency in one individual protein will stop the activity of the entire cascade. Functional tests, in particular different haemolytic assays that monitor a whole activation pathway from the recognition phase to MAC-formation (=lysis) can be used to detect both deficiencies in individual component as well as depression in complement function caused by consumption of intact complement components.

Activation of the CP of complement is monitored in haemolytic assays employing sheep erythrocytes coated with rabbit antibodies, preferably purified IgM (or mixed with IgG) to the Forssman antigen. Patient serum is added, C1q binds to the immunoglobulins which initiates formation of the CP C3 convertase and subsequent activation leads to assembly of the MAC which results in lysis of the erythrocytes, **Figure 4A** (21).

Activation of the AP of complement is monitored in haemolytic assays employing rabbit or guinea pig erythrocytes, which are spontaneous and potent activators of human AP. EGTA which chelates Ca^{2+} and thereby inhibits activation via the CP and LP, is added to the patient serum prior to incubation. Under these conditions the AP C3 convertase is formed on the target erythrocytes, leading to C3 activation and subsequent lysis (22).

A variety of haemolytic assays have been developed using different serum dilutions and amounts of erythrocytes. In the original haemolytic assays called CH50 and AH50, a specified limiting amount of erythrocytes are incubated with serum in serial dilution to determine the dilution of serum needed to lyse 50% of the cells during a certain time interval (**Figure 4B**) (21, 22). In samples with low function it is often necessary to repeat the analysis with additional dilution steps.

Unlike in the CH50 and AH50 assays, where incubation of erythrocytes and serum takes place in the fluid phase, an alternative approach is to cast the target erythrocytes in an agarose gel. The patient serum is then added into wells punched in the agarose and diffuses in the gel causing cell lysis. This haemolysis-in-gel technique is quick and very useful to screen for complement deficiencies but does not enable quantification (23).

Instead of using erythrocytes, which may cause problems due to individual variation of the animals that have donated the blood, systems using artificial liposomes have been developed. Assays which are commercially available is performed in a CH50-like way (24).

An alternative to the CH50 and AH50 assays is the considerably less laborious, and much quicker one-tube assay. The sample is here incubated in one tube for 20 min. These assays give similar results as CH50 and AH50 (21, 25) and are based on the fact that the "dose" of complement is proportional to the number of cells lysed and the assay is therefore performed in an excess of erythrocytes (**Figure 4C**).

All haemolytic assays have problems to detect properdin deficiencies. Normally they give intermediate to normal values, never low function as is seen in other deficiencies. Therefore, special arrangements need to be made. One way is to make a kinetic analysis of the sample in the AP haemolytic assay. In the example shown in **Figure 5A** it is seen that the curves for a properdin deficient patient and a healthy control merge at the same level after 20 min in the one-tube assay. Therefore, it is necessary to also incubate for shorter time to detect this deficiency (**Figure 5A**). Alternatively, the concentration of properdin is determined separately.

More recently, a method has been reported that makes use of parallel EIAs to quantify the function of the three activation pathways of complement (26). Target molecules for each pathway are coated on wells of microtitre plates; IgM for the CP, mannan or acetylated bovine serum albumin for the LP, and LPS for the AP. Patient serum is incubated in the wells in the presence of additions which enable specific activation of only one pathway at the time, since the activity of the other pathways are inhibited. The readout for each EIA is formation of C5b-9 which is detected by a mAb specific for a neo-epitope in C9 which is exposed in complex-bound but not in native C9 (17). These assays are commercially available (**Figure 6**).

The techniques described here are valuable to identify complement deficiencies and for the haemolytic assays (except the haemolysis-in-gel) also to monitor levels in complement function, for example in patients with SLE during exacerbations. A suspected deficiency can be confirmed by determination of the protein, using relevant assays as described above. Furthermore, since most plasma complement components are commercially available, it is possible to verify the deficiency by reconstituting the patient sample with the protein in question and then repeat the functional assay, where the activity should be normalized. i.e., by combining these techniques it is possible to distinguish between functional deficiency and lack of a single complement component (13).

EXAMPLES OF INDICATIONS FOR COMPLEMENT DIAGNOSTICS AND THE INTERPRETATION OF COMPLEMENT STATUS

The complement status of a patient cannot be determined using only one assay. In order to get a complete status, assays from all four categories of analyses have to be used (**Table 1**). Two major basic indications exist: identification of complement component deficiencies and monitoring of complement activation. In order to screen for complement deficiencies functional assays (haemolytic or EIA) are used. Here, both CP and AP assays are compulsory. For the LP, a commercial EIA to monitor activation via MBL exists, but it only covers MBL, MASP-1 and MASP-2. Also, C9 deficiencies may be missed depending on the erythrocytes used. For monitoring of the degree of complement activation a minimum set up is to use a functional assay triggered via the CP, C3 and an assay for activation products (iC3b, Ba, C3d,g etc.). Examples of add-on assays are the concentrations

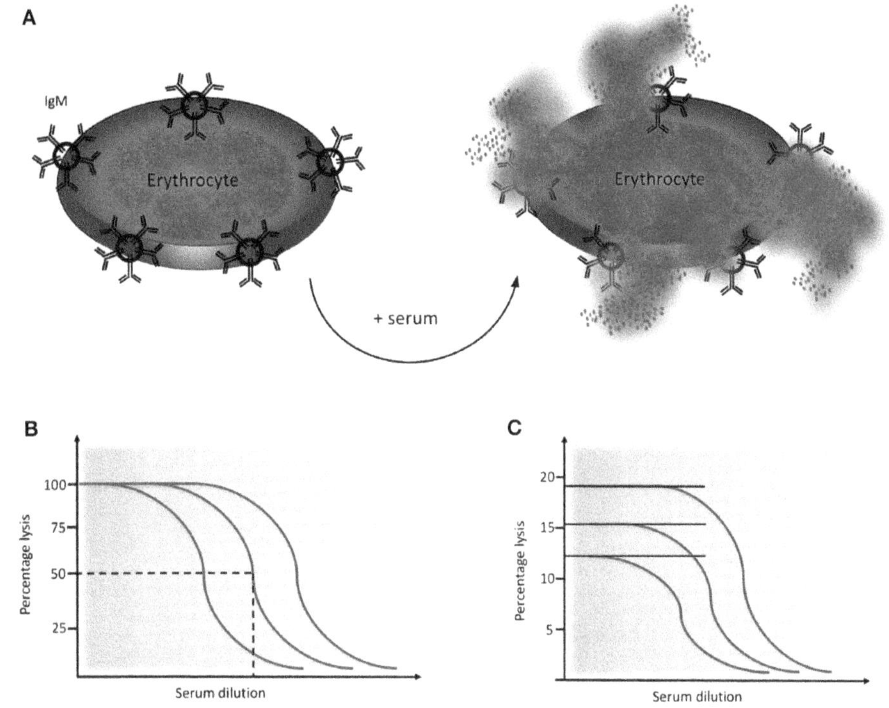

FIGURE 4 | Haemolytic assay for detection of complement classical pathway (CP) function. **(A)** CP haemolytic assay. Sheep erythrocytes coated with IgM antibodies are incubated with patient serum. The C1 complex binds and initiates formation of the CP convertase, leading to activation of C3, assembly of the C5b-9 complex, and subsequent erythrocyte lysis. **(B)** CH50 assay. Titration of the amount of serum needed to lyse 50% of a specified limited and fixed quantity of cells in the CH50 assay. The curves show three individuals with different levels of complement function. **(C)** One tube CP assay. Since the activity of complement is proportional to the quantity of cells that are lysed, this assay is performed in an excess of erythrocytes. The curves show three individuals with different levels of complement function. Assays for alternative pathway (AP) activation function similarly except that uncoated rabbit or guinea pig erythrocytes which spontaneously activate the AP, are used.

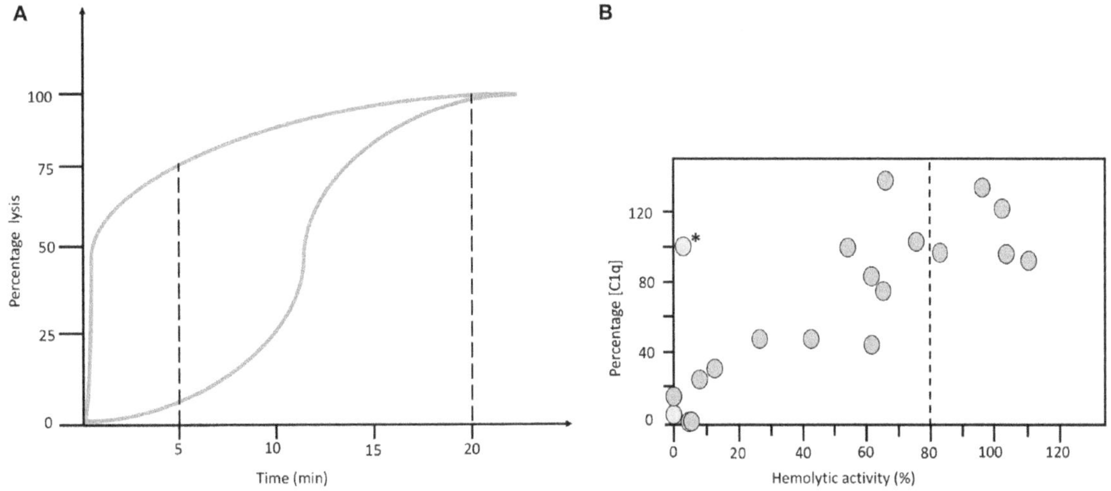

FIGURE 5 | Examples of specialized functional assays. **(A)** Time course alternative pathway (AP) haemolysis test. The left curve was obtained using serum form a complement sufficient individual and the right curve using serum form a properdin deficient patient. Since the curves merge at the same level after 20 min in the one tube assay it is necessary to also incubate for shorter time to locate this deficiency. **(B)** Correlation between functional test and individual analytes. Combination of haemolytic function via the classical pathway (CP) and an individual analyte (C1q) show a correlation in this material of systemic lupus erythematosus (SLE) patients. The exception, marked with (*) is a patient with total C2 deficiency. **(B)** reproduced from (15) with permission from the publisher.

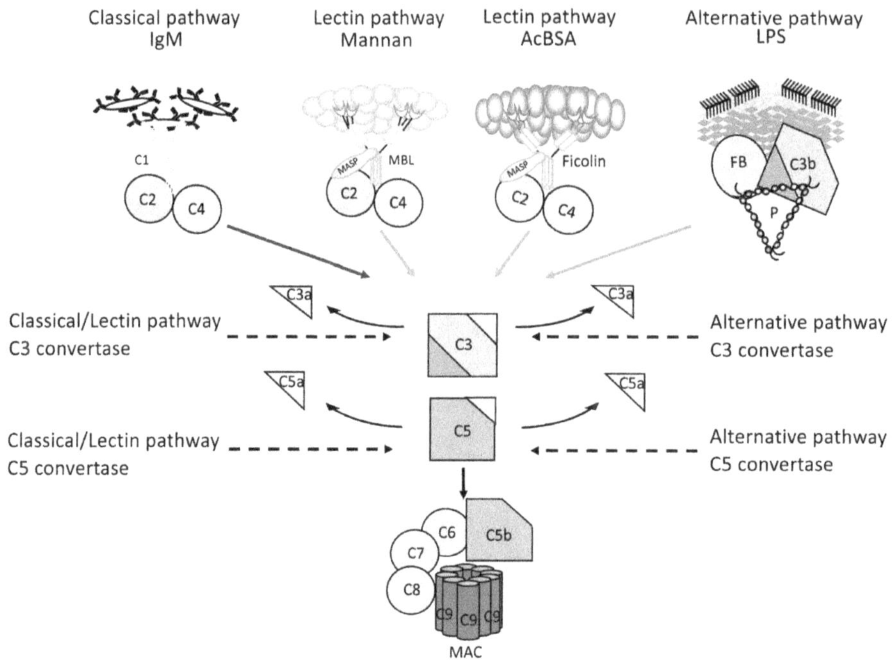

FIGURE 6 | Mechanism of action of microtitre plate based complement activation assays. Schematic representation of the mechanisms for commercially available enzyme immune assays (EIA) to monitor complement activation via the three different pathways. Wells of microtiter plates are coated with ligands for the recognition molecules within each pathway. For each assay, serum supplemented with inhibitors for the other two pathways is incubated. After complement activation, the readout for all assays is formation of the terminal complement complex C5b-9.

of, e.g., C1q, C4 and factor B, and a functional AP assay, e.g., a haemolytic assay (**Figure 5B**).

Inherited and Acquired Complement Component Deficiency

Complement Factor Deficiencies (General)

In general, complement deficiencies are rare, but when diagnosed, they are generally associated with recurrent bacterial infections (this applies to all activation pathways) (**Table 2**).

In addition, individuals deficient in MBL or MASPs of the LP are also susceptible to viral and protozoan infections and deficiencies in CP components are generally associated with an increased incidence of SLE or SLE-like disease. Most susceptible to autoimmune disease are patients with C1q deficiency while individuals with C2 deficiency are less predisposed to this type of diseases. C2 deficiency is the most common CP specific deficiency with a frequency of 1/20,000 (27, 28).

A deficiency is detected by functional assays and gives a very low to non-existing function via one (AP-, CP-, LP-specific deficiency) or all pathways (TP specific). In order to confirm that the functional defect is due to a specific deficiency, cryoglobulinemia has to be ruled out. Cryoglobulins can totally inactivate the CP+TP in serum (or lepuridin anticoagulated plasma) after the sample has been drawn. Also, severe consumption due to complement activation *in vivo* has to be excluded by measuring complement activation products, e.g., C3d,g. Identification of which component is lacking is established by performing measurements of individual factor concentration, by Western blotting, genetic screening etc. Confirmation of the deficiency (see above) can be done by reconstitution of the deficient serum with the purified identified complement component.

Monitoring of Complement Regulatory Drugs

Currently, there are only two complement inhibitors available in the clinic: C1-INH and eculizumab. Purified or recombinant C1-INH inactivates the proteases generated by the CP and LP (C1r, C1s, MASP-1, and MASP-2) as well as FXIIa, FXIa and kallikrein of the contact system (29). Eculizumab is a humanized mAb that binds to C5, preventing its activation to the anaphylatoxin C5a and C5b which initiates C5b-9 formation. Treatment with eculizumab is approved for treatment of aHUS, PNH, and refractory myasthenia gravis, but it is also currently undergoing clinical trials for the prevention of antibody-mediated rejection (AMR) in allogeneic kidney transplantation (30). In addition to these two drugs, a large number of complement-modulatory compounds that act at different control points are under development for various indications. Examples of compounds which are in clinical trials include mAbs against C1s (31), which inhibit the CP, the peptide CP40 of the compstatin family, which blocks C3 activation by the convertases of all three pathways (32), and APT070 (33), which inhibits the C3 convertases thereby blocking down-stream complement activation. In this field, there is a pressing need to monitor the complement status in all patients receiving treatment with complement-regulatory drugs, a need that is only expected to increase in the future. In most

TABLE 1 | Main indications for complement diagnostics.

DEFICIENCIES OF COMPLEMENT COMPONENTS
Increased susceptibility to bacterial infections
Repeated severe (invasive) bacterial infections
Meningococcal disease
Autoimmune disease (SLE and related diseases)
HAE (C1-INH deficiency)
AAE (C1-INH deficiency)
DISEASE ACTIVITY AND DIFFERENTIAL DIAGNOSIS
SLE
Antiphospholipid syndrome
Urticarial vasculitis
Cryoglobulinemia
Various (RA, GPA, Henoch Schönlein)
C3 glomerulopathy and other types of glomerulonephritis
Thrombotic microangiopathies (aHUS)
Transplantation (AMR)
ASSESSMENT OF THERAPEUTIC EFFECTS
C1-INH
Eculizumab

SLE, systemic lupus erythematosus; HAE, hereditary angioedema,; AAE, acquired angioedema; C1-INH, C1 inhibitor; RA, rheumatoid arthritis; GPA, granulomatous polyangiitis; antibody mediated rejection; aHUS, atypical haemolytic uremic syndrome.

TABLE 2 | Hereditary complement deficiencies.

LECTIN PATHWAY
MBL
Ficolins
MASPs 1-3
MBL, MASPs: increased susceptibility to bacterial, viral and protozoan infections MASPs1/3: 3MC syndrome
CLASSICAL PATHWAY
C1q, C1r, C1s
C4
C2
Bacterial infections, SLE
C2 deficiency: cardiovascular disease
ALTERNATIVE PATHWAY
Factor D
Factor B
C3
Properdin
Factor H
Factor I
Bacterial infections, e.g., *Neisseria, Haemophilus, Pneumococci*
TERMINAL PATHWAY
C5
C6
C7
C8
(C9)
Bacterial infections, e.g., *Neisseria*

MBL, mannan-binding lectin; MASPs, MBL associated serine proteases; 3MC syndrome Malpuech-Michels-Mingarelli-Carnevale syndrome; SLE, systemic lupus erythematosus.

cases monitoring can be achieved using CP and AP functional tests (either EIA or haemolytic), since an acquired deficiency of specific complement components is created. If the inhibitor is an antibody, direct binding assays to the specific antigen can supplement these assays. A comprehensive overview of the field of therapeutic complement inhibition is found in (34).

Disorders With Complement Activation (Table 3)

SLE, Antiphospholipid Syndrome and Urticarial Vasculitis

SLE, antiphospholipid syndrome and urticarial vasculitis are autoimmune immune complex diseases (35, 36). Other members of this group include rheumatoid arthritis with vasculitis, and cryoglobulinemia, as well as very rare cases of Henoch Schönlein disease and granulomatous polyangitiis (GPA) (37, 38). Complement analyses, in particular determination of CP function and analysis of components within the CP: C1q, C3, and C4 (C2 in some laboratories) are useful markers to monitor disease activity and for differential diagnosis (**Figure 7**). Furthermore, the detection of autoantibodies against C1q and C3 can be used to verify diagnosis (39–41). Hypocomplementemic urticarial vasculitis syndrome (HUVS) features anti-C1q antibodies with distinctive specificity as well as severe complement consumption via the CP (36, 42).

Antibody Mediated Rejection in Transplantation (AMR)

AMR is the leading cause of long-term kidney graft loss (43, 44). The presence or formation of antibodies directed against the vascular endothelium in the graft is a major trigger of complement activation in transplantation, leading to microvascular inflammation and thrombosis followed by ischemia, apoptosis, or necrosis, and finally graft failure. AMR leads to a CP activation, which is presented in biopsies as C4d deposition. The majority of antibodies are either anti-blood group ABO antibodies (so called natural antibodies) or antibodies against HLA, due to previous immunization. In blood in a severe AMR the typical signs of a CP activation are seen with low CP function, low levels of C1q, C4, and C3, and increased activation products (e.g., C3d,g/C3, sC5b-9 etc.). In less severe AMR only raised levels of activation products can be seen.

C3 Glomerulopathy (C3G)

C3 glomerulonephritis (C3GN) and dense deposit disease (DDD) are subsets of C3Gs that present a predominant C3 deposition in the glomerulus and is associated with C3NeF, other autoantibodies to complement, and in some cases mutations in complement protein genes (45). Since C3NeF binds to and stabilizes the AP C3 convertase, a profound C3 consumption occurs, that may lead to a functional C3 deficiency. The consumed C3 gives rise to C3d,g which is an indicator of substantial activation of C3. The level of

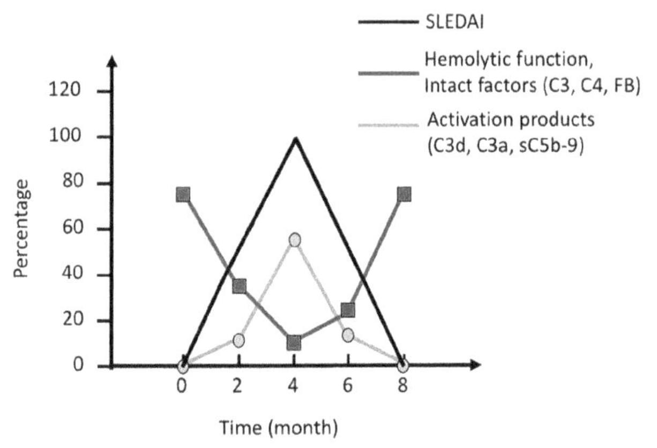

FIGURE 7 | Complement activation during an SLE (systemic lupus erythematosus) excacerbation. Clinically, the magnitude of an excacerbation of (SLE) is quantified as SLE disease index (SLEDAI; black line). During excacerbation, intact complement components C3, C4, factor B (FB), and other components are consumed, which results in a decline in haemolytic function by the classical pathway (CP) (red line). Complement activation markers e.g., C3d,g, C3a, and sC5b-9 (orange line), peak concomitantly with the SLEDAI. Figure adapted from (13).

factor B remains more or less unchanged. Since the stabilized convertase sometimes also cleaves C5, in some cases sC5b-9 can also be detected. Detection of C3NeF supports the diagnosis of C3G, in particular DDD. The severe C3 deficiency that results can, at least in theory increase the risk of bacterial infections.

Poststreptococcal Glomerulonephritis (PSGN)

Another type of glomerulopathy associated with AP activation is the post-streptococcal glomerulonephritis (PSGN) that may occur during the rehabilitation period in individuals that have suffered from Group A streptococcal disease. In particular C3, but also C5, is consumed and sC5b-9 is generated for typically 6–10 weeks following the infection (45). Since the levels of C3 and C5 can be depressed and, as is true for C3G with/without C3NeF, there is a theoretical risk of other bacterial infections. The levels of C3d,g are elevated resulting in a high ratio of C3d,g to C3. PSGN is associated with a concomitant consumption of properdin, which is the major complement-related diagnostic difference between these diseases (45).

Atypical Haemolytic Uremic Syndrome (aHUS) and Other Microangiopathies

aHUS is a disease that predominately appears in childhood and is characterized by thrombocytopenia, microangiopathic haemolytic anemia, and acute renal failure.

Affected cells in aHUS are endothelial cells, including those of the mesangium of the kidney as well as platelets and erythrocytes. aHUS is caused by uncontrolled complement activation due to combination of mutations of complement inhibitors, such as in factor H, but also factor I, factor H related proteins (FHR) 1, 3, 5, MCP, and thrombomodulin that impairs the function of these inhibitors (46). A deletion of the FHR-1/3 gene may lead to generation of anti-factor H antibodies which also is associated with aHUS. Gain of function mutations in C3 and factor B that lead to poorly controlled activation have also been reported (47, 48).

The most common cause of aHUS is mutations in the gene for factor H, and the majority of the mutations occur in the short consensus repeats (SCRs) 19 and 20 in the C-terminal of the molecule. These SCRs which interact with carbohydrates, e.g., heparan sulfate and sialic acid on the cell surface are important for binding factor H to the cell surface. Like in factor H dysfunction, other types of aHUS are also associated with AP activation, resulting in varying degrees of C3 consumption and the generation of C3d,g (and other C3 fragments) and sC5b-9. Factor H from aHUS patients may show different mobility compared to normal factor H when analyzed by SDS-PAGE, and western blotting. For a more precise diagnosis of AP components mutations, contact with a specialist laboratory is recommended.

In preeclampsia and other types of microangiopathy the levels of Bb and sC5b-9 are increased and various degrees of AP component consumption and low AP function can be seen (49).

Inherited and Acquired C1-INH Deficiency

C1-INH deficiency is the cause of the rare disorders hereditary angioedema (HAE) and acquired angioedema (AAE), but HAE may also, in some cases be caused by mutations in the gene coding for FXII (50). The hereditary form, HAE, is heterozygous autosomal dominant, whereas the acquired form, AAE, mainly occurs in patients with underlying disease but can also be idiopathic. Since the cause of these diseases is an unregulated generation of bradykinin by the contact system, these are not primarily complement-system related diseases, but their diagnosis is based on complement analysis. Both HAE and AAE are associated with recurrent attacks of bradykinin-mediated, non-pitting, local angioedema that are not responsive to antihistamine or steroids.

There are different types of HAE, which can be distinguished only by laboratory analysis. Two types of C1-INH-related forms exist, one with low concentration and function of C1-INH (Type I), and one with normal concentration, but dysfunctional C1-INH (Type II). In contrast, HAE with normal C1-INH levels, which is not associated with low C1-INH function is a heterogenous group and therefore less characterized than the other types. In this group, certain patients have a gain of function form of FXII (Type III), due to a mutation in the coding gene leading to defective glycosylation (50).

Acquired deficiencies of C1-INH can occur in lymphoproliferative and autoimmune diseases as a result of formation of autoantibodies against C1-INH, or paraproteins e.g., M-components (51–53). C4 concentrations are typically low in both HAE and AAE (54). AAE occurs as the result of the hypercatabolism of C1-INH; in AAE, as opposed to HAE, the serum concentration of C1q is low in ~70% of patients.

AUTOANTIBODIES TO COMPLEMENT PROTEINS (TABLE 4)

Anti-C1q Autoantibodies

Autoantibodies against C1q (anti-C1q) were first identified as low molecular weight C1q precipitins (55). Their immunoglobulin (Ig) nature was later confirmed, and the SLE-associated anti-C1q was shown to be specific for the collagenous region of the C1q molecule (56). Anti-C1q occurs in ~30% of unselected SLE patients but has a higher prevalence in lupus nephritis and is also associated with nephritis activity (57). In SLE, anti-C1q antibodies are often of the IgG2 subclass, but the reason for this selectivity is unknown. More than 95% of patients with HUVS are also positive for anti-C1q (58). However, anti-C1q antibodies are not specific for SLE and HUVS and may also be found in association with conditions such as primary glomerulonephritis and infectious diseases.

Anti-C1q is mainly analyzed by EIA. To avoid false-positive results in anti-C1q antibody analysis, it has been recommended that either only the collagenous part of C1q should be used as the antigen, or that high-salt buffer is used to abolish binding between the globular part of C1q and the Fc region of IgG in immune complexes (41). There are several commercially

TABLE 3 | Complement pathology.

Analyses	CP function (%)	AP function (%)	C1-INH conc (g/L)	C1-INH funct (%)	C1q conc (g/L)	C4 conc (g/L)	C3 conc (g/L)	C3d conc (mg/L)	C3d/C3	sC5b-9 (μg/L)
Reference interval	80–120	50–150	0.13–0.29	72–129	0.07–0.25	0.13–0.32	0.67–1.29	<5.3	<5.3	<25
Complement deficiencies CP, e.g., C2 deficiency	9	105	0.20	82	0.13	0.23	0.80	3.6	4.5	<25
Complement deficiencies AP, e.g., P deficiency	97	45	0.25	95	0.20	0.20	0.97	4.4	4.5	<25
Complement deficiencies TP, e.g., C6 deficiency	8	12	0.17	81	0.24	0.27	1.20	4.5	3.8	<25
SLE, urticarial vasculitis	10	109	0.17	79	0.06	0.08	0.65	6.3	9.7	75
Secondary phospholipid syndrome (SLE)	15	103	0.20	87	0.06	0.09	0.60	7.0	11.2	90
MPGN I	65	45	0.18	115	0.08	0.14	0.55	12	22	85
AMR	30	65	0.22	120	0.10	0.10	0.65	7	11	100
C3GN	15	10	0.26	122	0.22	0.15	0.10	18	180	200
PSGN	15	10	0.24	120	0.24	0.31	0.10	15	150	175
aHUS	95	105	0.19	103	0.20	0.21	0.75	6.5	8.7	75
HAE with low C1-INH conc	100	140	0.04	20	0.23	0.10	1.23	4.3	3.5	<25
HAE with dysfunct C1-INH	111	132	0.20	18	0.18	0.10	1.01	3.3	3.3	<25
AAE	93	94	0.03	11	0.05	0.09	0.80	3.9	4.9	<25
Eculizumab	5	10	0.23	79	0.25	0.26	1.17	4.2	3.6	<25

CP, classical pathway; AP alternative pathway; C1-INH, C1 inhibitor; TP, termial pathway; SLE, systemic lupus erythematosus; MPGN, membranoproliferative glomerulonephritis; AMR, antibody mediated rejection; C3GN, C3 glomerulonephritis; aHUS, atypical haemolytic uremic syndrome; PSGN, post-streptococcal glomerulonephritis; HAE, hereditary angioedema, AAE, acquired angioedema.

TABLE 4 | Autoantibodies against complement components.

Analyses	Anti-C1q[1]	Anti-C1q[2]	Anti-C1-INH	Anti-FH	C3NeF	C4NeF
SLE, Sjögrens	+	–	(+)	–	–/(+)	–
Hypocomplementary urticarial vasculitis	+	+	–	–	–	–
C3GN	–/+	–	–	–/(+)	+	+
aHUS	–	–	–	+	–	–
HAE Type I, Type II	–	–	–	–	–	–
AAE	–	–	+	–	–	–

Anti-C1q[1], antibodies against native C1q; Anti-C1q[2], antibodies against reduced chains of C1q; C3NeF, C3 nephritic factor; C4NeF, C4 nephritic factor; SLE, systemic lupus erythematosus; C3GN, C3 glomerulonephritis; aHUS, atypical haemolytic uremic syndrome; PSGN, post-streptococcal glomerulonephritis; HAE, hereditary angioedema, AAE, acquired angioedema.

available assays to detect anti-C1q. In addition, Western blot analysis of the separated C1q A, B, and C chains (after reduction) has been used to show that anti-C1q antibodies have different binding specificities in SLE than in (HUVS) (42, 59).

C3 Nephritic Factors and Other Convertase Autoantibodies

C3NeF are autoantibodies that bind to and stabilize the AP C3 convertase (C3bBb) to prevent its extrinsic or intrinsic decay (60), prolonging the half-life of the convertase and resulting in increased consumption of C3. C3NeF are frequent in patients with (C3G; hence the name "nephritic factor"), where they are found in ~80% of DDD cases and 40-50% of patients with C3GN (61). C3NeF can also be found in other conditions such as acquired partial lipodystrophy and an increased susceptibility to meningococcal infections secondary to persistently low C3 concentrations resulting from C3 consumption (62, 63).

Given the heterogeneity of C3NeF with regard to binding specificities and convertase-stabilizing effects, it is considered necessary to use more than one method for analysis (64, 65). Also, different methods are needed to demonstrate both the convertase-stabilizing capacity and the Ig nature of C3NeF. Most C3NeF have been shown to bind to the Bb part of the convertase (66). The heterogeneous nature of C3NeF was already described about 30 years ago in studies that showed differences regarding the dependency on properdin and the ability to activate the AP (67, 68). A recent study has also confirmed that some C3NeF are more efficient convertase stabilizers in the presence of properdin; these antibodies have been termed C5 nephritic factors (C5NeF) and shown to be associated with C5 consumption as well as low C3 (69).

C3NeF can be analyzed in several ways. The most widely used assays are (1) detection of fluid-phase C3 conversion after incubation of patient serum with normal serum at 37°C (70, 71) and (2) a simple haemolytic assay that utilizes unsensitized sheep erythrocytes (72). However, these functional assays are non-specific and do not establish that the C3NeF effects are caused by an antibody. Therefore, other types of EIA methods have been developed in which an AP C3 convertase is deposited in a microtiter plate (64, 73). Standardization of C3NeF analysis is as yet lacking, but recently an external quality assessment (EQA) program that includes C3NeF analysis has become available as the result of an international initiative to standardize complement analyses (74).

Rarely, patients will present autoantibodies against the CP convertase (C4b2a); these are known as C4 nephritic factors (C4NeF). Like C3NeF in the AP, these autoantibodies stabilize the CP convertase, leading to persistent C3 consumption. Also, like C3NeF, they are principally found in association with glomerulonephritis (75, 76). C4NeF can be identified via haemolytic assays in which the CP convertase is stabilized by C4NeF on sensitized sheep erythrocytes (75).

Anti-C1 Inhibitor Autoantibodies

Some patients with AAE have autoantibodies to C1-INH (anti-C1-INH), which can be of any Ig class. In AAE patients with monoclonal gammopathy, the Ig isotype of the M component is often identical to the anti-C1-INH isotype (77). Anti-C1-INH can increase the consumption of C1-INH or block its function, and AAE patients with anti-C1INH can benefit from treatment with B cell-inhibiting therapy (78). Although anti-C1-INH antibodies are much more common in AAE, they occur in a small fraction of patients with SLE, and anti-C1-INH IgM has also been reported in patients with HAE (79, 80). Anti-C1-INH antibodies are analyzed by EIA. Anti-C1-INH IgG, IgA, and IgM should all be determined, an unusual requirement in the context of autoantibody analysis. The assays may either detect the binding of anti-C1-INH to C1-INH or determine the capacity of the anti-C1-INH to block C1-INH function (81). Various in-house methods are used, since commercial methods are not available.

Anti-factor H Autoantibodies

Autoantibodies against factor H are detected in 6–10% of patients with aHUS and are also found in some patients with C3G. In aHUS, anti- factor H antibodies are mainly specific for the C-terminal part of factor H, and thus they block the ability of factor H to bind negatively charged carbohydrate residues on autologous cells. In C3G, anti- factor H may be directed toward other parts of factor H and may also be monoclonal or light chain-restricted (82–84). In aHUS, positivity for anti-factor H is strongly associated with a deletion of the genes for complement FHR-1/3 proteins, a deletion that is also common in the general population. aHUS with anti- factor H is considered a separate subgroup of aHUS for which the term "deficiency of CFHR plasma proteins and factor H autoantibody positive haemolytic uremic syndrome" (DEAP-HUS) has been proposed (85). Patients with anti- factor H -related aHUS will in most cases benefit from plasmapheresis and immunosuppressive treatment, unlike patients without anti- factor H, in whom C5-blocking therapy is mandatory (86). This difference implies that anti-factor H is an important diagnostic marker that needs to be analyzed rapidly.

Anti- factor H antibodies are analyzed by EIA. A multi-laboratory comparison of various in-house methods in 2014 established a recommended standard method, and a standard serum for calibration of arbitrary units is available (87). Commercial analysis kits are also available for anti- factor H determination.

Other Complement Autoantibodies

Anti-complement autoantibodies with several other specificities have been described in association with various diseases. For example, autoantibodies against factor B have been detected in C3 glomerulopathy and membranoproliferative glomerulonephritis (MPGN) (88, 89), antibodies against factor I in aHUS (90), antibodies against MBL in rheumatoid arthritis (91), and antibodies against ficolins in SLE (92, 93). However, the clinical significance of most of these antibodies is not clearly defined, and their analysis has not been adopted in regular clinical practice. Autoantibodies with specificity for C3 and C4 fragments, termed immunoconglutinins, are found in different inflammatory conditions and in SLE, where they can influence C3-mediated functions (39, 94). More recently, antibodies recognizing different C3 fragments were investigated in patients with lupus nephritis and were found to be more common in patients with more severe disease (95).

CONCLUSIONS

In summary, complement biomarkers can be used to follow the activity of a huge number of diseases and disorders in individual patients if they are compared with baseline values of the same individual. However, independent evaluations of the complement status in individuals without previous analyses are applicable on a relatively limited number of conditions due to low sensitivity and specificity of the existing assays and to preanalytical problems. Example profiles for a typical case of each condition are presented in **Table 3**. It is likely that introduction of new complement modulatory drugs with novel indications will increase the demand for complement monitoring in the near future.

AUTHORS CONTRIBUTIONS

KE, LS, and BN wrote the article. CM prepared the figures. BP and KS edited, and all authors approved the final manuscript.

ACKNOWLEDGMENTS

We thank Dr. Deborah McClellan for excellent editorial assistance. This work was supported by grant 2016-2075-5.1 and 2016-04519 from the Swedish Research Council (VR), and by faculty funding for from the Linnaeus university. The study was also supported by grants development and validation of complement assays provided by the University hospitals in Uppsala and Lund.

REFERENCES

1. Kemper C, Hourcade DE. Properdin: New roles in pattern recognition and target clearance. *Mol Immunol.* (2008) 45:4048–56. doi: 10.1016/j.molimm.2008.06.034
2. Nguyen HX, Galvan MD, Anderson AJ. Characterization of early and terminal complement proteins associated with polymorphonuclear leukocytes *in vitro* and *in vivo* after spinal cord injury. *J Neuroinflammation* (2008) 5:26. doi: 10.1186/1742-2094-5-26
3. Triantafilou K, Hughes TR, Triantafilou M, Morgan BP. The complement membrane attack complex triggers intracellular Ca^{2+} fluxes leading to NLRP3 inflammasome activation. *J Cell Sci.* (2013) 126:2903–13. doi: 10.1242/jcs.124388
4. Carroll MV, Sim RB. Complement in health and disease. *Adv Drug Delivery Rev.* (2011) 63:965–75. doi: 10.1016/j.addr.2011.06.005
5. Liszewski MK, Java A, Schramm EC, Atkinson JP. Complement dysregulation and disease: insights from contemporary genetics. *Annu Rev Pathol Mech Dis.* (2017) 12:25–52. doi: 10.1146/annurev-pathol-012615-044145
6. Banz Y, Rieben R. Role of complement and perspectives for intervention in ischemia-reperfusion damage. *Ann Med.* (2012) 44:205–17. doi: 10.3109/07853890.2010.535556
7. Hirose T, Ogura H, Takahashi H, Ojima M, Jinkoo K, Nakamura Y, et al. Serial change of C1 inhibitor in patients with sepsis: a prospective observational study. *J Intensive Care* (2018) 6:37. doi: 10.1186/s40560-018-0309-5
8. Charchaflieh J, Rushbrook J, Worah S, Zhang M. Activated complement factors as disease markers for sepsis. *Dis Markers* (2015) 2015:382463–9. doi: 10.1155/2015/382463
9. Howard JF. Myasthenia gravis: the role of complement at the neuromuscular junction. *Ann N Y Acad Sci.* (2018) 1412:113–28. doi: 10.1111/nyas.13522
10. Schick T, Steinhauer M, Aslanidis A, Altay L, Karlstetter M, Langmann T, et al. Local complement activation in aqueous humor in patients with age-related macular degeneration. *Eye* (2017) 31:810–3. doi: 10.1038/eye.2016.328
11. Giang J, Seelen MAJ, van Doorn MBA, Rissmann R, Prens EP, Damman J. Complement activation in inflammatory skin diseases. *Front Immunol.* (2018) 9:639. doi: 10.3389/fimmu.2018.00639
12. Crnogorac M, Horvatic I, Kacinari P, Ljubanovic DG, Galesic K. Serum C3 complement levels in ANCA associated vasculitis at diagnosis is a predictor of patient and renal outcome. *J Nephrol.* (2018) 31:257–62. doi: 10.1007/s40620-017-0445-3
13. Nilsson B, Ekdahl KN. Complement diagnostics: concepts, indications, and practical guidelines. *Clin Dev Immunol.* (2012) 2012:962702–11. doi: 10.1155/2012/962702
14. Bexborn F, Engberg AE, Sandholm K, Mollnes TE, Hong J, Ekdahl KN. Hirudin versus heparin for use in whole blood *in vitro* biocompatibility models. *J Biomed Mater Res A* (2009) 89:951–9. doi: 10.1002/jbm.a.32034
15. Ekdahl KN, Norberg D, Bengtsson AA, Sturfelt G, Nilsson UR, Nilsson B. Use of serum or buffer-changed EDTA-plasma in a rapid, inexpensive, and easy-to-perform hemolytic complement assay for differential diagnosis of systemic lupus erythematosus and monitoring of patients with the disease. *Clin Vaccine Immunol.* (2007) 14:549–55. doi: 10.1128/CVI.00486-06
16. Nilsson B, Hamad OA, Ahlstrom H, Kullberg J, Johansson L, Lindhagen L, et al. C3 and C4 are strongly related to adipose tissue variables and cardiovascular risk factors. *Eur J Clin Invest.* (2014) 44:587–96. doi: 10.1111/eci.12275
17. Mollnes TE, Lea T, Frøland SS, Harboe M. Quantification of the terminal complement complex in human plasma by an enzyme-linked immunosorbent assay based on monoclonal antibodies against a neoantigen of the complex. *Scand J Immunol.* (1985) 22:197–202.
18. Norda R, Schott U, Berseus O, Akerblom O, Nilsson B, Ekdahl KN, et al. Complement activation products in liquid stored plasma and C3a kinetics after transfusion of autologous plasma. *Vox Sanguin.* (2012) 102:125–33. doi: 10.1111/j.1423-0410.2011.01522.x
19. Teisner B, Brandslund I, Grunnet N, Hansen LK, Thellesen J, Svehag SE. Acute complement activation during an anaphylactoid reaction to blood transfusion and the disappearance rate of C3c and C3d from the circulation. *J Clin Lab Immunol.* (1983) 12:63–7.
20. Ekdahl KN, Hong J, Hamad OA, Larsson R, Nilsson B. Evaluation of the blood compatibility of materials, cells, and tissues: basic concepts, test models, and practical guidelines. *Adv Exp Med Biol.* (2013) 735:257–70. doi: 10.1007/978-1-4614-4118-2_18
21. Mayer MM. On the destruction of erythrocytes and other cells by antibody and complement. *Cancer Res.* (1961) 21:1262–9.
22. Platts-Mills TA, Ishizaka K. Activation of the alternate pathway of human complements by rabbit cells. *J Immunol.* (1974) 113:348–58.
23. Truedsson L, Sjöholm AG, Laurell AB. Screening for deficiencies in the classical and alternative pathways of complement by hemolysis in gel. *Acta Pathol Microbiol Scand C* (1981) 89:161–6.
24. Yamamoto S, Kubotsu K, Kida M, Kondo K, Matsuura S, Uchiyama S, et al. Automated homogeneous liposome-based assay system for total complement activity. *Clin Chem.* (1995) 41:586–90.
25. Nilsson UR, Nilsson B. Simplified assays of hemolytic activity of the classical and alternative complement pathways. *J Immunol Methods* (1984) 72:49–59.
26. Seelen MA, Roos A, Wieslander J, Mollnes TE, Sjöholm AG, Wurzner R, et al. Functional analysis of the classical, alternative, and MBL pathways of the complement system: standardization and validation of a simple ELISA. *J Immunol Methods* (2005) 296:187–98. doi: 10.1016/j.jim.2004.11.016
27. Jönsson G, Truedsson L, Sturfelt G, Oxelius VA, Braconier JH, Sjöholm AG. Hereditary C2 deficiency in Sweden: frequent occurrence of invasive infection, atherosclerosis, and rheumatic disease. *Medicine* (2005) 84:23–34. doi: 10.1097/01.md.0000152371.22747.1e

28. Skattum L, van Deuren M, van der Poll T, Truedsson L. Complement deficiency states and associated infections. *Mol Immunol.* (2011) 48:1643–55. doi: 10.1016/j.molimm.2011.05.001
29. Poppelaars F, Jager NM, Kotimaa J, Leuvenink HGD, Daha MR, van Kooten C, Seelen MA, Damman J. C1-inhibitor treatment decreases renal injury in an established brain-dead rat model. *Transplantation* (2017) 102:79–87. doi: 10.1097/TP.0000000000001895
30. Cornell LD, Schinstock CA, Gandhi MJ, Kremers WK, Stegall MD. Positive crossmatch kidney transplant recipients treated with eculizumab: outcomes beyond 1 year. *Am J Transplant.* (2015) 15:1293–302. doi: 10.1111/ajt.13168
31. Eskandary F, Jilma B, Mühlbacher J, Wahrmann M, Regele H, Kozakowski N, et al. Anti-C1s monoclonal antibody BIVV009 in late antibody-mediated kidney allograft rejection-results from a first-in-patient phase 1 trial. *Am J Transplant.* (2017) 8:670–926. doi: 10.1111/ajt.14528
32. Mastellos DC, Yancopoulou D, Kokkinos P, Huber-Lang M, Hajishengallis G, Biglarnia AR, et al. Compstatin: a C3-targeted complement inhibitor reaching its prime for bedside intervention. *Eur J Clin Invest.* (2015) 45:423–40. doi: 10.1111/eci.12419
33. Kassimatis T, Qasem A, Douiri A, Ryan EG, Rebollo-Mesa I, Nichols LL, et al. A double-blind randomised controlled investigation into the efficacy of Mirococept (APT070) for preventing ischaemia reperfusion injury in the kidney allograft (EMPIRIKAL): study protocol for a randomised controlled trial. *Trials* (2017) 18:2279–11. doi: 10.1186/s13063-017-1972-x
34. Ricklin D, Mastellos DC, Reis ES, Lambris JD. The renaissance of complement therapeutics. *Nat Rev Nephrol.* (2018) 14:26–47. doi: 10.1038/nrneph.2017.156
35. Spronk PE, Limburg PC, Kallenberg CG. Serological markers of disease activity in systemic lupus erythematosus. *Lupus* (1995) 4:86–94. doi: 10.1177/096120339500400202
36. Venzor J, Lee WL, Huston DP. Urticarial vasculitis. *Clinic Rev Allerg Immunol.* (2002) 23:201–16. doi: 10.1385/CRIAI:23:2:201
37. Rostoker G, Pawlotsky JM, Bastie A, Weil B, Dhumeaux D. Type I membranoproliferative glomerulonephritis and HCV infection. *Nephrol Dial Transplant.* (1996) 11(Suppl. 4):22–4.
38. Schneider HA, Yonker RA, Katz P, Longley S, Panush RS. Rheumatoid vasculitis: experience with 13 patients and review of the literature. *Semin Arthritis Rheum.* (1985) 14:280–6.
39. Nilsson B, Ekdahl KN, Sjoholm A, Nilsson UR, Sturfelt G. Detection and characterization of immunoconglutinins in patients with systemic lupus erythematosus (SLE): serial analysis in relation to disease course. *Clin Exp Immunol* (1992) 90:251–5.
40. Ronnelid J, Gunnarsson I, Nilsson Ekdahl K, Nilsson B. Correlation between anti-C1q and immune conglutinin levels, but not between levels of antibodies to the structurally related autoantigens C1q and type II collagen in SLE or RA. *J Autoimmun.* (1997) 10:415–23. doi: 10.1006/jaut.1997.0147
41. Mahler M, van Schaarenburg RA, Trouw LA. Anti-C1q autoantibodies, novel tests, and clinical consequences. *Front Immunol.* (2013) 4:117. doi: 10.3389/fimmu.2013.00117
42. Mårtensson U, Sjöholm AG, Sturfelt G, Truedsson L, Laurell AB. Western blot analysis of human IgG reactive with the collagenous portion of C1q: evidence of distinct binding specificities. *Scand J Immunol.* (1992) 35:735–44.
43. Einecke G, Sis B, Reeve J, Mengel M, Campbell PM, Hidalgo LG, et al. Antibody-mediated microcirculation injury is the major cause of late kidney transplant failure. *Am J Transplant.* (2009) 9:2520–31. doi: 10.1111/j.1600-6143.2009.02799.x
44. Halloran PF, Chang J, Famulski K, Hidalgo LG, Salazar IDR, Merino Lopez M, et al. Disappearance of T cell-mediated rejection despite continued antibody-mediated rejection in late kidney transplant recipients. *J Am Soc Nephrol.* (2015) 26:1711–20. doi: 10.1681/ASN.2014060588
45. Sethi S, Nester CM, Smith RJH. Membranoproliferative glomerulonephritis and C3 glomerulopathy: resolving the confusion. *Kidney Int.* (2011) 81:434–41. doi: 10.1038/ki.2011.399
46. Riedl M, Fakhouri F, Le Quintrec M, Noone DG, Jungraithmayr TC, Frémeaux-Bacchi V, et al. Spectrum of complement-mediated thrombotic microangiopathies: pathogenetic insights identifying novel treatment approaches. *Semin Thromb Hemost.* (2014) 40:444–64. doi: 10.1055/s-0034-1376153
47. Westra D, Vernon KA, Volokhina EB, Pickering MC, van de Kar NCAJ, van den Heuvel LP. Atypical hemolytic uremic syndrome and genetic aberrations in the complement factor H-related 5 gene. *J Hum Genet.* (2012) 57:459–64. doi: 10.1038/jhg.2012.57
48. Sartz L, Olin AI, Kristoffersson AC, Ståhl AL, Johansson ME, Westman K, et al. A novel C3 mutation causing increased formation of the C3 convertase in familial atypical hemolytic uremic syndrome. *J Immunol.* (2012) 188:2030–7. doi: 10.4049/jimmunol.1100319
49. Alrahmani L, Willrich MAV. The complement alternative pathway and preeclampsia. *Curr Hypertens Rep.* (2018) 20:40. doi: 10.1007/s11906-018-0836-4
50. Zuraw BL, Christiansen SC. Pathophysiology of hereditary angioedema. *Am J Rhinol Allergy* (2011) 25:373–8. doi: 10.2500/ajra.2011.25.3661
51. Cicardi M, Beretta A, Colombo M, Gioffré D, Cugno M, Agostoni A. Relevance of lymphoproliferative disorders and of anti-C1 inhibitor autoantibodies in acquired angio-oedema. *Clin Exp Immunol.* (1996) 106:475–80.
52. Cicardi M, Zanichelli A. The acquired deficiency of C1-inhibitor: lymphoproliferation and angioedema. *Curr Mol Med.* (2010) 10:354–60. doi: 10.2174/156652410791317066
53. Cicardi M, Aberer W, Banerji A, Bas M, Bernstein JA, Bork K, et al. Classification, diagnosis, and approach to treatment for angioedema: consensus report from the Hereditary Angioedema International Working Group. *Allergy* 602–16. doi: 10.1111/all.12380
54. Zanichelli A, Azin GM, Wu MA, Suffritti C, Maggioni L, Caccia S, et al. Diagnosis, course, and management of angioedema in patients with acquired C1-inhibitor deficiency. *J Allergy Clin Immunol Pract.* (2017) 5:1307–13. doi: 10.1016/j.jaip.2016.12.032
55. Agnello V, Koffler D, Eisenberg JW, Winchester RJ, Kunkel HG. C1q precipitins in the sera of patients with systemic lupus erythematosus and other hypocomplementemic states: characterization of high and low molecular weight types. *J Exp Med.* (1971) 134:228–41.
56. Uwatoko S, Mannik M. Low-molecular weight C1q-binding immunoglobulin G in patients with systemic lupus erythematosus consists of autoantibodies to the collagen-like region of C1q. *J Clin Invest.* (1988) 82:816–24. doi: 10.1172/JCI113684
57. Orbai A-M, Truedsson L, Sturfelt G, Nived O, Fang H, Alarcón GS, et al. Anti-C1q antibodies in systemic lupus erythematosus. *Lupus* (2015) 24:42–9. doi: 10.1177/0961203314547791
58. Wisnieski JJ, Jones SM. Comparison of autoantibodies to the collagen-like region of C1q in hypocomplementemic urticarial vasculitis syndrome and systemic lupus erythematosus. *J Immunol.* (1992) 148:1396–403.
59. Sjöwall C, Mandl T, Skattum L, Olsson M, Mohammad AJ. Epidemiology of hypocomplementaemic urticarial vasculitis (anti-C1q vasculitis). *Rheumatology* (2018) 65:1–1407. doi: 10.1093/rheumatology/key110
60. Daha MR, Fearon DT, Austen KF. C3 nephritic factor (C3NeF): stabilization of fluid phase and cell-bound alternative pathway convertase. *J Immunol.* (1976) 116:1–7.
61. Riedl M, Thorner P, Licht C. C3 Glomerulopathy. *Pediatr Nephrol.* (2017) 32:43–57. doi: 10.1007/s00467-015-3310-4
62. Misra A, Peethambaram A, Garg A. Clinical features and metabolic and autoimmune derangements in acquired partial lipodystrophy: report of 35 cases and review of the literature. *Medicine* (2004) 83:18–34. doi: 10.1097/01.md.0000111061.69212.59
63. Teisner B, Elling P, Svehag SE, Poulsen L, Lamm LU, Sjoholm A. C3 nephritic factor in a patient with recurrent Neisseria meningitidis infections. *Acta Pathol Microbiol Immunol Scand C* (1984) 92:341–9.
64. Paixão-Cavalcante D, López-Trascasa M, Skattum L, Giclas PC, Goodship TH, de Córdoba SR, et al. Sensitive and specific assays for C3 nephritic factors clarify mechanisms underlying complement dysregulation. *Kidney Int.* (2012) 82:1084–92. doi: 10.1038/ki.2012.250
65. Skattum L, Mårtensson U, Sjöholm AG. Hypocomplementaemia caused by C3 nephritic factors (C3 NeF): clinical findings and the coincidence of C3 NeF type II with anti-C1q autoantibodies. *J Intern Med.* (1997) 242:455–64.
66. Daha MR, Van Es LA. Stabilization of homologous and heterologous cell-bound amplification convertases, C3bBb, by C3 nephritic factor. *Immunology* (1981) 43:33–8.

67. Tanuma Y, Ohi H, Hatano M. Two types of C3 nephritic factor: properdin-dependent C3NeF and properdin-independent C3NeF. *Clin Immunol Immunopathol.* (1990) 56:226–38.
68. Mollnes TE, Ng YC, Peters DK, Lea T, Tschopp J, Harboe M. Effect of nephritic factor on C3 and on the terminal pathway of complement *in vivo* and *in vitro*. *Clin Exp Immunol.* (1986) 65:73–9.
69. Marinozzi MC, Chauvet S, Le Quintrec M, Mignotet M, Petitprez F, Legendre C, et al. C5 nephritic factors drive the biological phenotype of C3 glomerulopathies. *Kidney Int.* (2017) 92:1232–41. doi: 10.1016/j.kint.2017.04.017
70. Peters DK, Martin A, Weinstein A, Cameron JS, Barratt TM, Ogg CS, et al. Complement studies in membrano-proliferative glomerulonephritis. *Clin Exp Immunol.* (1972) 11:311–20.
71. Williams DG, Peters DK, Fallows J, Petrie A, Kourilsky O, Morel-Maroger L, et al. Studies of serum complement in the hypocomplementaemic nephritides. *Clin Exp Immunol.* (1974) 18:391–405.
72. Rother U. A new screening test for C3 nephritis factor based on a stable cell bound convertase on sheep erythrocytes. *J Immunol Methods* (1982) 51:101–7.
73. Seino J, vander Wall Bake WL, Van Es LA, Daha MR. A novel ELISA assay for the detection of C3 nephritic factor. *J Immunol Methods* (1993) 159:221–7.
74. Prohászka Z, Nilsson B, Frazer-Abel A, Kirschfink M. Complement analysis 2016: clinical indications, laboratory diagnostics and quality control. *Immunobiology* (2016) 221:1247–58. doi: 10.1016/j.imbio.2016.06.008
75. Halbwachs L, Leveillé M, Lesavre P, Wattel S, Leibowitch J. Nephritic factor of the classical pathway of complement: immunoglobulin G autoantibody directed against the classical pathway C3 convetase enzyme. *J Clin Invest.* (1980) 65:1249–56. doi: 10.1172/JCI109787
76. Zhang Y, Meyer NC, Fervenza FC, Lau W, Keenan A, Cara-Fuentes G, et al. C4 Nephritic factors in C3 glomerulopathy: a case series. *Am J Kidney Dis.* (2017) 70:834–43. doi: 10.1053/j.ajkd.2017.07.004
77. Castelli R, Deliliers DL, Zingale LC, Pogliani EM, Cicardi M. Lymphoproliferative disease and acquired C1 inhibitor deficiency. *Haematologica* (2007) 92:716–8. doi: 10.3324/haematol.10769
78. Bygum A, Vestergaard H. Acquired angioedema-occurrence, clinical features and associated disorders in a Danish nationwide patient cohort. *Int Arch Allergy Immunol.* (2013) 162:149–55. doi: 10.1159/000351452
79. Mészáros T, Füst G, Farkas H, Jakab L, Temesszentandrási G, Nagy G, et al. C1-inhibitor autoantibodies in SLE. *Lupus* (2010) 19:634–8. doi: 10.1177/0961203309357059
80. Varga L, Széplaki G, Visy B, Füst G, Harmat G, Miklós K, et al. C1-inhibitor (C1-INH) autoantibodies in hereditary angioedema. Strong correlation with the severity of disease in C1-INH concentrate naïve patients. *Mol Immunol.* (2007) 44:1454–60. doi: 10.1016/j.molimm.2006.04.020
81. Engel R, Rensink I, Roem D, Brouwer M, Kalei A, Perry D, et al. ELISA to measure neutralizing capacity of anti-C1-inhibitor antibodies in plasma of angioedema patients. *J Immunol Methods* (2015) 426:114–9. doi: 10.1016/j.jim.2015.08.011
82. Dragon-Durey MA, Loirat C, Cloarec S, Macher MA, Blouin J, Nivet H, et al. Anti-Factor H autoantibodies associated with atypical hemolytic uremic syndrome. *J Am Soc Nephrol.* (2005) 16:555–63. doi: 10.1681/ASN.2004050380
83. Blanc C, Togarsimalemath SK, Chauvet S, Le Quintrec M, Moulin B, Buchler M, et al. Anti-factor H autoantibodies in C3 glomerulopathies and in atypical hemolytic uremic syndrome: one target, two diseases. *J Immunol.* (2015) 194:5129–38. doi: 10.4049/jimmunol.1402770
84. Durey MAD, Sinha A, Togarsimalemath SK, Bagga A. Anti-complement-factor H-associated glomerulopathies. *Nat Rev Nephrol.* (2016) 12:563–78. doi: 10.1038/nrneph.2016.99
85. Józsi M, Licht C, Strobel S, Zipfel SLH, Richter H, Heinen S, et al. Factor H autoantibodies in atypical hemolytic uremic syndrome correlate with CFHR1/CFHR3 deficiency. *Blood* (2008) 111:1512–4. doi: 10.1182/blood-2007-09-109876
86. Loirat C, Fakhouri F, Ariceta G, Besbas N, Bitzan M, Bjerre A, et al. An international consensus approach to the management of atypical hemolytic uremic syndrome in children. *Pediatr Nephrol.* (2016) 31:15–39. doi: 10.1007/s00467-015-3076-8
87. Watson R, Lindner S, Bordereau P, Hunze EM, Tak F, Ngo S, et al. Standardisation of the factor H autoantibody assay. *Immunobiology* (2014) 219:9–16. doi: 10.1016/j.imbio.2013.06.004
88. Strobel S, Zimmering M, Papp K, Prechl J, Józsi M. Anti-factor B autoantibody in dense deposit disease. *Mol Immunol.* (2010) 47:1476–83. doi: 10.1016/j.molimm.2010.02.002
89. Marinozzi MC, Roumenina LT, Chauvet S, Hertig A, Bertrand D, Olagne J, et al. Anti-factor B and Anti-C3b autoantibodies in C3 glomerulopathy and Ig-associated membranoproliferative GN. *J Am Soc Nephrol.* (2017) 28:1603–13. doi: 10.1681/ASN.2016030343
90. Kavanagh D, Pappworth IY, Anderson H, Hayes CM, Moore I, Hunze EM, et al. Factor I autoantibodies in patients with atypical hemolytic uremic syndrome: disease-associated or an epiphenomenon? *Clin J Am Soc Nephrol.* (2012) 7:417–26. doi: 10.2215/CJN.05750611
91. Gupta B, Raghav SK, Agrawal C, Chaturvedi VP, Das RH, Das HR. Anti-MBL autoantibodies in patients with rheumatoid arthritis: prevalence and clinical significance. *J Autoimmun.* (2006) 27:125–33. doi: 10.1016/j.jaut.2006.07.002
92. Colliard S, Jourde-Chiche N, Clavarino G, Sarrot-Reynauld F, Gout E, Deroux A, et al. Autoantibodies targeting ficolin-2 in systemic lupus erythematosus patients with active nephritis. *Arthritis Care Res.* (2017) 6:280–1268. doi: 10.1002/acr.23449
93. Plawecki M, Lheritier E, Clavarino G, Jourde-Chiche N, Ouili S, Paul S, et al. Association between the presence of autoantibodies targeting ficolin-3 and active nephritis in patients with systemic lupus erythematosus. *PLoS ONE* (2016) 11:e0160879. doi: 10.1371/journal.pone.0160879
94. Nilsson B, Ekdahl KN, Svarvare M, Bjelle A, Nilsson UR. Purification and characterization of IgG immunoconglutinins from patients with systemic lupus erythematosus: implications for a regulatory function. *Clin Exp Immunol* (1990) 82:262–7.
95. Vasilev VV, Noe R, Dragon-Durey MA, Chauvet S, Lazarov VJ, Deliyska BP, et al. Functional characterization of autoantibodies against complement component C3 in patients with lupus nephritis. *J Biol Chem.* (2015) 290:25343–55. doi: 10.1074/jbc.M115.647008

10

Collectin-11 (CL-11) is a Major Sentinel at Epithelial Surfaces and Key Pattern Recognition Molecule in Complement-Mediated Ischaemic Injury

Christopher L. Nauser, Mark C. Howard, Giorgia Fanelli, Conrad A. Farrar and Steven Sacks*

MRC Centre for Transplantation, School of Immunology and Microbial Sciences, King's College London, Guy's and St. Thomas' NHS Foundation Trust, London, United Kingdom

***Correspondence:**
Christopher L. Nauser
christopher.nauser@kcl.ac.uk

The complement system is a dynamic subset of the innate immune system, playing roles in host defense, clearance of immune complexes and cell debris, and priming the adaptive immune response. Over the last 40 years our understanding of the complement system has evolved from identifying its presence and recognizing its role in the blood to now focusing on understanding the role of local complement synthesis in health and disease. In particular, the local synthesis of complement was found to have an involvement in mediating ischaemic injury, including following transplantation. Recent work on elucidating the triggers of local complement synthesis and activation in renal tissue have led to the finding that Collectin-11 (CL-11) engages with L-fucose at the site of ischaemic stress, namely at the surface of the proximal tubular epithelial cells. What remains unknown is the precise structure of the damage-associated ligand that participates in CL-11 binding and subsequent complement activation. In this article, we will discuss our hypothesis regarding the role of CL-11 as an integral tissue-based pattern recognition molecule which we postulate has a significant contributory role in complement-mediated ischaemic injury.

Keywords: collectin-11, lectin pathway, complement system, innate immunity, renal ischaemia, renal transplantation

INTRODUCTION

We have seen over many years that innate immune defense systems mounted at epithelial surfaces perform multiple and often non-immune roles. The toll-like receptor system is a classic example that has transformed our perception about the origins of innate immunity and its roles in insect development (1, 2), antimicrobial defense (3) and in the pathogenesis of some inflammatory conditions (4–6). The complement system **Figure 1** has been known about for longer (7), but the diversity of function and, in particular, its role at the interface between innate and adaptive immunity can now be re-visited as a typical model for innate immune function as well as a therapeutic target in a growing number of medical disorders.

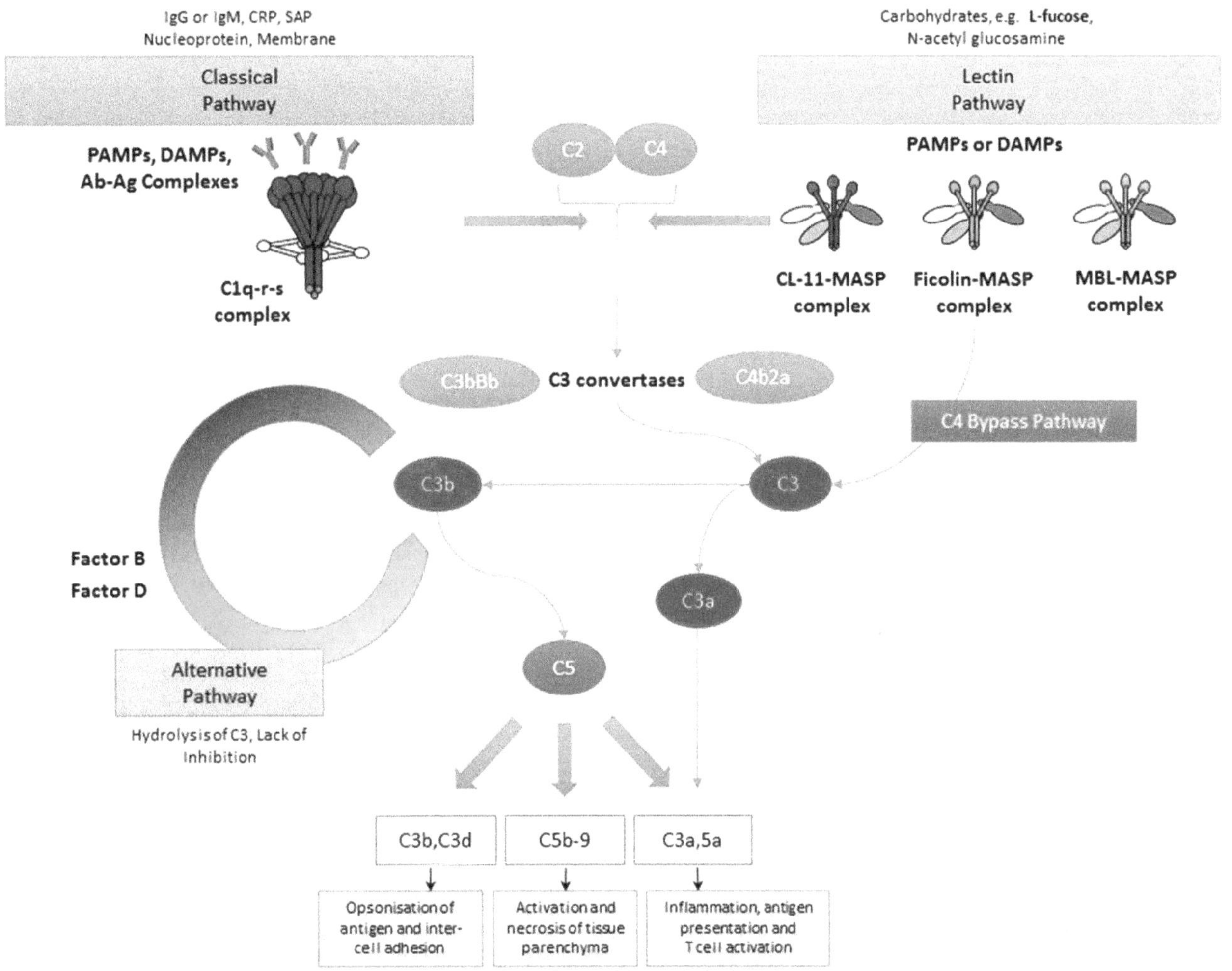

FIGURE 1 | The complement system. The complement system is activated through three main pathways: classical, lectin and alternative. The classical and lectin pathways are activated by pattern recognition molecules binding to pathogen cell surfaces as well as infected and/or damaged cells. In the case of the classical pathway this manifests as C1q binding, most commonly via immunoglobulin. However, C1q can also bind other immune surveillance molecules or directly to disrupted structures via pathogen-associated molecular patterns (PAMPs) or damage-associated molecular patterns (DAMPs). Meanwhile, the lectin pathway is initiated by binding of collectins, such as MBL and CL-11, as well as ficolins, to PAMPs or DAMPs expressing carbohydrate ligands. Also shown in the diagram is a C4-bypass mechanism in which MASP-2 in association with lectin molecules directly cleaves C3. The alternative pathway is activated by C3b binding to cell surfaces and acts as an amplification process for the central complement component, C3, upon which both the lectin and classical pathways converge upon. Recently, MASP-1/3 was also shown to trigger the alternative pathway as well. Through a number of complement convertases the effectors of the complement system are generated. These are the anaphylatoxins, C3a and C5a, the membrane attack complex (MAC, C5b-9) as well as C3b and its metabolite C3d which mediate antigen opsonisation and cell-cell adhesion *(NB This is a generalized overview of the complement system as it specifically relates to the focus of this manuscript and is not meant to be a comprehensive depiction of all parts of the complement system).*

EARLY BEGINNINGS—LOCAL COMPLEMENT SYNTHESIS

For us, the story begins with early reports detailing the significance of local complement synthesis. Colten et al. authored a number of publications that highlighted the capacity of macrophages for producing a wide range of complement components (8, 9). Well cited papers on skin cells, neural cells, gut cells, cardiac cells, and others came into vision, showing that the principle of local synthesis was almost universal in resident parenchymal cells and migratory leukocytes (10–17). Our interest, as a nephrology group starting up in the late 1980s, was caught by kidney expression of a number of complement genes in the context of inflammatory renal disease (18, 19).

It became apparent that among the variety of intrarenal cells studied, the renal tubule cells were a prolific source of complement components. The renal tubule supports vital functions in maintaining health and blocking invasive pathogens such as uropathogenic *Escherichia coli*. The capacity of renal tubule cells for complement synthesis was first characterized through the work of Daha and others (20–22) in Leiden and further confirmed through histological examination of both healthy and diseased tissue by several research groups (23–25). The link between inflammatory conditions primarily affecting the renal tubules and a high degree of intrarenal complement expression was striking. Notably, these diseases included ischaemic injury of the newly transplanted kidney and transplant rejection (26–28).

At the time, the techniques of tissue- or cell-specific gene deletion were not well enough established to allow interrogation of local complement gene function, in the way that would be pursued now. However, we found that we could harness skills in mouse kidney transplantation to swap kidneys between wild-type and gene-deleted mice, in both directions, to illuminate the relative importance of local complement synthesis (29–31). Our initial focus was on C3, the central and most abundant component of the complement cascade in blood. We had already shown, in human kidney transplantation, that C3 has a significant contribution to the systemic complement pool through intrarenal synthesis (32).

COMPLEMENT AND THE TRANSPLANTED KIDNEY

The summation of the research including knockout mouse transplant studies and clinical observational studies has demonstrated a number of important principles. Namely, it showed that local synthesis of C3 had a disproportionate influence on ischaemia-reperfusion injury relative to the systemic pool (30), and an impact was also observed in the process of cell mediated rejection of MHC mismatched kidney transplants (31). It was evident from the analyses that the renal tubule cell was the primary target for complement deposition in these conditions, and the tubule cell was also the primary site of C3 expression (30).

The evidence additionally highlighted the role of donor antigen-presenting cells (APCs) as a source of complement (33). These cells, also known as donor passenger cells, reside in the interstitial space of the donor kidney, specifically around the renal tubules. Within the first 24 h after transplantation, these cells migrate into the recipient lymphoid system where they immunize the recipient against donor MHC antigen (34). Local production of complement was shown to modify the capacity of the APC to prime the antigen-specific T cells that mediate rejection (31, 35–37).

Considerable work has gone into identifying the complement effectors generated downstream of C3 that mobilize the inflammatory and adaptive immune functions against the transplant [reviewed in (38)]. These investigations have resulted in a deeper understanding both of the roles of the anaphylatoxins, C3a and C5a, (39) and the membrane attack complex (C5b-9) on immune cells and parenchymal tissue (40).

In addition to expressing core complement components and activating enzyme-precursors, tissue-resident and migratory cells also display receptors that detect a range of biologically active complement products formed downstream of C3 cleavage (41–43). This emphasizes the ability for cross talk between tissue-resident and migratory cells within the transplant setting. It is helpful to think of the different cells that produce and detect complement as nodes in a local network, whose functions bring together and amplify the innate immune response and regulate adaptive immunity.

LOCAL TISSUE DEFENSE

Presumably, the local synthesis of complement components serves to enhance the defense against invasive organisms. For example, the synthesis of C3 by renal tract epithelium potentially increases the efficiency with which locally invasive organisms are opsonised and subsequently eliminated at the point of entry. There is strong evidence for such a role, as the renal tubular epithelium constitutively expresses complement, and the production is rapidly upregulated in the presence of infection (44, 45). Further testament to this mechanism is that many common urinary pathogens have developed resistance to complement, including clinically relevant strains of gram negative pathogens (46–48). Not only have these strains been found to resist complement mediated lysis but they can also utilize complement to invade complement receptor expressing tubular epithelial cells (44, 49, 50). The C3b receptor, CD46, is one such receptor used by uropathogenic *E. coli* to evade extracellular defenses (45, 51) and is an illustration of the means by which complement resistant strains can gain an advantage against the host. Thus, the local pool of complement can be both a protector against infection and a source of tissue injury.

EMERGENCE OF COLLECTIN-11

Whereas the last 20-years of research has taught us much about the effector functions of locally derived complement, our knowledge of the trigger mechanisms that localize tissue injury to a particular tissue compartment has lagged behind. This may be because the changes that induce complement activation are different for each organ and as such the studies in different organs have produced mixed and sometimes contradictory results [for more information refer to (52)]. Alternatively, it could be that the focus on circulating complement has not led us to the local mechanisms that drive complement-mediated disease. It is a common observation that measurement of circulating complement does not closely correlate with biopsy evidence of complement activation within an affected organ, and this may have delayed our understanding of local disease mechanisms. If only we understood more about the structures that triggered complement activation and how they are recognized in an organ such as the kidney, we would know more about how to detect and regulate harmful signals for health benefit.

We recently reviewed the evidence for the different pattern recognition molecules that could trigger complement activation in renal ischaemia-reperfusion injury and transplantation (52, 53). There, we considered whether the classical or lectin pathways could mediate the onset of ischaemia-reperfusion injury and found no conclusive evidence of a role for the classical pathway in the genesis of the renal injury within a murine model (54, 55). The lectin pathway also, at first, seemed not to have a key role in the induction of ischaemic renal injury, since the injury—at least in mice–was independent of C4, which is a component shared by both the classical and lectin pathways (56). However, we now believe that more recent findings on CL-11 and the coupled enzyme MBL associated serine protease-2 (MASP-2) reconcile these observations, both in the context of renal ischaemic epithelial cell damage and very possibly in retinal epithelial ischaemic damage (57–59).

CL-11 is a recently described member of the lectin family of pattern recognition molecules, with known antimicrobial functions and ability to trigger complement activation via the lectin pathway (60). Reported in 2006, CL-11 was at first named kidney collectin, or CL-K1, for its abundant expression in normal renal tissue (61, 62). The renaming of CL-11 is appropriate, since it is now known that the molecule is widely expressed (60). The most obvious expression site in the kidney is the renal tubule, for this structure encompasses the largest volume in the kidney, though CL-11 is also present in the glomerular mesangium and epithelium. Despite its strong presence in the kidney, the mean concentration of CL-11 in serum is just 284 ng/mL, by ELISA measurement. Furthermore, CL-11 is known to form heteromeric complexes with Collectin Liver 1 (CL-10) in the serum. Interestingly, this heterocomplex, CL-LK, has been shown to activate complement *in vitro* (63). However, we hypothesize that it is the local production of complement that accounts for tissue injury. Indeed, CL-11 has been shown to be produced by renal epithelial cells, whereas CL-10 has not been definitively shown to be expressed in the kidney (64) thereby making it less likely that the CL-LK heterocomplex is participating in renal injury.

CL-11 monomers have a similar structure to other C-type lectins such as MBL and consist of a globular head followed by a neck and a collagenous tail. The head contains a carbohydrate recognition domain (CRD), and the tail contains binding sites for MASPs which are required for complement activation. The CL-11 monomers form a triplet structure that self-combines to form oligomers with higher avidity of binding to ligand (65). Since hypoxia- or hypothermia-treated epithelial cells appear to bind CL-11 avidly (57–59), it is proposed that a change in presentation of the stress-induced cellular ligand for CL-11 underpins strong attachment of the oligomeric CL-11 complex. Whether this stress-induced pattern could involve a change in orientation or distribution of ligand, or increased expression or alteration of biochemical structure, is currently under investigation. However, clues to potential binding motifs or patterns can be gleaned from understanding the binding properties of other lectins. Mannose-Binding Lectin (MBL) is a well characterized C-type lectin similar to CL-11 in that it shares a similar structure with a CRD and collagenous tail, and binds oligosaccharide ligands in a calcium-dependent manner. In particular, MBL has a higher affinity for ligands that contain mannose or N-Acetyl-D-glucosamine residues (66). More recently, information has been gathered which further characterizes the MBL-oligosaccharide interaction, specifically in relation to MBL binding of lipopolysaccharide (67). Thus, our understanding of potential CL-11 ligands could be narrowed by considering and applying our knowledge of the glycan motifs that MBL recognizes.

Many molecules are normally glycosylated to some extent. In particular, fucosylated molecules are widely synthesized in normal tissues (68), and what is interesting to us is that L-fucose, the preferred monosaccharide recognized by CL-11, is also abundant in the proximal renal tubule (57). These are the very cells that express complement components in abundance. Therefore, the core components of the complement system including C3, C5 (23) and a lectin pathway trigger (CL-11) are expressed within the same hypoxia-sensitive segment of the renal tubule, where a potential binding ligand for CL-11 is also present. *In vivo* and *ex vivo* studies of epithelial cell injury suggest that hypoxia- or hypothermia-induced binding of CL-11 is followed by complement activation on the injured cell surface at sites that are specifically marked by CL-11. In a murine model of hypoxia-induced renal tubule cell stress, complement deposition was prevented by CL-11 deletion or by L-fucose blockade of the carbohydrate recognition domain of CL-11 (57). The protective effect of L-fucose blockade could also be demonstrated in wild type mice undergoing renal ischaemic insult (unpublished data). A similar injury mechanism also appears to occur in retinal pigmented epithelial cells, where hypoxia-induced membrane attack complex formation and CL-11 deposition correlate with sites of L-fucose expression (59). Thus, these findings may have potentially broad implications for diseases where complement mediated injury is thought to play a significant role.

CLOSING THE GAP

David and colleagues originally described the ability of renal tubule cells to spontaneously activate complement in the presence of normal human serum, and they attributed this to activation of the alternative complement pathway (69, 70). However, subsequent understanding of the lectin pathway and, in particular, the role of CL-11 now suggests another explanation (57). It points to a role for pattern recognition by CL-11 in contact with a damage-associated ligand on hypoxia-activated cells, and in turn the subsequent activation of the complement cascade by lectin-pathway associated serine proteases, i.e. MASPs. Although the alternative pathway may still play a role in hypoxia-mediated renal injury, the emerging data suggests that CL-11 is indispensable for triggering complement activation. Secondary activation of the alternative pathway could then occur either after the formation of C3b (which is an acceptor for factor B of the alternative pathway), or by MASP-1/3-mediated cleavage of complement factor D, which in turn cleaves factor B (60, 71). In the current model, CL-11 is expressed at physiological levels in the kidney and only substantially increases in binding to the tubule following cell stress. Complement activation then occurs at the sites where CL-11-MASP complexes form.

MASP-2 and its relationship with CL-11 are thought to play an essential role in this model. MASP-2 is one of the three MASPs that are physically linked with complement-activating lectins, including CL-11. MASP-2 differs from MASP-1 and MASP-3, in

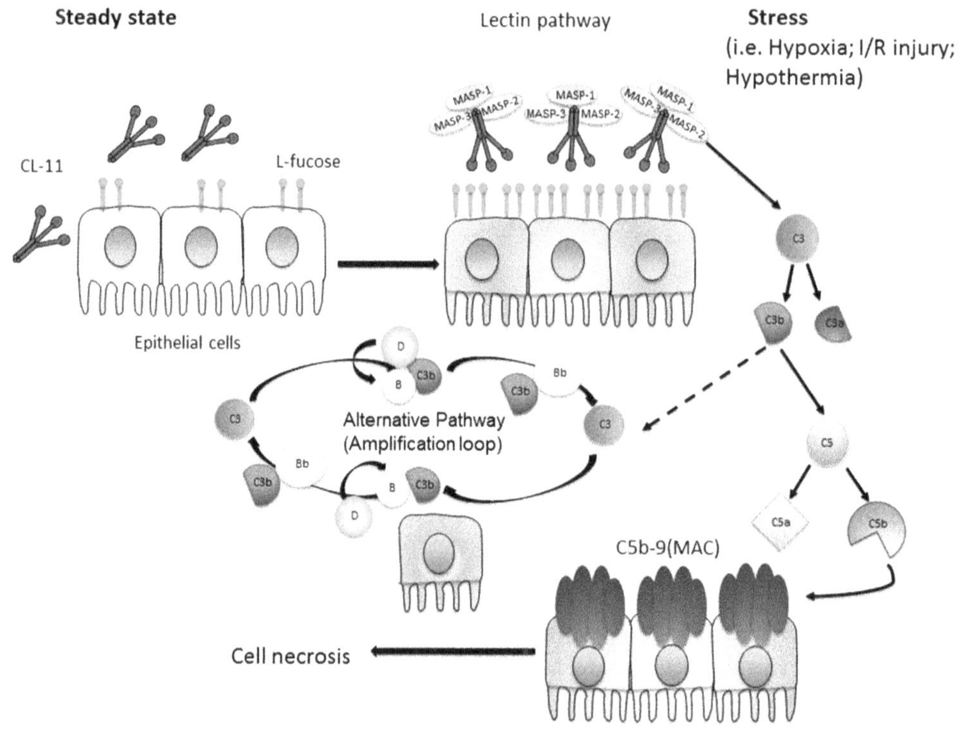

FIGURE 2 | Hypothesis of local complement activation triggered by CL-11 on stressed epithelial cells. We hypothesize that under steady state conditions, CL-11 is produced and released from the basolateral surface and likely the luminal surface of epithelial cells (e.g., renal tubular epithelial cells and retinal pigmented epithelial cells). Upon stress, damaged epithelial cells display an abnormal pattern of L-fucose resulting in CL-11 binding to cell surface. CL-11/MBL-associated serine protease (MASP 1, 2 & 3) complexes become activated promoting downstream complement activation. In particular, MASP-2 is a key player at the site of tissue injury cleaving C3 in a C4-independent manner. During this process, the anaphylatoxins C3a and C5a are generated and C5 cleavage initiates the terminal pathway that culminates in the formation of the membrane attack complex (MAC). C3b formed by the lectin pathway can covalently bind to target cells and initiate the alternative pathway. C3b bound to factor B (C3bB) is cleaved by factor D to form the alternative pathway C3 convertase.

that only MASP-2 can directly cleave C3 in human and murine sera (64, 72). It is only recently that studies in gene-deleted mice have not only confirmed the importance of MASP-2 in mediating renal, cardiac and intestinal ischaemic injuries, but have shown that the injury in each case was C4-independent (30, 58, 73). The evidence supports a pathway of injury in which stress-induced ligand presentation leads to CL-11 binding and subsequent MASP-2-mediated triggering of complement activation using a route that involves the direct cleavage of C3 by MASP-2 (60, 71, 74). As indicated above, MASP-1/3-mediated activation of the alternative complement pathway could be a supplementary mechanism of injury triggered by CL-11.

In total, the evidence suggests that the renal epithelial cell behaves as a unit of host defense and inflammation, in which CL-11 appears to integrate the detection of cell stress signals with activation of the complement system. We envisage that CL-11 is primarily a tissue-based pattern recognition molecule that binds damage associated molecular patterns (DAMPs) **Figure 2**. In the presence of tissue stress from non-infectious causes, the effector actions of CL-11 appear to be misdirected by glycan ligands that are inappropriately exposed on the renal tubule cell surface. Similar cellular responses to stress such as hypoxia probably exist at other surfaces, such as the retinal epithelium, where hypoxia-induced complement activation in the presence of CL-11 is also described (59). What remains unclear is the biochemical structure of the damage-related glycan ligands (and carrier molecules) recognized by CL-11. Future studies will need to elucidate the nature of the stress signal on cells and how it is induced by hypoxia to fully validate the hypothesis, and show whether the same or similar mechanism operates at other epithelial surfaces. As the identity of these DAMPs begin to emerge, it will be important to determine whether and how those exposed on renal tissue differ from the CL-11 ligands on other tissues and microbial structures, or indeed on developing tissues targeted by CL-11. There is little doubt that investigating CL-11 will provide new tools to prove the wider functions of immune surveillance at different sites, with the potential to develop new clinical agents for detecting or blocking specific patterns.

AUTHOR CONTRIBUTIONS

CN and MH participated in manuscript writing, editing, and figure development. GF contributed to figure development. CF and SS contributed to manuscript editing, and writing, respectively.

FUNDING

Some of the work described was supported by Medical Research Council grants MR/J006742/1, MR/L020254/1, G1001141, MR/J004553/1, MR/M007871/1, and MR/L012758/1, European Research Council (ERC-2012-ADG_20120314), UK Regenerative Medicine Platform, and by the National Institute for Health Research (NIHR) Biomedical Research Centre based at Guy's and St Thomas's NHS Foundation Trust and King's College London. The views expressed are those of the author(s) and not necessarily those of the NHS, the NIHR or the Department of Health.

REFERENCES

1. Imler JL, Zheng L. Biology of toll receptors: lessons from insects and mammals. *J Leukoc Biol.* (2004) 75:18–26. doi: 10.1189/jlb.0403160
2. Song X, Jin P, Qin S, Chen L, Ma F. The evolution and origin of animal Toll-like receptor signaling pathway revealed by network-level molecular evolutionary analyses. *PLoS ONE* (2012) 7:e51657. doi: 10.1371/journal.pone.0051657
3. Stocks CJ, Schembri MA, Sweet MJ, Kapetanovic R. For when bacterial infections persist: Toll-like receptor-inducible direct antimicrobial pathways in macrophages. *J Leukoc Biol.* (2018) 103:35–51. doi: 10.1002/JLB.4RI0917-358R
4. Lee YK, Kang M, Choi EY. TLR/MyD88-mediated innate immunity in intestinal graft-versus-host disease. *Immune Netw.* (2017) 17:144–51. doi: 10.4110/in.2017.17.3.144
5. Gao W, Xiong Y, Li Q, Yang H. Inhibition of toll-like receptor signaling as a promising therapy for inflammatory diseases: a journey from molecular to nano therapeutics. *Front Physiol.* (2017) 8:508. doi: 10.3389/fphys.2017.00508
6. Drexler SK, Foxwell BM. The role of toll-like receptors in chronic inflammation. *Int J Biochem Cell Biol.* (2010) 42:506–18. doi: 10.1016/j.biocel.2009.10.009
7. Nesargikar PN, Spiller B, Chavez R. The complement system: history, pathways, cascade and inhibitors. *Eur J Microbiol Immunol.* (2012) 2:103–11. doi: 10.1556/EuJMI.2.2012.2.2
8. Colten HR, Ooi YM, Edelson PJ. Synthesis and secretion of complement proteins by macrophages. *Ann N Y Acad Sci.* (1979) 332:482–90. doi: 10.1111/j.1749-6632.1979.tb47142.x
9. Einstein LP, Hansen PJ, Ballow M, Davis AE III, Davis JSt, Alper CA, et al. Biosynthesis of the third component of complement (C3) *in vitro* by monocytes from both normal and homozygous C3-deficient humans. *J Clin Invest.* (1977) 60:963–9. doi: 10.1172/JCI108876
10. Katz Y, Revel M, Strunk RC. Interleukin 6 stimulates synthesis of complement proteins factor B and C3 in human skin fibroblasts. *Eur J Immunol.* (1989) 19:983–8. doi: 10.1002/eji.1830190605
11. Katz Y, Cole FS, Strunk RC. Synergism between gamma interferon and lipopolysaccharide for synthesis of factor B, but not C2, in human fibroblasts. *J Exp Med.* (1988) 167:1–14. doi: 10.1084/jem.167.1.1
12. Barnum SR, Jones JL, Benveniste EN. Interleukin-1 and tumor necrosis factor-mediated regulation of C3 gene expression in human astroglioma cells. *Glia* (1993) 7:225–36. doi: 10.1002/glia.440070306
13. Halstensen TS, Mollnes TE, Brandtzaeg P. Persistent complement activation in submucosal blood vessels of active inflammatory bowel disease: immunohistochemical evidence. *Gastroenterology* (1989) 97:10–9. doi: 10.1016/0016-5085(89)91409-1
14. Ahrenstedt O, Knutson L, Nilsson B, Nilsson-Ekdahl K, Odlind B, Hallgren R. Enhanced local production of complement components in the small intestines of patients with Crohn's disease. *N Engl J Med.* (1990) 322:1345–9. doi: 10.1056/NEJM199005103221903
15. Witte DP, Welch TR, Beischel LS. Detection and cellular localization of human C4 gene expression in the renal tubular epithelial cells and other extrahepatic epithelial sources. *Am J Pathol.* (1991) 139:717–24.
16. Lappin D, Hamilton AD, Morrison L, Aref M, Whaley K. Synthesis of complement components (C3, C2, B and C1-inhibitor) and lysozyme by human monocytes and macrophages. *J Clin Lab Immunol.* (1986) 20:101–5.
17. Whaley K. Biosynthesis of the complement components and the regulatory proteins of the alternative complement pathway by human peripheral blood monocytes. *J Exp Med.* (1980) 151:501–16. doi: 10.1084/jem.151.3.501
18. Passwell J, Schreiner GF, Nonaka M, Beuscher HU, Colten HR. Local extrahepatic expression of complement genes C3, factor B, C2, and C4 is increased in murine lupus nephritis. *J Clin Invest.* (1988) 82:1676–84. doi: 10.1172/JCI113780
19. Couser WG. Mechanisms of glomerular injury in immune-complex disease. *Kidney Int.* (1985) 28:569–83. doi: 10.1038/ki.1985.167
20. Brooimans RA, Stegmann AP, van Dorp WT, van der Ark AA, van der Woude FJ, van Es LA, et al. Interleukin 2 mediates stimulation of complement C3 biosynthesis in human proximal tubular epithelial cells. *J Clin Invest.* (1991) 88:379–84. doi: 10.1172/JCI115314
21. Seelen MA, Brooimans RA, van der Woude FJ, van Es LA, Daha MR. IFN-gamma mediates stimulation of complement C4 biosynthesis in human proximal tubular epithelial cells. *Kidney Int.* (1993) 44:50–7. doi: 10.1038/ki.1993.212
22. Timmerman JJ, van der Woude FJ, van Gijlswijk-Janssen DJ, Verweij CL, van Es LA, Daha MR. Differential expression of complement components in human fetal and adult kidneys. *Kidney Int.* (1996) 49:730–40. doi: 10.1038/ki.1996.102
23. Khan TN, Sinniah R. Role of complement in renal tubular damage. *Histopathology* (1995) 26:351–6. doi: 10.1111/j.1365-2559.1995.tb00197.x
24. Welch TR, Beischel LS, Witte DP. Differential expression of complement C3 and C4 in the human kidney. *J Clin Invest.* (1993) 92:1451–8. doi: 10.1172/JCI116722
25. Welch TR, Beischel LS, Frenzke M, Witte D. Regulated expression of complement factor B in the human kidney. *Kidney Int.* (1996) 50:521–5. doi: 10.1038/ki.1996.344
26. Andrews PA, Finn JE, Lloyd CM, Zhou W, Mathieson PW, Sacks SH. Expression and tissue localization of donor-specific complement C3 synthesized in human renal allografts. *Eur J Immunol.* (1995) 25:1087-93. doi: 10.1002/eji.1830250434
27. Andrews PA, Pani A, Zhou W, Sacks SH. Local transcription of complement C3 in human allograft rejection. Evidence for a pathogenic role and correlation to histology and outcome. *Transplantation* (1994) 58:637–40. doi: 10.1097/00007890-199409150-00023
28. Sacks SH, Zhou W, Andrews PA, Hartley B. Endogenous complement C3 synthesis in immune complex nephritis. *Lancet* (1993) 342:1273–4. doi: 10.1016/0140-6736(93)92362-W
29. Sheerin NS, Springall T, Carroll MC, Hartley B, Sacks SH. Protection against anti-glomerular basement membrane (GBM)-mediated nephritis in C3- and C4-deficient mice. *Clin Exp Immunol.* (1997) 110:403–9. doi: 10.1046/j.1365-2249.1997.4261438.x
30. Farrar CA, Zhou W, Lin T, Sacks SH. Local extravascular pool of C3 is a determinant of postischemic acute renal failure. *FASEB J.* (2006) 20:217–26. doi: 10.1096/fj.05-4747com
31. Pratt JR, Basheer SA, Sacks SH. Local synthesis of complement component C3 regulates acute renal transplant rejection. *Nat Med.* (2002) 8:582–7. doi: 10.1038/nm0602-582
32. Tang S, Zhou W, Sheerin NS, Vaughan RW, Sacks SH. Contribution of renal secreted complement C3 to the circulating pool in humans. *J Immunol.* (1999) 162:4336–41.
33. Bartel G, Brown K, Phillips R, Peng Q, Zhou W, Sacks SH, et al. Donor specific transplant tolerance is dependent on complement receptors. *Transpl Int.* (2013) 26:99–108. doi: 10.1111/tri.12006

34. Marino J, Babiker-Mohamed MH, Crosby-Bertorini P, Paster JT, LeGuern C, Germana S, et al. Donor exosomes rather than passenger leukocytes initiate alloreactive T cell responses after transplantation. *Sci Immunol.* (2016) 1:aaf8759. doi: 10.1126/sciimmunol.aaf8759
35. Strainic MG, Liu J, Huang D, An F, Lalli PN, Muqim N, et al. Locally produced complement fragments C5a and C3a provide both costimulatory and survival signals to naive CD4+ T cells. *Immunity* (2008) 28:425–35. doi: 10.1016/j.immuni.2008.02.001
36. Lalli PN, Strainic MG, Yang M, Lin F, Medof ME, Heeger PS. Locally produced C5a binds to T cell-expressed C5aR to enhance effector T-cell expansion by limiting antigen-induced apoptosis. *Blood* (2008) 112:1759–66. doi: 10.1182/blood-2008-04-151068
37. Zhou W, Patel H, Li K, Peng Q, Villiers MB, Sacks SH. Macrophages from C3-deficient mice have impaired potency to stimulate alloreactive T cells. *Blood* (2006) 107:2461–9. doi: 10.1182/blood-2005-08-3144
38. Sacks SH, Zhou W. The role of complement in the early immune response to transplantation. *Nat Rev Immunol.* (2012) 12:431–42. doi: 10.1038/nri3225
39. Peng Q, Li K, Smyth LA, Xing G, Wang N, Meader L, et al. C3a and C5a promote renal ischemia-reperfusion injury. *J Am Soc Nephrol.* (2012) 23:1474–85. doi: 10.1681/ASN.2011111072
40. Zhou W, Farrar CA, Abe K, Pratt JR, Marsh JE, Wang Y, et al. Predominant role for C5b-9 in renal ischemia/reperfusion injury. *J Clin Invest.* (2000) 105:1363–71. doi: 10.1172/JCI8621
41. Wang YH, Zhang YG. Kidney and innate immunity. *Immunol Lett.* (2017) 183:73–8. doi: 10.1016/j.imlet.2017.01.011
42. Kemper C, Kohl J. Novel roles for complement receptors in T cell regulation and beyond. *Mol Immunol.* (2013) 56:181–90. doi: 10.1016/j.molimm.2013.05.223
43. Holers VM. Complement and its receptors: new insights into human disease. *Annu Rev Immunol.* (2014) 32:433–59. doi: 10.1146/annurev-immunol-032713-120154
44. Springall T, Sheerin NS, Abe K, Holers VM, Wan H, Sacks SH. Epithelial secretion of C3 promotes colonization of the upper urinary tract by *Escherichia coli*. *Nat Med.* (2001) 7:801–6. doi: 10.1038/89923
45. Li K, Zhou W, Hong Y, Sacks SH, Sheerin NS. Synergy between type 1 fimbriae expression and C3 opsonisation increases internalisation of *E. coli* by human tubular epithelial cells. *BMC Microbiol.* (2009) 9:64. doi: 10.1186/1471-2180-9-64
46. Li K, Sacks SH, Sheerin NS. The classical complement pathway plays a critical role in the opsonisation of uropathogenic *Escherichia coli*. *Mol Immunol.* (2008) 45:954–62. doi: 10.1016/j.molimm.2007.07.037
47. Kaca W, Arabski M, Fudala R, Holmstrom E, Sjoholm A, Weintraub A, et al. Human complement activation by smooth and rough *Proteus mirabilis* lipopolysaccharides. *Arch Immunol Ther Exp.* (2009) 57:383–91. doi: 10.1007/s00005-009-0043-8
48. Doorduijn DJ, Rooijakkers SH, van Schaik W, Bardoel BW. Complement resistance mechanisms of Klebsiella pneumoniae. *Immunobiology* (2016) 221:1102–9. doi: 10.1016/j.imbio.2016.06.014
49. Miller TE, Phillips S, Simpson IJ. Complement-mediated immune mechanisms in renal infection. II. Effect of decomplementation. *Clin Exp Immunol.* (1978) 33:115–21.
50. Abreu AG, Barbosa AS. How *Escherichia coli* circumvent complement-mediated killing. *Front Immunol.* (2017) 8:452. doi: 10.3389/fimmu.2017.00452
51. Li K, Feito MJ, Sacks SH, Sheerin NS. CD46 (membrane cofactor protein) acts as a human epithelial cell receptor for internalization of opsonized uropathogenic *Escherichia coli*. *J Immunol.* (2006) 177:2543–51. doi: 10.4049/jimmunol.177.4.2543
52. Nauser CL, Farrar CA, Sacks SH. Complement recognition pathways in renal transplantation. *J Am Soc Nephrol.* (2017) 28:2571–8. doi: 10.1681/ASN.2017010079
53. Howard M, Farrar CA, Sacks SH. Structural and functional diversity of collectins and ficolins and their relationship to disease. *Semin Immunopathol.* (2018) 40:75–85. doi: 10.1007/s00281-017-0642-0
54. Riedemann NC, Ward PA. Complement in ischemia reperfusion injury. *Am J Pathol.* (2003) 162:363–7. doi: 10.1016/S0002-9440(10)63830-8
55. Gorsuch WB, Chrysanthou E, Schwaeble WJ, Stahl GL. The complement system in ischemia-reperfusion injuries. *Immunobiology* (2012) 217:1026–33. doi: 10.1016/j.imbio.2012.07.024
56. Farrar CA, Zhou W, Sacks SH. Role of the lectin complement pathway in kidney transplantation. *Immunobiology* (2016) 221:1068–72. doi: 10.1016/j.imbio.2016.05.004
57. Farrar CA, Tran D, Li K, Wu W, Peng Q, Schwaeble W, et al. Collectin-11 detects stress-induced L-fucose pattern to trigger renal epithelial injury. *J Clin Invest.* (2016) 126:1911–25. doi: 10.1172/JCI83000
58. Asgari E, Farrar CA, Lynch N, Ali YM, Roscher S, Stover C, et al. Mannan-binding lectin-associated serine protease 2 is critical for the development of renal ischemia reperfusion injury and mediates tissue injury in the absence of complement C4. *FASEB J.* (2014) 28:3996–4003. doi: 10.1096/fj.13-246306
59. Fanelli G, Gonzalez-Cordero A, Gardner PJ, Peng Q, Fernando M, Kloc M, et al. Human stem cell-derived retinal epithelial cells activate complement via collectin 11 in response to stress. *Sci Rep.* (2017) 7:14625. doi: 10.1038/s41598-017-15212-z
60. Hansen S, Selman L, Palaniyar N, Ziegler K, Brandt J, Kliem A, et al. Collectin 11 (CL-11, CL-K1) is a MASP-1/3-associated plasma collectin with microbial-binding activity. *J Immunol.* (2010) 185:6096–104. doi: 10.4049/jimmunol.1002185
61. Keshi H, Sakamoto T, Kawai T, Ohtani K, Katoh T, Jang SJ, et al. Identification and characterization of a novel human collectin CL-K1. *Microbiol Immunol.* (2006) 50:1001–13. doi: 10.1111/j.1348-0421.2006.tb03868.x
62. Hogenkamp A, van Eijk M, van Dijk A, van Asten AJ, Veldhuizen EJ, Haagsman HP. Characterization and expression sites of newly identified chicken collectins. *Mol Immunol.* (2006) 43:1604–16. doi: 10.1016/j.molimm.2005.09.015
63. Henriksen ML, Brandt J, Andrieu JP, Nielsen C, Jensen PH, Holmskov U, et al. Heteromeric complexes of native collectin kidney 1 and collectin liver 1 are found in the circulation with MASPs and activate the complement system. *J Immunol.* (2013) 191:6117–27. doi: 10.4049/jimmunol.1302121
64. Garred P, Genster N, Pilely K, Bayarri-Olmos R, Rosbjerg A, Ma YJ, et al. A journey through the lectin pathway of complement-MBL and beyond. *Immunol Rev.* (2016) 274:74–97. doi: 10.1111/imr.12468
65. Selman L, Hansen S. Structure and function of collectin liver 1 (CL-L1) and collectin 11 (CL-11, CL-K1). *Immunobiology* (2012) 217:851–63. doi: 10.1016/j.imbio.2011.12.008
66. Drickamer K. Engineering galactose-binding activity into a C-type mannose-binding protein. *Nature* (1992) 360:183–6. doi: 10.1038/360183a0
67. Man-Kupisinska A, Swierzko AS, Maciejewska A, Hoc M, Rozalski A, Siwinska M, et al. Interaction of mannose-binding lectin with lipopolysaccharide outer core region and its biological consequences. *Front Immunol.* (2018) 9:1498. doi: 10.3389/fimmu.2018.01498
68. Ma B, Simala-Grant JL, Taylor DE. Fucosylation in prokaryotes and eukaryotes. *Glycobiology* (2006) 16:158R–84R. doi: 10.1093/glycob/cwl040
69. Biancone L, David S, Della Pietra V, Montrucchio G, Cambi V, Camussi G. Alternative pathway activation of complement by cultured human proximal tubular epithelial cells. *Kidney Int.* (1994) 45:451–60. doi: 10.1038/ki.1994.59
70. David S, Biancone L, Caserta C, Bussolati B, Cambi V, Camussi G. Alternative pathway complement activation induces proinflammatory activity in human proximal tubular epithelial cells. *Nephrol Dial Transplant.* (1997) 12:51–6. doi: 10.1093/ndt/12.1.51
71. Ma YJ, Skjoedt MO, Garred P. Collectin-11/MASP complex formation triggers activation of the lectin complement pathway–the fifth lectin pathway

initiation complex. *J Innate Immun.* (2013) 5:242–50. doi: 10.1159/000345356

72. Wallis R. Interactions between mannose-binding lectin and MASPs during complement activation by the lectin pathway. *Immunobiology* (2007) 212:289–99. doi: 10.1016/j.imbio.2006.11.004
73. Schwaeble WJ, Lynch NJ, Clark JE, Marber M, Samani NJ, Ali YM, et al. Targeting of mannan-binding lectin-associated serine protease-2 confers protection from myocardial and gastrointestinal ischemia/reperfusion injury. *Proc Natl Acad Sci USA.* (2011) 108:7523–8. doi: 10.1073/pnas.1101748108
74. Yaseen S, Demopulos G, Dudler T, Yabuki M, Wood CL, Cummings WJ, et al. Lectin pathway effector enzyme mannan-binding lectin-associated serine protease-2 can activate native complement C3 in absence of C4 and/or C2. *FASEB J.* (2017) 31:2210–9. doi: 10.1096/fj.201601306R

11

Self-Damage Caused by Dysregulation of the Complement Alternative Pathway: Relevance of the Factor H Protein Family

Pilar Sánchez-Corral[1†], Richard B. Pouw[2†], Margarita López-Trascasa[1,3†] and Mihály Józsi[4,5†]*

[1] Complement Research Group, Hospital La Paz Institute for Health Research (IdiPAZ), La Paz University Hospital, Center for Biomedical Network Research on Rare Diseases (CIBERER), Madrid, Spain, [2] Department of Pharmaceutical Sciences, University of Basel, Basel, Switzerland, [3] Department of Medicine, Universidad Autónoma de Madrid, Madrid, Spain, [4] Complement Research Group, Department of Immunology, ELTE Eötvös Loránd University, Budapest, Hungary, [5] MTA-SE Research Group of Immunology and Hematology, Hungarian Academy of Sciences and Semmelweis University, Budapest, Hungary

***Correspondence:**
Mihály Józsi
mihaly.jozsi@ttk.elte.hu

[†]These authors have contributed equally to this work.

The alternative pathway is a continuously active surveillance arm of the complement system, and it can also enhance complement activation initiated by the classical and the lectin pathways. Various membrane-bound and plasma regulatory proteins control the activation of the potentially deleterious complement system. Among the regulators, the plasma glycoprotein factor H (FH) is the main inhibitor of the alternative pathway and its powerful amplification loop. FH belongs to a protein family that also includes FH-like protein 1 and five factor H-related (FHR-1 to FHR-5) proteins. Genetic variants and abnormal rearrangements involving the FH protein family have been linked to numerous systemic and organ-specific diseases, including age-related macular degeneration, and the renal pathologies atypical hemolytic uremic syndrome, C3 glomerulopathies, and IgA nephropathy. This review covers the known and recently emerged ligands and interactions of the human FH family proteins associated with disease and discuss the very recent experimental data that suggest FH-antagonistic and complement-activating functions for the FHR proteins.

Keywords: age-related macular degeneration, atypical hemolytic uremic syndrome, C3 glomerulopathy, complement activation, complement de-regulation, factor H, factor H-related protein, opsonization

INTRODUCTION

While initially only regarded as a supporting factor for the effectivity of immunoglobulins, the complement system is nowadays widely recognized as a crucial part of the innate immune system involved in many different processes (1). In addition to acting as a first line of defense by directly targeting and killing invading pathogens, with or without the help of immunoglobulins, its role in inflammation, immune cell recruitment, and clearance of immune complexes, apoptotic cells, and necrotic cells places complement at the center of the human immune system. The relevant role of complement is corroborated by the variety of pathological situations associated with complement deficiency or dysfunction.

Three complement activation pathways have been defined, each comprised of various proteins forming an intricate cascade of activation events (**Figure 1**). Both the classical and the lectin pathways are initiated when pattern recognition molecules (PRMs) that are complexed with zymogens of serine proteases, bind to their ligand. The classical pathway is activated by the binding of the C1 complex to immunoglobulins and pentraxins, while the lectin pathway uses various PRMs, including mannose-binding lectin and ficolins, which bind to specific carbohydrate moieties. These ligands are normally not present on healthy human cells. In contrast, the alternative activation pathway is initiated through the constitutive low rate hydrolysis of the internal thioester bond of C3, allowing binding of various activating complement proteins. All three pathways lead to the cleavage of C3 into C3a and C3b. C3b contains a highly reactive thioester group that is exposed upon C3 cleavage, resulting in the deposition of C3b onto virtually any molecule or cell surface in close proximity. When left unchecked, C3b on its own will again initiate the alternative pathway. As both the classical and the lectin pathway will also activate the alternative pathway once C3b is formed, thus enhancing complement activation, the alternative pathway has a pivotal role as an amplification loop within the complement system. Up to 80% of total complement activation has been ascribed to this amplification loop (2). Due to the spontaneous nature of the alternative pathway, it must be tightly controlled to prevent unwarranted and dangerous complement activation.

Complement regulation takes places both on the human cell surface and in the fluid phase. Several regulators, like most complement components, are found in the circulation. In addition, human cells express a wide array of membrane-bound complement regulators that control the system at various steps. Especially due to the activating proteins of the alternative pathway, regulation in the fluid phase is crucial, as unchecked, spontaneous C3 activation would lead to complete consumption of C3 and loss of complement activity. The 155-kDa glycoprotein complement factor H (FH) is the major regulator of the alternative pathway, inhibiting C3 activation both in the fluid phase as well as on human cell surfaces (**Figure 1**) (3). Similar to other complement regulators encoded in the regulators of complement activation (RCA) gene cluster, FH is composed of complement control protein (CCP) domains, often also referred to as short consensus repeat domains. FH is composed of 20 CCPs (**Figure 2**) (4). The first four N-terminal domains contain the complement inhibiting activity, such as decay accelerating activity and co-factor activity (5). The two most C-terminal CCP domains (19 and 20), together with a region located in CCPs 6–8, are crucial for binding of FH to surfaces, such as human cell membranes, as well as for mediating binding to several host and non-host ligands (discussed below) (6, 7). FH is highly abundant in plasma, with circulating levels of 233–400 μg/mL on average, although it has to be noted that some of the assays used might detect other FH family members as well (8–11).

Factor H-like protein 1 (FHL-1) is a splice variant derived from the *CFH* gene. Serum levels of FHL-1 are estimated to be 10–50 μg/mL (12, 13). FHL-1 is identical to the first seven CCP domains of FH, with an unique, four amino acid long C-terminus (14, 15). Thus, FHL-1 shares the C3b binding and regulatory domains CCPs 1–4 with FH and, like FH, it has complement inhibiting activity (16). Likewise, due to the shared CCPs 6–7 domains, FHL-1 and FH bind some common ligands, such as heparin, the pentraxins C-reactive protein (CRP) and pentraxin 3 (PTX3), and malondialdehyde epitopes (**Figure 2**). However, there are also differences in ligand interactions between FHL-1 and FH, not only because of the extra domains in FH but also due to the difference in their conformation and the unique SFTL tail at the C-terminus of FHL-1. For example, it was recently reported that the SFTL tail increases the interaction of FHL-1 with CRP and PTX3 (17).

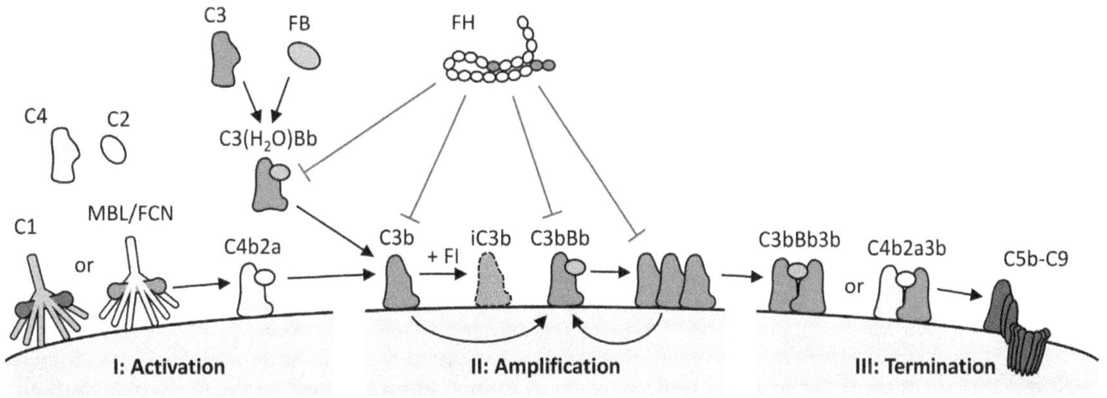

FIGURE 1 | Overview of the role of factor H (FH) within the complement system. (I) The complement system is activated *via* binding of C1q (classical pathway), or mannan binding lectin/ficolins (MBL/FCN) (lectin pathway) in complex with serine proteases to specific molecules, or through the spontaneous activation of C3 into C3(H_2O) (alternative pathway). Upon activation, the three pathways form C3 convertases (C4b2a or C3(H_2O)Bb) resulting in the generation and deposition of C3b on the activating surface. (II) C3b forms new C3 convertase molecules (C3bBb) that enhance C3b deposition and amplify complement activation. (III) C3b can also bind to C3 convertases to generate C5 convertases (C4b2a3b or C3bBb3b); this process initiates the terminal pathway of complement activation, and the formation of the lytic C5b–C9 complex. FH keeps the spontaneous activation of C3 under control, and it also inhibits the complement system at both the activation and amplification stages. FH binds to deposited C3b and C3bBb complexes on human cell surfaces and inhibits further activation by three mechanisms: it competes with factor B (FB) for C3b binding and C3bBb generation; it increases the decay of C3bBb complexes, and it acts as a cofactor for factor I (FI), which in turn cleaves C3b into inactive C3b (iC3b).

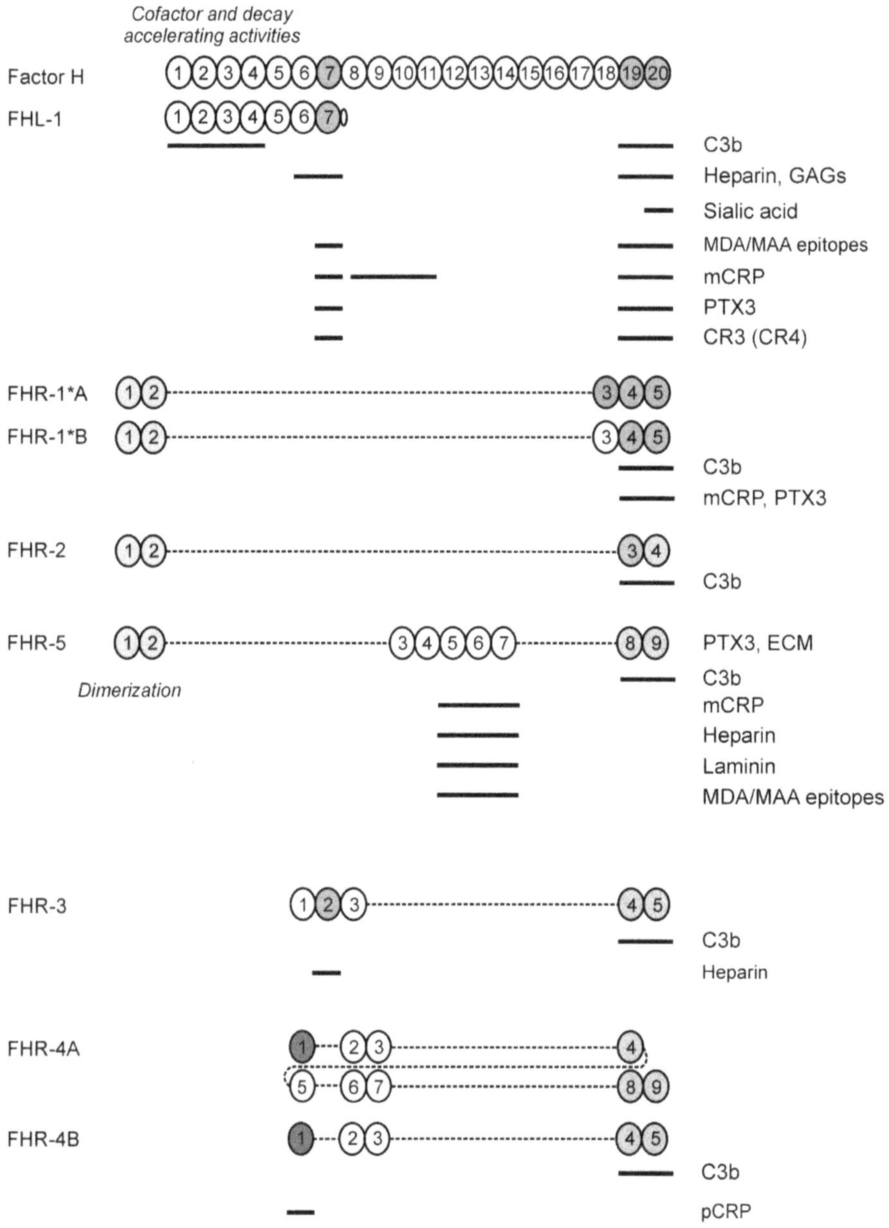

FIGURE 2 | Factor H (FH) family proteins and their ligands. The schematic complement control protein (CCP) domain structure of FH, FHL-1, and the FHR proteins is shown, with CCPs aligned vertically to the homologous domains in FH. The N-terminal CCPs 1–4 of FH and FHL-1 mediate the complement regulatory functions of these proteins (shown in yellow). CCPs 7 and 19–20 (shown in blue) harbor the main ligand- and host surface-recognition sites; selected ligand binding sites are indicated by horizontal lines. The CCPs 1–2 of factor H related protein 1 (FHR)-1, FHR-2, and FHR-5 are closely related to each other and mediate dimerization of these FHRs. The CCPs in FHRs with high sequence identity to the homologous FH domains are indicated by identical/similar colors.

Next to FH and FHL-1, humans (and several non-human species; not discussed here) possess FH-related (FHR) proteins, homologous to FH. They are encoded separately, with their genes (*CFHR1* to *CFHR5*) lying in tandem next to *CFH* at 1q31.3. The *CFHR* genes originate from *CFH* through gene duplication events (18). The *CFH–CFHRs* loci contain several segmental duplications, making them prone to genetic structural rearrangements due to nonallelic homologous recombination (NAHR) events. This has led to copy number polymorphisms (CNPs), with the very common 86.3-kb deletion (CNP147) that results in loss of *CFHR3–CFHR1* (Δ*CFHR3–CFHR1*), and the very rare 122-kb deletion (CNP148) resulting in loss of *CFHR1–CFHR4* (Δ*CFHR1–CFHR4*) (19). Like FH, the FHRs are entirely composed of CCP domains (**Figure 2**), which display high sequence similarity with CCP domains of FH known to be involved in ligand and surface binding. Remarkably, none of the human FHR proteins possess CCP domains homologous to FH CCPs 1–4. Thus, based on their primary structure, FHR proteins are not expected to have any direct complement inhibiting activity similar to FH. Nonetheless, several reports have observed direct complement inhibitory activity for some of the FHRs, albeit often weak compared to FH (20–24). However, other studies have not found such activity for FHRs, questioning whether this is truly the physiological role of the FHR proteins (25–30). Instead, the FHRs are currently hypothesized to have an antagonistic function over FH, competing with binding to FH ligands and cell surfaces. By lacking direct complement inhibiting activity, binding of FHRs instead of FH would allow complement activation to proceed (31). This process has also been termed complement de-regulation. Indeed, binding to various (FH) ligands has been reported for all FHRs, which will be discussed below. In addition, some FHRs were reported to promote alternative pathway activation by binding C3b and serving as a platform for the assembly of the C3 convertase (27, 32, 33). Recent characterization of some of the mouse FHRs supports a role of these proteins as positive regulators in the modulation of complement activation (34, 35).

In this review, we outline and provide an update on the recent developments regarding the FH protein family. New insights regarding circulating levels of FHRs, ligand binding, and disease associations allow re-assessing the role of FHRs in the complement system. Together, these results shed light on the balance of the FH–FHRs axis, and the role of FHRs in non-pathological and pathological conditions.

QUANTITATION OF FHR PROTEINS

Factor H, FHL-1, and the FHR proteins are mainly synthesized by hepatocytes, but synthesis by other cells and tissues has also been reported, particularly for FH and FHL-1 (36–38). FH production has been detected in endothelial cells, platelets, mesangial cells, keratinocytes, fibroblasts, retinal pigment epithelial cells, monocytes, and dendritic cells, among others (39–46). On the other hand, little information on the extrahepatic expression of the FHR proteins is available. Both *CFHR3* mRNA and FHR-3 protein have been identified in retinal macrophages, while no FHR-3 expression was found in other retinal cell types (47). Extrahepatic synthesis of FH/FHRs most likely contributes to an efficient control of complement activation locally, but a relevant contribution to the plasma levels of these proteins is unlikely, considering the relative low expression compared to the hepatic source.

Accurate quantification of the FHR proteins has been a great challenge since their discovery. Due to the high sequence similarity among FH and FHR proteins, it has proven to be very difficult to obtain specific reagents for each of the FHR proteins. For some time, only concentration estimates were available for most of the FHR proteins (21, 48). However, with recently renewed and successful efforts in generating highly specific antibodies, specific immunoassays for each of the FHR proteins are now becoming available, although some discrepancy about their actual physiological levels still remains (**Table 1**).

TABLE 1 | Reported serum levels of the factor H-related (FHR) proteins.

Protein measured	Gene copies	Levels (μg/mL)		N	Reference
Factor H (FH)	–	400	SD = 62	1,004	(8)
	–	319.9	SD = 71.4	358	(9)
	–	233.24	SD = 56.65	63	(10)
	–	232.7	SD = 74.5	1,514	(11)
FHL-1	–	47	SD = 11.3[a]	2	(12)
Total factor H-related protein 1 (FHR-1)	1*CFHR1*	61	SD = 31	24	(54)
	2*CFHR1*	122	SD = 26	44	(54)
	Not defined	94	IQR = 70.5–119.6	158	(55)
	Not defined	1.63	SD = 0.04	344	(66)
FHR-1 homodimers	1*CFHR1*	4.88	SD = 1.33	36	(53)
	2*CFHR1*	14.64	SD = 3.04	77	(53)
FHR-1/2 heterodimers	1*CFHR1*	5.01	SD = 1.49	36	(53)
	2*CFHR1*	5.84	SD = 2.41	77	(53)
FHR-2 homodimers	0*CFHR1*	3.1		Pool of four donors	(53)
	1*CFHR1*	0.85	SD = 0.41	36	(53)
	2*CFHR1*	0.65	SD = 0.41	77	(53)
Total FHR-2	Not defined	3.64	SD = 1.2	344	(66)
FHR-3	1*CFHR3*	0.38	SD = 0.23	26	(58)
	2*CFHR3*	0.83	SD = 0.48	69	(58)
	2*CFHR3*A*	0.55	SD = 0.15	16	(60)
	2*CFHR3*B*	0.82	SD = 0.08	4	(60)
	Not defined	1.06	SD = 0.53	21	(47)
	Not defined	0.020	SD = 0.001	344	(66)
FHR-4A	–	25.4	Range = 6.5–53.9	11	(27)
	–	2.42	SD = 0.18	344	(66)
	–	2.55	SD = 1.46	129	(63)
FHR-4B	–	Not detected		–	(63)
FHR-5 homodimers	–	5.5	Range = 3.4–10.1	13	(65)
	–	5.49	SD = 1.55	344	(66)
	–	2.46	IQR = 1.79–3.67	158	(55)
	–	1.66	SD = 0.43	115	(53)

[a]*FHL-1 levels were determined indirectly, by subtracting the values of FH measurements from those of FH + FHL-1 measurements. N: number of samples; SD: standard deviation; IQR: interquartile range.*

Factor H-Related Protein 1 (FHR-1)

Factor H-related protein 1 is composed of five CCP domains, and circulates in two forms (37 and 42 kDa), with either one or two *N*-linked carbohydrate moieties (30, 49, 50). Two genetic variants of FHR-1 have been described, FHR-1*A and FHR-1*B, the difference being three amino acids in CCP3 (51). FHR-1*B CCP3 is identical to FH CCP18, whereas FHR-1*A CCP3 shares 95% sequence identity with FH CCP18. FHR-1 CCPs 4 and 5 share high sequence identity (100 and 97%) with FH CCPs 19 and 20, respectively. FHR-1 has a dimerization motif located in CCPs 1–2 that are highly similar (>85% sequence identity) to CCPs 1–2 of FHR-2 and FHR-5, and allow the formation of FHR-1 homodimers and heterodimers with FHR-2 (26, 52, 53). While identified *in vitro*, the existence of FHR-1/FHR-5 heterodimers *in vivo* is still controversial (26, 52, 53). Similarly, FHR-1 quantification also remains controversial. In 2017, several groups determined FHR-1 levels. Tortajada et al. reported an average of 122 μg/mL in 44 healthy controls with two copies of *CFHR1*, and an overall average of 90.4 μg/mL in 76 controls (including eight homozygous Δ*CFHR3–CFHR1* carriers and 24 heterozygous Δ*CFHR3–CFHR1* carriers) (54). Using the same immunoassay, Medjeral-Thomas et al. reported 94.4 μg/mL FHR-1 in 158 controls (of whom 133 were genotyped: 3 Δ*CFHR3–CFHR1* homozygous, 45 Δ*CFHR3–CFHR1* heterozygous, and 85 without Δ*CFHR3–CFHR1*) (55). Of note, the immunoassay described by Tortajada et al. does not distinguish between FHR-1 homodimers or heterodimers. In contrast, using immunoassays specific for FHR-1 homodimers and FHR-1/-2 heterodimers, van Beek et al. reported ~10-fold lower levels (averages of 11.33 and 5.48 μg/mL, respectively), in 115 healthy donors (2 homozygous Δ*CFHR3–CFHR1*, 36 heterozygous Δ*CFHR3–CFHR1* carriers, and 77 without Δ*CFHR3–CFHR1*) (53).

Factor H-Related Protein 2

Factor H-related protein 2 is the smallest FHR protein, composed of four CCP domains (56). FHR-2 circulates either non-glycosylated (24 kDa) or with one *N*-linked carbohydrate moiety in CCP2 (29 kDa). FHR-2 CCP1 and CCP2 are nearly identical to FHR-1 CCP1 and CCP2 (100 and 98%), respectively, including all residues comprising the dimerization motif (26). Similar to the proposed FHR-1/FHR-5 dimers, FHR-2/FHR-5 dimers remain to be identified *in vivo*, while FHR-2 homodimers and FHR-1/FHR-2 heterodimers have been confirmed (52, 53). FHR-2 homodimer levels have been shown to be around 3 μg/mL; with these relatively low levels, FHR-2 seems to be the limiting factor in the formation of FHR-1/FHR-2 heterodimers and, indeed, most FHR-2 is found dimerized with FHR-1 (53).

Factor H-Related Protein 3

Factor H-related protein 3 is composed of five CCP domains, of which CCP1 and CCP2 have high sequence similarity with FH CCP6 and CCP7 (94 and 86%), respectively (57). The C-terminal CCPs 3–5 are virtually identical to the C-terminal domains of FHR-4A and FHR-4B (93–100%). FHR-3 contains four *N*-linked glycosylation sites, and it circulates in plasma as multiple glycosylation variants ranging from 37 to 50 kDa. A quantitative FHR-3-specific immunoassay was first described by Pouw et al., reporting levels of 0.38 and 0.83 μg/mL for healthy individuals carrying either one or two *CFHR3* copies, respectively (58). These results were later confirmed in a similar assay, reporting mean levels of 1.06 μg/mL (47). Two major genetic variants of *CFHR3* (*CFHR3*A* and *CFHR3*B*) have been described (59); interestingly, these are quantitative variants, with *CFHR3*B* determining higher FHR-3 levels than *CFHR3*A* (60). The FHR-3*A and FHR-3*B allotypes differ at aminoacid 241 in CCP3 (Pro/Ser), but its functional relevance has not been determined.

Factor H-Related Protein 4

CFHR4 is the only known *CFHR* gene that expresses two splice variants, FHR-4A and FHR-4B (61, 62). FHR-4A is composed of nine CCP domains (86 kDa), while FHR-4B has five CCP domains (43 kDa). All FHR-4B domains are also present in FHR-4A, with FHR-4B CCP1 being identical to FHR-4A CCP1, and FHR-4B CCPs 2–5 being identical to FHR-4A CCPs 6–9. FHR-4A CCPs 2–4 seems to have arisen from internal gene duplication, and have high sequence similarity (85–93% amino acid identity) with the other CCPs in FHR-4A/B (61). Thus, obtaining specific reagents to distinguish FHR-4A from FHR-4B is challenging on first sight. Quantification by using an immunoassay that in principle measures both FHR-4A and FHR-4B resulted in average levels of 25.4 μg/mL (27). However, FHR-4A-specific antibodies have been described recently and used in an FHR-4A-specific ELISA which shows 10-fold lower levels for FHR-4A (2.55 ± 1.46 μg/mL) (63). In line with the complete sequence identity of FHR-4B with several FHR-4A domains, no specific antibodies for FHR-4B could be obtained. Strikingly, FHR-4B was not detected in plasma using various antibodies that did react with recombinant FHR-4B (63). This indicates that free FHR-4B must be in an extremely low concentration or even absent from plasma.

Factor H-Related Protein 5

Factor H-related protein 5 is composed of nine CCPs and is the only FHR with domains (CCPs 3–7) homologous to FH CCPs 10–14 (64). FHR-5 CCPs 1–2 are highly similar (85–93% amino acid identity) to CCPs 1–2 of FHR-1 and FHR-2, although not all residues identified in the FHR-1/2 dimerization motif are present in FHR-5 (26). This could explain why the presence of FHR-5 heterodimers *in vivo* is still controversial (26, 52, 53). FHR-5 seems to circulate predominantly as homodimer *in vivo* (53), making quantification a bit more straightforward. FHR-5 serum levels were reported to be 3–6 μg/mL (24), which was later confirmed in 13 healthy individuals, with median levels of 5.5 μg/mL (65). Similar FHR-5 levels (median 2.46 μg/mL) were found in a larger group of 158 healthy controls using the same immunoassay (55). More recently, an average concentration of 1.66 μg/mL was shown in 115 controls by using a newly developed FHR-5 ELISA (53).

Other Quantifications

In addition to the specific immunoassays described above, mass spectrometry has also been used to quantify the FHR proteins (66). While this approach allows specific measurement of FHRs based on unique peptide sequences, quantification of FHR dimers is not possible. Results similar to the immunoassays were obtained for FHR-2 (3.64 ± 1.2 μg/mL), FHR-4A (2.42 ± 0.18 μg/mL), and FHR-5 (5.49 ± 1.55 μg/mL). However, much lower levels were found for FHR-1 (1.63 ± 0.04 μg/mL) and FHR-3 (0.020 ± 0.001 μg/mL). It is unclear why such lower concentrations were found for FHR-1 and FHR-3, although the frequency of Δ*CFHR3–CFHR1* in the studied population ($n = 344$, Icelandic origin) was not determined. Of note, the peptide used for FHR-4 quantification is only present in FHR-4A, thus providing no extra information whether FHR-4B exists *in vivo*.

Kopczynska et al. measured FHR-1, FHR-2, and FHR-5 altogether in one immunoassay, finding a total FHR-1/2/5 concentration of 10.67 μg/mL (±5.42) in 42 healthy individuals (67). This result is in great contrast to previously reported levels of approximately 100 μg/mL for FHR-1 (54, 55), but is comparable to a combined mean FHR-1/2/5 concentration of 19.27 (53) and 10.76 μg/mL (66).

The reasons for the huge differences in FHR levels outlined above are unclear. Moreover, the existence of homo- and heterodimers, and the fact that the frequency of the Δ*CFHR3–CFHR1* polymorphism is highly population-dependent (19, 68, 69), further complicate the accuracy and assessment of measurements. To exclude any possible cross-reactivity that interferes with FH or FHR quantifications, it is crucial to extensively characterize antibodies generated against FH or any of the FHRs. FH immunoassays should ideally use at least one antibody targeting an epitope located in domains absent from the FHRs, such as CCPs 15–17. Furthermore, when quantifying FHR proteins, it is highly recommended to stratify protein levels based on *CFHR* CNPs, as well as distinguishing between hetero- and homodimers. This would aid in comparison of control and patient groups, as CNP frequencies and dimer formation might be altered in patients. CNPs should be determined at the genetic level, as stratification based only on protein levels seems not to be possible due to the wide range in protein concentration within each CNP group (53, 58). CNPs are most commonly determined using multiplex ligation-dependent probe amplification (MLPA), although there is currently no commercial kit available that also covers *CFHR4*. In addition, while normal levels of FHR proteins are now being reported, further data are necessary to reach consensus on their actual concentrations in circulation.

LIGANDS OF FH AND THE FHR PROTEINS AND THEIR RELEVANCE

As outlined above, FH is a major inhibitor of the alternative pathway in plasma and when bound to cells and surfaces like the glomerular basement membrane. This complement regulatory activity is due to the interaction of FH with C3b (70). In addition, FH binds to several other ligands (**Figure 2**) and, when ligand-bound, in many cases maintains its complement inhibitory activity. These FH interactions ensure proper regulation of complement activation, as well as the resulting opsonization and inflammation.

Complement activation can be initiated on modified, dangerous self surfaces, which are recognized by PRMs within (C1q, ficolins, MBL, and properdin) and outside the complement system (e.g., pentraxins). FH along with other regulators may ensure targeted but restricted complement activation and an optimal degree of opsonization, while preventing overt inflammation and damage resulting from cascade over-activation (71, 72). The FHR proteins appear to counter-balance this activity of FH and enhance complement activation by binding to the same or similar ligands and outcompeting FH (**Figure 3**), and in some instances also by interacting with C3b and other ligands independent of FH (31). This section briefly summarizes the main ligand interactions of FH and the FHR proteins (**Figure 2**), and indicates their relevance in the regulation and modulation of complement activation.

We would like to briefly note that tumor cells and microbes can bind FH in an attempt to avoid their destruction by host complement. In addition, the main microbial ligand binding sites of FH are in CCPs 6–7 and 19–20, and homologous domains are conserved in the FHRs, thus these proteins may modulate opsonization/killing of microbes. These aspects have been reviewed in detail (6, 31, 73–75).

C3b

The main ligand of FH is the active C3 fragment C3b, which can be generated by fluid phase and surface-bound C3 convertases. Since C3b is the central component that promotes complement amplification *via* the alternative pathway, and is also required for the assembly of C5 convertases and the initiation of the terminal pathway, its regulation is key to maintain the proper balance of complement activation and inhibition. FH interacts with C3b at two main sites, harbored by CCPs 1–4 and 19–20 (76). The N-terminal C3b binding site is active when FH is in the fluid phase (e.g., in blood plasma) and also when FH is bound to cells or other surfaces [*via* glycosaminoglycans (GAGs), sialic acid, or a specific receptor—see below] (**Figure 3A**). FH may also bind C3b by CCPs 1–4 when already bound to other ligands, such as pentraxins, because these interactions typically involve CCPs 6–7 and 19–20 (74, 77–79). Thus, FH maintains its complement regulatory activity when bound to cells or other ligands.

Structural studies revealed that FH engages surface-deposited C3b in the context of host GAGs/sialic acid, i.e., CCPs 19–20 bind to these ligands at the same time, which allows avid interaction of FH with a host surface under complement attack. The FH C-terminal site also binds C3d, the final C3b degradation product that remains covalently attached to the surface (80, 81).

The FHR proteins also bind to C3b, but the nature of these interactions is inherently different from that of FH because FHRs lack domains homologous to FH CCPs 1–4. Thus, FHRs lack FH-like cofactor activity and decay accelerating activity, although some residual activity may be present due to the interaction of the C-terminal domains of these proteins with C3b. This should be investigated in detail in the future to clarify the currently contradicting reports in this regard (20, 23, 24, 26, 27, 32, 33).

In contrast to possible inhibitory activities, FHR-1, FHR-4, and FHR-5 were reported to activate the alternative pathway, by

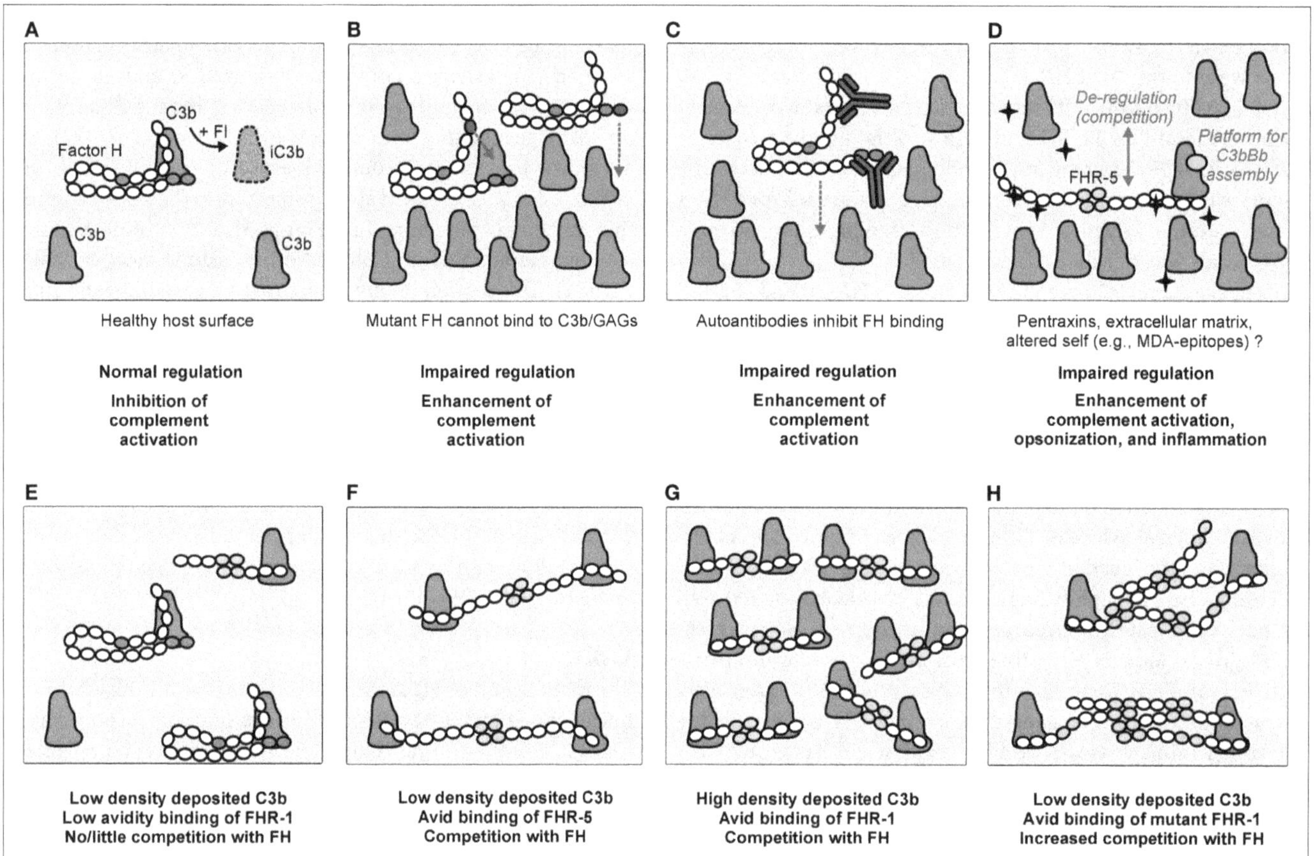

FIGURE 3 | The role of factor H (FH) and the FHRs under physiological and pathological conditions. **(A)** Normal complement control on a healthy host surface by FH bound to surface-deposited C3b. FH recognizes self surfaces under complement attack by binding to a complex of GAGs/sialic acid and C3b. This recognition is mediated by complement control proteins (CCPs) domain 19–20 indicated in blue. Through the activity of the N-terminal regulatory domains (CCPs 1–4, in yellow), FH assists factor I (FI) in the proteolytic cleavage of C3b into inactive C3b (iC3b). **(B)** Mutations in the regulatory or recognition domains, and **(C)** autoantibodies bound to these domains can cause functional FH defect and result in impaired surface complement control. **(D)** FHRs can also interact with similar surfaces and ligands as FH, and compete with FH for binding (de-regulation), and/or they can directly activate the alternative pathway by binding C3b and serving as a platform for the assembly of an active C3bBb convertase. The black star-shape indicates newly exposed ligand/altered self. **(E–H)** The relative FH/FHR concentrations, the ligand density (avidity), and the dimeric/oligomeric states of the FHRs influence surface complement regulation. **(E)** At low ligand (e.g., deposited C3b) density and relative FH surplus, FH can potently regulate complement activation on the surface. **(F)** Increased FHR levels and/or **(G)** ligand densities, and **(H)** formation of higher order oligomers (e.g., due to duplicated dimerization domains) can cause enhanced competition with FH and tip the balance to increased complement activation.

binding C3b through their C-terminal domains and forming a platform for the assembly of an active C3bBb convertase (27, 32, 33). This activity could take place on surfaces where these FHRs are bound directly, or *via* another ligand, such as pentraxins (33). FHR-1 and FHR-5 were shown to enhance complement activation on the extracellular matrix (ECM) and on the surface of apoptotic or necrotic cells (32, 33, 82).

Additionally, FHRs may compete with FH for binding to C3b deposited on surfaces, a process termed complement deregulation, because FHRs can enhance complement activation by inhibiting FH binding (**Figure 3D**). This activity of the FHRs may only be significant—considering their relative serum concentrations and avidity for C3b—if increased amounts of FHRs or altered FHR forms (such as higher order oligomers) are present (**Figures 3E–H**) (25, 26, 52, 83, 84). For FHR-2, it was described that, despite binding to C3b, it cannot effectively compete with FH for binding to surface-bound C3b (20).

Altogether, based on these data the FHRs can be regarded as positive complement regulators.

Other C3 Fragments

While interacting sites for other C3 fragments were described, current evidence strongly supports the physiologically relevant binding of FH to C3b *via* CCPs 1–4 and 19–20, as well as to C3d *via* CCPs 19–20 (76). Interaction of FHR-1 and FHR-2 with C3d was also shown, but without functional analyses (20, 84). Binding of FHR-3, but not of FHR-1, to C3d was shown to prevent the binding of C3d to its receptor on B cells, thus modulating B cell activation (85). FHR-5 was reported to bind to iC3b and C3d with affinities similar to C3b; in contrast, FH bound very weakly to iC3b and C3d compared with FHR-5, indicating that despite its lower serum concentration FHR-5 can be an efficient competitor of FH for binding to deposited C3 fragments (26).

Glycosaminoglycans (GAGs), Sialic Acid, and Heparin

Distinction between self, non-self, or altered self surfaces relies in part on the recognition of host-specific GAGs and sialic acid by FH (and FHL-1). This allows complement activation to proceed unhindered on microbial ("activator") surfaces, but prevents activation on host ("non-activator") surfaces (86). This has been a subject of intensive research, often using heparin as a model for polyanionic molecules. The main heparin-binding sites were identified in FH (and FHL-1) CCP7 and FH CCP20 (87, 88). This allows recognition of, and attachment to, host glycomatrix and cells, such as platelets and endothelial cells (89, 90). Recent studies revealed some functional differences indicating that while some GAGs are recognized by FH and FHL-1 *via* CCP7, the sialic acid binding site is in CCP20 (91), also targeting these host regulators to different surfaces and explaining the different consequences of mutations affecting these domains (89, 92, 93).

Factor H-related protein 1 can also bind to host surfaces *via* its FH-homologous C-terminus (22, 29), and FHR-3 binds heparin through CCP2, which is homologous to CCP7 of FH (23, 87). In addition, FHR-5 has a heparin-binding site in CCPs 5–7 (24, 94). The functional relevance of these interactions needs to be investigated further, but they could anchor these proteins on certain cells and surfaces.

ECM as a Non-Cellular Surface

Extracellular matrices occur in many tissues and can have different functions, the most important ones being the physical support of cells and acting as barriers and filters. The composition of ECMs differs at distinct anatomic sites and is dynamically regulated. Under certain conditions, e.g., endothelial cell activation or injury, ECMs can be exposed to body fluids and plasma proteins; in addition, the Bruch's membrane in the eye and the kidney glomerular basement membrane are also exposed because the lining cell layer is fenestrated. To prevent overt complement activation, such ECMs rely largely on soluble complement regulators, such as FH and FHL-1, which can bind *via* their GAG binding sites and locally regulate complement (95). As noted above, differences in ECMs and in domain composition of the FH family proteins may target FH and FHRs toward distinct sites, such as FH to the glomerular basement membrane (*via* CCPs 19–20) and FHL-1 to the Bruch's membrane (*via* CCP7) (95). FHR-5 was shown to bind to MaxGel, an ECM extract, and de-regulate complement on this surface (32); a recent study identified laminin as an ECM ligand of FHR-5 (94).

Ligands on Dead Cells

Complement is largely involved in the immunologically safe and silent disposal of apoptotic and necrotic cells *via* opsonophagocytosis (96). The soluble regulators FH and C4b-binding protein bind to dead cells and prevent excessive complement activation and potential deleterious effects when membrane-anchored regulators are down-regulated on the cells (97). FH can bind to Annexin-II, DNA, and histones (98), as well as malondialdehyde epitopes on apoptotic cells (94, 99). In addition, the pentraxins CRP and pentraxin 3 (PTX3) also bind to dead cells and recruit FH (77, 100). For FHR-1 and FHR-5, binding to necrotic cells and enhancement of complement activation have been shown (33, 82), suggesting that these FHRs modulate opsonization of dead cells.

Pentraxins

The pentraxins are soluble PRMs of the innate immune system and, based on their structure, categorized as short and long pentraxins. Pentraxins have numerous ligands and functions, reviewed in detail elsewhere (101); of note, they participate in the opsonization of microbes and dead cells, and they also bind to components of the ECM. For the prototypic short pentraxin CRP and the long pentraxin PTX3, interactions with both complement activators (C1q, MBL) and inhibitors (FH, C4b-binding protein) were described (74, 77, 79, 101–107).

C-reactive protein circulates in its native, pentameric form (pCRP) in body fluids, but it can adopt an altered conformation exposing neoepitopes upon pH change or binding to membranes, and it can even decay to its monomeric form (mCRP) *in vitro* by chelation of the Ca^{2+} ions or adsorption on plastic. FH was described to bind primarily to mCRP *via* CCPs 7, 8–11, and 19–20 (79, 108, 109), but interaction with pCRP *via* CCPs 7 and 19–20 at acute phase concentrations was also reported (110). The binding to mCRP allows targeting of the complement inhibitor FH to certain surfaces, including apoptotic cells (71, 100, 109). Among the FHRs, FHR-1 binds to mCRP *via* CCPs 4–5 (33) and FHR-5 *via* CCPs 5–7 (24, 32). The FHR-1/mCRP interaction enhanced classical and alternative pathway activation, and FHR-5 efficiently competed with FH for mCRP binding, resulting in enhanced complement activation on mCRP (32, 33). In contrast, FHR-4 binds to pCRP *via* CCP1, and this interaction results in enhanced classical pathway activation (111, 112).

PTX3 forms a complex, octameric structure stabilized in part by covalent bonds (113). PTX3 binds to FH *via* CCPs 7 and 19–20, and recruits it to apoptotic cells to downregulate complement activation (77). PTX3 also binds to FHR-1 (weaker than FH) and FHR-5 (stronger than FH); FHR-5 competes with FH and enhance complement activation on PTX3 (32, 33, 74).

Malondialdehyde Epitopes

Malondialdehyde (MDA) and malondialdehyde-acetaldehyde (MAA) adducts of proteins and lipids may be generated upon oxidation as oxidation-related neoepitopes, and induce inflammatory responses. FH was shown to bind to MDA/MAA epitopes and inhibit complement activation and the proinflammatory effects of such MDA/MAA epitopes (99). Two binding sites, within CCP7 and CCPs 19–20 of FH, were identified to bind to MDA/MAA epitopes (99, 114). Recently, FHR-5 was also shown to bind to MAA epitopes (MAA-BSA) *via* CCPs 5–7 and to compete with FH for MAA-BSA binding, thus increasing complement activation. In addition, binding of FHR-5 to necrotic cells was mediated by the same domains, possibly in part *via* the MDA/MAA epitopes that appear on dead cells (94).

Other, Less Characterized Ligand Interactions of FH

Factor H binds to other ligands that are implicated in certain diseases, particularly in the thrombotic microangiopathy atypical hemolytic uremic syndrome (aHUS). One of these ligands is thrombomodulin, a transmembrane glycoprotein present in endothelial cells, which is involved in the regulation of coagulation and inflammation; thrombomodulin soluble fragments can also be released upon endothelial cell activation or injury. Thrombomodulin was shown to bind to FH and the FH–C3b complex with nanomolar affinity and to enhance FH cofactor activity, which would be reduced in the case of thrombomodulin mutations in aHUS (115–117). These data suggest a role for thrombomodulin in inhibiting alternative pathway activation locally *via* its interaction with FH, but thrombomodulin was also found to inhibit complement hemolytic activity in a FH-independent mechanism (116). An additional, complement-activating function of thrombomodulin by enhancing C3 cleavage into C3b has also been described (117).

Similarly, binding of von Willebrand factor (vWF) to FH enhances FH cofactor activity and also modulates the vWF prothrombotic status (118–120). FH was found co-localized with vWF in the Weibel–Palade bodies in human umbilical vein endothelial cells, and the complex was also detected in human plasma. Purified FH and vWF were shown to interact with nanomolar affinity, and to influence their respective functions; vWF enhanced the cofactor activity of FH, whereas FH inhibited ADAMTS13-mediated cleavage of vWF and facilitated platelet aggregation (120). However, another investigation found that FH binds *via* its C-terminus to the vWF A2 domain, and enhances its cleavage by ADAMTS13 (118). FH was also reported to reduce large soluble vWF multimers (119). Thus, further studies are needed to clarify the functional relevance of the complex interaction between FH and vWF, and its potential role in disease.

Recently, hemolysis-derived heme was shown to activate the alternative pathway in serum and on endothelial cells, and to bind both C3 and FH. Heme-exposed C3 and endothelial cells displayed increased FH binding, and FH was shown to be a major serum factor that regulates C3 deposition on heme-treated endothelial cells (121).

Factor H was also reported to bind to apolipoprotein E *via* domains CCPs 5–7, and to regulate alternative pathway activation on high density lipoprotein particles (122). Complement regulation by FH on such lipoprotein particles could be potentially impaired in diseases characterized by immune deposits containing also apolipoprotein E, such as age-related macular degeneration (AMD) and dense deposit disease (DDD) (122).

In addition, FH binds to myeloperoxidase (MPO) released from activated neutrophil granulocytes, and FH and MPO colocalize in neutrophil extracellular traps. Interestingly, the binding site for MPO in FH was determined to be CCPs 1–4 and, thus, MPO inhibited FH binding to C3b, as well as FH decay accelerating activity and cofactor activity (123).

Binding to Cellular Receptors—Non-Canonical Roles of the FH Family Proteins

Factor H and some of the FHRs can also bind to cells *via* specific receptors, and may modulate the cell activation and response, as well as inflammatory processes. These aspects are reviewed in detail elsewhere (124); here, we summarize only some major FH/FHR-receptor interactions and their role, particularly those described very recently.

Complement receptor type 3 (CR3; CD11b/CD18; or integrin $\alpha_M\beta_2$) was identified as a main FH receptor on neutrophils and macrophages (125, 126). FH maintains its cofactor activity when receptor bound, but it also directly affects cellular functions, such as adhesion, cell spreading, migration, and cytokine production (125–127). Interestingly, FH was able to inhibit the release of extracellular traps by human neutrophils activated with immobilized fibronectin plus fungal β-glucan, or with phorbol 12-myristate 13-acetate (127). FH can also enhance the interaction of certain pathogens with human macrophages and neutrophils, and modulate the response of the phagocytes (128, 129). This was also shown for FHR-1 which, by binding to CR3, could enhance neutrophil responses to *Candida albicans* (129). In addition, FHL-1 was shown to mediate cell adhesion and spreading (129, 130).

Described functional effects of FH on monocytes include enhancement of IL-1β secretion, respiratory burst, and chemotactic effect (131–134). FH was shown to induce an anti-inflammatory and tolerogenic phenotype in monocyte-derived dendritic cells *in vitro* (135). Very recently, in the context of inflammation in AMD, FH, and its two variants Y402 and H402 were investigated in a mouse model. FH was shown to inhibit the resolution of inflammation by binding to CR3 and thus blocking thrombospondin-1–CD47 signaling that would normally promote the elimination of macrophages. The AMD-associated H402 FH variant displayed a stronger inhibitory effect compared to FH Y402, causing increased accumulation of macrophages in the inflamed tissue (136).

Factor H was shown to bind to B cells and may modulate some B cell functions, such as proliferation and immunoglobulin secretion, but no specific receptor has been identified to date (137–140). A recent report described an indirect modulation of B cell activation by FHR-3, which was shown to bind to C3d and inhibit its binding to complement receptor type 2, a co-receptor of the B cell receptor complex; FH and FHR-1 had no such effect (85).

These non-canonical functions of the FH family proteins deserve further investigation, because they may play roles in inflammation and anti-microbial defense that are currently underappreciated. Clarification of their cell-mediated effects may provide additional insights into disease mechanisms.

DISEASE ASSOCIATIONS

Studies in patients and controls have shown a variety of common *CFH/CFHRs* genetic variants that predispose to autologous damage, which is predominantly organ-specific. Prevalent kidney damage occurs in the rare diseases aHUS and C3 glomerulopathies (C3G), and in the more frequent IgA nephropathy (IgAN), while destruction of the retinal pigment epithelium by autologous complement contributes to AMD. A defective regulation of complement activation on the renal microvasculature endothelium occurs in aHUS, while in C3G uncontrolled complement activation in plasma gives rise to massive deposition of C3b breakdown products (iC3b, C3dg, and C3c) in the glomeruli (141–143). IgAN is characterized by mesangial cell proliferation and hypoglycosylated IgA1 deposits in the glomeruli, and it is likely that complement defects contribute, at least in part, to its clinical heterogeneity (144, 145). A defective control of complement activation in the retina is most relevant in AMD pathogenesis, and enhances the inflammatory response (146).

Extremely rare and pathogenic *CFH/CFHRs* variants have been mainly found in aHUS and C3G patients. Some of these variants result from gene conversion events between *CFH* and *CFHR1*, and they give rise to mutated FH or FHR-1. Other variants are intragenic duplications or hybrid genes resulting from gene rearrangements, and generate abnormal proteins; some of these proteins have distinct molecular weights and can be detected by Western blot analysis. It is interesting that abnormal rearrangements involving FH/FHRs associate with aHUS, while in C3G patients only FHR proteins are affected.

CFH Variants Associated With Renal or Ocular Damage

Common SNPs in *CFH* give rise to different haplotypes that can be disease neutral, predisposing, or protecting. Thus, haplotype *CFH(H1)* predisposes to membranoproliferative glomerulonephritis (MPGN) and AMD, haplotype *CFH(H3)* predisposes to aHUS, and haplotype *CFH(H2)* is protective against these three diseases (147–149). Haplotype *CFH(H2)* generates the FH_{62Ile} variant, which shows increased binding to C3b and cofactor activity in the fluid phase and on cellular surfaces (150), thus favoring protection against autologous complement damage.

The common variant FH_{402His}, which is present in FH and its shorter isoform FHL-1, is a major predisposing factor in AMD (151). The functional relevance of FH_{402His} in C3b, CRP, or heparin binding has been analyzed in several studies. Reduced binding of FH_{402His} to polyanionic surfaces has been found (152), but the pathogenic mechanism may also depend on FHL-1, which can regulate complement activation similarly to FH. It has been shown that FHL-1, but not FH, is present in the retinal Bruch's membrane, a major target in AMD pathogenesis, and that binding of the AMD-FHL-1_{402His} variant was lower than binding of the FHL-1_{402Tyr} variant (93). Nonetheless, *CFH* intronic variants show stronger association with AMD than FH_{402His} (153). In an analysis of seven common *CFH* haplotypes, haplotypes H1, H6, and H7 were found to confer increased risk to AMD; these haplotypes share a 32-kb region downstream of rs1061170 (FH Tyr402His) that must be critical for AMD development (19), and that includes a 12-kb block 89% similar to a noncoding region in CNP148 (see below).

Other disease-predisposing FH variants are very rare. One of the most relevant is Arg1210Cys (FH_{1210C}), which was initially identified in aHUS patients (154), and shown to be covalently bound to albumin in plasma (155); the presence of albumin most likely prevents the interaction of FH_{1210C} with its physiological ligands, generating a partial, pathogenic FH deficiency. FH_{1210C} has been also associated with C3G (156), and it highly increases AMD-risk and predisposes to early disease onset (157, 158). It has been suggested that in individuals with the FH_{1210C} variant it is the concurrence of other genetic predisposing factors what ultimately determines the clinical phenotype (159).

CFHR1 and *CFHR3* Variants Associated With Renal or Ocular Damage

As happens with the common *CFH* haplotypes, the two main *CFHR1* alleles show differential disease associations. *CFHR1*B*, displaying increased similarity with *CFH*, increases aHUS risk (51), and *CFHR1*A* predisposes to AMD (160). The molecular bases for these associations have not been determined, but they will most likely depend on subtle functional differences among the FHR-1*A and FHR-1*B allotypes. *CFHR1*A* is in strong linkage disequilibrium with the AMD-risk *CFH402His* allele, and *CFHR1* genotyping has similar predictive value of developing AMD as *CFH402His;ΔCFHR3–CFHR1* genotyping (160); these findings are suggestive of a direct role of FHR-1 in AMD pathogenesis, most likely by interfering with the interaction of FH with specific ligands and promoting complement activation (33).

The *CFHR3* gene also has two major variants, *CFHR3*A*, more frequent in healthy controls, and *CFHR3*B*, which predisposes to aHUS but not to C3G (59). Because the aHUS risk *CFHR3*B* allele generates higher FHR-3 levels than the non-risk *CFHR3*A* allele (60), it seems that increased competition of FHR-3 and FH for certain ligands could favor aHUS development. FHR-3 is also produced in the retina, and its contribution to retinal degeneration by inhibiting FH binding to C3b and modified surfaces has been suggested (47); nonetheless, the relevance of the *CFHR3*A* and *CFHR3*B* variants in AMD has not been addressed.

The two CNPs in the *CFHR* genes have been shown to be disease-relevant (19). The common variant *ΔCFHR3–CFHR1* is protective against AMD (161), and IgAN (162), but it predisposes to aHUS (163) and to systemic lupus erythematosus (SLE) (69) because it is associated with generation of anti-FH autoantibodies (discussed on page 13). The rare variant *ΔCFHR1–CFHR4* was initially identified in a few aHUS patients with anti-FH autoantibodies (51), and is present in 1.4% of aHUS patients and 0.9% of controls (164).

The protective effect of the *ΔCFHR3–CFHR1* haplotype against AMD was first described in 2006 (161), and it is the more common copy number variation in the *CFH/CFHRs* region (165). *ΔCFHR3–CFHR1* is tagged by *CFH* rs6677604A with 99% accuracy (166), and strongly correlates with the 86.4-kb deletion CNP147 and high FH levels (8). Because protection conferred by *ΔCFHR3–CFHR1* was independent of the FH Tyr402His polymorphism, a direct effect of FHR-1 and FHR-3 in AMD pathogenesis was suggested (21). Nonetheless, the strong association of *ΔCFHR3–CFHR1* with high FH levels, together with the finding that FHR-1 levels were lower in AMD patients than in control individuals, suggests that

Δ*CFHR3–CFHR1* is actually tagging an allele expressing high FH levels, but it is not causal in protection against AMD (8). The much rarer Δ*CFHR1–CFHR4* deletion (also referred to as CNP148) also confers protection against AMD independent of SNPs in *CFH* (19); because Δ*CFHR1–CFHR4* also removes non-coding flanking regions, its protective effect against AMD could either be due to the reduction of FHR-1 and/or FHR-4A levels, or to the absence of regulatory regions relevant for disease pathogenesis.

The first evidence for a direct complement role in IgAN pathogenesis was the finding that the common variant Δ*CFHR3–CFHR1* protects against IgAN when it is in homozygosis (162), pointing out to a possible role of FHR-3 and/or FHR-1 levels in the pathogenic mechanism. However, because the Δ*CFHR3–CFHR1* allele generates high FH levels which associate with lower mesangial C3 deposition, the actual contribution of FHR-1 and/or FHR-3 levels to IgAN is unclear (167). Two studies in different IgAN cohorts have recently shown that FHR-1 levels and FHR-1/FH ratios are increased in patients with disease progression, thus providing evidence for a direct role of FHR-1 in the disease mechanism. One of these studies reported that high FHR-5 levels were also slightly elevated in the IgAN patients, but without any correlation with progressive disease (55). The other study also reported low FH levels associated with *CFH* or *CFI* mutations in a few IgAN patients (54).

FH::FHR-1, FHR-1::FH, and FH::FHR-3 Hybrid Proteins Associate With aHUS

CFH exons 18–20 and *CFHR1* exons 4–6 have a high degree of sequence similarity, that result in only five amino acid difference between CCPs 18–20 of FH ($_{Y1040\text{-}V1042\text{-}Q1058\text{-}S1191\text{-}V1197}$) and CCPs 3–5 of FHR-1 ($_{H157\text{-}L159\text{-}E175\text{-}L290\text{-}A296}$). Studies in aHUS patients have revealed that these differences determine higher binding of FH than FHR-1 to cell surfaces. Amino acids S1191 and V1197 in FH seem to be particularly important, and single mutations involving these amino acids (FH_{S1191L} and FH_{V1197A}) have been found in a number of aHUS patients from different geographical origins. The double mutant ($FH_{S1191L\text{-}V1197A}$) was observed in two unrelated aHUS patients with early disease onset, showed a defective capacity to control complement activation on cellular surfaces, and had been generated by gene conversion (168).

$FH_{S1191L\text{-}V1197A}$ can also be generated by NAHR events that give rise to *CFH::CFHR1* hybrid genes. A *CFH(Ex1–21)::CFHR1(Ex5–6)* hybrid gene was first described in a family with many cases of aHUS along several generations, and a clinical history of disease recurrence in affected individuals (169), demonstrating that $FH_{S1191L\text{-}V1197A}$ is highly pathogenic. This hybrid gene has also been found in other non-related aHUS patients. A slightly different *CFH(Ex1–22):: CFHR1(Ex6)* gene which also generates $FH_{S1191L\text{-}V1197A}$ has been found in another patient with a prompt aHUS onset (170). The reverse situation (i.e., the existence of *CFHR1::CFH* hybrid genes) has also been reported. A *CFHR1(Ex1–3)::CFH(Ex19–20)* hybrid gene generated by "*de novo*" NAHR was identified in one sporadic case of aHUS (171), and a *CFHR1(Ex1–4)::CFH(Ex20)* hybrid gene was found in a family with two members affected with aHUS (172). These two *CFHR1::CFH* hybrid genes generated a double-mutated FHR-1 protein that carries the homologous amino acids in FH CCP20 domain ($FHR\text{-}1_{L290S\text{-}A296V}$); these amino acids most likely confer the mutated FHR-1 increased competition with FH for endothelial cell binding, and result in reduced protection against complement damage (173). Screening of *CFH::CFHR1* and *CFHR1::CFH* hybrid genes is normally done by MLPA analysis of copy number variations. The *CFH::CFHR1* alleles lack a normal copy of *CFHR3* and *CFHR1*, while the *CFHR1::CFH* allele contains two copies of *CFHR3*; it cannot be ruled out that these additional factors also contribute to the pathogenic mechanism.

A FH::FHR-3 hybrid protein containing CCPs 1–19 of FH and the five CCPs of FHR-3 was identified in a large family with aHUS (174). This protein resulted from an abnormal rearrangement that deleted the last exon of *CFH*, which was then fused to the adjacent *CFHR3* gene by the genetic mechanism microhomology mediated end joining (MMEJ). The absence of FH CCP20 domain in the hybrid protein and/or the presence of the FHR-3 CCPs does not affect complement regulation in the fluid phase, but cellular surface regulation seemed to be highly reduced. Estimation of aHUS penetrance in carriers of the hybrid gene is 33%. Another FH::FHR-3 hybrid protein containing CCPs 1–17 of FH and the five CCPs of FHR-3 was found in an aHUS patient with a very early disease onset (175). The hybrid protein resulted from a "*de novo*" 6.3 kb-deletion of exons 21–23 of the *CFH* gene through a MMEJ mechanism, and it showed impaired cell surface complement regulation.

Abnormal FHR Proteins in C3G

The abnormal rearrangements that predispose to C3G thus far described involve exclusively the *CFHR* genes, but not the *CFH* gene. This is a distinctive feature from aHUS that suggests a more important contribution of FHRs in the protection of the glomerular basement membrane and mesangium than in protection of endothelial cells. Abnormal rearrangements include intragenic duplications in *CFHR1* or *CFHR5*, and *CFHR2::CFHR5* and *CFHR3::CFHR1* hybrid genes.

FHR-5 and FHR-1 Proteins With Additional Dimerization Domains

Larger forms of FHR-1 and FHR-5 with duplicated dimerization domains have been observed in a few C3G patients. These proteins circulate in plasma together with the normal FHR-1 and FHR-5 proteins, but disease penetrance in mutation carriers is very high, strongly suggesting a dominant negative effect of the larger, abnormal protein. This is particularly evident for a partially duplicated FHR-5 protein initially observed in two families of Cypriot ancestry in which renal disease was consistent with autosomal dominant transmission (176). All affected individuals were heterozygous for a *CFHR5* gene in which exon 2 (coding for CCP1) and exon 3 (coding for CCP2) were duplicated, giving rise to an abnormal FHR-5 protein containing two extra dimerization domains ($FHR\text{-}5_{12123\text{-}9}$). *In vitro* studies with patient's sera showed reduced binding of the $FHR\text{-}5_{12123\text{-}9}$ to the cell surface, and increased FI cofactor activity, but the relevance of these findings for the pathogenic mechanism is unknown. Patients carrying $FHR\text{-}5_{12123\text{-}9}$ had a high risk of progressive renal disease, particularly males. This renal phenotype, which histologically corresponds to a C3 glomerulonephritis, is clinically characterized by continuous macroscopic hematuria, and was denominated as "CFHR5 nephropathy." These seminal observations were further extended to 16 pedigrees of Cypriot origin in a study that also provided a thorough description of histological, molecular, and clinical findings (177). Recurrence of CFHR5 nephropathy in a kidney allograft has been reported in one patient, although it did not occur in two other cases (178). The same duplicated FHR-5 protein observed in patients of Cypriot ancestry was found in a familial case of C3 glomerulonephritis with a different ethnic origin (179). Of note, this protein was generated from a different genomic rearrangement, reinforcing the relevance of the duplicated FHR-5 protein for the pathogenic mechanism, and the authors proposed that all patients with clinical suspicion of CFHR5 nephropathy should be screened for the abnormal protein by Western blot.

Another FHR-5 protein with two additional dimerization domains was found in a familial case of C3G with DDD (C3G-DDD) (83). In this family, a genomic 24.8 kb-deletion from intron III of the *CFHR2* gene to *CFHR5* gives rise to a hybrid *CFHR2::CFHR5* gene which generates a so-called FHR-$2_{1,2}$-FHR-5-hybrid protein very similar to the FHR-$5_{12123\text{-}9}$ protein previously described. This hybrid protein shows increased binding to C3b and stabilization of the AP C3 convertase, which would explain the low C3 and increased Ba levels detected in the patients' sera; in addition, reduced regulation of the AP C3 convertase by FH will result in increased generation of iC3b molecules which will deposit on the glomerular basement membrane and favor the pathogenic mechanism.

To understand how the presence of two extra dimerization domains in FHR-$5_{12123\text{-}9}$ has pathogenic consequences it is necessary to recapitulate that the dimerization domains in FHR-1, FHR-2, and FHR-5 confer these proteins the ability to generate homo- and hetero-dimers physiologically (26). Although a recent study has not found evidence of the presence of FHR-5 heterodimers with FHR-1 or FHR-2 (53), the additional dimerization domains in FHR-$5_{12123\text{-}9}$ and FHR-$2_{1,2}$-FHR-5 will most likely give rise to higher order oligomeric forms with increased avidity for surface-bound C3b, and these multimeric proteins will compete more efficiently with FH and favor autologous tissue damage, as illustrated in **Figure 3**. In this context, it is intriguing that two very similar FHR-5 proteins result in different clinical entities (CFHR5 nephropathy or DDD). FHR-$5_{12123\text{-}9}$ and FHR-$2_{1,2}$-FHR-5 contain the nine CCPs of FHR-5 preceded by the two dimerization domains of FHR-5 or FHR-2, respectively, that present 85% aminoacid identity. Functional studies with the recombinant forms of these two proteins (referred to as FHR-5_{Dup} and FHR-2-FHR-5_{Hyb}) revealed that they exacerbate local complement activation by recruiting the complement-activating protein properdin, and that properdin binding is mediated by the FHR-5 dimerization domains, and not by the FHR-2 dimerization domains (82). Therefore, local complement activation would be higher in patients with FHR-5_{Dup} than in patients with FHR-2-FHR-5_{Hyb}, and this could explain the different clinical phenotype. Another, non-exclusive, explanation is that the pathogenic mechanism is much dependent on the plasma levels of these FHR-5 proteins. In line with this hypothesis, Western blot analyses of patient serum samples showed that the FHR-5 band has similar intensity to a normal serum, while the intensity of the FHR-$5_{12123\text{-}9}$ (32) or the FHR-$2_{1,2}$-FHR-5 band is much higher, suggesting highly increased levels (82). The latter study also showed that FHR-5 binds to necrotic human endothelial cells, but not to normal endothelial cells, strongly suggesting a role for FHR-5 in complement-mediated elimination of damaged cells.

An abnormal, large FHR-1 protein was identified in a Spanish family with C3G by Western blot analysis (52). This protein was generated by an internal duplication of the *CFHR1* gene, and contains two copies of domains CCPs 1–4. Purification of the normal and the duplicated FHR-1 proteins allowed biochemical, functional, and structural studies that illustrated that normal FHR-1 circulates in plasma as homo- and hetero-oligomers (with FHR-2 and FHR-5), and that the duplicated FHR-1 (containing nine CCP domains) organized into much larger oligomers with increased binding to C3b, iC3b, and C3dg. These findings provided the first evidence for the existence of oligomeric forms of FHR-1, FHR-2, and FHR-5 in normal plasma, and confirmed that duplication of their homologous CCPs 1–2 is pathogenic and associates with C3G. The authors proposed that multimerization of FHR-1 strongly inhibits FH binding to certain cell surfaces, but not to endothelial cells, the target surface in aHUS. A different FHR-1 protein containing two copies of domains CCPs 1–2 has been described in another Spanish patient with a C3G clinical phenotype, but further characterization of this duplicated FHR-1 (containing seven domains) has not been provided (180).

FHR-3::FHR-1 Hybrid Protein

A hybrid *CFHR3::CFHR1* gene associated with C3G-MPGN III has been described in an Irish family (181). This hybrid gene contains exons 1–3 of *CFHR3* and exons 2–6 of *CFHR1*, and generates a protein containing CCPs 1–2 of FHR-3 followed by the five CCPs of FHR-1. The protein was detected in the patients' plasma by Western blot, and it was apparently at a much lower concentration than normal FHR-1. Because patients with the *CFHR3::CFHR1* gene also has two copies of *CFHR3* and *CFHR1*, the authors propose a dominant effect of the hybrid FHR-3::FHR-1 protein in the pathogenic mechanism. It is of note that plasma C3 levels in all affected individuals were normal, as opposed to the reduced levels observed in the C3G-DDD patient with FHR-$2_{1,2}$-FHR-5-hybrid protein (83); this fact suggests that the potential pathogenic effect of FHR-3::FHR-1 on complement activation or regulation is surface-restricted. The clinical data and outcome of the five patients from this family who received renal transplantation has been reported (182); disease recurrence in the kidney allograft was high, but the overall graft survival was good.

Anti-FH Autoantibodies Predispose to Renal Diseases

Disorders related with these autoantibodies are mainly present in aHUS and C3 glomerulonephritis patients and secondary in other autoimmune diseases. The anti-FH autoantibodies cause a functional FH defect, resulting in impaired complement regulation by FH (**Figure 3C**).

The existence of anti-factor H autoantibodies in aHUS and the resulting functional deficiency of FH were first described in 2005 (183). The frequency of the anti-FH antibodies associated with aHUS is approximately 10% of the pediatric patients in the European series and occasionally in patients with adult onset (184). These autoantibodies form complexes with FH and induce a functional FH deficiency. Characterization of these autoantibodies showed that they recognized the C-terminal region of FH, involved in the binding to cell surfaces (185, 186). Moreover, it has been shown that, especially in the acute phase, these antibodies are also capable of blocking the activity of FH as cofactor of FI and the acceleration of the dissociation of the convertases of the alternative pathway (187).

The presence of anti-FH autoantibodies is associated with homozygous Δ*CFHR3–CFHR1* in several aHUS cohorts (51, 164, 188, 189). The Δ*CFHR1–CFHR4* has also been found in a few patients (51, 164), suggesting a relevant role for the absence of FHR-1 in autoantibody generation. In this context, it has been found that most anti-FH autoantibodies also bind to FHR-1, which presents high similarity with FH CCPs 19–20 (29, 164).

The anti-FH autoantibodies in aHUS patients are able of forming immune complexes that can be detected in serum. The amount of these complexes correlates better with the clinical evolution than the total autoantibody titer (187), because FH bound to the complexes cannot regulate the AP on cell surfaces. The use of two monoclonal antibodies binding to different parts of FH allowed the quantitation of total and free FH, which depends on the concentration of circulating anti-FH immune complexes (29, 186, 190). In some cases, the concentration of total FH was within the normal range, but the amount of free FH was practically undetectable, indicating that the anti-FH autoantibodies almost completely blocked the ability of FH to protect cell surfaces from complement activation, although its regulatory activity in the fluid phase was conserved (190).

The epitope recognized by anti-FH autoantibodies has been defined more precisely using recombinant fragments of CCPs 19–20 containing point mutations (191). In this work, it was found that in patients with FHR-1 deficiency, anti-FH antibodies recognize a region that acquires a different conformation in FH and FHR-1 after binding to certain ligands, including various bacterial proteins. This suggests a model in which the absence of FHR-1 plays a role in the loss of tolerance to FH and in the generation of anti-FH autoantibodies, thus explaining the frequent association between the presence of anti-FH antibodies and homozygous Δ*CFHR3–CFHR1* in aHUS. By using the same mutated FH recombinant fragments in our series of patients with anti-FH autoantibodies, we have obtained concordant results, at least in the patients with FHR-1 deficiency, which supports the proposed model for the generation of autoantibodies in these patients (192). However, the mechanism of anti-FH autoantibody generation in aHUS patients without FHR-1 deficiency remains to be determined.

Anti-FH autoantibodies have also been described in patients with C3G (193–197). This association is much less frequent than in the case of aHUS despite having been described for the first time (196). In cases in which the effect of these anti-FH autoantibodies has been studied, it has been shown that they inhibit the regulatory activity of FH by recognizing and blocking its N-terminal region (193, 194, 197), which is a difference with the anti-FH autoantibodies from aHUS patients.

In patients with SLE and other autoimmune diseases, a greater frequency of anti-FH autoantibodies has been described with respect to healthy controls (198). Unlike the anti-FH autoantibodies present in aHUS, the epitopes that are recognized by the autoantibodies seem to be distributed throughout the entire protein, and they are not associated with FHR-1 deficiency.

CONCLUSION

The FH protein family remains an intriguing group of proteins. FH is well-known for its protecting role against self-damage from complement, and the FHRs are emerging as FH antagonists that act as an additional regulatory mechanism to control where and when FH protects human cells and/or surfaces. With the recent development of FHR-specific assays, quantification of the whole protein family has now become possible. This has elucidated the intricate balance between FH and the FHR proteins, showing that overall the balance is in favor of FH. However, this balance can shift on altered self, and also genetic variations have a major impact on FH and FHRs. This includes decreased FH function due to mutations, altered expression levels, as well as hybrid FH::FHR and FHR::FHR proteins and unusual FHR multimers with abnormal function that disturb complement regulation. Associations of increased FHR levels, as a result of genetic variations, with diseases like aHUS and IgAN are highly suggestive of a pathological role for the FHRs. It remains to be seen whether the FHRs are indeed causative in these diseases, but it is likely that they at least contribute to altered complement regulation on host surfaces.

AUTHOR CONTRIBUTIONS

PS-C, RBP, ML-T, and MJ prepared the text and the figures. All authors have revised and approved the manuscript.

FUNDING

PS-C and ML-T are funded by grants PI16/00723 and PI15/00255 (Spanish Ministerio de Economía y Competitividad/ISCIII, and European Program FEDER) and B2017/BMD3673 (Complement II-CM network from the Comunidad de Madrid). MJ is supported by the National Research, Development and Innovation Fund of Hungary (NKFIA grants K 109055 and K 125219), the Kidneeds Foundation, Iowa, US, and by the Institutional Excellence Program of the Ministry of Human Capacities of Hungary.

REFERENCES

1. Ricklin D, Mastellos DC, Reis ES, Lambris JD. The renaissance of complement therapeutics. *Nat Rev Nephrol* (2017) 14(1):26–47. doi:10.1038/nrneph.2017.156
2. Harboe M, Ulvund G, Vien L, Fung M, Mollnes TE. The quantitative role of alternative pathway amplification in classical pathway induced terminal complement activation. *Clin Exp Immunol* (2004) 138(3):439–46. doi:10.1111/j.1365-2249.2004.02627.x
3. Rodriguez de Cordoba S, Esparza-Gordillo J, Goicoechea de Jorge E, Lopez-Trascasa M, Sanchez-Corral P. The human complement factor H: functional roles, genetic variations and disease associations. *Mol Immunol* (2004) 41(4):355–67. doi:10.1016/j.molimm.2004.02.005
4. Ripoche J, Day AJ, Harris TJ, Sim RB. The complete amino acid sequence of human complement factor H. *Biochem J* (1988) 249(2):593–602. doi:10.1042/bj2490593
5. Gordon DL, Kaufman RM, Blackmore TK, Kwong J, Lublin DM. Identification of complement regulatory domains in human factor H. *J Immunol* (1995) 155(1):348–56.
6. Kopp A, Hebecker M, Svobodova E, Jozsi M. Factor h: a complement regulator in health and disease, and a mediator of cellular interactions. *Biomolecules* (2012) 2(1):46–75. doi:10.3390/biom2010046
7. Schmidt CQ, Herbert AP, Hocking HG, Uhrin D, Barlow PN. Translational mini-review series on complement factor H: structural and functional correlations for factor H. *Clin Exp Immunol* (2008) 151(1):14–24. doi:10.1111/j.1365-2249.2007.03553.x
8. Ansari M, McKeigue PM, Skerka C, Hayward C, Rudan I, Vitart V, et al. Genetic influences on plasma CFH and CFHR1 concentrations and their role in susceptibility to age-related macular degeneration. *Hum Mol Genet* (2013) 22(23):4857–69. doi:10.1093/hmg/ddt336
9. Esparza-Gordillo J, Soria JM, Buil A, Almasy L, Blangero J, Fontcuberta J, et al. Genetic and environmental factors influencing the human factor H plasma levels. *Immunogenetics* (2004) 56(2):77–82. doi:10.1007/s00251-004-0660-7
10. Hakobyan S, Harris CL, Tortajada A, Goicochea de Jorge E, Garcia-Layana A, Fernandez-Robredo P, et al. Measurement of factor H variants in plasma using variant-specific monoclonal antibodies: application to assessing risk of age-related macular degeneration. *Invest Ophthalmol Vis Sci* (2008) 49(5):1983–90. doi:10.1167/iovs.07-1523
11. Sofat R, Mangione PP, Gallimore JR, Hakobyan S, Hughes TR, Shah T, et al. Distribution and determinants of circulating complement factor H concentration determined by a high-throughput immunonephelometric assay. *J Immunol Methods* (2013) 390(1–2):63–73. doi:10.1016/j.jim.2013.01.009
12. Friese MA, Hellwage J, Jokiranta TS, Meri S, Muller-Quernheim HJ, Peter HH, et al. Different regulation of factor H and FHL-1/reconectin by inflammatory mediators and expression of the two proteins in rheumatoid arthritis (RA). *Clin Exp Immunol* (2000) 121(2):406–15. doi:10.1046/j.1365-2249.2000.01285.x
13. Zipfel PF, Skerka C. FHL-1/reconectin: a human complement and immune regulator with cell-adhesive function. *Immunol Today* (1999) 20(3):135–40. doi:10.1016/S0167-5699(98)01432-7
14. Misasi R, Huemer HP, Schwaeble W, Solder E, Larcher C, Dierich MP. Human complement factor H: an additional gene product of 43 kDa isolated from human plasma shows cofactor activity for the cleavage of the third component of complement. *Eur J Immunol* (1989) 19(9):1765–8. doi:10.1002/eji.1830190936
15. Schwaeble W, Zwirner J, Schulz TF, Linke RP, Dierich MP, Weiss EH. Human complement factor H: expression of an additional truncated gene product of 43 kDa in human liver. *Eur J Immunol* (1987) 17(10):1485–9. doi:10.1002/eji.1830171015
16. Kuhn S, Skerka C, Zipfel PF. Mapping of the complement regulatory domains in the human factor H-like protein 1 and in factor H1. *J Immunol* (1995) 155(12):5663–70.
17. Swinkels M, Zhang JH, Tilakaratna V, Black G, Perveen R, McHarg S, et al. C-reactive protein and pentraxin-3 binding of factor H-like protein 1 differs from complement factor H: implications for retinal inflammation. *Sci Rep* (2018) 8(1):1643. doi:10.1038/s41598-017-18395-7
18. Cantsilieris S, Nelson BJ, Huddleston J, Baker C, Harshman L, Penewit K, et al. Recurrent structural variation, clustered sites of selection, and disease risk for the complement factor H (CFH) gene family. *Proc Natl Acad Sci U S A* (2018) 115(19):E4433–42. doi:10.1073/pnas.1717600115
19. Sivakumaran TA, Igo RP Jr, Kidd JM, Itsara A, Kopplin LJ, Chen W, et al. A 32 kb critical region excluding Y402H in CFH mediates risk for age-related macular degeneration. *PLoS One* (2011) 6(10):e25598. doi:10.1371/journal.pone.0025598
20. Eberhardt HU, Buhlmann D, Hortschansky P, Chen Q, Bohm S, Kemper MJ, et al. Human factor H-related protein 2 (CFHR2) regulates complement activation. *PLoS One* (2013) 8(11):e78617. doi:10.1371/journal.pone.0078617
21. Fritsche LG, Lauer N, Hartmann A, Stippa S, Keilhauer CN, Oppermann M, et al. An imbalance of human complement regulatory proteins CFHR1, CFHR3 and factor H influences risk for age-related macular degeneration (AMD). *Hum Mol Genet* (2010) 19(23):4694–704. doi:10.1093/hmg/ddq399
22. Heinen S, Hartmann A, Lauer N, Wiehl U, Dahse HM, Schirmer S, et al. Factor H-related protein 1 (CFHR-1) inhibits complement C5 convertase activity and terminal complex formation. *Blood* (2009) 114(12):2439–47. doi:10.1182/blood-2009-02-205641
23. Hellwage J, Jokiranta TS, Koistinen V, Vaarala O, Meri S, Zipfel PF. Functional properties of complement factor H-related proteins FHR-3 and FHR-4: binding to the C3d region of C3b and differential regulation by heparin. *FEBS Lett* (1999) 462(3):345–52. doi:10.1016/S0014-5793(99)01554-9
24. McRae JL, Duthy TG, Griggs KM, Ormsby RJ, Cowan PJ, Cromer BA, et al. Human factor H-related protein 5 has cofactor activity, inhibits C3 convertase activity, binds heparin and C-reactive protein, and associates with lipoprotein. *J Immunol* (2005) 174(10):6250–6. doi:10.4049/jimmunol.174.10.6250
25. Caesar JJ, Lavender H, Ward PN, Exley RM, Eaton J, Chittock E, et al. Competition between antagonistic complement factors for a single protein on *N. meningitidis* rules disease susceptibility. *Elife* (2014) 3:e04008. doi:10.7554/eLife.04008
26. Goicoechea de Jorge E, Caesar JJ, Malik TH, Patel M, Colledge M, Johnson S, et al. Dimerization of complement factor H-related proteins modulates complement activation in vivo. *Proc Natl Acad Sci U S A* (2013) 110(12):4685–90. doi:10.1073/pnas.1219260110
27. Hebecker M, Jozsi M. Factor H-related protein 4 activates complement by serving as a platform for the assembly of alternative pathway C3 convertase via its interaction with C3b protein. *J Biol Chem* (2012) 287(23):19528–36. doi:10.1074/jbc.M112.364471
28. Meszaros T, Csincsi AI, Uzonyi B, Hebecker M, Fulop TG, Erdei A, et al. Factor H inhibits complement activation induced by liposomal and micellar drugs and the therapeutic antibody rituximab in vitro. *Nanomedicine* (2016) 12(4):1023–31. doi:10.1016/j.nano.2015.11.019
29. Strobel S, Abarrategui-Garrido C, Fariza-Requejo E, Seeberger H, Sanchez-Corral P, Jozsi M. Factor H-related protein 1 neutralizes anti-factor H autoantibodies in autoimmune hemolytic uremic syndrome. *Kidney Int* (2011) 80(4):397–404. doi:10.1038/ki.2011.152
30. Timmann C, Leippe M, Horstmann RD. Two major serum components antigenically related to complement factor H are different glycosylation forms of a single protein with no factor H-like complement regulatory functions. *J Immunol* (1991) 146(4):1265–70.
31. Jozsi M, Tortajada A, Uzonyi B, Goicoechea de Jorge E, Rodriguez de Cordoba S. Factor H-related proteins determine complement-activating surfaces. *Trends Immunol* (2015) 36(6):374–84. doi:10.1016/j.it.2015.04.008
32. Csincsi AI, Kopp A, Zoldi M, Banlaki Z, Uzonyi B, Hebecker M, et al. Factor H-related protein 5 interacts with pentraxin 3 and the extracellular matrix and modulates complement activation. *J Immunol* (2015) 194(10):4963–73. doi:10.4049/jimmunol.1403121
33. Csincsi AI, Szabo Z, Banlaki Z, Uzonyi B, Cserhalmi M, Karpati E, et al. FHR-1 binds to C-reactive protein and enhances rather than inhibits complement activation. *J Immunol* (2017) 199(1):292–303. doi:10.4049/jimmunol.1600483
34. Antonioli AH, White J, Crawford F, Renner B, Marchbank KJ, Hannan JP, et al. Modulation of the alternative pathway of complement by murine factor H-related proteins. *J Immunol* (2018) 200(1):316–26. doi:10.4049/jimmunol.1602017

35. Cserhalmi M, Csincsi AI, Mezei Z, Kopp A, Hebecker M, Uzonyi B, et al. The murine factor H-related protein FHR-B promotes complement activation. *Front Immunol* (2017) 8:1145. doi:10.3389/fimmu.2017.01145
36. de Cordoba SR, de Jorge EG. Translational mini-review series on complement factor H: genetics and disease associations of human complement factor H. *Clin Exp Immunol* (2008) 151(1):1–13. doi:10.1111/j.1365-2249.2007.03552.x
37. Friese MA, Hellwage J, Jokiranta TS, Meri S, Peter HH, Eibel H, et al. FHL-1/reconectin and factor H: two human complement regulators which are encoded by the same gene are differently expressed and regulated. *Mol Immunol* (1999) 36(13–14):809–18. doi:10.1016/S0161-5890(99)00101-7
38. Roumenina LT, Rayes J, Frimat M, Fremeaux-Bacchi V. Endothelial cells: source, barrier, and target of defensive mediators. *Immunol Rev* (2016) 274(1):307–29. doi:10.1111/imr.12479
39. Brooimans RA, van der Ark AA, Buurman WA, van Es LA, Daha MR. Differential regulation of complement factor H and C3 production in human umbilical vein endothelial cells by IFN-gamma and IL-1. *J Immunol* (1990) 144(10):3835–40.
40. Chen M, Forrester JV, Xu H. Synthesis of complement factor H by retinal pigment epithelial cells is down-regulated by oxidized photoreceptor outer segments. *Exp Eye Res* (2007) 84(4):635–45. doi:10.1016/j.exer.2006.11.015
41. Devine DV, Rosse WF. Regulation of the activity of platelet-bound C3 convertase of the alternative pathway of complement by platelet factor H. *Proc Natl Acad Sci U S A* (1987) 84(16):5873–7. doi:10.1073/pnas.84.16.5873
42. Dixon KO, O'Flynn J, Klar-Mohamad N, Daha MR, van Kooten C. Properdin and factor H production by human dendritic cells modulates their T-cell stimulatory capacity and is regulated by IFN-gamma. *Eur J Immunol* (2017) 47(3):470–80. doi:10.1002/eji.201646703
43. Katz Y, Strunk RC. Synthesis and regulation of complement protein factor H in human skin fibroblasts. *J Immunol* (1988) 141(2):559–63.
44. Timar KK, Pasch MC, van den Bosch NH, Jarva H, Junnikkala S, Meri S, et al. Human keratinocytes produce the complement inhibitor factor H: synthesis is regulated by interferon-gamma. *Mol Immunol* (2006) 43(4):317–25. doi:10.1016/j.molimm.2005.02.009
45. van den Dobbelsteen ME, Verhasselt V, Kaashoek JG, Timmerman JJ, Schroeijers WE, Verweij CL, et al. Regulation of C3 and factor H synthesis of human glomerular mesangial cells by IL-1 and interferon-gamma. *Clin Exp Immunol* (1994) 95(1):173–80. doi:10.1111/j.1365-2249.1994.tb06033.x
46. Whaley K. Biosynthesis of the complement components and the regulatory proteins of the alternative complement pathway by human peripheral blood monocytes. *J Exp Med* (1980) 151(3):501–16. doi:10.1084/jem.151.3.501
47. Schafer N, Grosche A, Reinders J, Hauck SM, Pouw RB, Kuijpers TW, et al. Complement regulator FHR-3 is elevated either locally or systemically in a selection of autoimmune diseases. *Front Immunol* (2016) 7:542. doi:10.3389/fimmu.2016.00542
48. Skerka C, Chen Q, Fremeaux-Bacchi V, Roumenina LT. Complement factor H related proteins (CFHRs). *Mol Immunol* (2013) 56(3):170–80. doi:10.1016/j.molimm.2013.06.001
49. Estaller C, Koistinen V, Schwaeble W, Dierich MP, Weiss EH. Cloning of the 1.4-kb mRNA species of human complement factor H reveals a novel member of the short consensus repeat family related to the carboxy terminal of the classical 150-kDa molecule. *J Immunol* (1991) 146(9):3190–6.
50. Skerka C, Horstmann RD, Zipfel PF. Molecular cloning of a human serum protein structurally related to complement factor H. *J Biol Chem* (1991) 266(18):12015–20.
51. Abarrategui-Garrido C, Martinez-Barricarte R, Lopez-Trascasa M, de Cordoba SR, Sanchez-Corral P. Characterization of complement factor H-related (CFHR) proteins in plasma reveals novel genetic variations of CFHR1 associated with atypical hemolytic uremic syndrome. *Blood* (2009) 114(19):4261–71. doi:10.1182/blood-2009-05-223834
52. Tortajada A, Yebenes H, Abarrategui-Garrido C, Anter J, Garcia-Fernandez JM, Martinez-Barricarte R, et al. C3 glomerulopathy-associated CFHR1 mutation alters FHR oligomerization and complement regulation. *J Clin Invest* (2013) 123(6):2434–46. doi:10.1172/JCI68280
53. van Beek AE, Pouw RB, Brouwer MC, van Mierlo G, Geissler J, Ooijevaar-de Heer P, et al. Factor H-related (FHR)-1 and FHR-2 Form homo- and heterodimers, while FHR-5 circulates only as homodimer in human plasma. *Front Immunol* (2017) 8:1328. doi:10.3389/fimmu.2017.01328
54. Tortajada A, Gutierrez E, Goicoechea de Jorge E, Anter J, Segarra A, Espinosa M, et al. Elevated factor H-related protein 1 and factor H pathogenic variants decrease complement regulation in IgA nephropathy. *Kidney Int* (2017) 92(4):953–63. doi:10.1016/j.kint.2017.03.041
55. Medjeral-Thomas NR, Lomax-Browne HJ, Beckwith H, Willicombe M, McLean AG, Brookes P, et al. Circulating complement factor H-related proteins 1 and 5 correlate with disease activity in IgA nephropathy. *Kidney Int* (2017) 92(4):942–52. doi:10.1016/j.kint.2017.03.043
56. Skerka C, Timmann C, Horstmann RD, Zipfel PF. Two additional human serum proteins structurally related to complement factor H. Evidence for a family of factor H-related genes. *J Immunol* (1992) 148(10):3313–8.
57. Skerka C, Kuhn S, Gunther K, Lingelbach K, Zipfel PF. A novel short consensus repeat-containing molecule is related to human complement factor H. *J Biol Chem* (1993) 268(4):2904–8.
58. Pouw RB, Brouwer MC, Geissler J, van Herpen LV, Zeerleder SS, Wuillemin WA, et al. Complement factor H-related protein 3 serum levels are low compared to factor H and mainly determined by gene copy number variation in CFHR3. *PLoS One* (2016) 11(3):e0152164. doi:10.1371/journal.pone.0152164
59. Bernabeu-Herrero ME, Jimenez-Alcazar M, Anter J, Pinto S, Sanchez Chinchilla D, Garrido S, et al. Complement factor H, FHR-3 and FHR-1 variants associate in an extended haplotype conferring increased risk of atypical hemolytic uremic syndrome. *Mol Immunol* (2015) 67(2 Pt B):276–86. doi:10.1016/j.molimm.2015.06.021
60. Pouw RB, Gomez Delgado I, Lopez Lera A, Rodriguez de Cordoba S, Wouters D, Kuijpers TW, et al. High complement factor H-related (FHR)-3 levels are associated with the atypical hemolytic-uremic syndrome-risk allele CFHR3*B. *Front Immunol* (2018) 9:848. doi:10.3389/fimmu.2018.00848
61. Jozsi M, Richter H, Loschmann I, Skerka C, Buck F, Beisiegel U, et al. FHR-4A: a new factor H-related protein is encoded by the human FHR-4 gene. *Eur J Hum Genet* (2005) 13(3):321–9. doi:10.1038/sj.ejhg.5201324
62. Skerka C, Hellwage J, Weber W, Tilkorn A, Buck F, Marti T, et al. The human factor H-related protein 4 (FHR-4). A novel short consensus repeat-containing protein is associated with human triglyceride-rich lipoproteins. *J Biol Chem* (1997) 272(9):5627–34. doi:10.1074/jbc.272.9.5627
63. Pouw RB, Brouwer MC, van Beek AE, Jozsi M, Wouters D, Kuijpers TW. Complement factor H-related protein 4A is the dominant circulating splice variant of CFHR4. *Front Immunol* (2018) 9:729. doi:10.3389/fimmu.2018.00729
64. McRae JL, Cowan PJ, Power DA, Mitchelhill KI, Kemp BE, Morgan BP, et al. Human factor H-related protein 5 (FHR-5). A new complement-associated protein. *J Biol Chem* (2001) 276(9):6747–54. doi:10.1074/jbc.M007495200
65. Vernon KA, Goicoechea de Jorge E, Hall AE, Fremeaux-Bacchi V, Aitman TJ, Cook HT, et al. Acute presentation and persistent glomerulonephritis following streptococcal infection in a patient with heterozygous complement factor H-related protein 5 deficiency. *Am J Kidney Dis* (2012) 60(1):121–5. doi:10.1053/j.ajkd.2012.02.329
66. Zhang P, Zhu M, Geng-Spyropoulos M, Shardell M, Gonzalez-Freire M, Gudnason V, et al. A novel, multiplexed targeted mass spectrometry assay for quantification of complement factor H (CFH) variants and CFH-related proteins 1-5 in human plasma. *Proteomics* (2017) 17(6):1600237. doi:10.1002/pmic.201600237
67. Kopczynska M, Zelek W, Touchard S, Gaughran F, Di Forti M, Mondelli V, et al. Complement system biomarkers in first episode psychosis. *Schizophr Res* (2017). doi:10.1016/j.schres.2017.12.012
68. Holmes LV, Strain L, Staniforth SJ, Moore I, Marchbank K, Kavanagh D, et al. Determining the population frequency of the CFHR3/CFHR1 deletion at 1q32. *PLoS One* (2013) 8(4):e60352. doi:10.1371/journal.pone.0060352
69. Zhao J, Wu H, Khosravi M, Cui H, Qian X, Kelly JA, et al. Association of genetic variants in complement factor H and factor H-related genes with systemic lupus erythematosus susceptibility. *PLoS Genet* (2011) 7(5):e1002079. doi:10.1371/journal.pgen.1002079
70. Xue X, Wu J, Ricklin D, Forneris F, Di Crescenzio P, Schmidt CQ, et al. Regulator-dependent mechanisms of C3b processing by factor I allow

differentiation of immune responses. *Nat Struct Mol Biol* (2017) 24(8):643–51. doi:10.1038/nsmb.3427
71. Riley-Vargas RC, Lanzendorf S, Atkinson JP. Targeted and restricted complement activation on acrosome-reacted spermatozoa. *J Clin Invest* (2005) 115(5):1241–9. doi:10.1172/JCI23213
72. Sjoberg AP, Trouw LA, Blom AM. Complement activation and inhibition: a delicate balance. *Trends Immunol* (2009) 30(2):83–90. doi:10.1016/j.it.2008.11.003
73. Jozsi M. Factor H family proteins in complement evasion of microorganisms. *Front Immunol* (2017) 8:571. doi:10.3389/fimmu.2017.00571
74. Kopp A, Strobel S, Tortajada A, Rodriguez de Cordoba S, Sanchez-Corral P, Prohaszka Z, et al. Atypical hemolytic uremic syndrome-associated variants and autoantibodies impair binding of factor h and factor h-related protein 1 to pentraxin 3. *J Immunol* (2012) 189(4):1858–67. doi:10.4049/jimmunol.1200357
75. Lambris JD, Ricklin D, Geisbrecht BV. Complement evasion by human pathogens. *Nat Rev Microbiol* (2008) 6(2):132–42. doi:10.1038/nrmicro1824
76. Schmidt CQ, Herbert AP, Kavanagh D, Gandy C, Fenton CJ, Blaum BS, et al. A new map of glycosaminoglycan and C3b binding sites on factor H. *J Immunol* (2008) 181(4):2610–9. doi:10.4049/jimmunol.181.4.2610
77. Deban L, Jarva H, Lehtinen MJ, Bottazzi B, Bastone A, Doni A, et al. Binding of the long pentraxin PTX3 to factor H: interacting domains and function in the regulation of complement activation. *J Immunol* (2008) 181(12):8433–40. doi:10.4049/jimmunol.181.12.8433
78. Hebecker M, Alba-Dominguez M, Roumenina LT, Reuter S, Hyvarinen S, Dragon-Durey MA, et al. An engineered construct combining complement regulatory and surface-recognition domains represents a minimal-size functional factor H. *J Immunol* (2013) 191(2):912–21. doi:10.4049/jimmunol.1300269
79. Jarva H, Jokiranta TS, Hellwage J, Zipfel PF, Meri S. Regulation of complement activation by C-reactive protein: targeting the complement inhibitory activity of factor H by an interaction with short consensus repeat domains 7 and 8–11. *J Immunol* (1999) 163(7):3957–62.
80. Kajander T, Lehtinen MJ, Hyvarinen S, Bhattacharjee A, Leung E, Isenman DE, et al. Dual interaction of factor H with C3d and glycosaminoglycans in host-nonhost discrimination by complement. *Proc Natl Acad Sci U S A* (2011) 108(7):2897–902. doi:10.1073/pnas.1017087108
81. Morgan HP, Schmidt CQ, Guariento M, Blaum BS, Gillespie D, Herbert AP, et al. Structural basis for engagement by complement factor H of C3b on a self surface. *Nat Struct Mol Biol* (2011) 18(4):463–70. doi:10.1038/nsmb.2018
82. Chen Q, Manzke M, Hartmann A, Buttner M, Amann K, Pauly D, et al. Complement factor H-related 5-hybrid proteins anchor properdin and activate complement at self-surfaces. *J Am Soc Nephrol* (2016) 27(5):1413–25. doi:10.1681/ASN.2015020212
83. Chen Q, Wiesener M, Eberhardt HU, Hartmann A, Uzonyi B, Kirschfink M, et al. Complement factor H-related hybrid protein deregulates complement in dense deposit disease. *J Clin Invest* (2014) 124(1):145–55. doi:10.1172/JCI71866
84. Hannan JP, Laskowski J, Thurman JM, Hageman GS, Holers VM. Mapping the complement factor H-related protein 1 (CFHR1):C3b/C3d interactions. *PLoS One* (2016) 11(11):e0166200. doi:10.1371/journal.pone.0166200
85. Buhlmann D, Eberhardt HU, Medyukhina A, Prodinger WM, Figge MT, Zipfel PF, et al. FHR3 blocks C3d-mediated coactivation of human B cells. *J Immunol* (2016) 197(2):620–9. doi:10.4049/jimmunol.1600053
86. Meri S. Self-nonself discrimination by the complement system. *FEBS Lett* (2016) 590(15):2418–34. doi:10.1002/1873-3468.12284
87. Blackmore TK, Hellwage J, Sadlon TA, Higgs N, Zipfel PF, Ward HM, et al. Identification of the second heparin-binding domain in human complement factor H. *J Immunol* (1998) 160(7):3342–8.
88. Blackmore TK, Sadlon TA, Ward HM, Lublin DM, Gordon DL. Identification of a heparin binding domain in the seventh short consensus repeat of complement factor H. *J Immunol* (1996) 157(12):5422–7.
89. Hyvarinen S, Meri S, Jokiranta TS. Disturbed sialic acid recognition on endothelial cells and platelets in complement attack causes atypical hemolytic uremic syndrome. *Blood* (2016) 127(22):2701–10. doi:10.1182/blood-2015-11-680009
90. Jokiranta TS, Cheng ZZ, Seeberger H, Jozsi M, Heinen S, Noris M, et al. Binding of complement factor H to endothelial cells is mediated by the carboxy-terminal glycosaminoglycan binding site. *Am J Pathol* (2005) 167(4):1173–81. doi:10.1016/S0002-9440(10)61205-9
91. Blaum BS, Hannan JP, Herbert AP, Kavanagh D, Uhrin D, Stehle T. Structural basis for sialic acid-mediated self-recognition by complement factor H. *Nat Chem Biol* (2015) 11(1):77–82. doi:10.1038/nchembio.1696
92. Clark SJ, Ridge LA, Herbert AP, Hakobyan S, Mulloy B, Lennon R, et al. Tissue-specific host recognition by complement factor H is mediated by differential activities of its glycosaminoglycan-binding regions. *J Immunol* (2013) 190(5):2049–57. doi:10.4049/jimmunol.1201751
93. Clark SJ, Schmidt CQ, White AM, Hakobyan S, Morgan BP, Bishop PN. Identification of factor H-like protein 1 as the predominant complement regulator in Bruch's membrane: implications for age-related macular degeneration. *J Immunol* (2014) 193(10):4962–70. doi:10.4049/jimmunol.1401613
94. Rudnick RB, Chen Q, Stea ED, Hartmann A, Papac-Milicevic N, Person F, et al. FHR5 binds to laminins, uses separate C3b and surface-binding sites, and activates complement on malondialdehyde-acetaldehyde surfaces. *J Immunol* (2018) 200(7):2280–90. doi:10.4049/jimmunol.1701641
95. Clark SJ, Bishop PN, Day AJ. The proteoglycan glycomatrix: a sugar microenvironment essential for complement regulation. *Front Immunol* (2013) 4:412. doi:10.3389/fimmu.2013.00412
96. Martin M, Blom AM. Complement in removal of the dead – balancing inflammation. *Immunol Rev* (2016) 274(1):218–32. doi:10.1111/imr.12462
97. Trouw LA, Bengtsson AA, Gelderman KA, Dahlback B, Sturfelt G, Blom AM. C4b-binding protein and factor H compensate for the loss of membrane-bound complement inhibitors to protect apoptotic cells against excessive complement attack. *J Biol Chem* (2007) 282(39):28540–8. doi:10.1074/jbc.M704354200
98. Leffler J, Herbert AP, Norstrom E, Schmidt CQ, Barlow PN, Blom AM, et al. Annexin-II, DNA, and histones serve as factor H ligands on the surface of apoptotic cells. *J Biol Chem* (2010) 285(6):3766–76. doi:10.1074/jbc.M109.045427
99. Weismann D, Hartvigsen K, Lauer N, Bennett KL, Scholl HP, Charbel Issa P, et al. Complement factor H binds malondialdehyde epitopes and protects from oxidative stress. *Nature* (2011) 478(7367):76–81. doi:10.1038/nature10449
100. Gershov D, Kim S, Brot N, Elkon KB. C-Reactive protein binds to apoptotic cells, protects the cells from assembly of the terminal complement components, and sustains an antiinflammatory innate immune response: implications for systemic autoimmunity. *J Exp Med* (2000) 192(9):1353–64. doi:10.1084/jem.192.9.1353
101. Bottazzi B, Doni A, Garlanda C, Mantovani A. An integrated view of humoral innate immunity: pentraxins as a paradigm. *Annu Rev Immunol* (2010) 28:157–83. doi:10.1146/annurev-immunol-030409-101305
102. Biro A, Rovo Z, Papp D, Cervenak L, Varga L, Fust G, et al. Studies on the interactions between C-reactive protein and complement proteins. *Immunology* (2007) 121(1):40–50. doi:10.1111/j.1365-2567.2007.02535.x
103. Braunschweig A, Jozsi M. Human pentraxin 3 binds to the complement regulator c4b-binding protein. *PLoS One* (2011) 6(8):e23991. doi:10.1371/journal.pone.0023991
104. Deban L, Jaillon S, Garlanda C, Bottazzi B, Mantovani A. Pentraxins in innate immunity: lessons from PTX3. *Cell Tissue Res* (2011) 343(1):237–49. doi:10.1007/s00441-010-1018-0
105. Ma YJ, Doni A, Skjoedt MO, Honore C, Arendrup M, Mantovani A, et al. Heterocomplexes of mannose-binding lectin and the pentraxins PTX3 or serum amyloid P component trigger cross-activation of the complement system. *J Biol Chem* (2011) 286(5):3405–17. doi:10.1074/jbc.M110.190637
106. Nauta AJ, Bottazzi B, Mantovani A, Salvatori G, Kishore U, Schwaeble WJ, et al. Biochemical and functional characterization of the interaction between pentraxin 3 and C1q. *Eur J Immunol* (2003) 33(2):465–73. doi:10.1002/immu.200310022
107. Sjoberg AP, Trouw LA, McGrath FD, Hack CE, Blom AM. Regulation of complement activation by C-reactive protein: targeting of the inhibitory activity of C4b-binding protein. *J Immunol* (2006) 176(12):7612–20. doi:10.4049/jimmunol.176.12.7612
108. Hakobyan S, Harris CL, van den Berg CW, Fernandez-Alonso MC, de Jorge EG, de Cordoba SR, et al. Complement factor H binds to denatured rather than to native pentameric C-reactive protein. *J Biol Chem* (2008) 283(45):30451–60. doi:10.1074/jbc.M803648200

109. Mihlan M, Stippa S, Jozsi M, Zipfel PF. Monomeric CRP contributes to complement control in fluid phase and on cellular surfaces and increases phagocytosis by recruiting factor H. *Cell Death Differ* (2009) 16(12):1630–40. doi:10.1038/cdd.2009.103
110. Okemefuna AI, Nan R, Miller A, Gor J, Perkins SJ. Complement factor H binds at two independent sites to C-reactive protein in acute phase concentrations. *J Biol Chem* (2010) 285(2):1053–65. doi:10.1074/jbc.M109.044529
111. Hebecker M, Okemefuna AI, Perkins SJ, Mihlan M, Huber-Lang M, Jozsi M. Molecular basis of C-reactive protein binding and modulation of complement activation by factor H-related protein 4. *Mol Immunol* (2010) 47(6):1347–55. doi:10.1016/j.molimm.2009.12.005
112. Mihlan M, Hebecker M, Dahse HM, Halbich S, Huber-Lang M, Dahse R, et al. Human complement factor H-related protein 4 binds and recruits native pentameric C-reactive protein to necrotic cells. *Mol Immunol* (2009) 46(3):335–44. doi:10.1016/j.molimm.2008.10.029
113. Inforzato A, Baldock C, Jowitt TA, Holmes DF, Lindstedt R, Marcellini M, et al. The angiogenic inhibitor long pentraxin PTX3 forms an asymmetric octamer with two binding sites for FGF2. *J Biol Chem* (2010) 285(23): 17681–92. doi:10.1074/jbc.M109.085639
114. Hyvarinen S, Uchida K, Varjosalo M, Jokela R, Jokiranta TS. Recognition of malondialdehyde-modified proteins by the C terminus of complement factor H is mediated via the polyanion binding site and impaired by mutations found in atypical hemolytic uremic syndrome. *J Biol Chem* (2014) 289(7):4295–306. doi:10.1074/jbc.M113.527416
115. Delvaeye M, Noris M, De Vriese A, Esmon CT, Esmon NL, Ferrell G, et al. Thrombomodulin mutations in atypical hemolytic-uremic syndrome. *N Engl J Med* (2009) 361(4):345–57. doi:10.1056/NEJMoa0810739
116. Heurich M, Preston RJ, O'Donnell VB, Morgan BP, Collins PW. Thrombomodulin enhances complement regulation through strong affinity interactions with factor H and C3b-Factor H complex. *Thromb Res* (2016) 145:84–92. doi:10.1016/j.thromres.2016.07.017
117. Tateishi K, Imaoka M, Matsushita M. Dual modulating functions of thrombomodulin in the alternative complement pathway. *Biosci Trends* (2016) 10(3):231–4. doi:10.5582/bst.2016.01052
118. Feng S, Liang X, Cruz MA, Vu H, Zhou Z, Pemmaraju N, et al. The interaction between factor H and Von Willebrand factor. *PLoS One* (2013) 8(8):e73715. doi:10.1371/journal.pone.0073715
119. Nolasco L, Nolasco J, Feng S, Afshar-Kharghan V, Moake J. Human complement factor H is a reductase for large soluble von Willebrand factor multimers – brief report. *Arterioscler Thromb Vasc Biol* (2013) 33(11):2524–8. doi:10.1161ATVBAHA.113.302280
120. Rayes J, Roumenina LT, Dimitrov JD, Repesse Y, Ing M, Christophe O, et al. The interaction between factor H and VWF increases factor H cofactor activity and regulates VWF prothrombotic status. *Blood* (2014) 123(1):121–5. doi:10.1182/blood-2013-04-495853
121. Frimat M, Tabarin F, Dimitrov JD, Poitou C, Halbwachs-Mecarelli L, Fremeaux-Bacchi V, et al. Complement activation by heme as a secondary hit for atypical hemolytic uremic syndrome. *Blood* (2013) 122(2):282–92. doi:10.1182/blood-2013-03-489245
122. Haapasalo K, van Kessel K, Nissila E, Metso J, Johansson T, Miettinen S, et al. Complement factor H binds to human serum apolipoprotein E and mediates complement regulation on high density lipoprotein particles. *J Biol Chem* (2015) 290(48):28977–87. doi:10.1074/jbc.M115.669226
123. Chen SF, Wang FM, Li ZY, Yu F, Chen M, Zhao MH. Myeloperoxidase influences the complement regulatory activity of complement factor H. *Rheumatology (Oxford)* (2018). doi:10.1093/rheumatology/kex529
124. Jozsi M, Schneider AE, Karpati E, Sandor N. Complement factor H family proteins in their non-canonical role as modulators of cellular functions. *Semin Cell Dev Biol* (2018). doi:10.1016/j.semcdb.2017.12.018
125. DiScipio RG, Daffern PJ, Schraufstatter IU, Sriramarao P. Human polymorphonuclear leukocytes adhere to complement factor H through an interaction that involves alphaMbeta2 (CD11b/CD18). *J Immunol* (1998) 160(8):4057–66.
126. Svoboda E, Schneider AE, Sandor N, Lermann U, Staib P, Kremlitzka M, et al. Secreted aspartic protease 2 of *Candida albicans* inactivates factor H and the macrophage factor H-receptors CR3 (CD11b/CD18) and CR4 (CD11c/CD18). *Immunol Lett* (2015) 168(1):13–21. doi:10.1016/j.imlet.2015.08.009
127. Schneider AE, Sandor N, Karpati E, Jozsi M. Complement factor H modulates the activation of human neutrophil granulocytes and the generation of neutrophil extracellular traps. *Mol Immunol* (2016) 72:37–48. doi:10.1016/j.molimm.2016.02.011
128. Agarwal V, Asmat TM, Luo S, Jensch I, Zipfel PF, Hammerschmidt S. Complement regulator Factor H mediates a two-step uptake of Streptococcus pneumoniae by human cells. *J Biol Chem* (2010) 285(30):23486–95. doi:10.1074/jbc.M110.142703
129. Losse J, Zipfel PF, Jozsi M. Factor H and factor H-related protein 1 bind to human neutrophils via complement receptor 3, mediate attachment to *Candida albicans*, and enhance neutrophil antimicrobial activity. *J Immunol* (2010) 184(2):912–21. doi:10.4049/jimmunol.0901702
130. Hellwage J, Kuhn S, Zipfel PF. The human complement regulatory factor-H-like protein 1, which represents a truncated form of factor H, displays cell-attachment activity. *Biochem J* (1997) 326(Pt 2):321–7. doi:10.1042/bj3260321
131. Iferroudjene D, Schouft MT, Lemercier C, Gilbert D, Fontaine M. Evidence for an active hydrophobic form of factor H that is able to induce secretion of interleukin 1-beta or by human monocytes. *Eur J Immunol* (1991) 21(4):967–72. doi:10.1002/eji.1830210416
132. Nabil K, Rihn B, Jaurand MC, Vignaud JM, Ripoche J, Martinet Y, et al. Identification of human complement factor H as a chemotactic protein for monocytes. *Biochem J* (1997) 326(Pt 2):377–83. doi:10.1042/bj3260377
133. Ohtsuka H, Imamura T, Matsushita M, Tanase S, Okada H, Ogawa M, et al. Thrombin generates monocyte chemotactic activity from complement factor H. *Immunology* (1993) 80(1):140–5.
134. Schopf RE, Hammann KP, Scheiner O, Lemmel EM, Dierich MP. Activation of human monocytes by both human beta 1H and C3b. *Immunology* (1982) 46(2):307–12.
135. Olivar R, Luque A, Cardenas-Brito S, Naranjo-Gomez M, Blom AM, Borras FE, et al. The complement inhibitor factor H generates an anti-inflammatory and tolerogenic state in monocyte-derived dendritic cells. *J Immunol* (2016) 196(10):4274–90. doi:10.4049/jimmunol.1500455
136. Calippe B, Augustin S, Beguier F, Charles-Messance H, Poupel L, Conart JB, et al. Complement factor H inhibits CD47-mediated resolution of inflammation. *Immunity* (2017) 46(2):261–72. doi:10.1016/j.immuni.2017.01.006
137. Erdei A, Sim RB. Complement factor H-binding protein of Raji cells and tonsil B lymphocytes. *Biochem J* (1987) 246(1):149–56. doi:10.1042/bj2460149
138. Hammann KP, Raile A, Schmitt M, Mussel HH, Peters H, Scheiner O, et al. beta 1H stimulates mouse-spleen B lymphocytes as demonstrated by increased thymidine incorporation and formation of B cell blasts. *Immunobiology* (1981) 160(3–4):289–301. doi:10.1016/S0171-2985(81)80055-1
139. Lambris JD, Dobson NJ, Ross GD. Release of endogenous C3b inactivator from lymphocytes in response to triggering membrane receptors for beta 1H globulin. *J Exp Med* (1980) 152(6):1625–44. doi:10.1084/jem.152.6.1625
140. Tsokos GC, Inghirami G, Tsoukas CD, Balow JE, Lambris JD. Regulation of immunoglobulin secretion by factor H of human complement. *Immunology* (1985) 55(3):419–26.
141. Goodship TH, Cook HT, Fakhouri F, Fervenza FC, Fremeaux-Bacchi V, Kavanagh D, et al. Atypical hemolytic uremic syndrome and C3 glomerulopathy: conclusions from a "kidney disease: improving global outcomes" (KDIGO) Controversies Conference. *Kidney Int* (2017) 91(3):539–51. doi:10.1016/j.kint.2016.10.005
142. Nester CM, Barbour T, de Cordoba SR, Dragon-Durey MA, Fremeaux-Bacchi V, Goodship TH, et al. Atypical aHUS: state of the art. *Mol Immunol* (2015) 67(1):31–42. doi:10.1016/j.molimm.2015.03.246
143. Noris M, Remuzzi G. Atypical hemolytic-uremic syndrome. *N Engl J Med* (2009) 361(17):1676–87. doi:10.1056/NEJMra0902814
144. Maillard N, Wyatt RJ, Julian BA, Kiryluk K, Gharavi A, Fremeaux-Bacchi V, et al. Current understanding of the role of complement in IgA nephropathy. *J Am Soc Nephrol* (2015) 26(7):1503–12. doi:10.1681/ASN.2014101000
145. Suzuki H, Kiryluk K, Novak J, Moldoveanu Z, Herr AB, Renfrow MB, et al. The pathophysiology of IgA nephropathy. *J Am Soc Nephrol* (2011) 22(10):1795–803. doi:10.1681/ASN.2011050464
146. Geerlings MJ, de Jong EK, den Hollander AI. The complement system in age-related macular degeneration: a review of rare genetic variants and implications for personalized treatment. *Mol Immunol* (2017) 84:65–76. doi:10.1016/j.molimm.2016.11.016

147. Hageman GS, Anderson DH, Johnson LV, Hancox LS, Taiber AJ, Hardisty LI, et al. A common haplotype in the complement regulatory gene factor H (HF1/CFH) predisposes individuals to age-related macular degeneration. *Proc Natl Acad Sci U S A* (2005) 102(20):7227–32. doi:10.1073/pnas.0501536102
148. Hageman GS, Hancox LS, Taiber AJ, Gehrs KM, Anderson DH, Johnson LV, et al. Extended haplotypes in the complement factor H (CFH) and CFH-related (CFHR) family of genes protect against age-related macular degeneration: characterization, ethnic distribution and evolutionary implications. *Ann Med* (2006) 38(8):592–604. doi:10.1080/07853890601097030
149. Pickering MC, de Jorge EG, Martinez-Barricarte R, Recalde S, Garcia-Layana A, Rose KL, et al. Spontaneous hemolytic uremic syndrome triggered by complement factor H lacking surface recognition domains. *J Exp Med* (2007) 204(6):1249–56. doi:10.1084/jem.20070301
150. Tortajada A, Montes T, Martinez-Barricarte R, Morgan BP, Harris CL, de Cordoba SR. The disease-protective complement factor H allotypic variant Ile62 shows increased binding affinity for C3b and enhanced cofactor activity. *Hum Mol Genet* (2009) 18(18):3452–61. doi:10.1093/hmg/ddp289
151. Zareparsi S, Branham KE, Li M, Shah S, Klein RJ, Ott J, et al. Strong association of the Y402H variant in complement factor H at 1q32 with susceptibility to age-related macular degeneration. *Am J Hum Genet* (2005) 77(1):149–53. doi:10.1086/431426
152. Clark SJ, Perveen R, Hakobyan S, Morgan BP, Sim RB, Bishop PN, et al. Impaired binding of the age-related macular degeneration-associated complement factor H 402H allotype to Bruch's membrane in human retina. *J Biol Chem* (2010) 285(39):30192–202. doi:10.1074/jbc.M110.103986
153. Li M, Atmaca-Sonmez P, Othman M, Branham KE, Khanna R, Wade MS, et al. CFH haplotypes without the Y402H coding variant show strong association with susceptibility to age-related macular degeneration. *Nat Genet* (2006) 38(9):1049–54. doi:10.1038/ng1871
154. Caprioli J, Bettinaglio P, Zipfel PF, Amadei B, Daina E, Gamba S, et al. The molecular basis of familial hemolytic uremic syndrome: mutation analysis of factor H gene reveals a hot spot in short consensus repeat 20. *J Am Soc Nephrol* (2001) 12(2):297–307.
155. Sanchez-Corral P, Perez-Caballero D, Huarte O, Simckes AM, Goicoechea E, Lopez-Trascasa M, et al. Structural and functional characterization of factor H mutations associated with atypical hemolytic uremic syndrome. *Am J Hum Genet* (2002) 71(6):1285–95. doi:10.1086/344515
156. Servais A, Noel LH, Roumenina LT, Le Quintrec M, Ngo S, Dragon-Durey MA, et al. Acquired and genetic complement abnormalities play a critical role in dense deposit disease and other C3 glomerulopathies. *Kidney Int* (2012) 82(4):454–64. doi:10.1038/ki.2012.63
157. Fritsche LG, Igl W, Bailey JN, Grassmann F, Sengupta S, Bragg-Gresham JL, et al. A large genome-wide association study of age-related macular degeneration highlights contributions of rare and common variants. *Nat Genet* (2016) 48(2):134–43. doi:10.1038/ng.3448
158. Raychaudhuri S, Iartchouk O, Chin K, Tan PL, Tai AK, Ripke S, et al. A rare penetrant mutation in CFH confers high risk of age-related macular degeneration. *Nat Genet* (2011) 43(12):1232–6. doi:10.1038/ng.976
159. Recalde S, Tortajada A, Subias M, Anter J, Blasco M, Maranta R, et al. Molecular basis of factor H R1210C association with ocular and renal diseases. *J Am Soc Nephrol* (2016) 27(5):1305–11. doi:10.1681/ASN.2015050580
160. Martinez-Barricarte R, Recalde S, Fernandez-Robredo P, Millan I, Olavarrieta L, Vinuela A, et al. Relevance of complement factor H-related 1 (CFHR1) genotypes in age-related macular degeneration. *Invest Ophthalmol Vis Sci* (2012) 53(3):1087–94. doi:10.1167/iovs.11-8709
161. Hughes AE, Orr N, Esfandiary H, Diaz-Torres M, Goodship T, Chakravarthy U. A common CFH haplotype, with deletion of CFHR1 and CFHR3, is associated with lower risk of age-related macular degeneration. *Nat Genet* (2006) 38(10):1173–7. doi:10.1038/ng1890
162. Gharavi AG, Kiryluk K, Choi M, Li Y, Hou P, Xie J, et al. Genome-wide association study identifies susceptibility loci for IgA nephropathy. *Nat Genet* (2011) 43(4):321–7. doi:10.1038/ng.787
163. Zipfel PF, Edey M, Heinen S, Jozsi M, Richter H, Misselwitz J, et al. Deletion of complement factor H-related genes CFHR1 and CFHR3 is associated with atypical hemolytic uremic syndrome. *PLoS Genet* (2007) 3(3):e41. doi:10.1371/journal.pgen.0030041
164. Moore I, Strain L, Pappworth I, Kavanagh D, Barlow PN, Herbert AP, et al. Association of factor H autoantibodies with deletions of CFHR1, CFHR3, CFHR4, and with mutations in CFH, CFI, CD46, and C3 in patients with atypical hemolytic uremic syndrome. *Blood* (2010) 115(2):379–87. doi:10.1182/blood-2009-05-221549
165. Kubista KE, Tosakulwong N, Wu Y, Ryu E, Roeder JL, Hecker LA, et al. Copy number variation in the complement factor H-related genes and age-related macular degeneration. *Mol Vis* (2011) 17:2080–92.
166. Schmid-Kubista KE, Tosakulwong N, Wu Y, Ryu E, Hecker LA, Baratz KH, et al. Contribution of copy number variation in the regulation of complement activation locus to development of age-related macular degeneration. *Invest Ophthalmol Vis Sci* (2009) 50(11):5070–9. doi:10.1167/iovs.09-3975
167. Zhu L, Zhai YL, Wang FM, Hou P, Lv JC, Xu DM, et al. Variants in complement factor H and complement factor H-related protein genes, CFHR3 and CFHR1, affect complement activation in IgA nephropathy. *J Am Soc Nephrol* (2015) 26(5):1195–204. doi:10.1681/ASN.2014010096
168. Heinen S, Sanchez-Corral P, Jackson MS, Strain L, Goodship JA, Kemp EJ, et al. De novo gene conversion in the RCA gene cluster (1q32) causes mutations in complement factor H associated with atypical hemolytic uremic syndrome. *Hum Mutat* (2006) 27(3):292–3. doi:10.1002/humu.9408
169. Venables JP, Strain L, Routledge D, Bourn D, Powell HM, Warwicker P, et al. Atypical haemolytic uraemic syndrome associated with a hybrid complement gene. *PLoS Med* (2006) 3(10):e431. doi:10.1371/journal.pmed.0030431
170. Maga TK, Meyer NC, Belsha C, Nishimura CJ, Zhang Y, Smith RJ. A novel deletion in the RCA gene cluster causes atypical hemolytic uremic syndrome. *Nephrol Dial Transplant* (2011) 26(2):739–41. doi:10.1093/ndt/gfq658
171. Eyler SJ, Meyer NC, Zhang Y, Xiao X, Nester CM, Smith RJ. A novel hybrid CFHR1/CFH gene causes atypical hemolytic uremic syndrome. *Pediatr Nephrol* (2013) 28(11):2221–5. doi:10.1007/s00467-013-2560-2
172. Valoti E, Alberti M, Tortajada A, Garcia-Fernandez J, Gastoldi S, Besso L, et al. A novel atypical hemolytic uremic syndrome-associated hybrid CFHR1/CFH gene encoding a fusion protein that antagonizes factor H-dependent complement regulation. *J Am Soc Nephrol* (2015) 26(1):209–19. doi:10.1681/ASN.2013121339
173. Goicoechea de Jorge E, Tortajada A, Garcia SP, Gastoldi S, Merinero HM, Garcia-Fernandez J, et al. Factor H competitor generated by gene conversion events associates with atypical hemolytic uremic syndrome. *J Am Soc Nephrol* (2018) 29(1):240–9. doi:10.1681/ASN.2017050518
174. Francis NJ, McNicholas B, Awan A, Waldron M, Reddan D, Sadlier D, et al. A novel hybrid CFH/CFHR3 gene generated by a microhomology-mediated deletion in familial atypical hemolytic uremic syndrome. *Blood* (2012) 119(2):591–601. doi:10.1182/blood-2011-03-339903
175. Challis RC, Araujo GS, Wong EK, Anderson HE, Awan A, Dorman AM, et al. A De Novo deletion in the regulators of complement activation cluster producing a hybrid complement factor H/complement factor H-related 3 gene in atypical hemolytic uremic syndrome. *J Am Soc Nephrol* (2016) 27(6):1617–24. doi:10.1681/ASN.2015010100
176. Gale DP, de Jorge EG, Cook HT, Martinez-Barricarte R, Hadjisavvas A, McLean AG, et al. Identification of a mutation in complement factor H-related protein 5 in patients of Cypriot origin with glomerulonephritis. *Lancet* (2010) 376(9743):794–801. doi:10.1016/S0140-6736(10)60670-8
177. Athanasiou Y, Voskarides K, Gale DP, Damianou L, Patsias C, Zavros M, et al. Familial C3 glomerulopathy associated with CFHR5 mutations: clinical characteristics of 91 patients in 16 pedigrees. *Clin J Am Soc Nephrol* (2011) 6(6):1436–46. doi:10.2215/CJN.09541010
178. Vernon KA, Gale DP, de Jorge EG, McLean AG, Galliford J, Pierides A, et al. Recurrence of complement factor H-related protein 5 nephropathy in a renal transplant. *Am J Transplant* (2011) 11(1):152–5. doi:10.1111/j.1600-6143.2010.03333.x
179. Medjeral-Thomas N, Malik TH, Patel MP, Toth T, Cook HT, Tomson C, et al. A novel CFHR5 fusion protein causes C3 glomerulopathy in a family without Cypriot ancestry. *Kidney Int* (2014) 85(4):933–7. doi:10.1038/ki.2013.348
180. Tortajada A, Gutierrez-Tenorio J, Saiz Gonzalez A, Marcen Letosa R, Bouthelier A, Sanchez-Corral P, et al. Novel duplication of the FHRs dimerization domain associated with C3G. *Mol Immunol* (2017) 89:181. doi:10.1016/j.molimm.2017.06.169
181. Malik TH, Lavin PJ, Goicoechea de Jorge E, Vernon KA, Rose KL, Patel MP, et al. A hybrid CFHR3-1 gene causes familial C3 glomerulopathy. *J Am Soc Nephrol* (2012) 23(7):1155–60. doi:10.1681/ASN.2012020166

182. Wong L, Moran S, Lavin PJ, Dorman AM, Conlon PJ. Kidney transplant outcomes in familial C3 glomerulopathy. *Clin Kidney J* (2016) 9(3):403–7. doi:10.1093/ckj/sfw020
183. Dragon-Durey MA, Loirat C, Cloarec S, Macher MA, Blouin J, Nivet H, et al. Anti-factor H autoantibodies associated with atypical hemolytic uremic syndrome. *J Am Soc Nephrol* (2005) 16(2):555–63. doi:10.1681/ASN.2004050380
184. Dragon-Durey MA, Blanc C, Garnier A, Hofer J, Sethi SK, Zimmerhackl LB. Anti-factor H autoantibody-associated hemolytic uremic syndrome: review of literature of the autoimmune form of HUS. *Semin Thromb Hemost* (2010) 36(6):633–40. doi:10.1055/s-0030-1262885
185. Jozsi M, Oppermann M, Lambris JD, Zipfel PF. The C-terminus of complement factor H is essential for host cell protection. *Mol Immunol* (2007) 44(10):2697–706. doi:10.1016/j.molimm.2006.12.001
186. Strobel S, Hoyer PF, Mache CJ, Sulyok E, Liu WS, Richter H, et al. Functional analyses indicate a pathogenic role of factor H autoantibodies in atypical haemolytic uraemic syndrome. *Nephrol Dial Transplant* (2010) 25(1):136–44. doi:10.1093/ndt/gfp388
187. Blanc C, Roumenina LT, Ashraf Y, Hyvarinen S, Sethi SK, Ranchin B, et al. Overall neutralization of complement factor H by autoantibodies in the acute phase of the autoimmune form of atypical hemolytic uremic syndrome. *J Immunol* (2012) 189(7):3528–37. doi:10.4049/jimmunol.1200679
188. Dragon-Durey MA, Blanc C, Marliot F, Loirat C, Blouin J, Sautes-Fridman C, et al. The high frequency of complement factor H related CFHR1 gene deletion is restricted to specific subgroups of patients with atypical haemolytic uraemic syndrome. *J Med Genet* (2009) 46(7):447–50. doi:10.1136/jmg.2008.064766
189. Jozsi M, Licht C, Strobel S, Zipfel SL, Richter H, Heinen S, et al. Factor H autoantibodies in atypical hemolytic uremic syndrome correlate with CFHR1/CFHR3 deficiency. *Blood* (2008) 111(3):1512–4. doi:10.1182/blood-2007-09-109876
190. Nozal P, Garrido S, Alba-Dominguez M, Espinosa L, Pena A, Cordoba SR, et al. An ELISA assay with two monoclonal antibodies allows the estimation of free factor H and identifies patients with acquired deficiency of this complement regulator. *Mol Immunol* (2014) 58(2):194–200. doi:10.1016/j.molimm.2013.11.021
191. Bhattacharjee A, Reuter S, Trojnar E, Kolodziejczyk R, Seeberger H, Hyvarinen S, et al. The major autoantibody epitope on factor H in atypical hemolytic uremic syndrome is structurally different from its homologous site in factor H-related protein 1, supporting a novel model for induction of autoimmunity in this disease. *J Biol Chem* (2015) 290(15):9500–10. doi:10.1074/jbc.M114.630871
192. Nozal P, Bernabeu-Herrero ME, Uzonyi B, Szilagyi A, Hyvarinen S, Prohaszka Z, et al. Heterogeneity but individual constancy of epitopes, isotypes and avidity of factor H autoantibodies in atypical hemolytic uremic syndrome. *Mol Immunol* (2016) 70:47–55. doi:10.1016/j.molimm.2015.12.005
193. Blanc C, Togarsimalemath SK, Chauvet S, Le Quintrec M, Moulin B, Buchler M, et al. Anti-factor H autoantibodies in C3 glomerulopathies and in atypical hemolytic uremic syndrome: one target, two diseases. *J Immunol* (2015) 194(11):5129–38. doi:10.4049/jimmunol.1402770
194. Goodship TH, Pappworth IY, Toth T, Denton M, Houlberg K, McCormick F, et al. Factor H autoantibodies in membranoproliferative glomerulonephritis. *Mol Immunol* (2012) 52(3–4):200–6. doi:10.1016/j.molimm.2012.05.009
195. Jokiranta TS, Solomon A, Pangburn MK, Zipfel PF, Meri S. Nephritogenic lambda light chain dimer: a unique human miniautoantibody against complement factor H. *J Immunol* (1999) 163(8):4590–6.
196. Meri S, Koistinen V, Miettinen A, Tornroth T, Seppala IJ. Activation of the alternative pathway of complement by monoclonal lambda light chains in membranoproliferative glomerulonephritis. *J Exp Med* (1992) 175(4):939–50. doi:10.1084/jem.175.4.939 Epub 1992/04/01.,
197. Nozal P, Strobel S, Ibernon M, López D, Sánchez-Corral P, Rodriguez de Cordoba S, et al. Anti-factor H antibody affecting factor H cofactor activity in a patient with dense deposit disease. *Clin Kidney J* (2012) 5:133–6. doi:10.1093/ckj/sfs002
198. Foltyn Zadura A, Zipfel PF, Bokarewa MI, Sturfelt G, Jonsen A, Nilsson SC, et al. Factor H autoantibodies and deletion of complement factor H-related protein-1 in rheumatic diseases in comparison to atypical hemolytic uremic syndrome. *Arthritis Res Ther* (2012) 14(4):R185. doi:10.1186/ar4016

12

Functional Characterization of Alternative and Classical Pathway C3/C5 Convertase Activity and Inhibition Using Purified Models

Seline A. Zwarthoff[1], Evelien T. M. Berends[1], Sanne Mol[1], Maartje Ruyken[1], Piet C. Aerts[1], Mihály Józsi[2], Carla J. C. de Haas[1], Suzan H. M. Rooijakkers[1†] and Ronald D. Gorham Jr.[1†]*

[1] Department of Medical Microbiology, University Medical Center Utrecht, Utrecht University, Utrecht, Netherlands,
[2] Department of Immunology, ELTE Eötvös Loránd University, Budapest, Hungary

***Correspondence:**
Suzan H. M. Rooijakkers
s.h.m.rooijakkers@umcutrecht.nl

†These authors have contributed equally to this work.

Complement is essential for the protection against infections; however, dysregulation of complement activation can cause onset and progression of numerous inflammatory diseases. Convertase enzymes play a central role in complement activation and produce the key mediators of complement: C3 convertases cleave C3 to generate chemoattractant C3a and label target cells with C3b, which promotes phagocytosis; C5 convertases cleave C5 into chemoattractant C5a, and C5b, which drives formation of the membrane attack complex. Since convertases mediate nearly all complement effector functions, they are ideal targets for therapeutic complement inhibition. A unique feature of convertases is their covalent attachment to target cells, which effectively confines complement activation to the cell surface. However, surface localization precludes detailed analysis of convertase activation and inhibition. In our previous work, we developed a model system to form purified alternative pathway (AP) C5 convertases on C3b-coated beads and quantify C5 conversion *via* functional analysis of released C5a. Here, we developed a C3aR cell reporter system that enables functional discrimination between C3 and C5 convertases. By regulating the C3b density on the bead surface, we observe that high C3b densities are important for conversion of C5, but not C3, by AP convertases. Screening of well-characterized complement-binding molecules revealed that differential inhibition of AP C3 convertases (C3bBb) and C5 convertases [C3bBb(C3b)$_n$] is possible. Although both convertases contain C3b, the C3b-binding molecules Efb-C/Ecb and FHR5 specifically inhibit C5 conversion. Furthermore, using a new classical pathway convertase model, we show that these C3b-binding proteins not only block AP C3/C5 convertases but also inhibit formation of a functional classical pathway C5 convertase under well-defined conditions. Our models enable functional characterization of purified convertase enzymes and provide a platform for the identification and development of specific convertase inhibitors for treatment of complement-mediated disorders.

Keywords: innate immunity, inflammatory disease, convertase enzymes, complement, complement therapeutics, multi-molecular proteases

INTRODUCTION

The human complement system comprises a family of proteins that are essential to the human immune response against infections (1). Complement recognizes microbes or damaged host cells and subsequently triggers an enzymatic cascade that mainly serves to (a) label target cells for phagocytosis by immune cells, (b) produce chemoattractants, and (c) directly kill target cells *via* pore formation (2). Unwanted complement activation on the body's own cells is a key pathological driver in a wide spectrum of immune diseases including autoimmune, inflammatory, and degenerative diseases (3–5). For current and future development of therapeutic complement inhibitors, knowledge of complement activation and how it can be regulated is of great importance.

Convertase enzymes fulfill a central role in the complement cascade as they cleave C3 and C5, which mediate nearly all complement effector functions. C3 convertases cleave C3 into C3a, a chemoattractant molecule, and C3b, which covalently binds to target surfaces and triggers phagocytosis. C5 convertases cleave C5 into C5a, a potent mediator of leukocyte recruitment and inflammation, and C5b, the initiator of the membrane attack complex and cell lysis. The complement cascade begins *via* specific recognition of target cells in the classical (CP) and lectin (LP) pathways. In the CP, antibodies bind epitopes on the target cell and subsequently recruit the C1 complex ($C1qr_2s_2$). Upon binding to the antibody platforms (6), C1q-associated protease C1s converts C4 and C2 to generate a C3 convertase enzyme (C4b2a) on the cell surface (**Figure 1A**). Similarly, the lectin

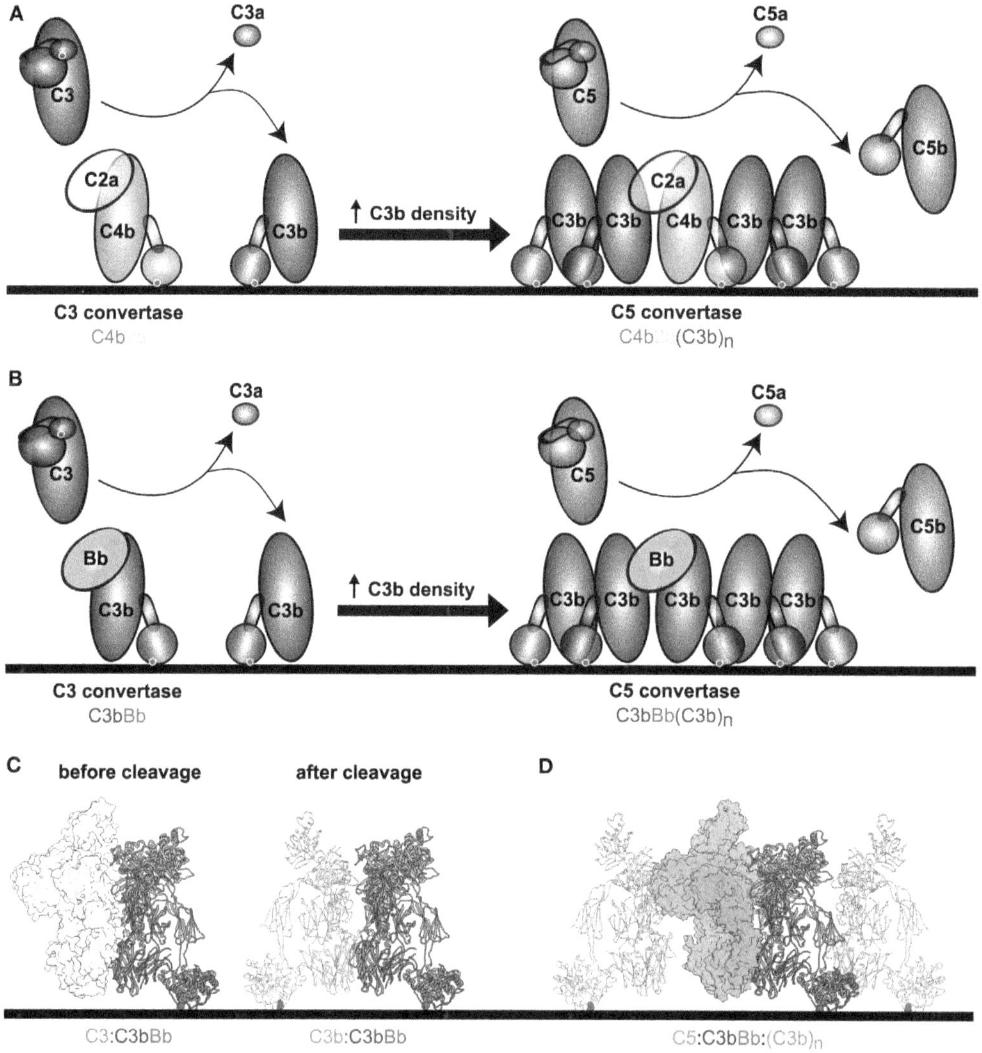

FIGURE 1 | Complement convertases mediate C3 and C5 conversion. **(A)** Upon complement activation, C3 convertases consisting of either C4b2a (CP and LP) or **(B)** C3bBb [alternative pathway (AP)] form on the cell surface. Conversion of C3 results in deposition of C3b molecules *via* the thioester (red dot), which form the basis for new AP convertases (amplification loop) or associate with existing C3 convertases to form C5 convertases. These accessory C3b molecules ($C3b_n$) enable efficient C5 conversion, however, the molecular mechanisms underlying this process are not clear. Shown are C4b (purple), C2a (blue), C3 and cleavage products C3b/C3a (gray), Factor B (orange), C5 and cleavage products C5b/C5a (green). **(C)** Structural models of the C3 convertase C3bBb with its substrate C3 before and after cleavage. Models are based on structures of the C3bBb-SCIN dimer (PDB: 2WIN). The convertase is shown in ribbon representation, with C3b in dark gray and Bb in orange. On the left, the substrate C3 (light gray surface) is shown before cleavage. On the right, the product C3b (light gray licorice) is shown after cleavage. The red dots highlight the thioester. **(D)** Structural model of the previously proposed AP C5 convertase with its substrate C5. At a high density of C3b molecules, C5 is recruited to the target surface and can be cleaved after binding of Bb to C3b. The exact molecular arrangement of the C5 convertases remains unknown. This structural model is based on the CVF-C5 crystal structure (PDB: 3PVM), with accessory C3b molecules added manually surrounding the convertase and C5. CVF (cobra venom factor) is a C3b homolog that lacks the thioester domain and forms stable C5 convertases when associated with Bb in solution. Structure is shown in ribbon representation with C3b (dark gray), Bb (orange), accessory C3b molecules (light gray licorice), and C5 (green surface).

pathway also forms C4b2a *via* activation of mannose-binding lectin-associated serine proteases. The resulting CP/LP C4b2a convertases cleave C3 into C3a and C3b. Following cleavage, a reactive thioester in C3b is exposed, which enables its covalent attachment to target cell surfaces, leading to recognition of the cells by phagocytes. The labeling of target cells with C3b is amplified by the alternative pathway (AP) in which surface-bound C3b binds factor B (FB). The proconvertase C3bB is then cleaved by factor D (FD) to form an active C3 convertase complex that consists of C3b and the protease fragment Bb (C3bBb) (**Figure 1B**). Since the resulting active AP C3 convertase (C3bBb) is comprised of C3b itself, substrate cleavage results in generation of additional convertases, further propagating C3b deposition (**Figure 1B**). When the density of C3b molecules on the cell surface becomes sufficiently high, the existing C3 convertases (C4b2a and C3bBb) gain the ability to cleave C5, leading to formation of C5a and C5b (**Figures 1A,B**) (7, 8).

Selective inhibition of C3 and C5 convertases is of great therapeutic interest. Most complement inhibitors currently used in the clinic or in clinical development target precursor (not yet activated) complement proteins, that circulate through the body and do not mediate complement effector functions (4). Due to high concentrations of these precursor proteins, effective therapeutic concentrations of complement inhibitors are often quite high, and clearance of these molecules is enhanced due to rapid turnover of complement proteins. Furthermore, saturation of precursor proteins is more likely to systemically suppress complement activation, leading to increased susceptibility to infection (4). Such therapies would be more effective if they specifically targeted active protein complexes like convertases that are primarily formed during complement activation on target cell surfaces. While some therapeutic molecules inhibit convertase function, these likely inhibit multiple convertase enzymes and block all effector functions of complement (4). In some cases, specific inhibition of C5 convertases is desirable for complement therapy, since blocking these would prevent unwanted formation of the major inflammatory trigger C5a but leave C3b deposition *via* C3 convertases intact and thus phagocytosis of bacteria. However, the molecular details of C5 convertase formation and C5 cleavage remain poorly understood, largely due to the transient nature of convertases and the fact that efficient C5 conversion is constrained to cell surfaces (7, 9). Several earlier studies successfully investigated individual convertases in purified or semi-purified environments (10–14), however, no single model can fully characterize activity and inhibition of both AP and CP C3 and C5 convertases in a purified and controlled environment. Herein, we extended our recently developed model system for AP C5 convertases (7) to also study surface-bound AP C3 convertases, in order to screen for specific inhibitors of convertase enzymes. Furthermore, we developed functional analyses to study CP C3 and C5 convertases using purified complement proteins. Using these models, we can evaluate how known complement inhibitors affect C3/C5 conversion. In these analyses, we included bacterial and therapeutic complement inhibitors, and human complement regulatory proteins that protect healthy tissue from complement attack (8, 15–18). The analyses reveal that several C3b-binding molecules can discriminate between C3 and C5 convertases, suggesting that it is possible to develop more specific convertase inhibitors in the future. Through comparison of our inhibitory data with previously reported structural and biochemical data, we further postulate molecular models of convertase formation.

MATERIALS AND METHODS

Complement Proteins

C3 and C5 were prepared from human plasma as previously described (7). For CP assays and inhibitor dose-response assays, recombinant C5 was used. C5 with a C-terminal His-tag was therefore cloned from gBlocks (Integrated DNA Technologies) using Gibson assembly (Gibco), expressed in HEK293 cells (U-Protein Express, Utrecht, The Netherlands) and purified on a HisTrap column (GE Healthcare). $C3b_{H2O}$ and C3b-PEG11-biotin were prepared as previously described using 180 μg/ml maleimide-PEG11-biotin for the latter (Thermo Scientific Pierce Protein Research, IK, USA) (7). Methylamine-treated C3 ($C3_{MA}$) was prepared by mixing 2.7 μM C3 with 300 mM methylamine hydrochloride (Sigma Aldrich) in VBS^{++} buffer (Veronal Buffered Saline pH 7.4, 0.25 mM $MgCl_2$, 0.5 mM $CaCl_2$). This reaction was incubated at 37°C for 1 h and dialyzed overnight to VBS^{++} buffer at 4°C. FB with N-terminal His-tag and FD were expressed recombinantly as previously described (U-Protein Express, Utrecht, The Netherlands) (7). C4 was isolated from blood from a healthy individual that was anti-coagulated with 20 mM EDTA. Plasma was collected and protease inhibitors (10 mM benzamidine, 1 mM PMSF, 7.5 μM SBTI, EDTA 5 mM, 2.1 mM Pefabloc SC, 30 μM NPGB) were added quickly, while stirring the plasma at 4°C. To remove large complexes, plasma was precipitated with 4% PEG 6000, which was added slowly to the plasma for 45 min. After centrifugation, the supernatant was isolated from which plasminogen was removed by adding 20 mM EDTA and Lysine-Sepharose and incubation for 1 h at 4°C. From the supernatant, C4 was isolated by SourceQ anion exchange. Loading was performed in 50 mM Tris–HCl, 100 mM NaCl, pH 8.0 (containing 1 mM benzamidine, 1 mM PMSF, 30 mM EACA, and 5 mM EDTA) after which C4 was eluted in a gradient of 100–500 mM NaCl in 50 mM Tris–HCl, 100 mM NaCl, pH 8.0 (containing 1 mM benzamidine, 1 mM PMSF, 30 mM EACA, and 5 mM EDTA). Fractions were analyzed by 10% SDS-PAGE following Instant Blue (Roche) protein staining according to the manufacturer's instructions. C2 with a N-terminal His-tag was expressed in HEK293 cells stably expressing EBNA1 (HEK293E) as described (U-Protein Express, Utrecht, The Netherlands) (19). C2 was purified from expression medium *via* immobilized metal affinity chromatography using a HisTrap column (GE Healthcare). C1 was obtained from Complement Technology Inc. (TX, USA).

Complement-Binding Molecules and Proteins

FH and C4b-binding protein (C4BP) were ordered *via* Complement Technology Inc. (Tyler, TX, USA). FHR5 was purchased at R&D systems (Minneapolis, MN, USA). Eculizumab was obtained *via* Genmab (Utrecht, The Netherlands). Cp40 was kindly provided by John Lambris. CRIg was kindly provided by Genentech (South San Francisco, CA, USA). OmCI was produced in HEK293E cells and purified as described previously (20). Efb-C and Efb-C mutant (Efb-C-R131E/N138E) were prepared as previously described (21, 22), as well as Ecb, Ecb mutant (Ecb-N63E/R75E/N82E) (23), and SSL7 (24).

Human Monoclonal Antibodies

Monoclonal human anti-DNP-IgG1 was produced recombinantly in human Expi293F cells (Life Technologies). Therefore, the variable region of the heavy chain (>VH7007-DNP-G2a2: DVRLQESGPGLVKPSQSLSLTCSVTGYSITNSYYWNWIRQF PGNKLEWMVYIGYDGSNNYNPSLKNRISITRDT SKNQFFLKLNSVTTEDTATYYCARATYYGNYRGFAYWGQ GTLVTVSA) and light chain (>VL7007-DNP-G2a2: DIRMTQT TSSLSASLGDRVTISCRASQDISNYLNWYQQKPDGTVKLLIY YTSRLHSGVPSRFSGSGSGTDYSLTISNLEQEDIATYFCQQG NTLPWTFGGGTKLEIK) (25) were cloned in the pFUSE-CHIg-hG1 and pFUSE2-CLIg-hk vector, respectively, according to the manufacturer's description (Invivogen). A KOZAK sequence and the HAVT20 signal peptide (MACPGFLWALVISTCLEFSMA) were included upstream each variable region. Human codon optimized sequences were ordered as gBlocks (Integrated DNA Technologies) for Gibson assembly (Bioke). TOP10F′ *E. coli* were used for propagation of the plasmids. After sequence, verification plasmids were isolated using NucleoBond Xtra Midi plasmid DNA purification (Macherey-Nagel). Transfection of EXPI293F cells was performed using ExpiFectamine 293 reagent according to the manufacturer's description (Life Technologies). 1 μg DNA/ml cells was used in a 3:2 (hk:hG1) ratio. Cell supernatant was collected after 4 days of transfection and antibodies were isolated using a HiTrap protein A column (GE Healthcare).

U937 Cell Lines

U937 human monocyte cells and 293 T human embryonic kidney cells were obtained from American Type Culture Collection and grown (37°C, 5% CO_2) in RPMI (Lonza) supplemented with penicillin and streptomycin (Gibco) and 10% FCS (Gibco). For stable expression of human C3aR in U937 cells, a lentiviral expression system was used. The human C3aR cDNA was cloned in a dual promoter lentiviral vector, derived from no. 2025.pCCLsin.PPT.pA.CTE.4x-scrT.eGFP.mCMV.hPGK. NGFR.pre (kindly provided by Dr. Luigi Naldini, San Raffaele Scientific Institute, Milan, Italy) as previously described (26). This altered lentiviral vector (BIC-PGK-Zeo-T2a-mAmetrine; EF1A) uses the human EF1A promoter to facilitate potent expression in immune cells and expresses the fluorescent protein mAmetrine and selection marker ZeoR. Virus was produced in 24-well plates using standard lentiviral production protocols and the third-generation packaging vectors pMD2G-VSVg, pRSV-REV, and pMDL/RRE. Briefly, 0.25 μg lentiviral vector and 0.25 μg packaging vectors were co-transfected in 293 T cells by using 1.5 μl Mirus LT1 tranfection reagent (Sopachem, Ochten, The Netherlands). After 72 h, 100 μl viral supernatant adjusted to 8 mg/ml polybrene was used to infect ~50,000 U937 cells by spin infection at 1,000 g for 2 h at 33°C. U937-C5aR cells were a generous gift from Eric Prossnitz (University of New Mexico, Albuquerque, NM, USA).

C3 and C5 Conversion in AP Model

Streptavidin-coated magnetic beads (Dynabeads M-270 Streptavidin, Invitrogen) were washed once in VBS-T/Mg [Veronal Buffered Saline pH 7.4, 2.5 mM $MgCl_2$, 0.05% (v/v) Tween]. To prepare fully loaded C3b-beads, beads (4 μl/sample) were resuspended in 0.4 ml VBS-T/Mg per sample with C3b-PEG11-biotin (1 μg/ml) and incubated for 1 h at 4°C on roller. To load beads with different amounts of C3b, five different amounts of beads per sample (4, 8, 16, 32, or 64 μl beads) were incubated in 0.4 ml VBS-T/Mg with 0.6 μg/ml C3b-PEG11-biotin. After C3b-labeling, beads were washed three times and incubated in 100 μl VBS-T/Mg per sample with FB (50 μg/ml) for 30 min at room temperature on roller. After FB incubation, beads were washed three times and incubated in 100 μl VBS-T/Mg per sample with FD (5 μg/ml) and either C3 (20 μg/ml) or C5 (20 μg/ml) and with or without inhibitor at the desired concentration (1 μM or threefold dilution starting from 1 μM) for 1 h at 37°C on shaker. After incubation, supernatant of each sample was collected and kept at −20°C until measurement in calcium mobilization assay.

C3 and C5 Conversion in CP Model

Streptavidin-coated magnetic beads (Dynabeads M-270 Streptavidin, Invitrogen) were washed once in PBS-TH [Phosphate Buffered Saline pH 7.4, 0.05% (v/v) Tween, 0.5% HSA]. Beads (4 μl/sample) were resuspended in 0.4 ml PBS-TH per sample with 1 μg/ml biotinylated 2,4-dinitrophenol [DNP-PEG2-GSGS GSGK(Biotin)-NH2; 1,186 Da; obtained from Pepscan Therapeutics B.V., The Netherlands] and incubated for 30 min at 4°C on roller. Beads were washed once in PBS-TH and incubated in 0.2 ml PBS-TH per sample with 10 nM human monoclonal anti-DNP-IgG1 for 30 min at 4°C on roller.

After one wash in PBS-TH, beads were incubated in 0.1 ml VBS^{++}-TH [Veronal Buffered Saline pH 7.4, 0.25 mM $MgCl_2$, 0.5 mM $CaCl_2$, 0.05% (v/v) Tween, 0.5% HSA] per sample with 0.8 μg/ml C1 for 30 min at 37°C, shaking. Beads were washed three times in VBS^{++}-TH and incubated in 0.1 ml VBS^{++}-TH per sample with 10 μg/ml C4 for 30 min at 37°C, shaking. After three washes in VBS^{++}-TH, beads were incubated in 0.1 ml VBS^{++}-TH per sample with 10 μg/ml C2, 10 μg/ml C3, and 0.5 μg/ml C5 with or without 1 μM inhibitor for 5 min at 37°C on shaker. After incubation, the supernatant of each sample was collected and kept at −20°C until measurement in calcium mobilization assay.

In some CP experiments, the amount of deposited C3b was influenced by adding lower concentrations of C3 (threefold decrease starting from 10 μg/ml). In one condition, C3 and C5 conversion were separated by incubating beads first in 0.1 ml VBS^{++}-TH per sample with 10 μg/ml C2 and 10 μg/ml C3 for 5 min at 37°C and subsequently, after washing, in 0.1 ml VBS^{++}-TH with 10 μg/ml C2 and 0.5 μg/ml C5 for 5 min at 37°C. Supernatant of both C2 + C3 and C2 + C5 incubation were here collected and used for calcium mobilization in U937-C3aR and U937-C5aR cells, respectively. Controls were carried out with 10 μg/ml $C3b_{H2O}$ or 10 μg/ml $C3_{MA}$.

Calcium Mobilization Assay With U937 Cells

U937-C3aR and U937-C5aR cells were washed in RPMI/0.05% HSA and diluted to 5×10^6 cells/ml. Cells were incubated with 0.5 μM Fluo-3-AM (Invitrogen) on roller in dark at room temperature for 20 min, washed and resuspended in RPMI/1% HSA to a final concentration of 1×10^6 cells/ml. For calcium mobilization measurements, the labeled cells were stimulated with sample supernatant (ratio cells to supernatant is 9:1) while cell fluorescence is measured by flow cytometry (BD FACSVerse) from 10 s before until 40 s after addition of the sample. The absolute calcium mobilization was calculated by subtracting the cell mean fluorescence intensity (MFI) before cell activation (t = 5–15 s) from the MFI after stimulation (t = 30–50 s) using FlowJo software. Standard curves were obtained using 10-fold dilutions starting from 1 μM of C3a (Complement Technology Inc., TX, USA) or C5a (Bachem, Switzerland) as stimuli for the cells. As negative controls the calcium mobilization in U937-C3aR and U937-C5aR cells induced by 0.1 μM C3 or C5 was measured.

C3b Binding to Beads

To determine the level of C3b-biotin bound to streptavidin-coated beads in the AP model or the level of actively deposited C3b in the CP model, beads were washed three times in PBS-T (AP) or PBS-TH (CP) after the C3b-biotin or C3 incubation and incubated (4 μl beads/sample) in 100 μl PBS-TH per sample with 1:100 FITC-conjugated goat-anti-human C3 (Protos) for 30 min at 4°C. Subsequently, beads were washed three times in PBS-T (AP) or PBS-TH (CP) and C3b binding was analyzed by flow cytometry (BD FACSVerse).

Statistical Analysis

Statistical analysis was performed with GraphPad Prism 6 software. All calcium flux data are presented as mean ± SD from three independent experiments. C3b binding data are presented as geometric mean ± SD from three independent experiments.

RESULTS

Functional Analysis of C3 Conversion *via* Purified AP Convertases

Previously, we described the development of a model system to study C5 convertases of the AP using purified components (7). The AP C5 convertase is formed when C3 convertases (C3bBb) cleave C3 into nascent C3b that covalently binds to target surfaces *via* the thioester (structural model in **Figure 1C**) (27). At a critical density of C3b molecules, multimeric $C3b_n$ complexes arise that have a high affinity for C5. These $C3b_n$ complexes, together with FB and FD, generate C5 convertases that bind and cleave C5 (**Figure 1D**). We recently set out to mimic surface-bound high C3b-density using purified proteins. To establish this, we first labeled C3b with biotin *via* the thioester by activating plasma-purified C3 into C3b in the presence of a biotinylation agent that reacts with the cysteine residue of the C3b thioester (28). These biotinylated C3b molecules were subsequently loaded onto small magnetic streptavidin (SA) beads (2.8 μm diameter) and incubated with FB and FD to form surface-bound convertases. C5 conversion was examined by quantifying the release of C5a using a flow cytometry-based calcium mobilization assay (29, 30). In short, U937 cells transfected with the C5a receptor (U937-C5aR) were exposed to sample supernatants containing C5a. Binding of C5a to the C5a receptor mediates intracellular calcium release, which is detected by a fluorescent indicator. To get more insights into convertase formation and inhibition, we here extended this model to also study C3 conversion by purified AP convertases. First, we transfected U937 cells with the C3a receptor (U937-C3aR) and showed that purified C3a, but not C3, successfully triggers the mobilization of intracellular calcium in U937-C3aR cells (**Figure 2A**). Low-level activation by purified C5a is likely due to low levels of endogenous C5aR expression in these cells (**Figure 2A**). Second, C3b-coated beads were incubated with FB, FD and C3 and release of C3a was determined in supernatants *via* calcium mobilization in U937-C3aR (**Figure 2B**). C3a-dependent calcium flux specifically required all convertase components. In our previous study, we determined that high C3b-density is essential to effectively convert C5 (7). By maintaining a constant concentration of C3b in each sample while increasing the number of beads, we artificially lowered the local concentration of C3b on the surface (Figure S1 in Supplementary Material). Here, we find that while lowering C3b surface density reduces C5 conversion by AP convertases, it does not lead to less C3 conversion (**Figure 2C**). These results demonstrate key differences in the conditions required for C3 and C5 conversion on a surface in the AP.

Select C3b-Binding Molecules Inhibit AP C5 but Not C3 Conversion

Having established a system to study both C3 and C5 conversion by AP convertases, we could now dissect whether known convertase inhibitory molecules block cleavage of both substrates. We focused on studying C3b- or C5-binding molecules for which the binding sites to C3b/C5 have been determined. Each of these molecules has been extensively characterized in previous studies and is known to influence convertase activity in physiological environments (**Table 1**). The structures of the C3b-binding molecules in complex with the C3bBb convertase are shown in **Figure 3A**. The inhibitors include naturally occurring complement inhibitors derived from humans [C3b-binders CRIg (31, 32), FH (33, 34), and FHR5 (35)], bacteria [homologous C3b-binders Efb-C (36) and Ecb (16, 23) and C5-binder SSL7 (37)], and ticks [C5-binder OmCI (20)], or therapeutic inhibitors eculizumab [Soliris, a clinically approved antibody against C5 (38)] and Cp40 [a compstatin analog, strong C3- and C3b-binding molecule (39)]. As expected, we observed that the three C5-binding molecules SSL7, OmCI, and eculizumab specifically interfered with C5 conversion but not C3 conversion (**Figure 3B**). C4BP (40) was included as a negative control for inhibition, as it should not have an effect on AP C3 or C5 convertases, since these convertases lack C4b (**Figure 3B**). Next, we analyzed the activity of C3b-binding molecules on C3 versus

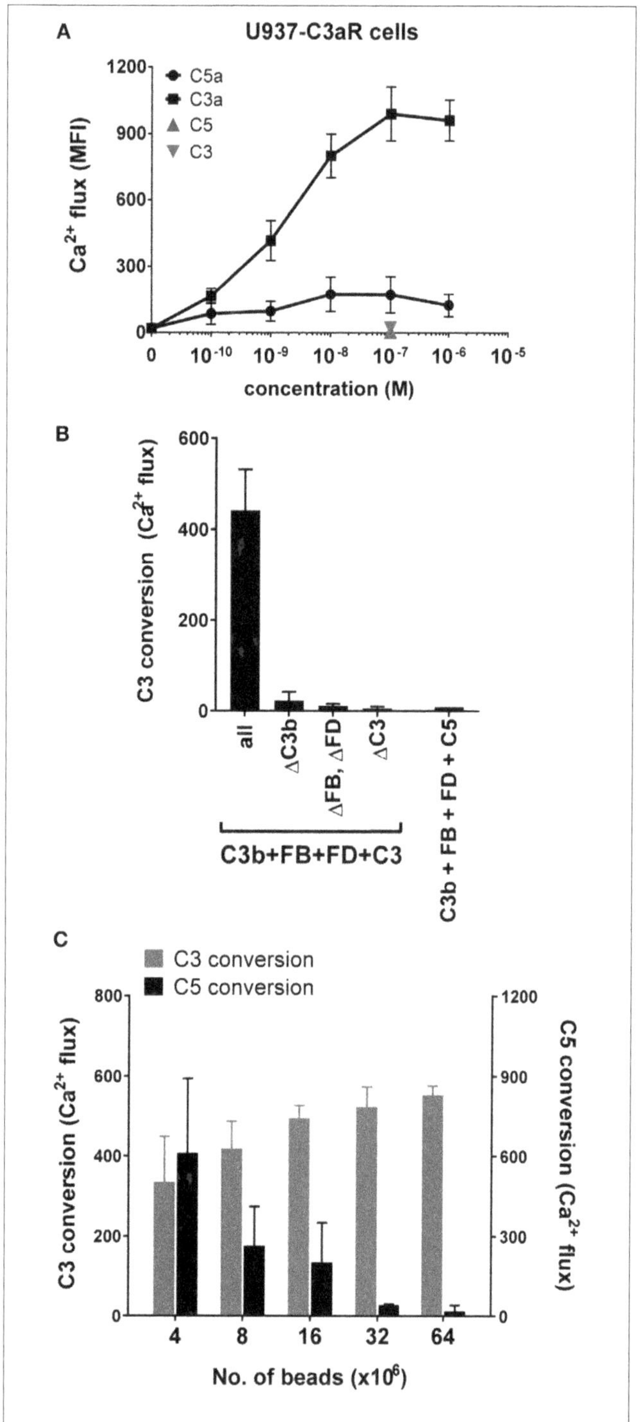

FIGURE 2 | Development of an alternative pathway (AP) C3 convertase model. **(A)** C3a specifically induces calcium mobilization in U937-C3aR cells, while C3 and C5 do not. **(B)** C3 conversion by AP convertases on beads was analyzed in a calcium mobilization assay with U937-C3aR cells. C3a could only be detected in the sample supernatant in the presence of all AP components. C5 conversion in the AP model did not induce calcium flux in the U937-C3aR cells. **(C)** AP C3 and C5 conversion were performed on beads coated with different densities of C3b and analyzed by calcium mobilization assay with U937-C3aR and -C5aR cells, respectively. A high density of C3b molecules on the target surface enhances C5 but not C3 conversion. **(A–C)** Data of three independent experiments, presented as mean ± SD.

TABLE 1 | Overview of complement inhibitors used in this study.

Inhibitor		Type	Key references
C3b-binding molecules			
Cp40	Compstatin (analog Cp40)	Cyclic peptide	(39, 41, 42)
CRIg	Complement receptor of immunoglobulin family	Human complement regulator protein	(31, 32)
FH	Factor H	Human complement regulator protein	(33, 34, 43, 44)
FHR5	Factor H related-protein 5	Human complement regulator protein	(35, 45)
Efb-C	(C-terminal region of) Extracellular fibrinogen binding protein	*Staphylococcus aureus* immune evasion protein	(21, 36, 46)
Ecb	Extracellular complement binding protein (also known as Ehp)	*Staphylococcus aureus* immune evasion protein	(16, 23)
C5-binding molecules			
SSL7	Staphylococcal superantigen-like protein 7	*Staphylococcus aureus* immune evasion protein	(37, 47, 48)
OmCI	Ornithodoros moubata complement inhibitory protein	*Ornithodoros moubata* immune evasion protein	(20, 49, 50)
Eculizumab	Also known as Soliris	Humanized monoclonal antibody	(38, 51, 52)
C4b-binding molecules			
C4BP	C4b-binding protein	Human complement regulator protein	(40, 53, 54)

C5 conversion. While C3b-binding molecules Cp40, CRIg, and FH blocked both C3 and C5 conversion by AP convertases, host regulatory protein FHR5, and staphylococcal immune evasion proteins Efb-C and Ecb specifically blocked C5 conversion, while leaving C3 conversion unaffected (**Figure 3C**). Mutants of Efb-C/Ecb proteins that cannot bind C3b could not inhibit C5 conversion, confirming that the observed inhibition is mediated through interaction with C3b (**Figure 3C**) (21, 23). Furthermore, Efb-C, Ecb, and FHR5 all inhibit AP C5 conversion in a concentration-dependent manner (**Figure 3E**), but do not affect C3 conversion (**Figure 3D**). As a control, we observed that Cp40, which showed inhibition of both AP C3 and C5 conversion at 1 μM concentration, also inhibits both C3 and C5 conversion in a concentration-dependent manner (**Figures 3D,E**). Thus, these data suggest that by binding C3b, selective inhibition of AP C5 convertases is possible. AP C5 convertases are similar to AP C3 convertases, but contain accessory C3b molecules ($C3b_n$) that enable efficient C5 conversion on surfaces. Since Efb-C, Ecb, and FHR5 only affect C5 (and not C3) conversion, they likely inhibit through affecting accessory C3b molecules on the bead surface. However, the fact that AP C3 and C5 convertases both contain C3b confounds the ability to independently study the role of accessory C3b molecules in C5 conversion.

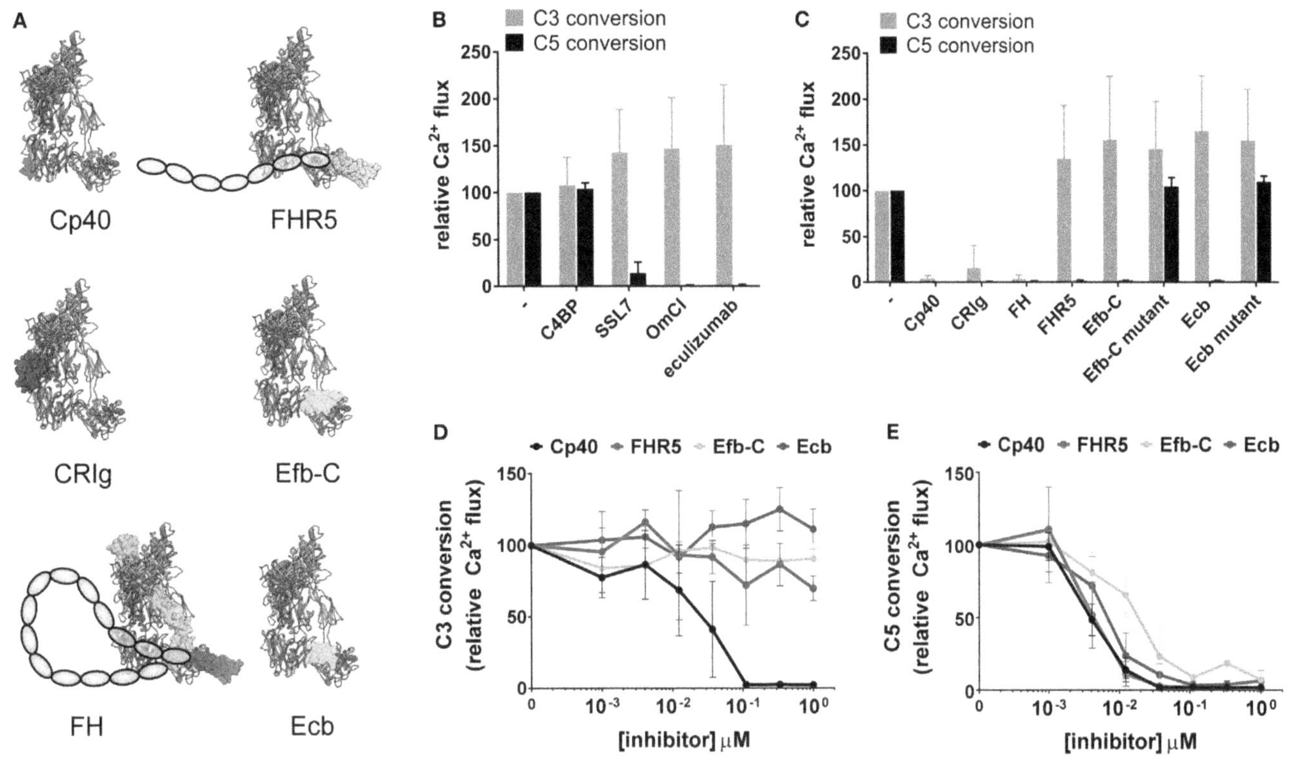

FIGURE 3 | C3b-binding molecules FHR5 and Efb-C/Ecb selectively inhibit C5 conversion by alternative pathway (AP) convertases. **(A)** Structural models of the C3bBb convertase with C3b-binding molecules. The structure of C3bBb [from the C3bBb-SCIN dimer structure, PDB 2WIN (55)] is identical to the convertase shown in **Figures 1C,D** with C3b (gray) and Bb (orange) shown as ribbons, and in the same orientation, with the C3b–C3b dimerization site (as shown in **Figure 1C**, right) on the left side of the convertase. C3b-binding molecules are shown as molecular surfaces; Cp40 (magenta) is based on the C3c–compstatin complex structure [PDB 2QKI (41)], CRIg (dark red) is based on the C3b–CRIg complex structure [PDB 2ICF (31)], FH is based on the C3b–FH (1–4) structure [light blue, PDB 2WII (43)] and the C3d–FH (19–20) structure [dark blue, PDB 2XQW (44)], FHR5 (yellow) is modeled from the C3d–FH (19–20) structure [PDB 2XQW (44)], Efb-C (spring green) is based on the C3d–Efb-C structure [PDB 2GOX (21)], and Ecb (spring green) is based on the C3d–Ehp structure [PDB 2NOJ (23)]. For FH and FHR5 only some domains are structurally resolved. Additional domains are represented by colored ovals. **(B–E)** Conversion of C3 and C5 (0.1 μM) in the AP convertase model in the presence of complement-binding molecules measured by calcium mobilization in U937-C3aR and U937-C5aR cells, respectively. Conversion is shown as a percentage relative to the control without inhibitor. Data of three independent experiments, presented as mean ± SD. **(B)** C5-binding molecules SSL7, OmCI, and eculizumab (all 1 μM) inhibit AP C5 but not C3 conversion. C4b-binding protein has no effect in the AP model. **(C)** C3b-binding molecules Cp40, CRIg, and FH prevent both C3 and C5 conversion, while FHR5, Efb-C, and Ecb selectively inhibit C5 conversion. Mutant Efb-C and mutant Ecb are unable to bind C3b and thus do not exhibit inhibition. **(D)** FHR5, Efb-C, and Ecb do not affect C3 conversion, but **(E)** selectively inhibit C5 conversion in a dose-dependent manner. Cp40 was used as positive control, inhibiting both C3 and C5 conversion.

Development of a Purified Classical Pathway C3/C5 Convertase Model

To more closely investigate convertase inhibitory mechanisms of complement inhibitors, we next developed a model to study C3/C5 conversion *via* purified CP convertases. In this pathway, modulation of accessory C3b molecules can be better analyzed since the CP C3 convertase (C4b2a) does not contain C3b. We have used a model that fully recapitulates the CP activation pathway using purified complement components. Streptavidin beads were labeled with biotinylated DNP antigen (**Figure 4A**) and sequentially incubated with recombinant human IgG1 recognizing DNP, C1, C4, C2 and substrates C3 and C5. Similar to the AP, we detected the release of C3a and C5a in the sample supernatant *via* calcium mobilization in U937-C3aR and U937-C5aR cells, respectively. The lack of calcium mobilization by the sample supernatants in the absence of DNP, IgG or the individual complement proteins demonstrates the necessity of functional CP convertases on the bead surface for C3/C5 cleavage (**Figure 4B**). Our results also showed that there was no cross-reactivity between mismatched ligands and receptors. The absence of calcium flux in U937-C5aR cells by samples lacking C5 (and thus C5a) showed that C3a generated in these samples does not interfere with C5a detection. As calcium mobilization levels in U937-C3aR cells were not affected by the presence of C5, interference of C5a with C3a-specific detection could be excluded, as well. Unlike our AP C5 convertase model where we artificially coupled C3b to the bead surface, deposition of C3b in the CP could only be established by natural C3 conversion *via* C4b2a. By adding different concentrations of C3 to beads with naturally formed C4b2a convertases, we influenced the level of C3 conversion and thus C3b deposition on the bead surface (**Figures 4C,D**). Indeed, CP C5 conversion was highly dependent on the level of deposited C3b (**Figure 4E**). As a control, we showed that C5 conversion specifically depends

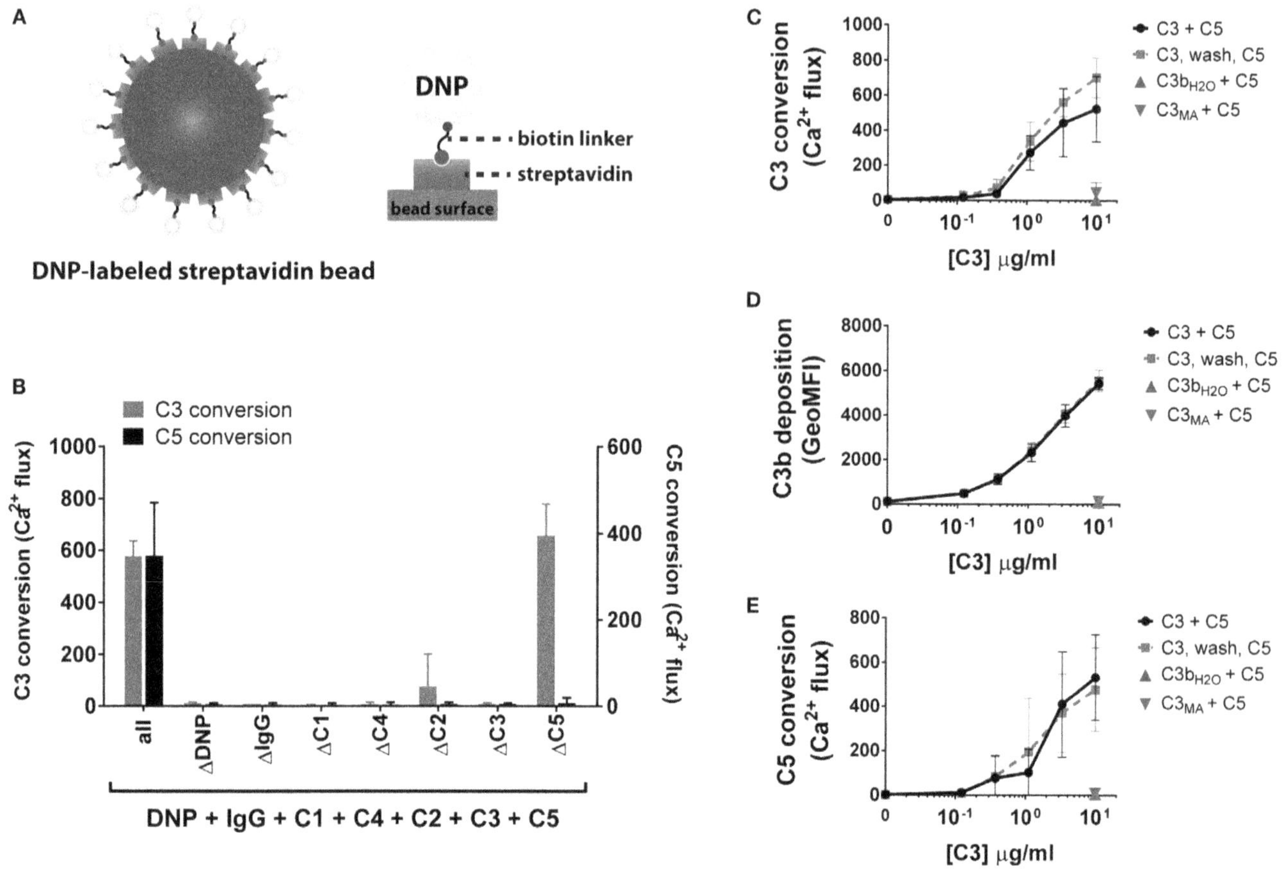

FIGURE 4 | Development of a classical pathway C3 and C5 convertase model. **(A)** In the CP convertase model, streptavidin beads are labeled with biotinylated DNP which serves as a model antigen. Addition of IgG1 recognizing DNP and complement proteins results in formation of C4b2a and C4b2a(C3b)$_n$ convertases on the bead surface, which convert C3 and C5. **(B)** Only in the presence of all CP components (antigen, IgG, and CP proteins) C3 and C5 are converted, as measured by calcium mobilization in U937-C3aR and U937-C5aR cells, respectively. **(C)** C3 conversion *via* CP convertases results in release of C3a in the supernatant (as shown by calcium mobilization) and **(D)** C3b deposition on the bead surface (as shown by flow cytometry). Identical amounts of the non-reactive C3 variants C3b$_{H2O}$ and C3$_{MA}$ do not bind to the bead surface. **(E)** C5 convertase activity increases with the level of deposited C3b molecules on the beads surface, but is not affected by C3b$_{H2O}$ or C3$_{MA}$ in solution. Uncoupling C3 and C5 conversion by introduction of an extra washing step does not alter C5 conversion, indicating that CP C5 conversion only depends on deposited C3b molecules around existing C3 convertases. **(B–E)** Data of three independent experiments, presented as mean ± SD.

on covalently deposited C3b since addition of non-reactive C3 variants [C3b$_{H2O}$ in which the thioester had already reacted with water or methylamine-treated C3 (C3$_{MA}$) (7, 56)] did not induce the convertase to cleave C5 (**Figures 4C–E**). In addition, introducing a washing step in between C3b deposition and C5 conversion confirmed that only deposited C3b and not C3 or the active process of C3 cleavage is required for C5 conversion (**Figure 4E**). These results demonstrate the specificity of our CP convertase models in measuring the activity of CP C3 and C5 conversion.

C3b-Binding Molecules Inhibit Classical Pathway C5 Conversion by Modulating Accessory C3b

Next, we examined the effect of the above-tested C3b- and C5-binding molecules in the CP convertase model. Beads with actively formed C4b2a convertases were incubated with C2, C3, and C5 in the presence of complement binding molecules at a concentration of 1 μM and the C3a/C5a generated in the sample supernatant was measured. The known CP convertase inhibitor C4BP effectively inhibited both CP C3 and C5 conversion, confirming the validity of our model (**Figure 5A**). Furthermore, C5-binding molecules OmCI and eculizumab potently inhibited CP C5 conversion but left C3 conversion unaffected (**Figure 5A**). SSL7 also inhibits CP C5 conversion, but to a lesser extent, which could arise from differences in the models or in the C5-binding sites involved in convertase recognition. Since C3b is not part of the CP C3 convertase, we hypothesized that C3b-binding molecules would not influence C3 conversion in the CP model. Accordingly, most C3b-binding molecules did not affect C3 conversion, with the exception of Cp40, which showed potent inhibition (**Figure 5B**). The lack of C3 conversion in the presence of Cp40 can be explained by its strong affinity for uncleaved C3 causing steric hindrance during C3 recognition by the convertase (57). Efb-C and Ecb, which can also bind C3, do not inhibit

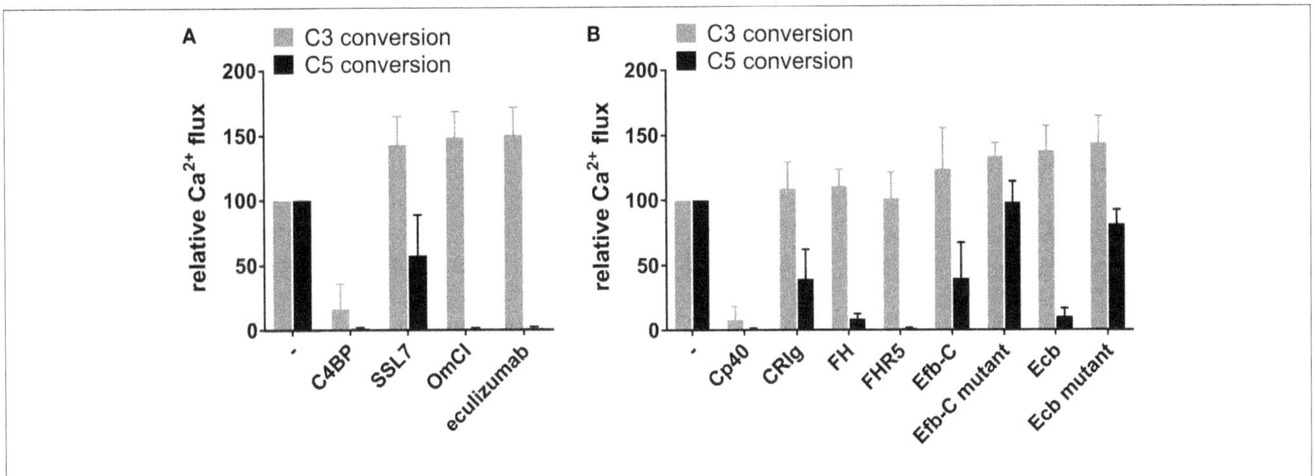

FIGURE 5 | The effect of inhibitors on classical pathway C3 and C5 conversion. Conversion of C3 (50 nM) or C5 (2.5 nM) in the CP model in the absence or presence of 1 μM complement-binding molecule measured by calcium mobilization in U937-C3aR and U937-C5aR cells, respectively. Conversion is shown as a percentage relative to the control without inhibitor. **(A)** C5-binding molecules OmCI and eculizumab inhibit CP C5 but not C3 conversion. SSL7 inhibits C5 conversion, as well, but less efficiently. C4b-binding protein (C4BP) inhibits both CP C3 and C5 convertases. **(B)** None of the C3b-binding molecules, except for Cp40, affect CP C3 conversion, whereas all inhibit C5 conversion. Mutant Efb-C and mutant Ecb are unable to bind C3b and thus do not exhibit inhibition. **(A,B)** Data of three independent experiments, presented as mean ± SD.

convertase activity in that manner, as further evidenced by lack of inhibition of AP C3 conversion. Interestingly, we found that all C3b-binding molecules can prevent C5 conversion in the CP model (**Figure 5B**). This establishes an important role for accessory C3b in the formation and activity of CP C5 convertases. Moreover, the fact that FHR5, Efb-C, and Ecb exhibited similar effects on C5 conversion by the AP and CP convertases, indicates a similar role for accessory C3b in C5 conversion in both pathways. The CP model provides more detail about their inhibitory mechanism by showing that they can act specifically *via* accessory C3b molecules. Similarly, the CP inhibition data show that CRIg and FH can inhibit C5 conversion specifically *via* accessory C3b. Overall, our data suggest that all C3b-binding molecules tested can inhibit C5 conversion (in both AP and CP) through interaction with accessory C3b molecules, but only some can inhibit the core convertase enzyme (C3bBb) itself.

DISCUSSION

Since C3 and C5 convertase enzymes play such a vital role in propagating the cascade but also driving unwanted complement effector functions, it is essential to better understand mechanisms of convertase activation and inhibition. Since C5 convertases are largely constrained to cell surfaces, it has been difficult to study these enzymes with highly purified complement components. Here, we developed bead-based models to functionally characterize both C3 and C5 convertases on a surface using purified components and in the absence of confounding factors from serum. These models serve several important purposes: (1) to understand the molecular biology of convertases, (2) to characterize the mode of action of known complement inhibitors, (3) to characterize the role of disease-associated deficiencies and mutations of complement proteins, and (4) to screen for novel and specific convertase inhibitors.

In the past, several models have been developed to study convertase activation and inhibition. One of the most common models employs erythrocytes to serve as a platform for complement activation, using either serum or stepwise addition of purified complement components. Other studies have employed non-cellular surfaces, including SPR chips, to examine stepwise assembly and dissociation of convertases. While each of these models differ in many aspects, each has inherent advantages and disadvantages in addressing various aspects of complement function, and no single model can capture all molecular and physiological details of convertases or inhibition thereof. Our models offer the ability to (1) quantitatively compare activity and inhibition of AP and CP C3 and C5 convertases independently and (2) enable controlled formation and distribution of convertases in a highly purified environment in the absence of complement regulators found in serum and on cells. In our model, we chose to quantify C3 and C5 cleavage through measurement of chemoattractants C3a and C5a, molecules that are released into solution and can be selectively and sensitively detected in a functional cell-based calcium mobilization assay using flow cytometry. Alternatively, C3a and C5a can be quantified by ELISA, however, this is not a direct functional readout, and one should exercise caution in selecting antibodies with high specificity for each chemoattractant molecule (58). Measurement of C3a *via* calcium responses allows a more accurate quantification of C3 convertase activity than antibody detection of deposited C3b molecules. During C3 cleavage, the thioester of newly formed C3b molecules becomes exposed and can react with molecules on the cell surface. Rapid amplification results in dense clusters of C3b, which may deposit on top of each other, making accurate quantification difficult (59). Furthermore, many newly formed C3b molecules never attach to the surface (60). Therefore, immunodetection of deposited C3b is not the best measure of C3 conversion. In addition, since C3a and C5a are hallmarks of complement-mediated inflammation, detection of these chemoattractants is a critical readout when screening for convertase inhibitors as potential therapeutic molecules and disease-associated mutants of complement factors *in vitro*. It is important to note that in more complex environments (i.e., serum or *in vivo*), measurement of functionally active C3a/C5a is challenging due to proteolytic cleavage and scavenging by receptors. In addition, our bead-based models enable additional readouts, including quantification of surface complement deposition and breakdown of complement opsonins through cofactor activity of inhibitory molecules (Figure S2 in Supplementary Material).

The models presented in this work may assist in obtaining better insights into the structural organization of convertase enzymes. While significant progress has been made in understanding the structural organization of C3 convertases and C3 cleavage (**Figure 1C**) (55), the molecular details of C5 convertase formation remain poorly understood. Molecular models of C5 convertase activation have been proposed (**Figure 1D**) (47, 49, 61) but the exact organization of this complex remains unknown. It is known that C5 convertases form when C3 convertases (C4b2a and C3bBb) deposit high densities of C3b molecules on the target surface (9). The non-catalytic subunits of C3 convertases (C4b or C3b) are thought to associate with extra C3b molecules and form multimeric C4b-C3b$_n$ or C3b-C3b$_n$ complexes that have an increased affinity for C5 (62, 63). In this study, we verified the requirement of high C3b densities for C5 conversion. In line with previous data, we also find that C3b density affects C5, but not C3 conversion by AP convertases (7). Interestingly, our data for Efb-C/Ecb and FHR5 also suggest that the orientation of C3b molecules on the surface is particularly important for conversion of C5, but not C3. We previously demonstrated that the (natural) surface attachment of C3b molecules *via* the thioester is crucial for efficient conversion of C5 (7). Here, we found that three molecules that interact with the C3b thioester domain (TED) (Efb-C, Ecb, and FHR5) selectively inhibit AP and CP C5 convertases, while leaving C3 conversion unaffected. Among examined C3b-binding molecules, this selective inhibition of C5 conversion in the AP was specific for molecules interacting with the TED of C3b. Several crystallographic structures of C3b revealed interdomain interactions between TED and the MG1 domain, which facilitate the prototypical "upright" conformation of C3b attached to surfaces *via* its thioester (31, 43, 55, 64–69). However, recent electron microscopy data reveal conformational flexibility of C3b under different conditions, and in particular, TED can exhibit markedly different positions (70–74). Hydrogen-deuterium exchange experiments demonstrated a conformational change in C3b upon Efb-C binding to TED, suggesting that Efb-C acts as a wedge to disrupt the TED–MG1 interaction and affects the orientation of C3b on the surface (71). Although the exact binding interface of C3b and FHR5 is unknown, it does interact with TED (75), and therefore it is possible that FHR5 acts through a similar mechanism. It is unclear whether FHR5 also interacts with other regions of C3b. Binding of C3b by FHR5 is different from that by FH, because FHR5 lacks domains homologous to the FH N-terminal C3b binding and complement regulatory domains. The results reported here confirm the previously reported lack of solid phase C3 convertase inhibition by FHR5 (45, 76), although inhibition of fluid phase C3 convertase was described (45). Why the C3b orientation is critical for C5 conversion but not C3 conversion remains to be determined. Potentially it supports the recently proposed model in which C5 needs to be "sandwiched" in between the C3 convertase and the accessory C3b molecule in order to be primed for convertase cleavage (49). One could envision that such "sandwiching" is affected by differently oriented C3b's. Alternatively, C3b orientation may determine how closely C3b molecules can pack together. If tightly packed and aligned accessory C3b molecules are required for efficient C5 conversion, altered orientation may result in decreased conversion of C5 (**Figure 6**). The fact that Efb/Ecb and FHR5 also inhibit C5 conversion in the CP suggests that the accessory C3b molecules have a similar function in the activation of both the CP and AP C5 convertases.

Functional analyses of well-defined complement inhibitors also reveal other important binding interfaces of C3/C5 convertases.

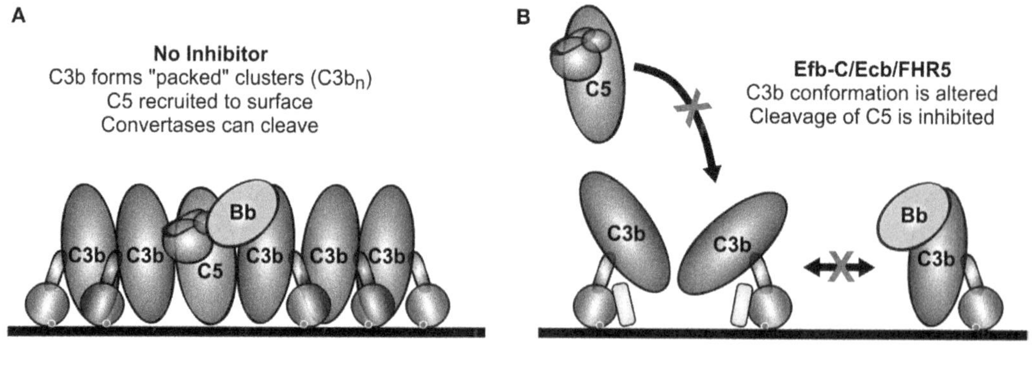

FIGURE 6 | Model for selective inhibition of C5 conversion. **(A)** Under normal conditions, high levels of accessory C3b (C3b$_n$) deposition on a cell surface around existing C3 convertases enables binding and conversion of C5. All C3b molecules are tightly packed and aligned in the same vertical orientation, both of which are necessary for efficient C5 conversion. **(B)** Thioester domain (TED)-binding molecules (i.e., Efb-C and Ecb) act as a wedge to separate TED from the rest of C3b, which alters its surface conformation and prevents efficient C5 conversion. Colors of molecules correspond to **Figures 1C,D** and **3A**, with Efb-C/Ecb shown in spring green. The red crosses indicate inhibition of C5 and C3bBb binding to surface-bound accessory C3b molecules (C3b$_n$).

Our model demonstrates that the C3b–C3b dimerization site (**Figure 1C**, right) is important for activity of all C3b-containing convertases, including AP C3 and C5 convertases, as well as the CP C5 convertase. The C3b-binding molecules Cp40 and CRIg, which bind at this interface (**Figure 3A**), universally inhibit activity of C3b-containing convertases. These molecules likely interfere with convertase-substrate binding (as in **Figures 1C,D**) and/or surface-bound accessory C3b molecules (as in **Figure 1D**). Unlike CRIg, Cp40 inhibits all convertases, including the CP C3 convertase, which lacks C3b. Since Cp40 can bind to both C3b and uncleaved C3, it could inhibit CP C3 conversion by binding to the substrate (C3) and preventing recognition by the CP C3 convertase (57, 77). Substrate C3 binding can also explain the difference in inhibition of AP C3 and C5 conversion by Cp40 (**Figures 3D,E**). In the AP C3 conversion assay, Cp40 can bind to both C3 and C3b, and therefore the concentration required to block C3 conversion is higher than for in the AP C5 conversion assay, where C3 is not present. Next to CRIg, we also found that FH inhibits CP C5 convertases. Although FH is known as an inhibitor of AP C3/C5 convertases because it dissociates Bb from C3b, the mechanism of FH-mediated inhibition of CP C5 conversion is not known. Since FH is a large molecule with several distant binding sites on C3b (43, 44, 78) it likely interferes with binding C5 (79). Thus, our data for FH demonstrate that not only the C3b–C3b dimerization site, but also other sites on C3b, are important for its interaction with C5. Overall, C3b-binding molecules illustrate several key properties of convertase assembly and inhibition. While much of the data here are in line with previous inhibitor studies (**Table 1**), more extensive and complementary studies are required to fully understand the physiological modes of inhibition of these molecules.

Finally, the tools developed in this study can be used for identification of effective therapeutic convertase inhibitors. The ability to examine each convertase separately affords the opportunity to identify selective convertase inhibitors. The complement therapeutics landscape is rapidly expanding, as new roles for complement in disease continue to be uncovered. It is clear that not all complement-mediated diseases are created equal, and it is necessary to design therapeutics that target different points in the complement cascade. For example, diseases mediated primarily by C5a or MAC may benefit from selective inhibition of C5 conversion. Blocking the complement cascade upstream of the terminal pathway (i.e., inhibition of C3 cleavage) may unnecessarily increase patient susceptibility to infections by effectively inhibiting all complement effector functions. Our work now demonstrates the characterization of inhibitors that selectively inhibit C5 conversion, which may prove useful in treatment of MAC-mediated and inflammatory disorders of the complement system. Thus, these models provide a platform for the identification of tailored next-generation complement therapeutics.

AUTHOR CONTRIBUTIONS

SZ, EB, and SR designed and developed convertase models. SZ, EB, SR, and RG designed the study and experiments. SZ, SM, MR, and RG performed the experiments and analyzed data. CH developed cell lines. CH and PA cloned and produced monoclonal antibodies. SZ, SM, SR, and RG wrote the manuscript. SZ, MJ, SR, and RG contributed to critical analysis and discussion of the results. All authors read and reviewed the manuscript.

ACKNOWLEDGMENTS

We would like to acknowledge John Lambris for providing Cp40, Menno van Lookeren Campagne (Genentech) for providing CRIg, Genmab for providing eculizumab, Brian Geisbrecht for providing constructs for Efb-C and Ecb mutants, U-Protein Express BV (Utrecht, The Netherlands) for help with protein expression, and Kaila Bennett, Bart Bardoel, and Julia Kolata for cloning advice. The work was funded by Marie-Skłodowska Curie Fellowship (659633, to RG); ERC Starting grant (639209-ComBact, to SR), the EMBO Young Investigator Program (to SR); Kidneeds Foundation, Iowa, US (to MJ). MJ was also supported by the Institutional Excellence Program of the Ministry of Human Capacities of Hungary.

REFERENCES

1. Walport MJ. Complement. First of two parts. *N Engl J Med* (2001) 344:1058–66. doi:10.1056/NEJM200104053441406
2. Ricklin D, Hajishengallis G, Yang K, Lambris JD. Complement: a key system for immune surveillance and homeostasis. *Nat Immunol* (2010) 11:785–97. doi:10.1038/ni.1923
3. Ricklin D, Lambris JD. Complement in immune and inflammatory disorders: pathophysiological mechanisms. *J Immunol* (2013) 190:3831–8. doi:10.4049/jimmunol.1203487
4. Ricklin D, Mastellos DC, Reis ES, Lambris JD. The renaissance of complement therapeutics. *Nat Rev Nephrol* (2017) 14:26–47. doi:10.1038/nrneph.2017.156
5. Morgan BP, Harris CL. Complement, a target for therapy in inflammatory and degenerative diseases. *Nat Rev Drug Discov* (2015) 14:857–77. doi:10.1038/nrd4657
6. Diebolder CA, Beurskens FJ, de Jong RN, Koning RI, Strumane K, Lindorfer MA, et al. Complement is activated by IgG hexamers assembled at the cell surface. *Science* (2014) 343:1260–3. doi:10.1126/science.1248943
7. Berends ETM, Gorham RD, Ruyken M, Soppe JA, Orhan H, Aerts PC, et al. Molecular insights into the surface-specific arrangement of complement C5 convertase enzymes. *BMC Biol* (2015) 13:93. doi:10.1186/s12915-015-0203-8
8. Merle NS, Church SE, Fremeaux-Bacchi V, Roumenina LT. Complement system part I: molecular mechanisms of activation and regulation. *Front Immunol* (2015) 6:262. doi:10.3389/fimmu.2015.00262
9. Pangburn MK, Rawal N. Structure and function of complement C5 convertase enzymes. *Biochem Soc Trans* (2002) 30:1006–10. doi:10.1042/bst030a098c
10. Medof ME, Kinoshita T, Nussenzweig V. Inhibition of complement activation on the surface of cells after incorporation of decay-accelerating factor (DAF) into their membranes. *J Exp Med* (1984) 160:1558–78. doi:10.1084/jem.160.5.1558
11. Krych-Goldberg M, Hauhart RE, Subramanian VB, Yurcisin BM, Crimmins DL, Hourcade DE, et al. Decay accelerating activity of complement receptor type 1 (CD35). *J Biol Chem* (1999) 274:31160–8. doi:10.1074/jbc.274.44.31160
12. Harder MJ, Anliker M, Höchsmann B, Simmet T, Huber-Lang M, Schrezenmeier H, et al. Comparative analysis of novel complement-targeted inhibitors, MiniFH, and the natural regulators factor H and factor H-like

protein 1 reveal functional determinants of complement regulation. *J Immunol* (2016) 196:866–76. doi:10.4049/jimmunol.1501919
13. Harris CL, Abbott RJM, Smith RA, Morgan BP, Lea SM. Molecular dissection of interactions between components of the alternative pathway of complement and decay accelerating factor (CD55). *J Biol Chem* (2005) 280:2569–78. doi:10.1074/jbc.M410179200
14. Okroj M, Holmquist E, King BC, Blom AM. Functional analyses of complement convertases using C3 and C5-depleted sera. *PLoS One* (2012) 7: e47245. doi:10.1371/journal.pone.0047245
15. Bajic G, Degn SE, Thiel S, Andersen GR. Complement activation, regulation, and molecular basis for complement-related diseases. *EMBO J* (2015) 34:2735–57. doi:10.15252/embj.201591881
16. Jongerius I, Köhl J, Pandey MK, Ruyken M, van Kessel KPM, van Strijp JAG, et al. Staphylococcal complement evasion by various convertase-blocking molecules. *J Exp Med* (2007) 204:2461–71. doi:10.1084/jem.20070818
17. Rooijakkers SHM, van Strijp JAG. Bacterial complement evasion. *Mol Immunol* (2007) 44:23–32. doi:10.1016/j.molimm.2006.06.011
18. Ricklin D, Lambris JD. Complement in immune and inflammatory disorders: therapeutic interventions. *J Immunol* (2013) 190:3839–47. doi:10.4049/jimmunol.1203200
19. Durocher Y, Perret S, Kamen A. High-level and high-throughput recombinant protein production by transient transfection of suspension-growing human 293-EBNA1 cells. *Nucleic Acids Res* (2002) 30:E9. doi:10.1093/nar/30.2.e9
20. Nunn MA, Sharma A, Paesen GC, Adamson S, Lissina O, Willis AC, et al. Complement inhibitor of C5 activation from the soft tick *Ornithodoros moubata*. *J Immunol* (2005) 174:2084–91. doi:10.4049/jimmunol.174.4.2084
21. Hammel M, Sfyroera G, Ricklin D, Magotti P, Lambris JD, Geisbrecht BV. A structural basis for complement inhibition by *Staphylococcus aureus*. *Nat Immunol* (2007) 8:430–7. doi:10.1038/ni1450
22. Geisbrecht BV, Bouyain S, Pop M. An optimized system for expression and purification of secreted bacterial proteins. *Protein Expr Purif* (2006) 46: 23–32. doi:10.1016/j.pep.2005.09.003
23. Hammel M, Sfyroera G, Pyrpassopoulos S, Ricklin D, Ramyar KX, Pop M, et al. Characterization of Ehp, a secreted complement inhibitory protein from *Staphylococcus aureus*. *J Biol Chem* (2007) 282:30051–61. doi:10.1074/jbc.M704247200
24. Bestebroer J, Aerts PC, Rooijakkers SHM, Pandey MK, Köhl J, Van Strijp JAG, et al. Functional basis for complement evasion by staphylococcal superantigen-like 7. *Cell Microbiol* (2010) 12:1506–16. doi:10.1111/j.1462-5822.2010.01486.x
25. Gonzales N. Minimizing immunogenicity of the SDR-grafted humanized antibody CC49 by genetic manipulation of the framework residues. *Mol Immunol* (2003) 40:337–49. doi:10.1016/S0161-5890(03)00166-4
26. van de Weijer ML, Bassik MC, Luteijn RD, Voorburg CM, Lohuis MAM, Kremmer E, et al. A high-coverage shRNA screen identifies TMEM129 as an E3 ligase involved in ER-associated protein degradation. *Nat Commun* (2014) 5:3832. doi:10.1038/ncomms4832
27. Rawal N, Pangburn MK. C5 convertase of the alternative pathway of complement. *J Biol Chem* (1998) 273:16828–35. doi:10.1074/jbc.273.27.16828
28. Sarrias MR, Franchini S, Canziani G, Argyropoulos E, Moore WT, Sahu A, et al. Kinetic analysis of the interactions of complement receptor 2 (CR2, CD21) with its ligands C3d, iC3b, and the EBV glycoprotein gp350/220. *J Immunol* (2001) 167:1490–9. doi:10.4049/jimmunol.167.3.1490
29. Kew RR, Peng T, DiMartino SJ, Madhavan D, Weinman SJ, Cheng D, et al. Undifferentiated U937 cells transfected with chemoattractant receptors: a model system to investigate chemotactic mechanisms and receptor structure/function relationships. *J Leukoc Biol* (1997) 61:329–37. doi:10.1002/jlb.61.3.329
30. Veldkamp KE, Heezius HC, Verhoef J, van Strijp JA, van Kessel KP. Modulation of neutrophil chemokine receptors by *Staphylococcus aureus* supernate. *Infect Immun* (2000) 68:5908–13. doi:10.1128/IAI.68.10.5908-5913.2000
31. Wiesmann C, Katschke KJ, Yin J, Helmy KY, Steffek M, Fairbrother WJ, et al. Structure of C3b in complex with CRIg gives insights into regulation of complement activation. *Nature* (2006) 444:217–20. doi:10.1038/nature05263
32. Helmy KY, Katschke KJ, Gorgani NN, Kljavin NM, Elliott JM, Diehl L, et al. CRIg: a macrophage complement receptor required for phagocytosis of circulating pathogens. *Cell* (2006) 124:915–27. doi:10.1016/j.cell.2005.12.039
33. Józsi M. Factor H family proteins in complement evasion of microorganisms. *Front Immunol* (2017) 8:571. doi:10.3389/fimmu.2017.00571
34. Kopp A, Hebecker M, Svobodová E, Józsi M. Factor H: a complement regulator in health and disease, and a mediator of cellular interactions. *Biomolecules* (2012) 2:46–75. doi:10.3390/biom2010046
35. McRae JL, Cowan PJ, Power DA, Mitchelhill KI, Kemp BE, Morgan BP, et al. Human factor H-related protein 5 (FHR-5): a new complement-associated protein. *J Biol Chem* (2001) 276:6747–54. doi:10.1074/jbc.M007495200
36. Lee LYL, Höök M, Haviland D, Wetsel RA, Yonter EO, Syribeys P, et al. Inhibition of complement activation by a secreted *Staphylococcus aureus* protein. *J Infect Dis* (2004) 190:571–9. doi:10.1086/422259
37. Langley R, Wines B, Willoughby N, Basu I, Proft T, Fraser JD. The staphylococcal superantigen-like protein 7 binds IgA and complement C5 and inhibits IgA-Fc RI binding and serum killing of bacteria. *J Immunol* (2005) 174:2926–33. doi:10.4049/jimmunol.174.5.2926
38. Rother RP, Rollins SA, Mojcik CF, Brodsky RA, Bell L. Discovery and development of the complement inhibitor eculizumab for the treatment of paroxysmal nocturnal hemoglobinuria. *Nat Biotechnol* (2007) 25:1256–64. doi:10.1038/nbt1344
39. Qu H, Ricklin D, Bai H, Chen H, Reis ES, Maciejewski M, et al. New analogs of the clinical complement inhibitor compstatin with subnanomolar affinity and enhanced pharmacokinetic properties. *Immunobiology* (2013) 218: 496–505. doi:10.1016/j.imbio.2012.06.003
40. Gigli I, Fujita T, Nussenzweig V. Modulation of the classical pathway C3 convertase by plasma proteins C4 binding protein and C3b inactivator. *Proc Natl Acad Sci U S A* (1979) 76:6596–600. doi:10.1073/pnas.76.12.6596
41. Janssen BJC, Halff EF, Lambris JD, Gros P. Structure of compstatin in complex with complement component C3c reveals a new mechanism of complement inhibition. *J Biol Chem* (2007) 282:29241–7. doi:10.1074/jbc.M704587200
42. Sahu A, Kay BK, Lambris JD. Inhibition of human complement by a C3-binding peptide isolated from a phage-displayed random peptide library. *J Immunol* (1996) 157:884–91.
43. Wu J, Wu YQ, Ricklin D, Janssen BJC, Lambris JD, Gros P. Structure of complement fragment C3b-factor H and implications for host protection by complement regulators. *Nat Immunol* (2009) 10:728–33. doi:10.1038/ni.1755
44. Kajander T, Lehtinen MJ, Hyvarinen S, Bhattacharjee A, Leung E, Isenman DE, et al. Dual interaction of factor H with C3d and glycosaminoglycans in host-nonhost discrimination by complement. *Proc Natl Acad Sci U S A* (2011) 108:2897–902. doi:10.1073/pnas.1017087108
45. McRae JL, Duthy TG, Griggs KM, Ormsby RJ, Cowan PJ, Cromer BA, et al. Human factor H-related protein 5 has cofactor activity, inhibits C3 convertase activity, binds heparin and C-reactive protein, and associates with lipoprotein. *J Immunol* (2005) 174:6250–6. doi:10.4049/jimmunol.174.10.6250
46. Lee LYL, Liang X, Höök M, Brown EL. Identification and characterization of the C3 binding domain of the *Staphylococcus aureus* extracellular fibrinogen-binding protein (Efb). *J Biol Chem* (2004) 279:50710–6. doi:10.1074/jbc.M408570200
47. Laursen NS, Andersen KR, Braren I, Spillner E, Sottrup-Jensen L, Andersen GR. Substrate recognition by complement convertases revealed in the C5-cobra venom factor complex. *EMBO J* (2011) 30:606–16. doi:10.1038/emboj.2010.341
48. Laursen NS, Gordon N, Hermans S, Lorenz N, Jackson N, Wines B, et al. Structural basis for inhibition of complement C5 by the SSL7 protein from *Staphylococcus aureus*. *Proc Natl Acad Sci U S A* (2010) 107:3681–6. doi:10.1073/pnas.0910565107
49. Jore MM, Johnson S, Sheppard D, Barber NM, Li YI, Nunn MA, et al. Structural basis for therapeutic inhibition of complement C5. *Nat Struct Mol Biol* (2016) 23:378–86. doi:10.1038/nsmb.3196
50. Fredslund F, Laursen NS, Roversi P, Jenner L, Oliveira CLP, Pedersen JS, et al. Structure of and influence of a tick complement inhibitor on human complement component 5. *Nat Immunol* (2008) 9:753–60. doi:10.1038/ni0808-945
51. Kaplan M. Eculizumab (Alexion). *Curr Opin Investig Drugs* (2002) 3:1017–23.
52. Schatz-Jakobsen JA, Zhang Y, Johnson K, Neill A, Sheridan D, Andersen GR. Structural basis for eculizumab-mediated inhibition of the complement terminal pathway. *J Immunol* (2016) 197:337–44. doi:10.4049/jimmunol.1600280
53. Scharfstein J. Human C4-binding protein. I. Isolation and characterization. *J Exp Med* (1978) 148:207–22. doi:10.1084/jem.148.1.207

54. Rawal N, Rajagopalan R, Salvi VP. Stringent regulation of complement lectin pathway C3/C5 convertase by C4b-binding protein (C4BP). *Mol Immunol* (2009) 46:2902–10. doi:10.1016/j.molimm.2009.07.006
55. Rooijakkers SHM, Wu J, Ruyken M, van Domselaar R, Planken KL, Tzekou A, et al. Structural and functional implications of the alternative complement pathway C3 convertase stabilized by a staphylococcal inhibitor. *Nat Immunol* (2009) 10:721–7. doi:10.1038/ni.1756
56. Pangburn MK. Spontaneous reformation of the intramolecular thioester in complement protein C3 and low temperature capture of a conformational intermediate capable of reformation. *J Biol Chem* (1992) 267:8584–90.
57. Ricklin D, Lambris JD. Compstatin: a complement inhibitor on its way to clinical application. *Adv Exp Med Biol* (2008) 632:273–92. doi:10.1016/j.biotechadv.2011.08.021.Secreted
58. Nilsson PH, Thomas AM, Bergseth G, Gustavsen A, Volokhina EB, van den Heuvel LP, et al. Eculizumab-C5 complexes express a C5a neoepitope in vivo: consequences for interpretation of patient complement analyses. *Mol Immunol* (2017) 89:111–4. doi:10.1016/j.molimm.2017.05.021
59. Rawal N, Pangburn MK. Formation of high-affinity C5 convertases of the alternative pathway of complement. *J Immunol* (2001) 166:2635–42. doi:10.4049/jimmunol.166.4.2635
60. Sim RB, Twose TM, Paterson DS, Sim E. The covalent-binding reaction of complement component C3. *Biochem J* (1981) 193:115–27. doi:10.1042/bj1930115
61. Mortensen S, Kidmose RT, Petersen SV, Szilágyi Á, Prohászka Z, Andersen GR. Structural basis for the function of complement component C4 within the classical and lectin pathways of complement. *J Immunol* (2015) 194:5488–96. doi:10.4049/jimmunol.1500087
62. Kinoshita T, Takata Y, Kozono H, Takeda J, Hong KS, Inoue K. C5 convertase of the alternative complement pathway: covalent linkage between two C3b molecules within the trimolecular complex enzyme. *J Immunol* (1988) 141:3895–901.
63. Kim YU, Carroll MC, Isenman DE, Nonaka M, Pramoonjago P, Takeda J, et al. Covalent binding of C3b to C4b within the classical complement pathway C5 convertase. *J Biol Chem* (1992) 267:4171–6.
64. Katschke KJ, Stawicki S, Yin J, Steffek M, Xi H, Sturgeon L, et al. Structural and functional analysis of a C3b-specific antibody that selectively inhibits the alternative pathway of complement. *J Biol Chem* (2009) 284:10473–9. doi:10.1074/jbc.M809106200
65. Forneris F, Ricklin D, Wu J, Tzekou A, Wallace RS, Lambris JD, et al. Structures of C3b in complex with factors B and D give insight into complement convertase formation. *Science* (2010) 330:1816–20. doi:10.1126/science.1195821
66. Janssen BJC, Christodoulidou A, McCarthy A, Lambris JD, Gros P. Structure of C3b reveals conformational changes that underlie complement activity. *Nature* (2006) 444:213–6. doi:10.1038/nature05172
67. Garcia BL, Ramyar KX, Tzekou A, Ricklin D, McWhorter WJ, Lambris JD, et al. Molecular basis for complement recognition and inhibition determined by crystallographic studies of the staphylococcal complement inhibitor (SCIN) bound to C3c and C3b. *J Mol Biol* (2010) 402:17–29. doi:10.1016/j.jmb.2010.07.029
68. Forneris F, Wu J, Xue X, Ricklin D, Lin Z, Sfyroera G, et al. Regulators of complement activity mediate inhibitory mechanisms through a common C3b-binding mode. *EMBO J* (2016) 35:1133–49. doi:10.15252/embj.201593673
69. Xue X, Wu J, Ricklin D, Forneris F, Di Crescenzio P, Schmidt CQ, et al. Regulator-dependent mechanisms of C3b processing by factor I allow differentiation of immune responses. *Nat Struct Mol Biol* (2017) 24:643–51. doi:10.1038/nsmb.3427
70. Nishida N, Walz T, Springer TA. Structural transitions of complement component C3 and its activation products. *Proc Natl Acad Sci U S A* (2006) 103:19737–42. doi:10.1073/pnas.0609791104
71. Chen H, Ricklin D, Hammel M, Garcia BL, McWhorter WJ, Sfyroera G, et al. Allosteric inhibition of complement function by a staphylococcal immune evasion protein. *Proc Natl Acad Sci U S A* (2010) 107:17621–6. doi:10.1073/pnas.1003750107
72. Alcorlo M, Tortajada A, Rodriguez de Cordoba S, Llorca O. Structural basis for the stabilization of the complement alternative pathway C3 convertase by properdin. *Proc Natl Acad Sci U S A* (2013) 110:13504–9. doi:10.1073/pnas.1309618110
73. Rodriguez E, Nan R, Li K, Gor J, Perkins SJ. A revised mechanism for the activation of complement C3 to C3b. *J Biol Chem* (2015) 290:2334–50. doi:10.1074/jbc.M114.605691
74. López-Perrote A, Harrison RES, Subías M, Alcorlo M, Rodríguez de Córdoba S, Morikis D, et al. Ionic tethering contributes to the conformational stability and function of complement C3b. *Mol Immunol* (2017) 85:137–47. doi:10.1016/j.molimm.2016.12.015
75. Goicoechea de Jorge E, Caesar JJE, Malik TH, Patel M, Colledge M, Johnson S, et al. Dimerization of complement factor H-related proteins modulates complement activation in vivo. *Proc Natl Acad Sci U S A* (2013) 110:4685–90. doi:10.1073/pnas.1219260110
76. Csincsi ÁI, Szabó Z, Bánlaki Z, Uzonyi B, Cserhalmi M, Kárpáti É, et al. FHR-1 binds to C-reactive protein and enhances rather than inhibits complement activation. *J Immunol* (2017) 199:292–303. doi:10.4049/jimmunol.1600483
77. Sfyroera G, Ricklin D, Reis ES, Chen H, Wu EL, Kaznessis YN, et al. Rare loss-of-function mutation in complement component C3 provides insight into molecular and pathophysiological determinants of complement activity. *J Immunol* (2015) 194:3305–16. doi:10.4049/jimmunol.1402781
78. Morgan HP, Schmidt CQ, Guariento M, Blaum BS, Gillespie D, Herbert AP, et al. Structural basis for engagement by complement factor H of C3b on a self surface. *Nat Struct Mol Biol* (2011) 18:463–71. doi:10.1038/nsmb.2018
79. DiScipio RG. The binding of human complement proteins C5, factor B, beta 1H and properdin to complement fragment C3b on zymosan. *Biochem J* (1981) 199:485–96. doi:10.1042/bj1990485

13

CL-L1 and CL-K1 Exhibit Widespread Tissue Distribution with High and Co-Localized Expression in Secretory Epithelia and Mucosa

Soren W. K. Hansen[1], Josephine B. Aagaard[1], Karen B. Bjerrum[1], Eva K. Hejbøl[2], Ole Nielsen[2], Henrik D. Schrøder[2], Karsten Skjoedt[1], Anna L. Sørensen[1], Jonas H. Graversen[1] and Maiken L. Henriksen[1]*

[1] Institute of Cancer and Inflammation Research, University of Southern Denmark, Odense, Denmark, [2] Department of Pathology, Odense University Hospital, Odense, Denmark

***Correspondence:**
Soren W. K. Hansen
shansen@health.sdu.dk

Collectin liver 1 (CL-L1, alias collectin 10) and collectin kidney 1 (CL-K1, alias collectin 11) are oligomeric pattern recognition molecules associated with the complement system, and mutations in either of their genes may lead to deficiency and developmental defects. The two collectins are reportedly localized and synthesized in the liver, kidneys, and adrenals, and can be found in the circulation as heteromeric complexes (CL-LK), which upon binding to microbial high mannose-like glycoconjugates activates the complement system *via* the lectin activation pathway. The tissue distribution of homo- vs. heteromeric CL-L1 and -K1 complexes, the mechanism of heteromeric complex formation and in which tissues this occurs, is hitherto incompletely described. We have by immunohistochemistry using monoclonal antibodies addressed the precise cellular localization of the two collectins in the main human tissues. We find that the two collectins have widespread and almost identical tissue distribution with a high expression in epithelial cells in endo-/exocrine secretory tissues and mucosa. There is also accordance between localization of mRNA transcripts and detection of proteins, showing that local synthesis likely is responsible for peripheral localization and eventual formation of the CL-LK complexes. The functional implications of the high expression in endo-/exocrine secretory tissue and mucosa is unknown but might be associated with the activity of MASP-3, which has a similar pattern of expression and is known to potentiate the activity of the alternative complement activation pathway.

Keywords: collectin, complement system, 3MC syndrome, mucosal immunology, innate immunity

INTRODUCTION

The innate immune system is a first line of defense and plays major roles in preventing microorganisms in settling and becoming pathogens, and also in the mounting of suitable immune responses against eventual pathogens. It often relies on recognition and binding to pathogen-associated molecular patterns by host pattern recognition molecules (PRMs). Based on an often observed association between microbial evasion of the complement system and pathogenicity (1), the complement system appears to play substantial roles in the innate immune system. The overall antimicrobial functions of the complement system are to tag microorganisms for elimination by phagocytes, to initiate inflammation and to lyse the microorganisms. The complement system is a "self-amplificative" cascade system, mainly found in the blood, and includes several PRMs; among which some activate a pathway known as the lectin activation pathway, *via* activation of serine proteases known as MBL-associated serine protease (MASP-1, -2, and -3) (2, 3). Mannan-binding lectin (MBL) is probably the most studied PRM of the lectin activation pathway and binds to mannose-rich glycoconjugates on the surface of microorganisms, initiating complement activation. In humans, MBL deficiency may increase susceptibility toward infections in certain situations but not in general (4), most likely contributed by coincidental activation of different complement activation pathways by a given microorganism.

Collectin liver 1 (CL-L1) and collectin kidney 1 (CL-K1) are "MBL-like" proteins that also are found in the circulation in association with MASPs and with specificity toward mannose-rich glycoconjugates and negatively charged molecules (5–10). In the circulation they can be found as heteromeric molecules, referred to as CL-LK, with superior complement abilities *via* MASP-2 in comparison with their respective homomers (11). They are both synthesized in the liver by hepatocytes, in the adrenal glands and in the tubules of the kidney, in addition to other tissues as well (5–7). On the protein level, human CL-K1 has been associated with the same tissues, while human CL-L1 in the original study only was associated with hepatocytes, however, without examination or exclusion of other tissues and cells (6, 7). Among normal healthy populations of different origins, they both constitute average serum concentrations of 250–450 ng/ml, with a clear correlation between levels of CL-L1 and CL-K1, supportive of heteromeric complexes between the two or similar regulation (7, 12–15). The liver and adrenals are due to their endocrine nature and a relative high synthesis of mRNA believed to be the major organs contributing to the CL-L1 and CL-K1 found in the circulation. Partly due to the recently described characterization and association with complement, little is known about their roles *in vivo*. In a recent work using mice deficient of CL-K1, Wakamiya and colleagues showed that CL-K1 protected mice against *Streptococcus pneumonia* infections induced *via* nasal inoculation (16). However, in another work there was no protective effect of CL-K1/CL-LK in a mouse model for infection by *Mycobacterium tuberculosis* (17). CL-K1 has been shown to bind with relative high affinity to the disaccharide Man(α1-2) and to negatively charged molecules, including nucleic acid ligands, and may also play a role in the opsonization of apoptotic cells by recognizing a combination of carbohydrate and nucleic ligands (10, 18).

Recently, it was demonstrated that CL-K1-deficient mice partly were protected against destructive complement-mediated inflammatory responses in post ischemic kidneys and that CL-K1 further promoted development of renal fibrosis in the tubules (19, 20).

CL-K1 and CL-L1 are not regulated significantly by inflammatory stimuli. Their plasma/serum levels do not correlate with increased levels of traditional inflammatory mediators, including CRP and TNF-alpha (8, 9).

The two collectins play apparently also important roles for embryogenesis. Deficiency of CL-K1 or CL-L1 leads in humans to a rare congenital developmental syndrome known as 3MC (alias Malpuech facial clefting syndrome), an effect that the two collectins share with MASP-3. It has been shown that CL-K1 and CL-L1 may act as attractants and guidance cue for neural crest cells, although the precise mechanism for embryonic involvement remains to be elucidated (21, 22).

A functional and complete activation of the complement system involves many complement factors and is in general only associated with the effect in the circulation or at inflamed sites, where blood components gain access. Most tissue expresses certain complement components, e.g., the lung and the intestinal system (23, 24). At such sites the complement system is believed to be partially functional or to mediate activation when inflammation progresses. In the quest of elucidating the function of CL-L1 and CL-K1, we characterized their localization in human tissues. It appears that the previously characterized sites of localization in the circulation, adrenals, liver, and kidney, may have disparaged a compelling localization in especially exocrine/endocrine tissues and mucosa, suggestive of that CL-L1, CL-K1, and CL-LK may play roles in the periphery as well.

MATERIALS AND METHODS

General Reagents and Buffers

Unless otherwise stated, reagents were obtained from Sigma-Aldrich, Denmark. Phosphate-buffered saline: 10 mM Na_2HPO_4, 140 mM NaCl, and 2.7 mM KCl pH 7.4. Tris-buffered saline (TBS): 10 mM Tris and 145 mM NaCl. TNT buffer: 0.10 M Tris, 0.15 M NaCl, and 0.05% Tween 20 pH 7.5.

Generation of MAbs Against CL-L1 and CL-K1

CL-LK was purified from outdated plasma by calcium sensitive immunoaffinity chromatography as previously described (25). Purified CL-LK (50 μg) was used for *s.c.* immunizations of outbred NMRI female mice using Gerbu as adjuvant. Three days before the fusion, mice were boosted (i.p.) with the same amount of CL-LK. The fusion between spleen cells obtained from the CL-LK immunized mice and myeloma cells (Sp2) was performed using polyethylene glycol essentially as described previously in Ref. (26). Positive clones were identified by ELISA using microtiter plates coated with either purified recombinant CL-K1 or CL-L1 expressed in CHO cells as full-length molecules without any tags. Cells from the positive wells were recloned at least thrice by the limiting dilution method. For antibody production and subsequent purification, hybridomas were grown and allowed to express the MAb in Hybridoma-SFM (Invitrogen). Monoclonal antibodies were purified by means of affinity chromatography using a HiTrap Protein G HP column (GE Healthcare) under previously described conditions and elution with 50 mM glycine, pH 2.3 (27). The two antibodies, MAb 11-1 (anti-CL-K1) and MAb 16-13 (CL-L1), which were superior in specificity and IHC sensitivity and applied in the following studies, were both of the isotype IgG1kappa.

SDS-PAGE and Western Blotting

SDS-PAGE was performed according to the method of Laemmli (1970) using pre-casted NuPAGE 4–12% Bis-Tris gels

(Invitrogen) and MES or MOPS SDS running buffer (Invitrogen) (28). Proteins were transferred to the Hybond-P polyvinylidene fluoride membrane (GE Healthcare) (29). The membrane was blocked in 5% non-fat dried milk and 0.1% HSA, and incubated with primary monoclonal antibodies (0.5 μg/ml). Subsequently, the membrane was washed and incubated with HRP-conjugated rabbit anti-mouse antibody diluted (1:20,000) accordingly to the manufacturer's recommendation (Dako, Denmark) and developed by means of the ECL plus Western blotting detection kit (GE Healthcare). For specificity testing of applied antibodies, 1 μl of serum was applied to the gel per 4 mm well width.

Surface Plasmon Resonance

Binding characteristics of the monoclonal antibodies, 11-1 and 16-13, was investigated by SPR on a Biacore 3000 instrument (Biacore, Sweden) with immobilized CL-K1, CL-L1, and CL-LK on a CM5 chip. The proteins were immobilized on EDC/NHS-activated flow cells by injecting the collectin (10 μg/ml) in 10 mM acetate pH 5.0 to a surface density ranging from 0.028 to 0.042 pmol/mm^2. One M of ethanolamine, pH 8.5 was used for capping. For binding experiments antibodies were diluted in running buffer (10 mM HEPES, 150 mM $NaCl_2$, 5 mM EDTA, and 0.005% Tween-20 pH 7.4) in a range from 2.08 to 166 nM. Each sample (40 μl) was injected with a flow rate of 5 μl/min. Regeneration was obtained for antibody 11-1 by injection of two cycles of 10 μl: 10 mM glycine, 20 mM EDTA, 500 mM NaCl, and 0.005% Tween-20 pH 4.0. Regeneration was obtained for antibody 16-13 by injection of two cycles of 10 μl: 100 mM glycine, 5 mM EDTA, 500 mM NaCl, and 0.05% Tween-20 pH 3.0. BIAevaluation software 4.0.1 was used for analysis of the data. The apparent dissociation constants were found by fitting the curves to a 1:1 binding model. All experiments were as a minimum conducted as triplicates of duplicates.

mAbs' Impact on Ligand Binding and Complement Activation

MaxiSorpTM 96-well plate were coated with DNA (2 μg/ml, cat. no. D2001, Sigma-Aldrich) or mannan (20 μg/ml, cat. no. M3640, Sigma-Aldrich) in 1 M NaCl. Purified native CL-LK (0.25 μg/ml) was pre-incubated in non-adsorbent wells for 1 h at RT in the presence of serum, mannose, or mAbs, diluted twofold from 10%, 200 mM, or 2 μg/ml respectively, and subsequently incubated on ligand-coated plates for 4 h. Bound CL-LK was detected using biotin-labeled anti-CL-K1 mAb (0.5 μg/ml, Hyb 14-29, N-terminal specific) and streptavidin-HRP (0.1 μg/ml). Samples were diluted in TBS (20 mM Tris, 125 mM NaCl, pH 7.4) with 2 mM CaCl2, 0.05% Tween 20, and 0.1% BSA. For assessing CL-LK-mediated complement activation plates were prepared

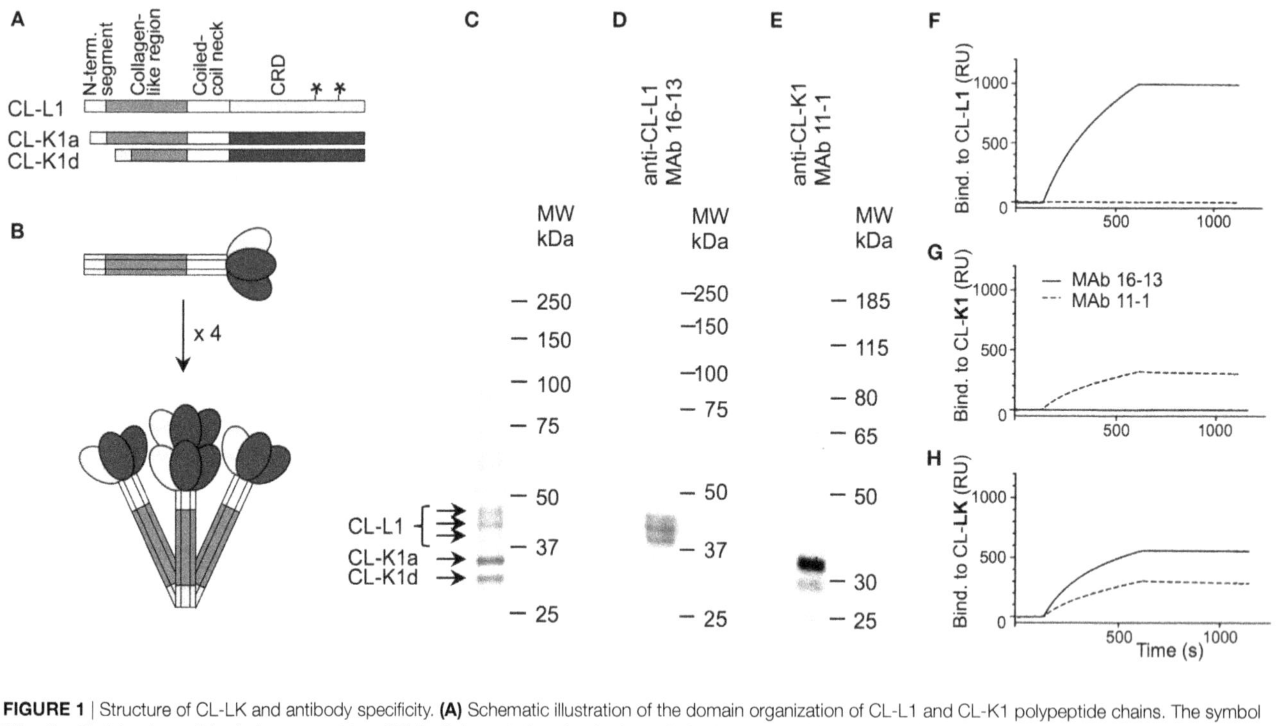

FIGURE 1 | Structure of CL-LK and antibody specificity. **(A)** Schematic illustration of the domain organization of CL-L1 and CL-K1 polypeptide chains. The symbol "*"on the CL-L1 polypeptide chain represent two N-linked glycosylation sites in the carbohydrate recognition domain. CL-K1 is found in the circulation in the form of two isoforms: CL-K1a represents full-length and CL-K1d represents an alternative spliced form devoid of a part of the collagen-like region. **(B)** Subunit of CL-LK and oligomeric structures. A total of three polypeptide chains of CL-K1 and CL-L1 join to form a heteromeric subunit, which may further oligomerize into structures ranging from dimers to hexamers of subunits, here illustrated by a tetramer. **(C)** Analysis of purified CL-LK by SDS-PAGE and visualization by silver staining. The three bands of CL-L1 represent non-, partially, and fully glycosylated forms of CL-L1. **(D,E)** Specificity of monoclonal antibodies by Western blotting of serum under reducing conditions and visualization by ECL. **(F–H)** SPR analyses of monoclonal antibodies with immobilized CL-K1, CL-L1, and CL-LK as antigen, respectively. MAbs 16-13 (--) and 11-1 (---) were analyzed for binding to immobilized purified CL-L1 **(F)**, CL-K1 **(G)**, or CL-KL **(H)** MAb using concentrations ranging from 0.1 to 10 μg/ml.

as above. Purified native CL-LK (2 μg/ml) was pre-incubated in non-adsorbent wells with mAbs (0.5 or 4 μg/ml) or mannose (50 or 200 mM) at 37°C for 1 h, and subsequently incubated on ligand-coated plates at 37°C overnight. Wells were washed and incubated with recombinant MASP-2 (0.25 μg/ml for 3 h) followed by incubation with purified C4 (4 μg/ml, CompTech, Tyler, TX, USA, for 1 h) at 37°C. C4b deposition was detected using biotinylated anti-C4 mAb (0.5 μg/ml, HYB 162-02, BioPorto, Gentofte, Denmark). Samples were diluted in VBS (5 mM barbital, 142 mM NaCl, pH 7.4) with 2 mM $CaCl_2$, 1 mM $MgCl_2$, 0.05% Tween 20, and 0.1% BSA.

Human Tissue Samples

Human tissue samples were obtained from the tissue bank at the Department of Pathology, Odense University Hospital (Odense, Denmark) and derived from surgically removed specimens fixed 4% phosphate buffered formaldehyde for 12–48 h. Samples were conventionally dehydrated, and subsequently embedded in paraffin before sectioning (4–5 μm) and mounting on slides.

Immunohistochemistry

Paraffin-embedded, formalin-fixed human tissue sections were deparaffinized and rehydrated through serial wash in xylene and decreasing concentrations of ethanol. Endogen peroxidase activity was blocked by incubation with 1.5% H_2O_2 for 10 min. Antigen retrieval was performed by microwave boiling in 10 mM Tris base, 0.5 mM EDTA, and pH 9.0 buffer for 15 min. The tissue sections were washed in TNT buffer and incubated with primary antibodies MAb 16-13 (2 μg/ml), 11-1 (0.5 μg/ml), and mouse MAb anti-chicken IgY (1 μg/ml) for 1 h. The tissue sections were washed in TNT buffer and incubated with EnVision + System HRP-labeled polymer (Dako) for 30 min. After wash in TNT buffer, the tissue sections were incubated with DAB+ (Dako) for 10 min followed by staining with hematoxylin. The final immunohistochemical analysis was carried out using "multi block" sections comprising the following normal tissues: the cerebellum, esophagus, fetal and adult liver, gall bladder, kidney, large intestine, lung, skeletal muscle, pancreas, parotid gland, placenta, prostate, pylorus, spleen, tonsils, thymus, thyroid gland, rectum, small intestine, testis, and urinary bladder. The adrenal gland was derived from a patient diagnosed with pheochromocytoma.

Image Acquisition

Histology slides were scanned at 20× (controls) or 40× magnification using a NanoZoomer-XR (Hamamatsu Photonics, Japan). Image sections were acquired using NDP.view2 software (NanoZoomer Digital Pathology; Hamamatsu Photonics) and final JPG images were all uniformly adjusted for color saturation (+25) and light (−1) in Adobe Photoshop.

RESULTS

Antibody Specificity, Affinities, and Impact on Complement Activation

The reactivity of the applied MAbs was demonstrated by Western blotting using serum as source of antigens (**Figure 1**). This analysis showed that the applied MAbs 16-13 (anti-CL-L1) and 11-1 (anti-K1) only reacted with protein bands correlating with the molecular weight of CL-L1 and CL-K1, respectively (**Figure 1**) (7). There was no cross-reactivity of the two antibodies, and both MAbs recognized all isoforms, ensuring detection

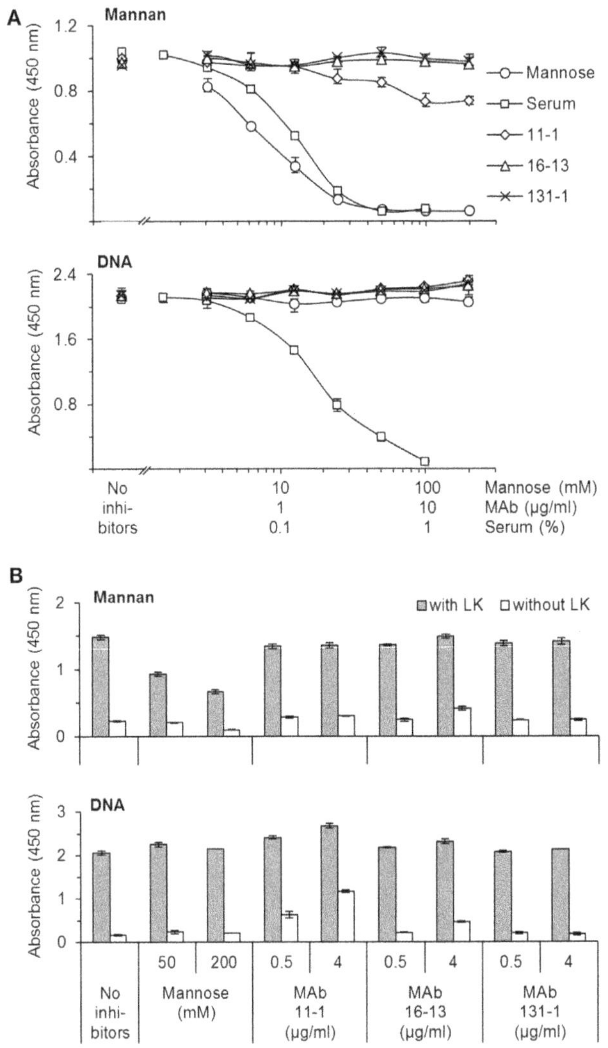

FIGURE 2 | Characterization of mAbs' impact on the ligand-binding and complement activity mediated by CL-LK. **(A)** Impact on ligand-binding. CL-LK was incubated on ligand-coated plates (mannan or DNA) in the presence or absence of the mAbs used for IHC (mAb 11-1 and mAb 16-13), mannose, or serum (known to interfere with the binding of CL-LK to ligands). mAb 131-1 (anti-MBL) was included as control. Bound CL-LK was detected with biotinylated mAb-anti-CL-K1 (compatible with the applied mAbs) and HRP-streptavidin. **(B)** Impact on CL-LK-mediated complement activation. Prior to incubation with MASP-2 and C4, plates were prepared with CL-LK and coated ligands (mannan or DNA) as above. Deposition of C4b was detected with biotin-labeled anti-C4b mAb and HRP-streptavidin. The results shown are representative of three independent experiments. Error bars refer to max and min of triplicate measurements. None of the tested mAbs interfered with ligand binding or complement activation. CL-LK binding to mannan and DNA occurs *via* two separate binding site, and the latter is not inhibited by mannose, whereas uncharacterized blood components inhibit both types of interaction (10, 11).

of all forms of CL-K1 and CL-L1 in the tissue sections. To further validate the specificity and reactivity, the two monoclonal antibodies were analyzed by SPR using immobilized purified collectins and antibodies in fluid phase. MAb16-13 bound to CL-L1 (K_D = 0.16 ± 0.007 nM, means ± SD) and to CL-LK (K_D = 0.14 ± 0.003 nM) but not to CL-K1. MAb 11-1 bound to CL-K1 (K1 K_D = 5.4 ± 1.8 nM) and to CL-LK (K_D = 4.6 ± 1.9 nM) but not to CL-L1. Again, cross-reactivity was undetectable and binding affinities/avidities were of satisfactory strengths. In the characterization of the two applied MAbs, we found that they neither interfered with the binding activity of CL-LK to suitable ligands nor did they modulate or inhibit the CL-LK-mediated complement activation *via* MASP-2 (**Figure 2**).

Immunohistochemical Localization of CL-L1 and CL-K1

In the majority of the tested tissues we observed identical localization of CL-K1 and CL-L1, both in terms of tissue and cell types. Unless the difference in immunoreactivity between the two was striking, the co-localization is not commented further, neither is the absence of staining of the tissues incubated with isotype matched control antibody. Frequently, the immunoreactivity of the CL-K1 MAb (11-1) was stronger than that of the CL-L1 MAb (16-13). This may not necessarily reflect an increase in CL-K1 quantity in comparison with CL-L1 but may originate from the nature of the antibodies (also discussed further below).

In the liver, immunoreactivity for CL-K1 and CL-L1 was associated with hepatocytes with absent staining of Kupffer cells. Staining intensities of CL-L1 was pronounced in the centrilobular hepatocytes (**Figure 3**).

In the kidney, immunoreactivity for CL-K1 and CL-L1 was especially associated with the tubular system, with the most pronounced staining of the distal tubules (**Figure 3**), in comparison with proximal tubules. CL-L1 immunoreactivity was for some distal tubules distinctly associated with the brush border. Immunoreactivity for both collectins was also associated with the epithelial cells lining the Bowman's capsules, whereas immunoreactivity in the glomerulus itself mainly was associated with CL-K1 and only minimally with CL-L1. CL-K1 immunoreactivity in the glomerulus was associated morphologically appeared to include both podocytes and mesangial cells.

In the lung, CL-K1 immunoreactivity was associated with alveolar macrophages, type I and II pneumocytes (**Figure 3**). CL-L1 immunoreactivity appeared only to be associated with alveolar macrophages.

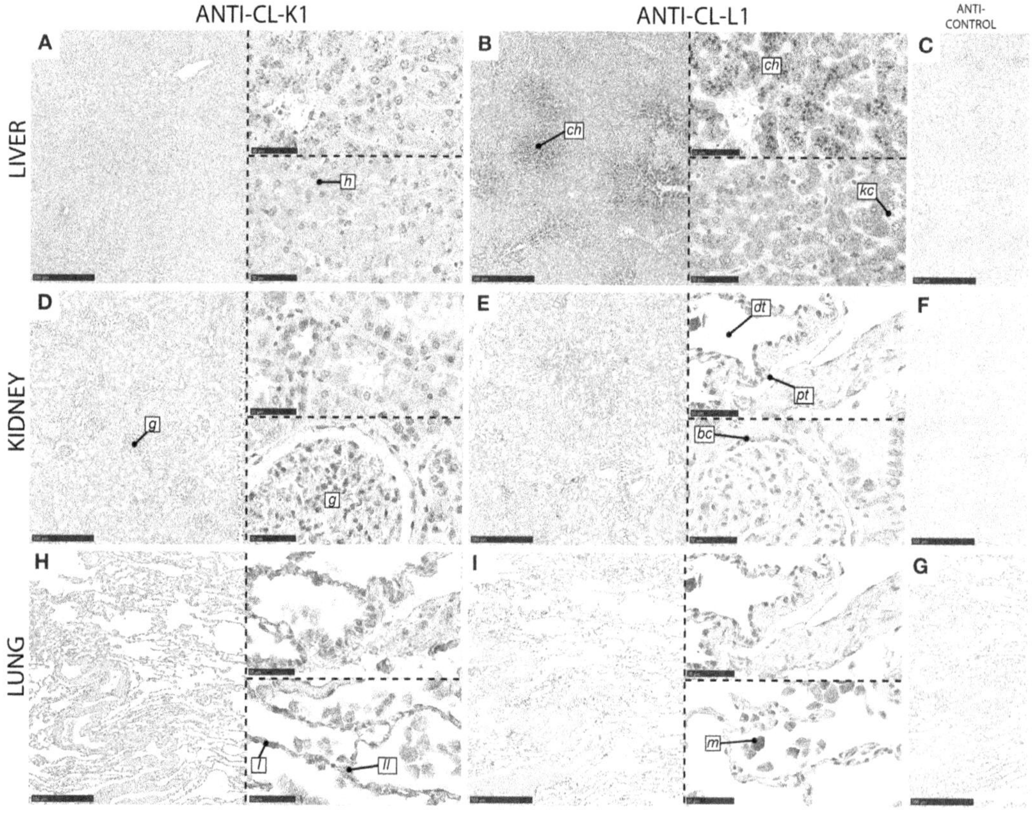

FIGURE 3 | Immunohistochemical localization of CL-K1 and CL-L1 in formalin fixed and paraffin embedded sections of the liver **(A,B)**, kidney **(D,E)**, and lung **(H,I)**. Italic letters within images refer to: for the **liver** *h*: hepatocytes, *ch*: centrilobular hepatocytes, and *kc*: Kupffer cells; **kidney** *g*: glomerulus, *dt*: distal tubules, *pt*: proximal tubules, and *bc*: Bowman's capsule; **lung** *I*: type I pneumocytes, *II*: type II pneumocytes, and *m*: alveolar macrophages. Scale bars in large sections and in isotype control sections **(C,F,G)** correspond to 500 μm and in small sections to 50 μm.

In the thyroid gland, cuboidal epithelial cells lining the base membrane of thyroid follicles and parafollicular cells (C-cells) were associated with immunoreactivity for both CL-K1 and CL-L1 (**Figure 4**). Most pronounced staining was observed for CL-K1.

In the pancreas CL-K1 and CL-L1 immunoreactivity was associated with the islets of Langerhans and the pancreatic epithelial acinar cells and ducts (**Figure 4**). Within the islets, the vast majority of cells stained positive, indicating for sure that insulin-producing cells (beta cells) were associated with immunoreactivity and also most likely glucagon-producing cells (alpha cells) as well.

In the adrenal tissue section (**Figure 4**), derived from a patient diagnosed with pheochromocytoma, the histology was slightly unclear. However, as immunoreactivity for both CL-K1 and CL-L1 was associated with nearly all cells, it was deducted that the majority of adrenal cells, including both medullary and cortical cells, are associated with the two collectins, similar with previous findings for the localization of CL-K1 (7).

In the gall bladder, immunoreactivity for both CL-K1 and CL-L1 was associated with columnar epithelial cells of the mucosal folds, with increasing intensity toward the luminal side of the folds (**Figure 5**). Various cell types in the lamina propria stained weakly positive. We observed only scattered staining of cells in the muscularis and serosa layers.

In the duodenum, immunoreactivity for CL-K1 and CL-L1 was associated with epithelial cells in both the mucosa and submucosa. In the mucosal luminal membrane of the villi, especially columnar cells (enterocytes) stained positive (**Figure 5**). Further and intense immunoreactivity of the mucosa was associated with the crypts of Lieberkuhn, whereas the muscularis externa was only weakly positive for staining. In the submucosa, immunoreactivity was associated with cells of the Brunner's glands.

In the colon, CL-K1 and CL-L1 immunoreactivity was dominantly associated with mucosa and especially with columnar epithelial cells in the crypts of Lieberkuhn (tubular glands) (**Figure 5**). In the lamina propria, the staining was scattered and associated with various cells types. Within the layers of the muscularis externa and submucosa, staining was also associated with endothelial cells, best illustrated for the localization of CL-K1.

In the testis, CL-K1 immunoreactivity was associated with germinal epithelial cells lining the tunica propria of the seminiferous tubules, spermatogonia (type A and B), and spermatocytes (primary and secondary) (**Figure 6**). These cells were embedded in the less immunoreactive Sertoli cells. In the interstitium between seminiferous tubules, Leydig cells and endothelial cells of capillaries stained weakly positive. CL-L1 immunoreactivity was weak in comparison with that of CL-K1, but the pattern of the two collectins followed each other.

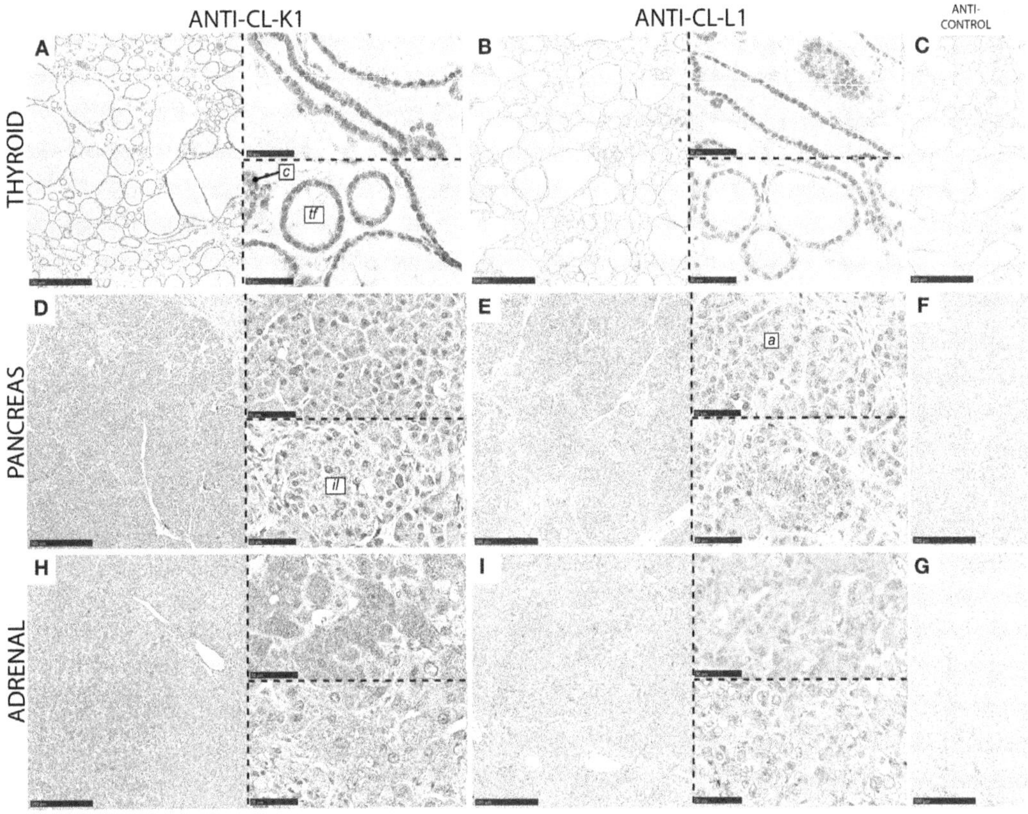

FIGURE 4 | Immunohistochemical localization of CL-K1 and CL-L1 in formalin fixed and paraffin embedded sections of the thyroid gland **(A,B)**, pancreas **(D,E)**, and adrenal gland from a patient diagnosed with pheochromocytoma, **(H,I)**. Italic letters within images refer to: for the **thyroid gland** *tf*, thyroid follicles and *c*, parafollicular C cells; **pancreas** *il*: islets of Langerhans and *a*: acinar epithelial cells. Scale bars in large sections and in isotype control sections **(C,F,G)** correspond to 500 μm and in small sections to 50 μm.

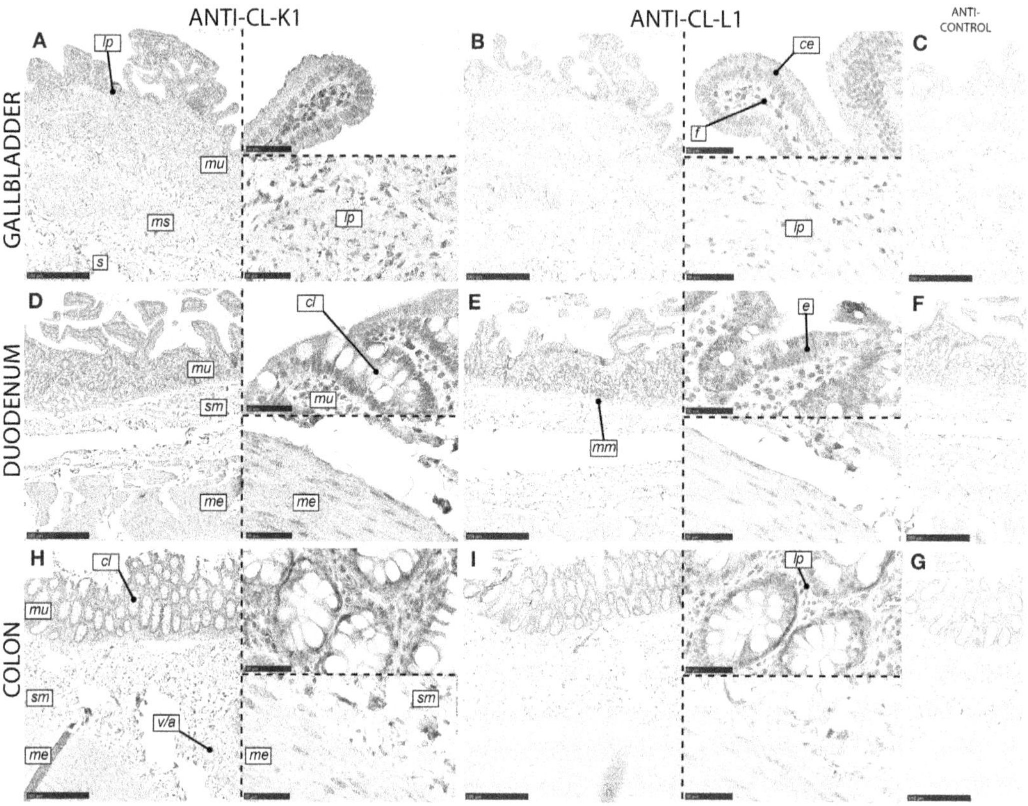

FIGURE 5 | Immunohistochemical localization of CL-K1 and CL-L1 in formalin-fixed and paraffin-embedded sections of the gallbladder **(A,B)**, duodenum **(D,E)**, and colon **(H,I)**. Italic letters within images refers to: for the **gallbladder** *s*: serosa layer, *ms*: muscularis layer, *m*: mucosa layer, *lp*: lamina propria, *ce*: columnar epithelial cells, and *f*: fibroblasts; **duodenum** and **colon** *me*: muscularis externica layers, *sm*: submucosa, *mu*: mucosa, *cl*: crypts of Lieberkuhn (tubular glands), *mm*: muscularis mucosa, and *v/a*: vein/artery. Scale bars in large sections and in isotype control sections **(C,F,G)** correspond to 500 μm and in small sections to 50 μm.

In the prostate, CL-K1 and CL-L1 immunoreactivity was associated with epithelial cells of the prostatic glands, with staining of both acini and ducts (**Figure 6**). The staining was associated with both columnar pseudostratified and involuted luminal epithelial cells; however, with most intense staining of the basal epithelial cells. In the stroma, scattered staining was observed in various cells types, including staining of endothelial cells. In the ducts, secretory vesicles and concretized material stained weakly positive, especially for CL-K1.

In the corpus uterus, CL-K1 and CL-L1 immunoreactivity was localized to the epithelial cells in the endometrial glands, glandular ducts, and at luminal surface, with comparable staining of glandular structures in both the stratum functionalis (compactum and spongiosum) and stratum basale (**Figure 6**). Both stratified columnar and ciliated cells in the glands stained intensely. In the stroma, the immunoreactivity was moderate but associated with the majority of cells, with a pronounced staining of endothelial cells of the capillaries.

In the skin, CL-K1 and CL-L1 immunoreactivity was associated with the sweat glands and ducts (**Figure 7**). CL-K1 staining was further associated with the basal layer of the epidermis. In the sweat glands and ducts, especially epithelial cells, stained positive, while myoepithelial cells only stained weakly positive. Within the inner duct, staining was associated with the luminal part and eventual content in the duct. Staining of sporadically distributed and non-identifiable cells in the dermis was also observed.

In the partoid salivary glands, immunoreactivity for CL-L1 and CL-K1 was associated with both epithelial glandular (acini) and epithelial ductal cells (**Figure 7**). Immunoreactivity was localized dominantly to the epithelial cells constituting the salivary ducts and less with the secretory acini. However, the majority of serous-producing epithelial cells were associated with immunoreactivity. Basal epithelial cells of mucin producing stained weakly positive. All three kinds of ducts: intercalated (minor), intralobulated (striated), and major showed equal and dominant immunoreactivity. The immunoreactivity of CL-L1 in the salivary serous glands was superior to that of CL-K1.

In the full-term (mature) placenta, CL-K1 and CL-L1 immunoreactivity was mainly associated with the syncytiotrophoblast layer, at the border of maternal and fetal circulation, and weakly with the underlying cytotrophoblasts associated with a villus (**Figure 7**).

Various levels of CL-K1 and CL-L1 immunoreactivity were also found to be associated with the following tissues: the thymus, spleen, tonsil (Figure S1 in Supplementary Material), esophagus,

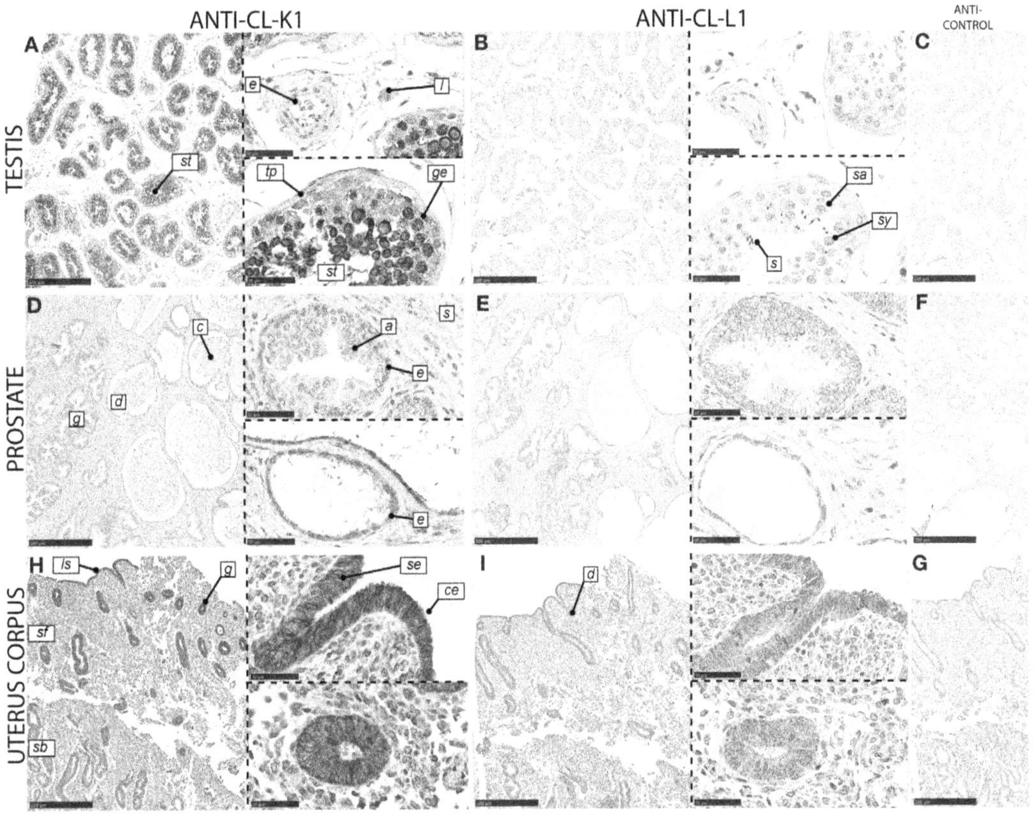

FIGURE 6 | Immunohistochemical localization of CL-K1 and CL-L1 in formalin-fixed and paraffin-embedded sections of the testis **(A,B)**, prostate **(D,E)**, and uterus corpus **(H,I)**. Italic letters within images refers to: for the **testis** st: seminiferous tubules, *e*: endothelial cells, *l*: Leydig cell, *tp*: tunicapropria, *ge*: germinal epithelial cells, *s*: spermatogonia, *sy*: spermatocytes, and *s*: spermatids; **prostate** *g*: gland, *d*: duct, *c*: "concretized" material: *a*: acininar cells/acinus, *s*: stroma, and *e*: basal epithelial cells; **uterus corpus** *sb*: stratum basale, *sf*: stratum functionalis, *ls*: luminal surface, *g*: gland, *d*: duct, *se*: stratified columnar epithelial cells, and *ce*: ciliated epithelial cells. Scale bars in large sections and in isotype control sections **(C,F,G)** correspond to 500 μm and in small sections to 50 μm.

stomach (Figure S2 in Supplementary Material), cervix uterus, portio uterus, abortus (Figure S3 in Supplementary Material), skeletal muscle, cerebellum, and urinary bladder (Figure S4 in Supplementary Material). A description of their detailed localizations is provided in the associated figure legends.

CL-K1 and CL-L1 mRNA Abundancies

To compare protein localization by IHC with site of synthesis for the two collectins, data were retrieved from the three major RNA expression databases HPA, GTEx, and FANTOM5 RNA. For comparison, expression levels were normalized and graduated into four categories based on a logarithmic division (Tables S1 and S2 in Supplementary Material). Levels of immunoreactivity were visually validated by three independent persons and categorized similarly (**Table 1**).

mRNA transcripts encoding CL-K1 was detectable in all tested tissues and the major sites of synthesis, grouped in the "high" category, comprised the adrenals, gallbladder, and liver. In all the tested tissues, there was only minimal variance, in terms of a single category shift, i.e., "high" to "medium," between CL-K1 mRNA levels and immunoreactivity, therefore we considered there to be an excellent accordance between site of CL-K1 synthesis and protein localization. mRNA transcript encoding CL-L1 was not detected in as many tissues as CL-K1. Some tissues were categorized with "extremely low/absent" number of CL-L1 transcripts. However, by IHC quite a lot of these tissues were found to be associated with immunoreactivity, albeit in a "low" degree. The major site of CL-L1 mRNA synthesis was the liver and placenta and in these tissues the protein was also readily detected. Similar to the observations for CL-K1 and using the same criteria, there appeared in general to be accordance between site of CL-L1 synthesis and protein localization (discussed further below).

To associate the protein localization with an eventual local functionality of the two collectins, mediated *via* the presence of MASPs, localization of MASPs (and MAps), and synthesis of their respective mRNAs were evaluated by the same approach. As the major RNA expression databases currently do not take alternatively splicing of the MASP genes into consideration, data were retrieved and gathered from the previous work by Thiel and colleagues and Garred and colleagues (30–33). MASP-3 expression appeared to both overlap and being as widely distributed as the two collectins, whereas the other MASPs and MAp had a restricted pattern of tissue localization, with the liver being a tissue of major synthesis and/or detection: an observation, which also applied for MBL.

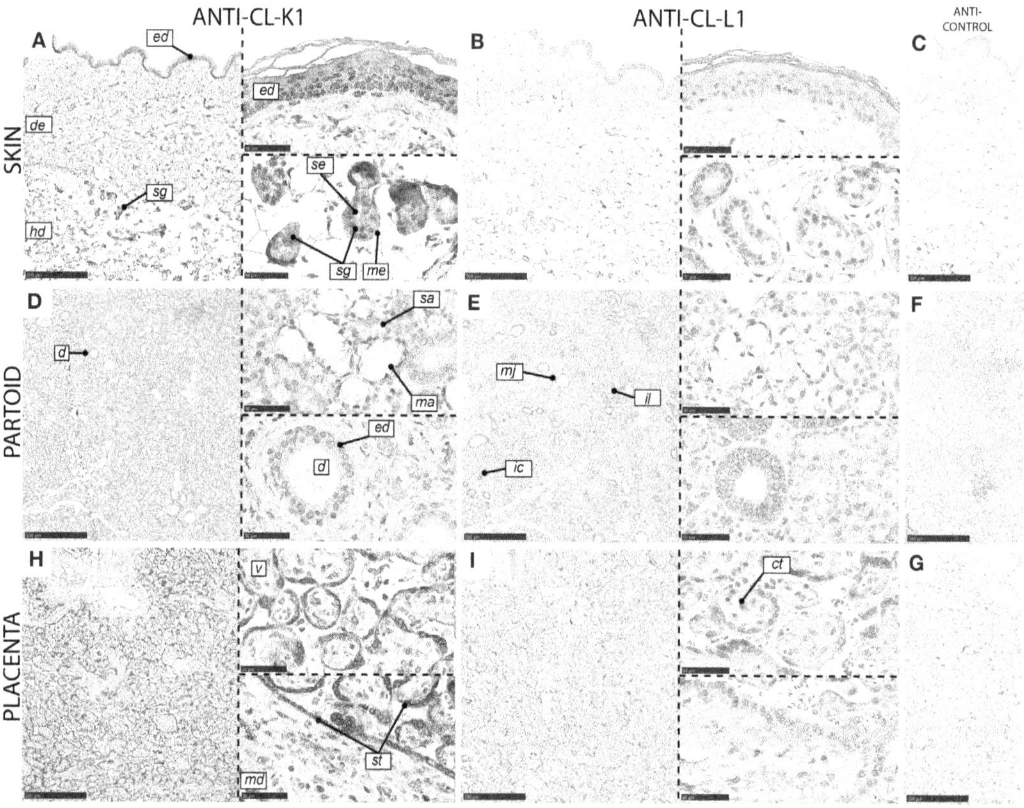

FIGURE 7 | Immunohistochemical localization of CL-K1 and CL-L1 in formalin fixed and paraffin embedded sections of the skin **(A,B)**, parotid gland **(D,E)**, and placenta **(H,I)**. Italic letters within images refers to: for the **skin** *ed*: epidermis, *de*: dermis, *hd*: hypodermis, *sg*: sweat glands, *me*: myoepithelial cells, and *se*: stratified cuboidal epithelia cells; **partoid salivary gland** *d*: duct, *ed*: epithelial ductal cells, *sa*: serous acini, *ma*: mucous acini, *mj*: major duct, *il*: intralobulated duct, and *ic*: intercalated duct; **placenta** *v*: villus, st: syncytiotrophoblast, *ct*: cytotrophoblast, and *md*: mesoderm. Scale bars in large sections and in isotype control sections **(C,F,G)** correspond to 500 µm and in small sections to 50 µm.

DISCUSSION

The present work describes the localization of CL-L1 and CL-K1 in human tissues as determined by immunohistochemistry and summarizes further their mRNA tissue profiles derived from transcriptome databases. Both CL-L1 and CL-K1 were demonstrated in epithelial cells in a variety of tissue throughout the human body.

Of all the tested MAbs, MAbs 16-13 (anti-CL-L1) and 11-1 (anti-CL-K1) had the best sensitivity and specificity. The two MAbs demonstrated excellent immunoreactivity in the three tissues, the liver, kidney, and adrenals, wherein human CL-K1 and CL-L1 localization previously have been demonstrated (6, 7). The major positive cell types comprised, hepatocytes, renal epithelial cells of tubules, and medullary and cortical cells of the adrenals. In addition to the adrenals, tissues from other endocrine glands, i.e., pancreas, demonstrated a similar convincing excellent immunoreactivity for both collectins, derived from cells in the islets of Langerhans and epithelial cells of the ducts. Exocrine tissues of the digestive system comprising the gallbladder, duodenum, colon, and also partly the stomach and esophagus were also associated with epithelial and mucosal immunoreactivity for generally both collectins. Other exocrine tissues, comprising sex-specific organs, such as the testis, prostate, and uterus, had also excellent to moderate immunoreactivity for both collectins. Among all the analyzed tissues, the testis and uterus appeared to be the two tissues with the relative highest CL-K1 immunoreactivity. Again, epithelial cells and mucosa in the uterus were the major source of immunoreactivity, whereas immunoreactivity in testis was associated with germinal epithelial cells of the tubules. Among the tissues analyzed, the highest CL-L1 immunoreactivity was observed in the liver, followed by the kidney and parotid gland, wherein immunoreactivity was also associated with epithelial cells. Our observation of CL-K1 synthesis in various tissues falls in line with previous work by Wakamiya and colleagues, who by immunofluorescence techniques demonstrated partly overlapping localization of CL-K1 in murine tissues, using a polyclonal anti-mouse-CL-K1 antibody (34). In general, we observed a stronger staining of CL-K1 than of CL-L1. This may reflect that CL-K1 is more abundant than CL-L1, although their levels in the circulation are approximately the same (12), or it may simply be a matter of affinities of the applied MAbs in combination with availability of antigen epitopes on the fixed and embedded tissue sections.

Retrieval and normalization of mRNA levels from three transcriptome databases demonstrated accordance between site

TABLE 1 | Levels of RNA expression: The symbols "+++," "++," "+," and "− "denote high, medium, low, and absent/extremely low expression, respectively, based on the criteria established in Figures S1 and S2 in Supplementary Material.

	***CL-K1* IHC/ RNA[a]**	***CL-L1* IHC/ RNA[a]**	***MASP-1* IHC/ RNA[b]**	***MASP-3* IHC/ RNA[b]**	***MAp44* IHC[c]/ RNA[d]**	***MASP-2* IHC[e]/ RNA[f]**	***MAp19* IHC[e]/ RNA[e]**	***MBL* IHC[g]/ RNA[a]**
Abortus	++/	+/						
Adrenal	+++/+++	++/+						−/−
Cerebellum	++/+	+/−					+/	−/−
Cervix uterus	++/+	+/−	/+	/+++	/++	/−	/−	−/−
Colon	++/+	+/−	/−	/+++	/+	+/−	/−	−/−
Corpus uterus	+++/	+/						
Esophagus	++/+	−/−	/++	/+	/−	/−	/−	−/−
Fetal liver	+/	++/						
Fetal muscle	++/	++/						
Gallbladder	+++/+++	++/+						+/−
Heart	/++	/+	/++	/+++	+++/+++	/−	/−	+/−
Kidney	++/++	++/+	/++	/++	/−	++/−	++/++	+/−
Liver	++/+++	+++/+++	/+++	/+++	+++/++	+++/+++	+++/+++	+++/+++
Lung	++/+	+/+	/++	/+++	/++	+/+	++/−	−/−
Muscle	+/+	−/−	/−	/+++	++/+++	/−	/−	−/−
Pancreas	++/++	+/-	/−	/+++	/−	+/−		−/−
Placenta	+++/++	+/+++	/++	/+++	/−	/−	/−	−/−
Portio uterus	+/	−/						
Prostate	++/+	+/+	/−	/+++	/−	/−	+/−	−/−
Salivary gland	+/+	++/−						−/−
Skin	++/+	+/−						−/−
Small intestine	++/++	+/+	/++	/+++	/−	/++	/−	−/−
Spleen	++/++	+/−	/−	/++	/−	/−	/−	−/−
Stomach	++/+	+/−					+/	+/−
Testis	+++/++	+/−	/−	/++	/−	/++	/−	−/−
Thymus	+/	−/	/−	/++	/−	/−	/−	
Thyroid	+++/++	+/+	/−	/−	/−	/−	+/+++	−/−
Tonsil	+/+	−/−						−/−
Urinary bladder	++/++	−/+	/−	/++	/−	/−	/−	−/−

IHC immunoreactivity levels were judged arbitrarily into the same categories by three independent validations (persons). Missing symbols reflect that the tissue has not been analyzed. MASP-1, MASP-3, and Map44 derive all from the MASP1 gene. MASP-2 and MAp19 derive both from the MASP2 gene.
[a]*Relative and normalized data from HPA, GTEx, and FANTOM5 RNA expression databases (Tables S1–S3 in Supplementary Material).*
[b]*Relative and normalized data from Seyfarth et al. (30) and Degn et al. (31) (Tables S4 and S5 in Supplementary Material).*
[c]*Skjoedt et al. (32).*
[d]*Relative and normalized data from Degn et al. (31) and Skjoedt et al. (32) (Table S6 in Supplementary Material).*
[e]*Degn et al. (33) (Table S7 in Supplementary Material).*
[f]*Relative and normalized data from Seyfarth et al. (30) and Degn et al. (33) (Table S8 in Supplementary Material).*
[g]*The Human Protein Atlas Project (antibody CAB016782).*

of synthesis and protein localization. The only tissue, wherein there appeared to be a notable difference, was for CL-L1 in the salivary gland. By IHC CL-L1 localization was judged to be medium, whereas CL-L1 mRNA appeared to be absent. Other CL-L1-specific antibodies showed varying staining of particular the salivary gland (data not shown), making us hypothesize that the observed disagreement could reflect some sort of uncharacterized alternative splicing of CL-L1 in this tissue.

Throughout the IHC staining it was evident that within the majority of the tissues, the localization pattern of two collectins was identical; meaning that exactly the same cells in a given tissue demonstrated immunoreactivity for both collectins. This is best exemplified when two neighbor sections were mounted and processed, as illustrated, e.g., with the corpus uterus (**Figure 6**). Thus, in the majority of tissues there is opportunity for the making of CL-LK heteromeric complexes, and as previously described, this structure also appears to be the most thermodynamic stabile conformation (11). In some of the tissues, comprising the thyroid gland, skeletal muscle, skin, urinary bladder, and partly the testis and esophagus, CL-K1 appeared to be present in large excess in comparison with CL-L1, as judged by immunoreactivity; it is likely that CL-K1 homomers will be the dominating form in these tissues. The precise distribution of homomers vs. heteromers in different tissues should not be judged by immunoreactivity and remains thus to be characterized in detail. Although the heteromers are eminent in their association with MASP-2 and C4b deposition, in comparison with the homomers, it is worth emphasizing that both types of homomers interact well with MASP-1/-3, and may mediate downstream complement activation *via* those alone (8, 11).

To further illustrate the presence of heteromers in different tissues we tried to establish a proximity ligation assay using antibodies usable on formalin fixed sections but without convincing results. By using purified and fixed CL-LK it appeared that even the best combination of antibodies partly shadowed for each other in proximity ligation assays and were only capable of detecting the very high oligomers of CL-LK, with a sensitivity of only 0.2 μg of purified CL-LK per ml immobilized onto polylysine-treated object glasses (data not shown).

The overlapping localization of the two collectins in the same cells justifies, with a few exceptions, possible assembly and presence of the heteromeric CL-LK in most tissues. Based on a combination of previous observations and unpublished results by our laboratory, it appears that the oligomeric state of CL-LK depends on the relative content of CL-L1 and the ratio of the CL-K1a/d isotypes (11). As all of our anti-CL-K1 MAbs recognize the two isotypes equally well, the immunohistochemical results does not *per se* allow us to deduct any final conclusions on the variability of oligomers in different tissues. However, tissues with a relative large expression of CL-L1 could potentially favor assembly of CL-LK into large oligomers, ranging from 2 to 6 subunits.

We have previously demonstrated that the binding activity of CL-K1 and CL-LK, and hence also their complement activating ability, in serum/plasma is inhibited by unknown factors (11). This has made it difficult to comprehend the role of the two collectins as *bona fida* activators of complement. In the light of the widespread presence of CL-K1 and CL-L1 in various tissues, it is possible that binding activity in the periphery, in the absence of inhibitory blood components, may be more efficient.

As the hitherto described biological functions of CL-K1 and CL-L1, in terms of complement activation or involvement in embryogenesis, appear to rely on MASPs it is relevant to investigate co-localization with MASPs in the periphery. However, there is a lack of suitable antibodies specific for the three products of the MASP-1 gene, MASP-1/-3, and MAp44, but the summarized mRNA profile presented in **Table 1** shows that MASP-3 synthesis, in contrast with all other MASPs and MAps, appears to overlap greatly with the localization of CL-K1 and CL-L1. Thus, it is likely that the role of CL-K1 and CL-L1 in the periphery is mainly mediated *via* MASP-3, which was recently shown to activate profactor D to factor D, and thereby potentiate the alternative pathway and amplification loop (35–37). Although (pro) factor D mainly is synthesized in adipose tissue (hence the alias "adipsin") various tissues synthesize minor amounts of profactor D, which could be a target for MASP-3 in complex with CL-K1/-L1/-LK, and thereby potentiate the complement amplification loop in the periphery, upon encounter and binding of collectins to suitable (microbial) ligands. Alternatively, the two collectins may in the periphery, and in parallel with MBL and C1q, exert some of their functions by interacting with the metalloproteases bone morphogenic protein 1 and tolloid-like proteases, involved in extracellular matrix assembly and growth factor signaling (38). Interactions between CL-K1, -L1, or -LK with these metalloproteases remain to be investigated.

In the light of our (co-)localization of CL-K1 and CL-L1 to peripheral tissues it appears that the previously focus on their roles in the circulation, liver, and kidney, may have disparaged a compelling localization in especially exocrine/endocrine tissues and mucosa, suggestive of that CL-L1, CL-K1, and CL-LK may lay roles on epithelial surfaces in general and in tissue characterized by a high degree of exocytosis. The localization of CL-K1 and CL-L1 reminds also in many ways of the localization of the collectin surfactant protein D (39).

AUTHOR CONTRIBUTIONS

SH and MH designed the study and carried out: antibody development, characterization, immunohistochemistry, data analysis, computational bioinformatics, and wrote the paper, on which all authors commented. JA and KB carried out antibody development, characterization, and immunohistochemistry. EH, ON, and HS participated in designing and performing the immunohistochemistry and analyzing data. KS carried out development of antibodies. AS and JG carried out SPR analysis and analyzed data.

ACKNOWLEDGMENTS

The authors thank Anette Holck Draborg, Department of Cancer and Inflammation Research, University of Southern Denmark for critical reading of the manuscript and for giving valuable comments. The authors thank Lisbeth Mortensen, Department of Pathology, Odense University Hospital for technical advice relating to immunohistochemistry.

FUNDING

This work was in part supported by the A. P. Møller Foundation, Augustinus Foundation, and Dagmar Marshall Foundation.

REFERENCES

1. Zipfel PF, Hallstrom T, Riesbeck K. Human complement control and complement evasion by pathogenic microbes – tipping the balance. *Mol Immunol* (2013) 56(3):152–60. doi:10.1016/j.molimm.2013.05.222
2. Thiel S, Vorup-Jensen T, Stover CM, Schwaeble W, Laursen SB, Poulsen K, et al. A second serine protease associated with mannan-binding lectin that activates complement. *Nature* (1997) 386(6624):506–10. doi:10.1038/386506a0
3. Dobo J, Pal G, Cervenak L, Gal P. The emerging roles of mannose-binding lectin-associated serine proteases (MASPs) in the lectin pathway of complement and beyond. *Immunol Rev* (2016) 274(1):98–111. doi:10.1111/imr.12460
4. Heitzeneder S, Seidel M, Forster-Waldl E, Heitger A. Mannan-binding lectin deficiency – good news, bad news, doesn't matter? *Clin Immunol* (2012) 143(1):22–38. doi:10.1016/j.clim.2011.11.002
5. Keshi H, Sakamoto T, Kawai T, Ohtani K, Katoh T, Jang SJ, et al. Identification and characterization of a novel human collectin CL-K1. *Microbiol Immunol* (2006) 50(12):1001–13. doi:10.1111/j.1348-0421.2006.tb03868.x
6. Ohtani K, Suzuki Y, Eda S, Kawai T, Kase T, Yamazaki H, et al. Molecular cloning of a novel human collectin from liver (CL-L1). *J Biol Chem* (1999) 274(19):13681–9. doi:10.1074/jbc.274.19.13681
7. Hansen S, Selman L, Palaniyar N, Ziegler K, Brandt J, Kliem A, et al. Collectin 11 (CL-11, CL-K1) is a MASP-1/3-associated plasma collectin with

microbial-binding activity. *J Immunol* (2010) 185(10):6096–104. doi:10.4049/jimmunol.1002185

8. Axelgaard E, Jensen L, Dyrlund TF, Nielsen HJ, Enghild JJ, Thiel S, et al. Investigations on collectin liver 1. *J Biol Chem* (2013) 288(32):23407–20. doi:10.1074/jbc.M113.492603
9. Hansen SW, Ohtani K, Roy N, Wakamiya N. The collectins CL-L1, CL-K1 and CL-P1, and their roles in complement and innate immunity. *Immunobiology* (2016) 221(10):1058–67. doi:10.1016/j.imbio.2016.05.012
10. Henriksen ML, Brandt J, Iyer SS, Thielens NM, Hansen S. Characterization of the interaction between collectin 11 (CL-11, CL-K1) and nucleic acids. *Mol Immunol* (2013) 56(4):757–67. doi:10.1016/j.molimm.2013.07.011
11. Henriksen ML, Brandt J, Andrieu JP, Nielsen C, Jensen PH, Holmskov U, et al. Heteromeric complexes of native collectin kidney 1 and collectin liver 1 are found in the circulation with MASPs and activate the complement system. *J Immunol* (2013) 191(12):6117–27. doi:10.4049/jimmunol.1302121
12. Troldborg A, Hansen A, Hansen SW, Jensenius JC, Stengaard-Pedersen K, Thiel S. Lectin complement pathway proteins in healthy individuals. *Clin Exp Immunol* (2017) 188(1):138–47. doi:10.1111/cei.12909
13. Yoshizaki T, Ohtani K, Motomura W, Jang SJ, Mori K, Kitamoto N, et al. Comparison of human blood concentrations of collectin kidney 1 and mannan-binding lectin. *J Biochem* (2012) 151(1):57–64. doi:10.1093/jb/mvr114
14. Bayarri-Olmos R, Hansen S, Henriksen ML, Storm L, Thiel S, Garred P, et al. Genetic variation of COLEC10 and COLEC11 and association with serum levels of collectin liver 1 (CL-L1) and collectin kidney 1 (CL-K1). *PLoS One* (2015) 10(2):e0114883. doi:10.1371/journal.pone.0114883
15. Selman L, Henriksen ML, Brandt J, Palarasah Y, Waters A, Beales PL, et al. An enzyme-linked immunosorbent assay (ELISA) for quantification of human collectin 11 (CL-11, CL-K1). *J Immunol Methods* (2012) 375(1–2):182–8. doi:10.1016/j.jim.2011.10.010
16. Hwang I, Mori K, Ohtani K, Matsuda Y, Roy N, Kim Y, et al. Collectin kidney 1 plays an important role in innate immunity against *Streptococcus pneumoniae* infection. *J Innate Immun* (2017) 9(2):217–28. doi:10.1159/000453316
17. Troegeler A, Lugo-Villarino G, Hansen S, Rasolofo V, Henriksen ML, Mori K, et al. Collectin CL-LK is a novel soluble pattern recognition receptor for *Mycobacterium tuberculosis*. *PLoS One* (2015) 10(7):e0132692. doi:10.1371/journal.pone.0132692
18. Venkatraman Girija U, Furze CM, Gingras AR, Yoshizaki T, Ohtani K, Marshall JE, et al. Molecular basis of sugar recognition by collectin-K1 and the effects of mutations associated with 3MC syndrome. *BMC Biol* (2015) 13:27. doi:10.1186/s12915-015-0136-2
19. Farrar CA, Tran D, Li K, Wu W, Peng Q, Schwaeble W, et al. Collectin-11 detects stress-induced L-fucose pattern to trigger renal epithelial injury. *J Clin Invest* (2016) 126(5):1911–25. doi:10.1172/JCI83000
20. Wu W, Liu C, Farrar CA, Ma L, Dong X, Sacks SH, et al. Collectin-11 promotes the development of renal tubulointerstitial fibrosis. *J Am Soc Nephrol* (2018) 29(1):168–81. doi:10.1681/ASN.2017050544
21. Munye MM, Diaz-Font A, Ocaka L, Henriksen ML, Lees M, Brady A, et al. COLEC10 is mutated in 3MC patients and regulates early craniofacial development. *PLoS Genet* (2017) 13(3):e1006679. doi:10.1371/journal.pgen.1006679
22. Rooryck C, Diaz-Font A, Osborn DP, Chabchoub E, Hernandez-Hernandez V, Shamseldin H, et al. Mutations in lectin complement pathway genes COLEC11 and MASP1 cause 3MC syndrome. *Nat Genet* (2011) 43(3):197–203. doi:10.1038/ng.757
23. Bolger MS, Ross DS, Jiang H, Frank MM, Ghio AJ, Schwartz DA, et al. Complement levels and activity in the normal and LPS-injured lung. *Am J Physiol Lung Cell Mol Physiol* (2007) 292(3):L748–59. doi:10.1152/ajplung.00127.2006
24. Andoh A, Fujiyama Y, Sakumoto H, Uchihara H, Kimura T, Koyama S, et al. Detection of complement C3 and factor B gene expression in normal colorectal mucosa, adenomas and carcinomas. *Clin Exp Immunol* (1998) 111(3):477–83. doi:10.1046/j.1365-2249.1998.00496.x
25. Henriksen ML, Madsen KL, Skjoedt K, Hansen S. Calcium-sensitive immunoaffinity chromatography: gentle and highly specific retrieval of a scarce plasma antigen, collectin-LK (CL-LK). *J Immunol Methods* (2014) 413:25–31. doi:10.1016/j.jim.2014.07.006
26. Kohler G, Milstein C. Continuous cultures of fused cells secreting antibody of predefined specificity. *Nature* (1975) 256(5517):495–7. doi:10.1038/256495a0
27. Akerstrom B, Bjorck L. A physicochemical study of protein G, a molecule with unique immunoglobulin G-binding properties. *J Biol Chem* (1986) 261(22):10240–7.
28. Laemmli UK. Cleavage of structural proteins during the assembly of the head of bacteriophage T4. *Nature* (1970) 227(5259):680–5. doi:10.1038/227680a0
29. Towbin H, Staehelin T, Gordon J. Electrophoretic transfer of proteins from polyacrylamide gels to nitrocellulose sheets: procedure and some applications. *Proc Natl Acad Sci U S A* (1979) 76(9):4350–4. doi:10.1073/pnas.76.9.4350
30. Seyfarth J, Garred P, Madsen HO. Extra-hepatic transcription of the human mannose-binding lectin gene (mbl2) and the MBL-associated serine protease 1-3 genes. *Mol Immunol* (2006) 43(7):962–71. doi:10.1016/j.molimm.2005.06.033
31. Degn SE, Hansen AG, Steffensen R, Jacobsen C, Jensenius JC, Thiel S. MAp44, a human protein associated with pattern recognition molecules of the complement system and regulating the lectin pathway of complement activation. *J Immunol* (2009) 183(11):7371–8. doi:10.4049/jimmunol.0902388
32. Skjoedt MO, Hummelshoj T, Palarasah Y, Honore C, Koch C, Skjodt K, et al. A novel mannose-binding lectin/ficolin-associated protein is highly expressed in heart and skeletal muscle tissues and inhibits complement activation. *J Biol Chem* (2010) 285(11):8234–43. doi:10.1074/jbc.M109.065805
33. Degn SE, Thiel S, Nielsen O, Hansen AG, Steffensen R, Jensenius JC. MAp19, the alternative splice product of the MASP2 gene. *J Immunol Methods* (2011) 373(1–2):89–101. doi:10.1016/j.jim.2011.08.006
34. Motomura W, Yoshizaki T, Ohtani K, Okumura T, Fukuda M, Fukuzawa J, et al. Immunolocalization of a novel collectin CL-K1 in murine tissues. *J Histochem Cytochem* (2008) 56(3):243–52. doi:10.1369/jhc.7A7312.2007
35. Pihl R, Jensen L, Hansen AG, Thogersen IB, Andres S, Dagnaes-Hansen F, et al. Analysis of factor D isoforms in Malpuech-Michels-Mingarelli-Carnevale patients highlights the role of MASP-3 as a maturase in the alternative pathway of complement. *J Immunol* (2017) 199:2158–70. doi:10.4049/jimmunol.1700518
36. Dobo J, Szakacs D, Oroszlan G, Kortvely E, Kiss B, Boros E, et al. MASP-3 is the exclusive pro-factor D activator in resting blood: the lectin and the alternative complement pathways are fundamentally linked. *Sci Rep* (2016) 6:31877. doi:10.1038/srep31877
37. Takahashi M, Ishida Y, Iwaki D, Kanno K, Suzuki T, Endo Y, et al. Essential role of mannose-binding lectin-associated serine protease-1 in activation of the complement factor D. *J Exp Med* (2010) 207(1):29–37. doi:10.1084/jem.20090633
38. Lacroix M, Tessier A, Dumestre-Perard C, Vadon-Le Goff S, Gout E, Bruckner-Tuderman L, et al. Interaction of complement defence collagens C1q and mannose-binding lectin with BMP-1/tolloid-like proteinases. *Sci Rep* (2017) 7(1):16958. doi:10.1038/s41598-017-17318-w
39. Madsen J, Kliem A, Tornoe I, Skjodt K, Koch C, Holmskov U. Localization of lung surfactant protein D on mucosal surfaces in human tissues. *J Immunol* (2000) 164(11):5866–70. doi:10.4049/jimmunol.164.11.5866

14

Interaction of Mannose-Binding Lectin with Lipopolysaccharide Outer Core Region and its Biological Consequences

*Aleksandra Man-Kupisinska[1], Anna S. Swierzko[2], Anna Maciejewska[1], Monika Hoc[1], Antoni Rozalski[3], Malgorzata Siwinska[4], Czeslaw Lugowski[1], Maciej Cedzynski[2] and Jolanta Lukasiewicz[1]**

[1] Laboratory of Microbial Immunochemistry and Vaccines, Department of Immunochemistry, Ludwik Hirszfeld Institute of Immunology and Experimental Therapy, Polish Academy of Sciences, Wroclaw, Poland, [2] Laboratory of Immunobiology of Infections, Institute of Medical Biology, Polish Academy of Sciences, Lodz, Poland, [3] Department of Biology of Bacteria, Faculty of Biology and Environmental Protection, Institute of Microbiology, Biotechnology and Immunology, University of Lodz, Lodz, Poland, [4] Laboratory of General Microbiology, Faculty of Biology and Environmental Protection, Institute of Microbiology, Biotechnology and Immunology, University of Lodz, Lodz, Poland

***Correspondence:**
Jolanta Lukasiewicz
jolanta.lukasiewicz@iitd.pan.wroc.pl

Lipopolysaccharide (LPS, endotoxin), the main surface antigen and virulence factor of Gram-negative bacteria, is composed of lipid A, core oligosaccharide, and O-specific polysaccharide (O-PS) regions. Each LPS region is capable of complement activation. We have demonstrated that LPS of *Hafnia alvei*, an opportunistic human pathogen, reacts strongly with human and murine mannose-binding lectins (MBLs). Moreover, MBL–LPS interactions were detected for the majority of other Gram-negative species investigated. *H. alvei* was used as a model pathogen to investigate the biological consequences of these interactions. The core oligosaccharide region of *H. alvei* LPS was identified as the main target for human and murine MBL, especially L-*glycero*-D-*manno*-heptose (Hep) and *N*-acetyl-D-glucosamine (GlcNAc) residues within the outer core region. MBL-binding motifs of LPS are accessible to MBL on the surface of bacterial cells and LPS aggregates. Generally, the accessibility of outer core structures for interaction with MBL is highest during the lag phase of bacterial growth. The LPS core oligosaccharide–MBL interactions led to complement activation and also induced an anaphylactoid shock in mice. Unlike *Klebsiella pneumoniae* O3 LPS, robust lectin pathway activation of *H. alvei* LPS *in vivo* was mainly the result of outer core recognition by MBL; involvement of the O-PS is not necessary for anaphylactoid shock induction. Our results contribute to a better understanding of MBL–LPS interaction and may support development of therapeutic strategies against sepsis based on complement inhibition.

Keywords: lipopolysaccharide, endotoxin, anaphylactoid shock, complement, mannose-binding lectin, *Hafnia*

Abbreviations: Ab, antibody; AP, alternative pathway; CP, classical pathway; DS, disaccharide; LP, lectin pathway; LPS, lipopolysaccharide, endotoxin; MBL, mannose-binding lectin; MASP, MBL-associated serine proteases; MHP, mannose homopolymer; NHS; normal human serum; OS, oligosaccharide; O-PS, O-specific polysaccharide; PAMP, pathogen-associated molecular pattern; R-LPS, rough LPS; S-LPS; smooth LPS; TS, trisaccharide.

INTRODUCTION

Mannose-binding lectin (MBL) is one of several pattern recognition molecules forming complexes with MBL-associated serine proteases (MASP) able to activate complement *via* the lectin pathway (LP). That process contributes to clearance of infection, but when excessive may be detrimental to the host (1).

Humans synthesize one type of MBL (hMBL), whereas mice (like the majority of mammals) synthesize two forms, MBL-A and -C, differing slightly in their specificity, serum concentration, activity, and local expression (2–5). Generally, hMBL recognizes carbohydrate patterns present on pathogens that are rich in D-mannose (D-Man), *N*-acetyl-D-glucosamine (D-GlcNAc), *N*-acetyl-D-mannosamine (D-ManNAc), or L-fucose (L-Fuc).

Lipopolysaccharide (LPS, endotoxin), the main surface antigen of Gram-negative bacteria, may be a ligand of MBL. LPS is composed of lipid A linked to a core oligosaccharide (OS) consisting of inner and outer regions that is further substituted with O-specific polysaccharide (O-PS) comprising oligosaccharide repeating units. O-PS is a very variable region that determines O-serotype, whereas core OS and lipid A are characterized by moderate structural variability. Smooth bacterial strains synthesize highly heterogeneous LPS being the mixture of S-LPS built of all three regions and short R-LPS (devoid of the O-PS) (**Figure 1**). Rough bacteria synthesize exclusively R-LPS. Such factors as bacterial growth phase and temperature influence LPS heterogeneity (6).

Each LPS region may induce synthesis of specific antibodies (Ab), able to activate the classical pathway (CP) of complement activation. However, in the absence of Ab, lipid A may activate CP *via* direct binding of C1, while core OS-LP (MBL-dependent) and O-PS may activate the alternative pathway (AP) and/or LP (involving MBL or ficolins) (7–10). Recently, MASP-1 (crucial for activating MASP-2 and therefore initiation of the LP cascade) was shown to participate in LPS-induced AP activation (11). Regarding core OS, L-*glycero*-D-*manno*-heptose (Hep) in the inner core region (characteristic for majority of LPS) and D-GlcNAc in the outer core region end (in *Salmonella enterica* serovar Minnesota) were reported as hMBL-binding motifs in R-LPS (12, 13). Although lipid A is considered the toxic principle of LPS, responsible for CD14–TLR-4–MD-2 complex-dependent immune cell response, the contribution of LPS polysaccharide-induced complement activation seems to be important for development of septic shock. Unlike lipid A-dependent endotoxic shock, polysaccharide-induced anaphylactoid reactions can be evoked in LPS-hyporesponsive mice (14, 15). Intravenous injection of certain S-LPS (but not isolated lipid A or R-type LPS) leads to rapid accumulation of platelets in the lungs and liver, followed by their degradation and release of serotonin, and death within 15–60 min, preceded by characteristic symptoms like convulsions and unconsciousness (16). Complement activated by LPS–MBL may be responsible for the degradation of platelets (16). LPS having mannose homopolymers (MHP) as O-PS (e.g., *Klebsiella pneumoniae* O3) (17) are potent inducers of anaphylaxis-like endotoxic shock in mice (16, 18). Some smooth bacteria (including *Proteus vulgaris* O25, *S. enterica* ser. Minnesota, and Abortusequi) have MBL-binding motifs within the core OS only and are capable of inducing a lethal early-phase shock (19, 20).

Hafnia alvei is an opportunistic human pathogen responsible for nosocomial mixed infections and sepsis (21). Most *H. alvei* LPS possesses smooth forms. So far, 40 O-serotypes (O-PS structures), and 4 types of core OS have been identified. *H. alvei* LPS is also an example of endotoxin having the *E. coli*-type structure of lipid A (22–24). A few strains of *H. alvei* synthesize LPS containing *E. coli* R4 [strains Polish Collection of Microorganisms (PCM) 23 or 1222] or *Salmonella* Ra (strain PCM 1212) core types (**Figure 1**) (25, 26). The OS1 hexasaccharide is the predominant core OS for this species, with Hep and Kdo residues in its inner core region like most Gram-negative bacteria (**Table 1**, footnote f) (24, 27).

A peculiarity of *H. alvei* LPS is the presence of Hep-Kdo-containing motifs also in the outer core region (24) (**Figure 1**). Branched trisaccharide (TS1), L-α-D-Hep*p*-(1→4)-[α-D-Gal*p*6 OAc-(1→7)]-α-Kdo*p*-(2→, was identified, for example, at the outer core region of *H. alvei* 32 and PCM 1192 LPS (OS1-TS1 core) (24, 31). Linear trisaccharide α-D-Gal*p*-(1→2)-L-α-D-Hep*p*-(1→4)-α-Kdo*p*-(2→ (TS2) is characteristic for *H. alvei* PCM 1196 (OS1-TS2 core) (32). The disaccharide (DS), L-α-D-Hep*p*3OAc-(1→4)-α-Kdo*p*-(2→ was identified in *H. alvei* PCM 1200 and 1209 (OS1-DS type core) (29). The presence of Hep-Kdo-containing motifs in the outer core region makes *H. alvei* LPS similar to *K. pneumoniae* and *P. vulgaris* O25 LPS (28, 33). This similarity prompted us to examine the ability of *H. alvei* LPS to bind MBL, activate human and murine complement systems and induce anaphylactoid reactions in mice.

Here, we explicate the structural basis of interactions between MBL and core OS of a variety of *H. alvei* LPS. These interactions lead to the activation of complement *via* the LP. Moreover, complexes of *H. alvei* LPS with MBL were able to induce anaphylactoid shock in BALB/c mice. LPS from 10 different species of opportunistic pathogens were tested to identify other examples of such interactions. We suggest that common interactions between core OS of LPS and MBL triggering LP activation might influence the course of Gram-negative infections, including nosocomial infections and sepsis. Therefore, consideration of surface antigen structure should be helpful in understanding pathogenicity and may influence development of new therapeutic strategies in Gram-negative sepsis.

MATERIALS AND METHODS

Animals

BALB/c mice (males, 7–8 weeks old) were purchased from the animal facility of the Polish Mother's Memorial Hospital, Research Institute, Lodz, Poland. The BALB/c mice were housed at the animal facility of the Ludwik Hirszfeld Institute of Immunology and Experimental Therapy (Wroclaw, Poland) and *in vivo* experiments were approved by the Local Ethical Commission for Animal Experimentation (Wroclaw, Poland).

Bacteria

Hafnia alvei strains PCM 537, 1188, 1190, 1191, 1192, 1195, 1196, 1200, 1203, 1204, 1205, 1206, 1207, 1208, 1209, 1210,

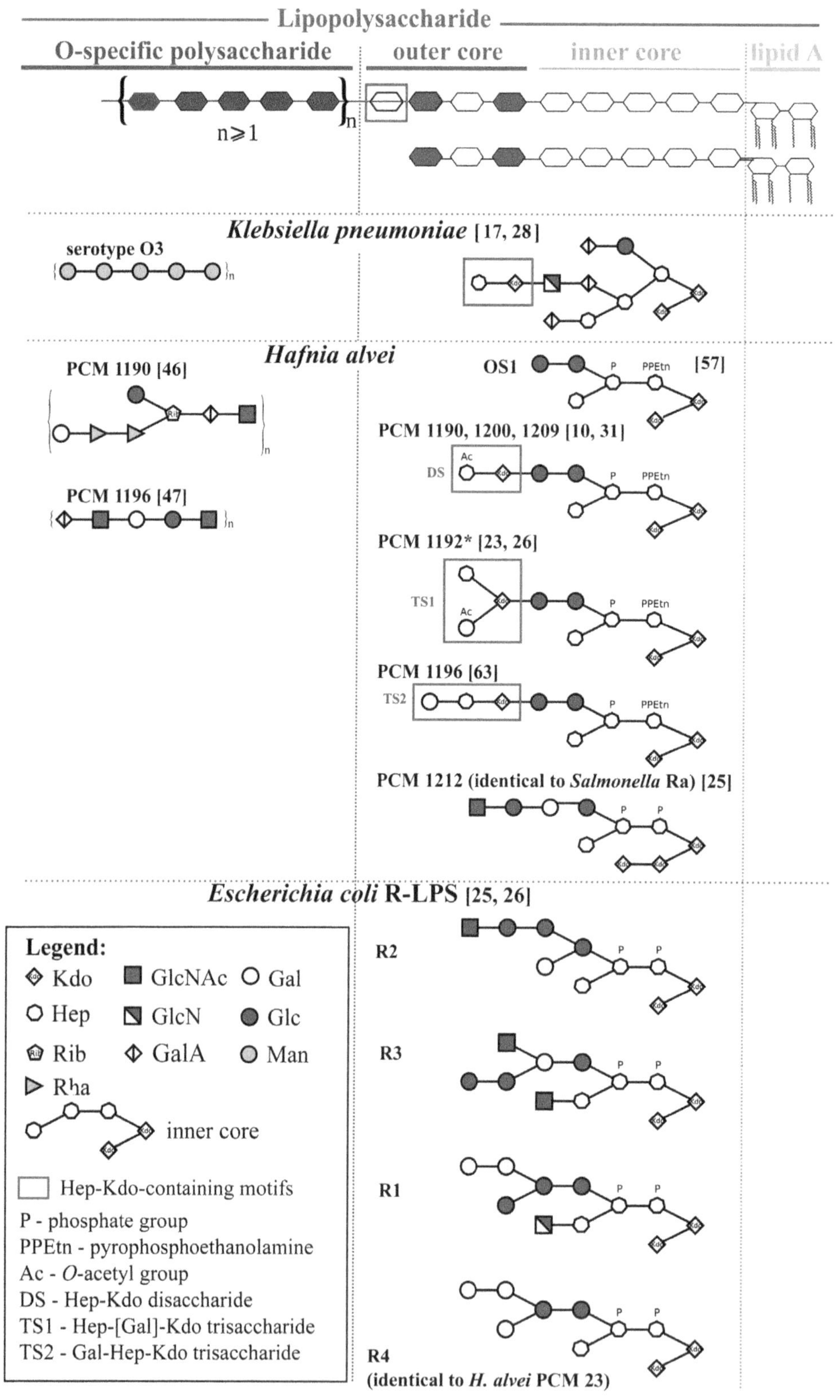

FIGURE 1 | Schematic structures of selected *Klebsiella pneumoniae*, *Hafnia alvei*, and *E. coli*, and *Salmonella* spp. lipopolysaccharides (LPSs) relevant for an interpretation of human mannose-binding lectin–LPS interactions. All structures are grouped according to the schematic diagram of an LPS molecule (upper panel) built of lipid A, core oligosaccharide (inner and outer), and O-specific polysaccharide consisting of a varying number of oligosaccharide repeating units. Information about linkages and isomers was hidden to simplify an interpretation of structures and may be found in details in references (numbers in brackets).

TABLE 1 | Structural characteristics of LPS and lectin blotting results of SDS-PAGE separated *Hafnia alvei* LPS with serum-derived hMBL.[a]

LPS	Region of interaction		Outer core OS motifs
	O-PS	Core OS/lipid A (core OS type)	
Klebsiella pneumoniae O3	+	+ (OS *K. pneumoniae*)	α-GlcN, α-Kdo, α-Hep[b]
H. alvei 23	–	– (R4)	nd
H. alvei 1190	+	+ (OS1[f])	Hep-Kdo[c](DS)
H. alvei 1192	–	+ (OS1[f])	Hep-[Gal-]-Kdo[d](TS1)
H. alvei 1196	+	+ (OS1[f])	Gal-Hep-Kdo[e](TS2)
H. alvei 1200	–	+ (OS1[f])	Hep-Kdo[c](DS)
H. alvei 1209	–	+ (OS1[f])	Hep-Kdo[c](DS)
H. alvei 1212	–	+ (Ra)	nd
H. alvei 1222	–	– (R4)	nd

[a]*All LPS represent smooth type molecules. "+" or "–" indicate positive or negative interaction with hMBL, respectively. R4, Ra, and OS1 indicate core oligosaccharides present in LPS of E. coli R4, Salmonella spp. Ra, and typical H. alvei core OS, respectively (26, 27).*
[b]*Terminal residues present in outer core OS region (28).*
[c]*L-α-D-Hepp3OAc-(1→4)-α-Kdop (10, 23, 29).*
[d]*L-α-D-Hepp-(1→4)-[α-D-Galp6OAc-(1→7)]-α-Kdop (24).*
[e]*α-D-Galp-(1→2)-L-α-D-Hepp-(1→4)-α-Kdop (30).*
[f]*α-D-Glcp-(1→3)-α-D-Glcp-(1→3)-[L-α-D-Hepp-(1→7)]-L-α-D-Hepp4P-(1→3)-L-α-D-Hepp4PPEtn-(1→5)-α-Kdo (27).*
nd, not determined; LPS, lipopolysaccharide; hMBL, human MBL.
Schematic structures are presented in ***Figure 1***.

1211, 1212, 1213, 1214, 1218, 1220, 1221, 1222, 1224, and *E. coli* O55 were obtained from the PCM at the Ludwik Hirszfeld Institute of Immunology and Experimental Therapy (Wroclaw, Poland). *Proteus* spp. strains (*P. mirabilis*, *P. vulgaris*, *P. penneri*, *P. myxofaciens*, and *P. genomospecies*) came from the collection of the Laboratory of General Microbiology, University of Lodz (Poland). *K. pneumoniae* O3:K55$^-$ (strain 5505Δ*cps*) was kindly provided by Prof. S. Kaluzewski (National Institute of Hygiene, Warsaw, Poland). *H. alvei*, *E. coli*, and *K. pneumoniae* were grown till exponential phase (8 h) in Davis medium as described (34), and *Proteus* spp. strains were grown in liquid nutrient broth containing 1% glucose (35). They were stored in a glycerol mixture at −75°C.

Sera

Sera obtained from BALB/c mice were used as a source of murine MBL and ficolins. Pooled normal human serum (NHS) was used as a source of hMBL and came from the collection of the Laboratory of Immunobiology of Infections, Institute of Medical Biology, Polish Academy of Sciences. Polyclonal rabbit sera anti-*H. alvei* core OS (OS1) conjugated with tetanus toxoid (OS1-TT) came from Laboratory of Microbial Immunochemistry and Vaccines (Ludwik Hirszfeld Institute of Immunology and Experimental Therapy, Wroclaw, Poland). Polyclonal rabbit immunoglobulins specific for TS (Hep-[Gal]-Kdo) were isolated from antisera using an adsorption on bacterial mass as previously described (24). DS-specific Ab were isolated by two-step affinity chromatography of anti-*H. alvei* 1209 serum (immunization with killed bacteria, DS-positive strain) on: (i) *H. alvei* 1209 core OS1-Sepharose 4B gel and (ii) *H. alvei* 1209 O-PS-Sepharose 4B gel. Both resins were prepared as previously described (10, 36, 37). Eluates containing anti-DS Ab were collected in sterile vials and stored at −20°C.

Preparation of LPS

Lipopolysaccharide were extracted from bacterial cells by the hot phenol/water method (38) and purified by ultracentrifugation as previously described (34, 35). *Proteus* spp. LPS were extracted from dried bacterial cells, as previously described (39), by the phenol–water procedure according to the method of Westphal and Jann (38) and purified with aqueous 50% trichloroacetic acid. For analyses of growth phase dependence of hMBL–bacteria interactions (SDS-PAGE and lectin blotting), LPS was isolated from bacteria by Tri-Reagent method (40). LPS of *H. alvei* strains 1, 2, 17, 23, 31, 32, 37, 38, 39, 114/60, 481L, 600, 744, 981, *Edwardsiella anguillimortifera*, *Citrobacter* (kindly provided by Prof. E. Katzenellenbogen), and *E. coli* came from the collection of the Laboratory of Microbial Immunochemistry and Vaccines (Ludwik Hirszfeld Institute of Immunology and Experimental Therapy, Wroclaw, Poland).

O-PSs, Core Oligosaccharides, and Lipid A Isolation

Polysaccharides, oligosaccharides, and lipids A were isolated by mild acidic hydrolysis of *H. alvei* PCM 1190, 1192, and 1200 LPS at 100°C for 45 min. Poly- and oligosaccharides were fractionated and purified as previously described using Bio-Gel P-10 (10). The Hep-Kdo-containing fraction was isolated from the heterogeneous core OS fraction and analyzed by the use of liquid chromatography-electrospray ionization-tandem mass spectrometry (LC-ESI-MS) on SeQuant®ZIC®-HILIC column as previously described (41). Fractions 3 and 4 were pooled and used for surface plasmon resonance (SPR) analysis. Lipid A was isolated as a water-insoluble fraction of the LPS hydrolyzate. Prior to lectin blotting, lipids A were purified by extraction with 2:1:3 chloroform/methanol/water mixture (v/v/v) to remove membrane phospholipids and remains of LPS. Both water phase (w) and chloroform (ch) phase lipids A were collected (23).

SDS-PAGE

The LPS and lipids A were analyzed by SDS-PAGE. Briefly, 4.5 and 15.4% polyacrylamide-bisacrylamide gels were used as the stacking and resolving gels, respectively. Glycolipids (3 µg) were mixed with sample buffer (65 mM Tris, pH 6.8, 2% SDS, 35% glycerol, 0.6 M DTT, ~0.1% bromophenol blue) in ratio 1:1 (v/v). LPS/lipid A bands were visualized by the silver staining method (42).

Lectin Blotting

SDS-PAGE-separated LPS were transferred onto polyvinylidene fluoride membranes (Bio-Rad, USA). Membranes were blocked with SuperBlock® Blocking Buffer (Thermo Scientific, USA) for 2 h, followed by overnight incubation at 4°C, with 25-fold diluted human or murine serum as previously described (10). Bound proteins were detected by immunostaining with different primary Ab: (i) monoclonal mouse anti-hMBL Ab (clone HYB 131-01, BioPorto, Denmark), (ii) monoclonal rat anti-MBL-A (clone 2B4) and (iii) anti-MBL-C Ab (clone 16A8) (both from Hycult Biotech, The Netherlands), (iv) rabbit anti-ficolin-A kindly provided by Dr. Yuichi Endo (Fukushima Medical University, Fukushima, Japan), and (v) reactions were detected with HRP-conjugated rabbit anti-mouse, anti-rat secondary IgG Ab (Dako, Denmark) or anti-rabbit IgG secondary Ab, and visualized with Immun-Star HRP Chemiluminescent Substrate Kit (Bio-Rad, USA) and G:Box chemiluminescent imaging system (Syngene, UK). Nonspecific interactions of secondary Ab were excluded by controls without the primary Ab or the serum as a source of hMBL.

ELISA for Lectin Binding

Interactions of hMBL, MBL-A, MBL-C, and murine ficolins A and B with *H. alvei* LPS were tested as previously described (10). Briefly, NUNC Maxisorp U96 plates were coated with 2 μg of LPS/well. After blocking with 0.1% BSA in TBS-Ca^{2+} buffer (10 mM Tris, 120 mM NaCl, 1 mM $CaCl_2$, pH 7.4), NHS or murine serum (prediluted in 0.1% BSA/20 mM Tris, 1 M NaCl, 10 mM $CaCl_2$, pH 7.4) was added. After overnight incubation at 4°C, the bound proteins were detected by using specific primary antibodies (mentioned in the lectin blotting procedure) and HPR-conjugated anti-mouse, anti-rat, or anti-rabbit corresponding anti-IgG antibodies (Dako, Denmark). As substrate for peroxidase, 2,2′-azino-bis(3-ethylbenz-thiazoline-6-sulfonic)acid (ABTS) (Sigma, USA) was employed. Absorbance values were measured at 405 nm using Benchmark Plus microplate spectrophotometer (Bio-Rad).

Determination of hMBL–MASP-2 and MBL–MASP-1 Complex Activity

Activity of lectin(s)-MASP-2 complexes was determined as previously described (43) with modification (44). LPS from various bacteria were used for coating of microtiter plates (Maxisorp U96, Nunc). The products of C4 activation were detected with rabbit anti-hC4c and HRP-conjugated anti-rabbit Ig (Dako). To test MBL-MASP-1 complex activity, VPR-AMC (Val-Pro-Arg-aminomethylcoumarin) peptide (Bachem, Switzerland), as the substrate for MASP-1 was used as previously described (45) and the fluorescence was read using a Varioskan Flash reader (Thermo Scientific, USA).

Flow Cytometry Analysis of Binding of hMBL to Formaldehyde-Inactivated Bacteria

Flow cytometry analysis was performed as previously described (10). Depending on experiment, bacteria were cultured and harvested at lag phase (3 h), log phase (6 h), or stationary phase (24 h) of growth. The growth phase of culture was determined on the basis of optical density measurement at 600 nm and the appropriate growth curve. Immediately before each experiment, bacterial cells were centrifuged, washed with PBS, and suspended in 10-fold diluted NHS (pool), used as a source of hMBL. Monoclonal anti-hMBL Ab (clone HYB 131-01) and fluorescein isothiocyanate-labeled anti-mouse IgG Ab (Dako) were used as detection system. The analysis of the FITC-labeled bacteria was performed using a Cytomics FC 500 MPL Beckman-Coulter (USA) flow cytometer. Bacteria were detected using log-forward and log-side scatter dot plot. Gating region was set to exclude debris and larger aggregates of bacteria. A total of 10,000 events were acquired.

Induction of Anaphylaxis-Like Endotoxic Shock in muramyldipeptide (MDP)-Primed Mice

The BALB/c mice were treated i.p. with 100 μg of MDP in PBS (20), and after 4 h, animals received i.v. 100 μg of LPS. *K. pneumoniae* O3 and *E. coli* O55 LPS were used as a positive and negative control, respectively. Incidence, severity, and scoring of the anaphylaxis-like shock were recorded within 30 min: 0, no signs of shock; 1, staggering; 2, crawling and prostration; 3, prostration and weak convulsions; 4, prostration and strong convulsions (16). Subsequent mortality was recorded within 1 h and after 24 h after LPS injection.

Surface Plasmon Resonance

Surface plasmon resonance studies were assessed with a Biacore T200 system (GE Healthcare Bio-Science AB, Sweden). Carrier free recombinant hMBL (R&D Systems, USA) was immobilized in 10 mM sodium acetate, pH 4.0 on the CM5 series S sensor chip (GE Healthcare Bio-Science AB) at a flow rate 5 μl/min, to the level of 16,000 RU using the amine coupling chemistry. A flow cell with immobilized 240 RU of ethanolamine was used as a reference surface. HBS-P buffer (GE Healthcare Bio-Science AB) supplemented with Ca^{2+}, Mg^{2+} ions (5 mM $MgCl_2$, 5 mM $CaCl_2$) was used as a running buffer. *H. alvei* O-PS (PCM 1190, 1196, 1200, and 1209) and core hexasaccharides from *H. alvei* PCM 1200 LPS at various concentrations were injected at a flow rate 30 μl/min. 0.5% SDS injected for 30 s was used as a regenerator in all SPR experiments.

RESULTS

H. alvei LPS Core Oligosaccharide Is a Common MBL Target

Screening for the presence of structural motifs recognized by hMBL was performed by lectin blotting for LPS isolated from 39 different O-serotypes of *H. alvei* (**Figure 2**). LPS isolated from smooth strains gave a characteristic ladder-like multiband pattern after SDS-PAGE reflecting natural heterogeneity of LPS on the cell wall surface and facilitating core OS accessibility (**Figure 2A**). The fast-migrating fractions originate from lipid A substituted with core OS, whereas the slow-migrating fractions show the length distribution of the polymer built up of lipid A-core OS substituted with varying numbers of O-PS repeating units. LPS isolated from *K. pneumoniae* O3 strain 5505 (MHP as O-PS) was used as a positive control, where interactions were observed both in the core OS/lipid A and O-PS regions. hMBL recognized 34 out of 39 *H. alvei* LPS. Generally, reactivity was related to the fast-migrating fractions of the core OS-lipid A region. No interactions were

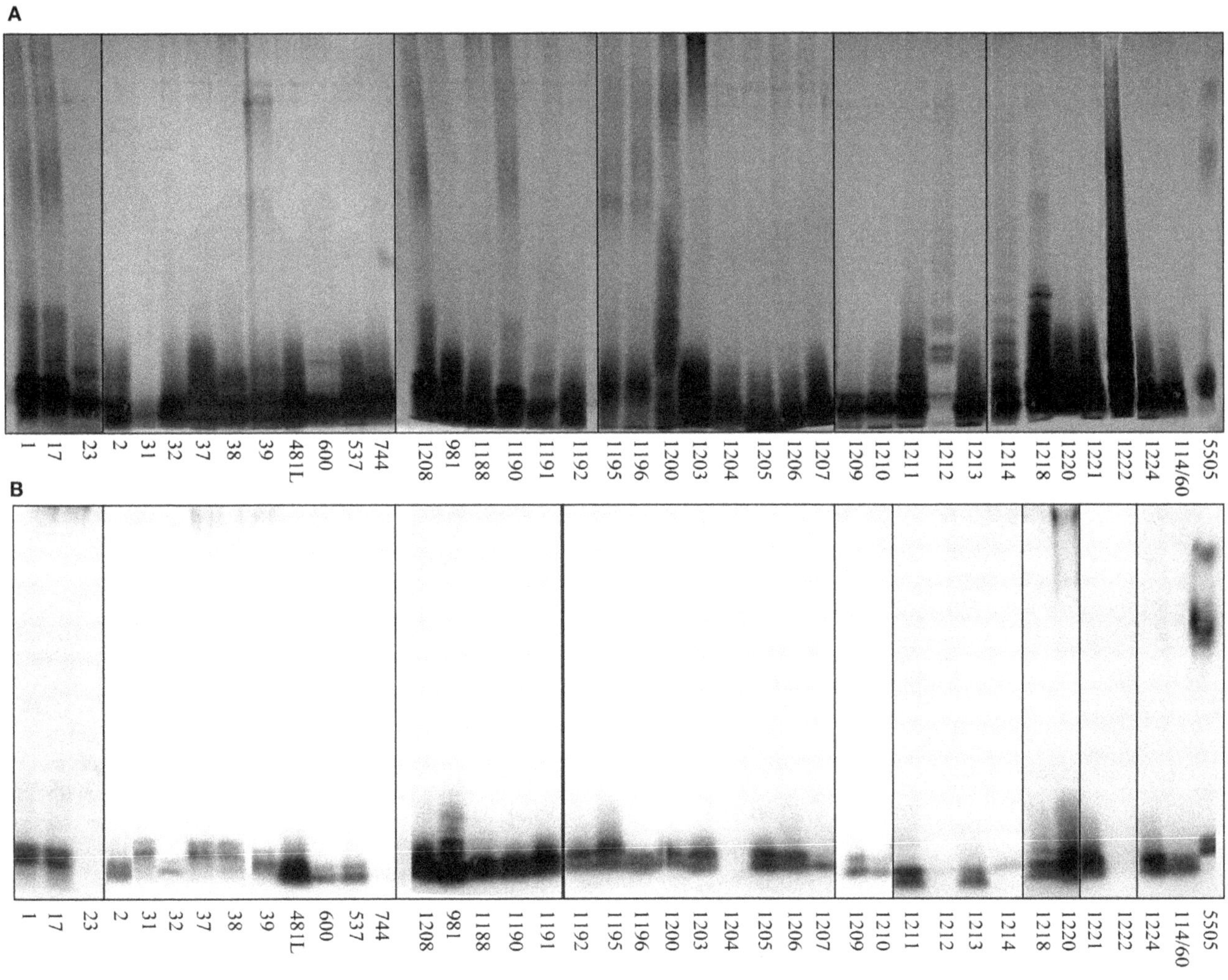

FIGURE 2 | Silver stained SDS-PAGE **(A)** and lectin blotting analysis **(B)** of the interaction of human MBL (hMBL) with *Hafnia alvei* lipopolysaccharides (LPSs). Normal human serum (pool) was used as a source of hMBL. Lanes are depicted with the strain number in Polish Collection of Microorganisms. The number 5505 represents *Klebsiella pneumoniae* O3:K55^{-} LPS used as a positive control.

observed for *H. alvei* 23, PCM 744, 1204, 1212, and 1222 LPS (**Figure 2B**).

Nine representative LPS, chosen on the basis of well-characterized structure (**Figure 1**) and different hMBL-binding patterns (**Figure 2B**; **Table 1**), were selected for further experiments to explore human and murine MBL specificity (**Figure 3**). For *H. alvei* PCM 1192, 1200, 1209, and 1212, hMBL bound within the core OS region only. For *H. alvei* PCM 1190 and 1196, hMBL bound within both the core OS and O-PS regions. For *H. alvei* 23 and PCM 1222, no binding was observed. These LPS–hMBL interactions were confirmed by ELISA (**Figure 4**). Eight *H. alvei* LPS (and *K. pneumoniae* O3 LPS as positive control) were used as solid-phase antigens. The strongest reactions of serum hMBL were observed for LPS *K. pneumoniae* O3 and *H. alvei* PCM 1190, 1196, and 1209 LPS. In contrast to the lectin blotting, no reaction with *H. alvei* PCM 1200 LPS was observed, what might be explained by competition between strong binding of O-PS-reactive ficolin-3 (10) and moderate binding of core OS-reactive hMBL. In addition, long O-PS chains of LPS 1200 might also hinder hMBL access to core OS.

Since murine model was chosen for further studies to test *in vivo* activity of LPS on complement-mediated anaphylaxis-like endotoxic shock, the reactivity of LPS with murine MBL-A and MBL-C (as well as with ficolin A and ficolin B) was analyzed by lectin blotting (**Figure 3**). Murine MBL-C showed binding pattern very similar to hMBL within the core OS region. Strong reactions with *H. alvei* PCM 1190, 1196, 1200, 1209, 1212, and *K. pneumoniae* O3 LPS and negligible reactions with LPS 23, PCM 1192 and 1222 were noted. In addition, interactions with high molecular weight fractions (O-PS region) were easily visible for *H. alvei* 1190 and *K. pneumoniae* O3 LPS. For MBL-A, no reactivity was observed for PCM 1192 and 1222 and very weak reactivity for 23 (within O-PS). Binding of this lectin to LPS *K. pneumoniae* O3 and PCM 1209 strains was attributed to core OS only. Reactivity within both core OS and O-PS region

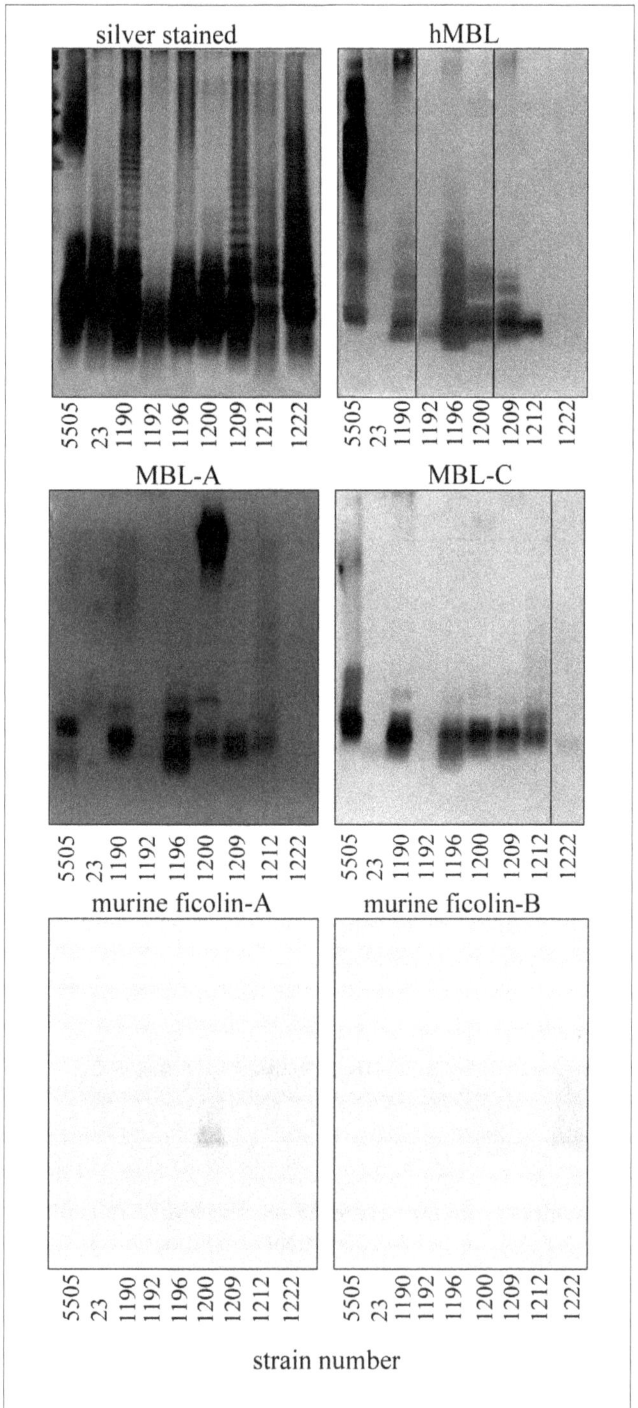

FIGURE 3 | Silver stained SDS-PAGE of representative *Hafnia alvei* lipopolysaccharides (LPSs) and lectin blotting of their interactions with human MBL (hMBL) and murine mannose-binding lectin (MBL)-A, MBL-C, ficolin-A, and ficolin-B. Normal human serum and BALB/c mice sera were used as a source of hMBL or murine MBL-A, MBL-C, ficolin A, and B, respectively. Lanes are depicted with the strain number in Polish Collection of Microorganisms. Strain 5505 represents *Klebsiella pneumoniae* O3:K55⁻ LPS used as a positive control.

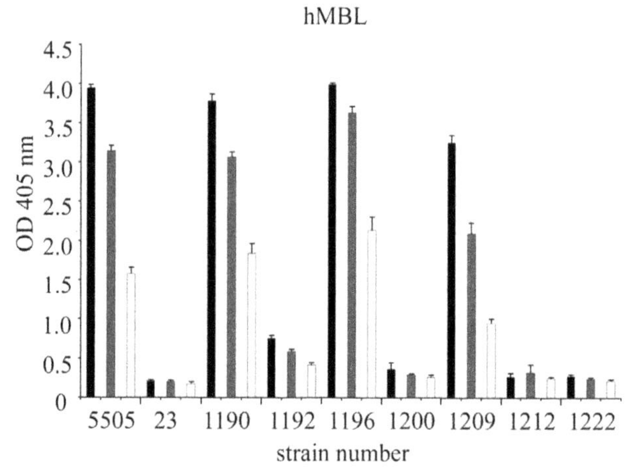

FIGURE 4 | Recognition of selected *Hafnia alvei* lipopolysaccharides (LPSs) by human MBL. Microtiter plates were coated with LPS, incubated with NHS to measure interactions with hMBL. Black, gray, and white bars represent 200-, 400-, and 800-fold dilutions, respectively. Data represent the mean values of four replicates and are marked by PCM strain number. Strain 5505 represents *Klebsiella pneumoniae* O3:K55⁻ LPS used as a positive control. Abbreviations: OD, optical density measured at λ = 405 nm; hMBL, human MBL; NHS, normal human serum; PCM, Polish Collection of Microorganisms.

were observed for *H. alvei* PCM 1190, 1196, 1212, and 1200. Especially strong recognition of PCM 1200 LPS was unique for MBL-A, whereas MBL-C (similarly to hMBL) were devoid of such activity. Moreover, only traces of signal related to O-PS region were observed for interactions of ficolin A with PCM 1200 and ficolin B with PCM 1222 (**Figure 3**). Interactions of MBL-A and MBL-C with *H. alvei* lipid A was excluded by lectin blotting (**Figure 5B**).

Hep-Kdo Motifs in *H. alvei* LPS Inner and Outer Core Are Recognized by MBL

From lectin blotting (**Figures 2** and **3**), it was suggested that most *H. alvei* LPS were bound by hMBL *via* the core OS/lipid A region. SPR analyses confirmed interactions of hMBL with O-PS regions of PCM 1190 (46) and 1196 (47) and excluded O-PS of PCM 1209 and 1200 LPS as targets for the lectin (**Figure 5A**). Data from lectin blotting with the use of purified lipid A fractions of *H. alvei* PCM 1190 and 1192 confirmed the lack of hMBL reactivity with that part of LPS (**Figure 5B**).

Next, we identified the core OS regions involved. Immunostaining with the use of OS1, DS- and TS1-specific Ab revealed four bands of low molecular weight fractions of migrating LPS (**Figure 5C**) attributed to lipid A-OS1 (two bands), lipid A-OS1-TS1, and lipid A-OS1-DS molecules. Two bands marked by lipid A-OS1 reflected OS1 heterogeneity related to ethanolamine, phosphate groups, and glycine substituents and are common for all three studied LPS (PCM 1192, 1200, and 1209). The band assigned as lipid A-OS1-DS was present in DS-expressing LPS of *H. alvei* PCM 1200 and 1209, while the lipid A-OS1-TS1 band in LPS of *H. alvei* PCM 1192 LPS.

The ability of recombinant hMBL to bind different core OS fractions of *H. alvei* LPS was further investigated by SPR on Biacore T200 (**Figure 5D**). Core OS isolated from PCM 1200 LPS were used as analytes. Both isolated OS1 and low molecular

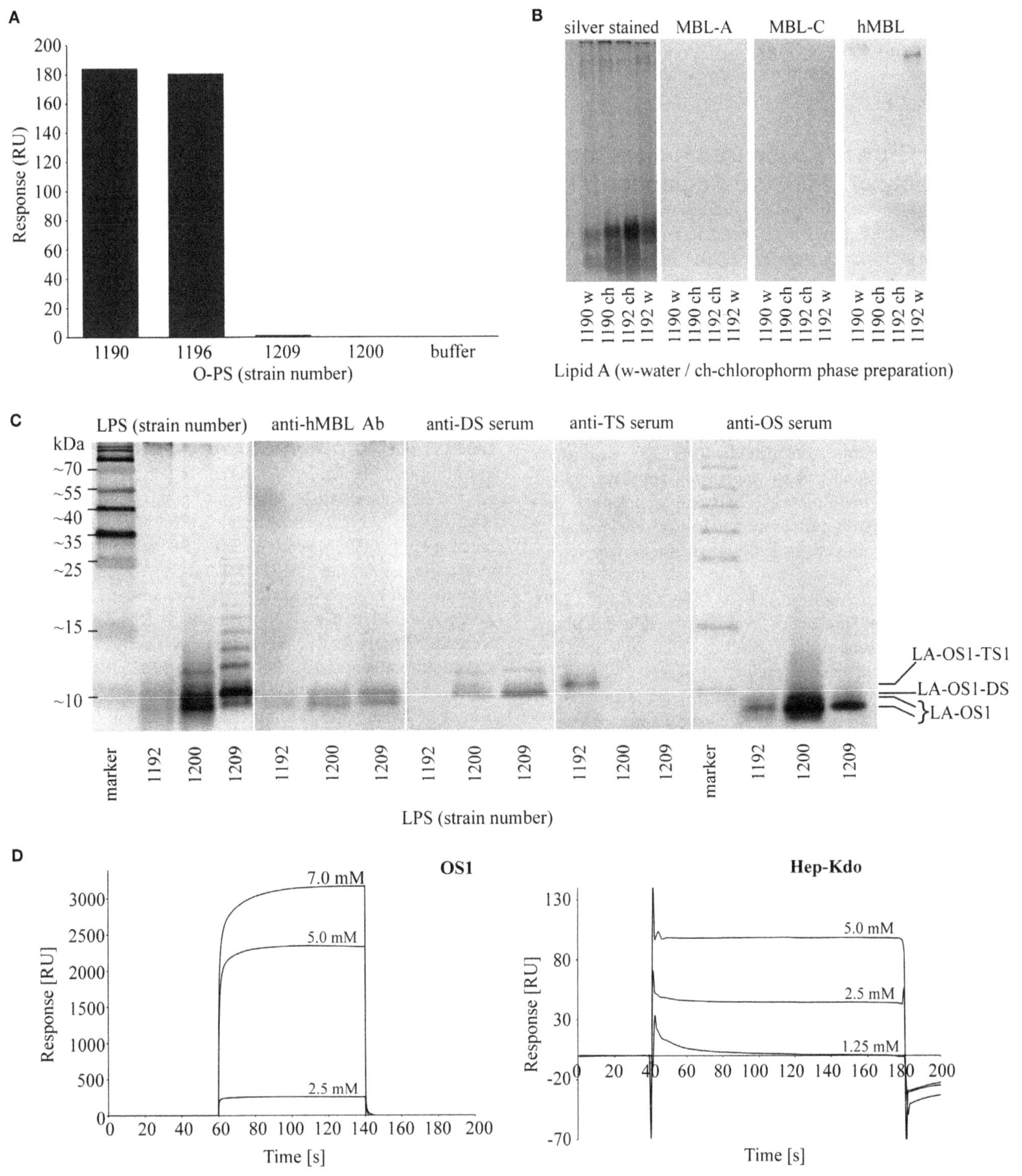

FIGURE 5 | Identification of hMBL-binding regions in *Hafnia alvei* lipopolysaccharides (LPSs). **(A)** Surface plasmon resonance (SPR) analysis of interactions between recombinant hMBL and O-specific polysaccharides (O-PSs) of *H. alvei* PCM 1190, 1196, 1200, and 1209 LPS. The bars represent binding response of immobilized recombinant hMBL (immobilization level: 16,000 RU) to O-PS (0.5 mg/ml) in running buffer HBS-P supplemented with $MgCl_2$ and $CaCl_2$. **(B)** Silver stained SDS-PAGE and lectin blotting analysis of the interaction between *H. alvei* lipids A [water phase (w) and chloroform phase (ch) preparations] and serum-derived murine MBL-A, MBL-C, and hMBL. Lanes are depicted with the strain PCM number. **(C)** Silver stained SDS-PAGE and lectin blotting analyses of the interactions between LPS of *H. alvei* PCM 1192 (TS1-positive), 1200 (DS-positive), 1209 (DS-positive) and serum-derived hMBL, DS-specific rabbit serum, TS1-specific rabbit serum, and OS1-specific rabbit serum. M—molecular weight markers. Marked bands corresponded to different forms of R-LPS: LA-OS1, LA-OS1-DS, LA-OS1-TS1, where LA stands for lipid A. **(D)** SPR sensograms for interactions of recombinant hMBL and OS1 and Hep-Kdo-containing OS isolated from *H. alvei* 1200 LPS. Sensor chip: CM5; Abbreviations: RU, response units; hMBL, human MBL; PCM, Polish Collection of Microorganisms; MBL, mannose-binding lectin.

weight fraction of Hep-Kdo interacted with immobilized recombinant hMBL in a concentration-dependent manner, with higher affinity observed for OS1. It was also confirmed by ELISA inhibition assay with the use of both analytes (data not shown).

Bacterial Growth Phase Determines the Accessibility of LPS Core Region for MBL

Binding of hMBL to LPS on bacterial surface was further investigated by flow cytometry. Since bacterial growth phase may be associated with changes in LPS expression, accessibility of core OS regions for hMBL was examined using microbial cells collected at lag (3 h), log (6 h), and stationary phase (24 h) (**Figure 6**). Four strains were chosen for this study: (i) *H. alvei* PCM 1190 recognized by hMBL within DS-carrying core OS and O-PS regions, (ii) *H. alvei* PCM 1192 and 1209 with hMBL targets located in low molecular weight fraction of LPS (core OS1 decorated with TS1 or DS, respectively), and (iii) *H. alvei* PCM 1222 expressing LPS not recognized by hMBL. *K. pneumoniae* O3 grown to the stationary phase was used as a positive control. The percentage of hMBL-labeled cells was confronted with R-LPS and S-LPS distribution examined by SDS-PAGE analysis of LPS extracted from cells at lag, log, and stationary phases (**Figure 6**, inset).

For all hMBL-reacting strains (PCM 1190, 1192, and 1209), the highest values of labeled cells were recorded for lag phase, where R-LPS represented the prevailing LPS population. The low content of O-PS chains facilitated access of hMBL to outer core regions of R-LPS (OS1 and DS). For strains PCM 1190 and 1192, the proportions of labeled cells were inversely associated with the expression of the S-LPS population. The highest values, at each growth phase, were recorded for the PCM 1190 strain. This was expected since its LPS has MBL-binding motifs not only in the core but also in O-PS region. PCM 1192 and 1209 LPS were recognized by hMBL within the core OS region only, whereby the most efficient binding was observed for bacteria at the lag phase (10.4 and 27.7% positive cells, respectively). In contrast to other strains, PCM 1209 bacteria showed the lowest accessibility for hMBL at log but not stationary phase. That might be explained by a higher content of R-LPS forms with accessible OS1 and DS motifs at stationary phase contrary to log phase (as evidenced by SDS-PAGE). Performed experiments demonstrated that observed relationships clearly resulted from LPS structure, i.e., the length of O-PS chains that hindered structural motifs recognized by hMBL (OS1 and DS).

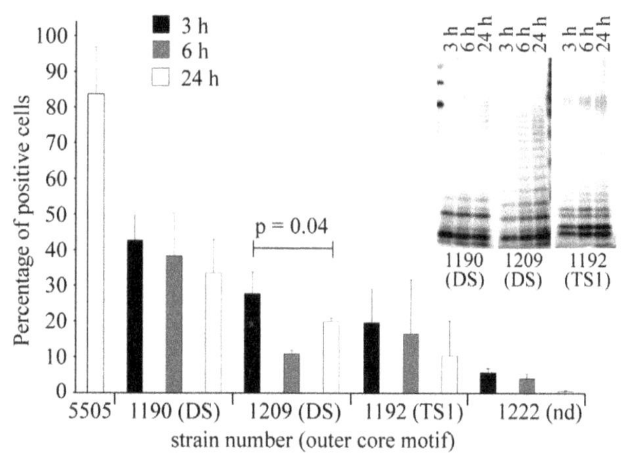

FIGURE 6 | Growth phase-dependence of hMBL–*Hafnia alvei* interactions observed in FACS analyses. Binding of hMBL to inactivated smooth *H. alvei* PCM 1190, 1192, and 1209 bacterial cells at the lag (black bars), exponential (gray bars), and the stationary phases (white bars) of growth. Silver stained SDS-PAGE (inset) of LPS 1190, 1209, and 1192 isolated from bacterial mass collected at lag, log, and stationary phases. Data represent the mean values ± SD from three independent experiments. DS and TS1 stand for the disaccharide and trisaccharide outer core motif in LPS of selected *H. alvei* strains. Abbreviations: Nd, not determined; hMBL, human MBL; PCM, Polish Collection of Microorganisms; LPS, lipopolysaccharide.

Interaction of hMBL With *H. alvei* LPS Leads to Complement Activation

The ability of selected LPS to initiate the complement cascade *via* the LP was tested by investigating activation of MASP-1 (cleavage of synthetic substrate, VPR-AMC) and MASP-2 (cleavage of C4) dependent on LPS recognition by LP molecules, especially hMBL. MBL–MASP-1 concentration-dependent activation was triggered by *H. alvei* 23, PCM 1190, 1192, 1196, 1200, 1209 LPS, as well as *K. pneumoniae* O3 (control) (**Figure 7**). The deposition of C4 activation products was additionally noted for PCM 1212 and 1222 LPS. It is worth mentioning that procedure employed does not exclude activation of LP by complexes of ficolin-3 with MASP (as described previously for 23 and PCM 1200 LPS) (10) or other than MBL collectins. Contribution of ficolin-1 and -2 was excluded (10). The influence of CP was excluded by high ionic strength of the buffer that inhibits the binding of C1q to immune complexes and disrupts the C1 complex, whereas MBL complexes integrity is maintained (48). The variations in reactivity profiles (**Figures 4** and **7**) may reflect differences in serum dilution used and sensitivity of assays.

Interaction of MBL With *H. alvei* LPS Core Oligosaccharide Induces Anaphylactoid Shock

The biological consequences of *in vivo* MBL interaction with *H. alvei* PCM 1190, 1192, 1200, 1209, and 1212 LPS were tested by ability to induce an anaphylactoid reaction in mice. *K. pneumoniae* O3 and *E. coli* O55 as well as *H. alvei* PCM 1222 LPS were used as positive and negative controls, respectively (14).

Intravenous injection of *H. alvei* PCM 1190, 1200, 1209, or 1212 LPS-induced rapid shock (within 30 min, score 3–4) leading to death of MDP-sensitized BALB/c mice (**Table 2**). The distinctive effect was observed for LPS of *H. alvei* PCM 1200 that was strongly recognized by MBL-A within the O-PS region and moderately within the OS1-DS core region (**Figure 3**). The reaction, comparable to that provoked by *K. pneumoniae* O3 LPS, was also induced by *H. alvei* PCM 1190 (OS1-DS core type) and 1212 (*Salmonella* Ra core type)

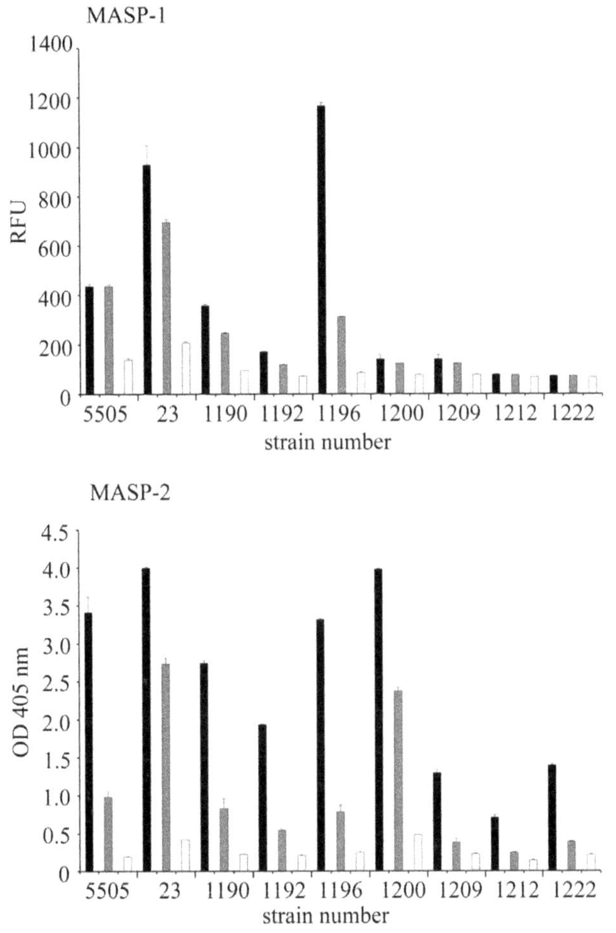

FIGURE 7 | Activation of the human lectin pathway of complement by *Hafnia alvei* LPS. (Top) Human LPS-MASP-1 activity (ability to cleave a VPR-AMC peptide). Black, gray, and white bars represent 5-, 20-, and 40-fold dilutions, respectively. (Bottom) Human LPS–MASP-1/2 complex-dependent C4c deposition. Black, gray, and white bars represent 50-, 200-, and 800-fold dilution, respectively. Each dilution series is described by the strain number on the *X*-axis. Pattern recognition molecule states for MBL or other complement-activating collectin/ficolin present in serum. Data represent the mean values of four replicates. LPS were used as solid phase. Abbreviations: RFU, relative fluorescence units; OD, optical density measured at $\lambda = 405$ nm; LPS, lipopolysaccharide; MBL, mannose-binding lectin; MASP, MBL-associated serine proteases.

moderately bound by MBL-A and MBL-C within the O-PS and core OS regions. *H. alvei* PCM 1209 LPS (OS1-DS core type) that was reactive for murine MBL-A and MBL-C within the core OS region only (**Figure 3**), still had a powerful ability to induce an anaphylactoid shock similar to *K. pneumoniae* O3. By contrast, mice treated with *H. alvei* PCM 1192 (OS1-TS1 core type) or 1222 (*E. coli* R4 core type) LPS developed mild or no characteristic symptoms within the first hour and died in the late phase of endotoxic shock (lipid A-dependent) (**Table 2**), similar to animals injected with *E. coli* O55 LPS (negative control).

LPS Core Oligosaccharide Is a Common MBL Target in Many Gram-Negative Bacteria

Screening for LPS from a variety of opportunistic pathogens (Table S1 in Supplementary Material), recognized by serum hMBL was performed with the use of lectin blotting. False positive reactions of primary and secondary detecting Ab were excluded. We found interactions between hMBL and LPS core regions to be very common: 13 of 15 *K. pneumoniae*, 11/22 *P. vulgaris*, 10/33 *P. mirabilis*, 7/15 *P. penneri*, 1/1 *P. myxofaciens*, 5/10 *E. coli* (including R-LPS containing R2 and R3 core types), 1/5 *Citrobacter* spp., and all of 4/4 *Edwardsiella anguillimortifera* LPS gave positive results.

DISCUSSION

Lipopolysaccharide is a major pathogen-associated molecular pattern (PAMP) and virulence factor of Gram-negative bacteria, responsible for development of sepsis and septic shock. Whereas the role of lipid A in those life-threatening events is well-documented (49), the influence of the polysaccharide region is poorly characterized. It is known that the carbohydrate moiety influences endotoxin clearance and biological activity of lipid A (50, 51). Recognition of LPS polysaccharide by a variety of pattern recognition molecules may lead to complement activation *via* CP, AP, and/or LP, all involved in sepsis development (52).

The core OS-lipid A region is a target for such plasma proteins as LPS-binding protein, BPI (bactericidal/permeability-increasing protein), CAP18 (cationic antimicrobial protein), and lysozyme. Consequently, bactericidal and inflammatory processes are induced by the host immune system. Due to the high structural heterogeneity of O-PS, the number of innate immunity factors interacting with that region is much lower. One example is ficolin-3, recognizing *H. alvei* PCM 1200 O-PS resulting in LP activation (10). Ficolin-3 was also demonstrated to enhance agglutination, phagocytosis, and killing of *H. alvei* PCM 1200 bacteria (53). Another example is pulmonary surfactant collectin SP-D binding mannose-rich O-PS of *K. pneumoniae* O3 and O5 (54).

This study provided well-documented evidence that core OS is the main target for human and murine MBL. Depending on the assay, the binding of recombinant (SPR) or NHS or murine serum MBL (lectin blotting, ELISA, flow cytometry) was detected in presented studies. Thus, it is worth noting that the oligomer distribution may vary for recombinant and NHS-derived MBL according to purification procedure (55), what may influences binding affinity between MBL and target ligand. Notwithstanding similar oligomer distribution patterns were reported for both forms (55, 56), including trimeric and tetrameric forms. Even though proposed oligomerization models indicated a polypeptide dimer as the basic unit in this process for MBL (57), higher oligomeric states are usually detected in rMBL and NHS-derived MBL preparations that ensure complement activation (56).

Performing screening analysis, we have shown that interactions of serum hMBL with different core OS regions were prevalent among LPS isolated from numerous opportunistic pathogens, such as *H. alvei, E. coli, K. pneumoniae, Proteus* spp., *Citrobacter*

TABLE 2 | Ability of LPS from smooth strains of *Hafnia alvei*, *E. coli*, and *Klebsiella pneumoniae* to induce anaphylactoid shock and death in BALB/c mice.[a]

LPS (core OS type)	LPS region recognized by		Shock[b]		
	MBL-A	MBL-C	Incidence	Score[c] 30 min	Mortality
H. alvei 1200 (OS1-DS)	O-PS/core OS	Core OS	5/5	10 min: 4	0.5 h: 5/5
H. alvei 1209 (OS1-DS)	Core OS	Core OS	5/5	3–4	0.5 h: 4/5 1 h: 5/5
H. alvei 1212 (Ra)	O-PS/core OS	Core OS	4/4	3–4	0.5 h: 4/4
H. alvei 1190 (OS1-DS)	O-PS/core OS	Core OS	5/5	3	0.5 h: 5/5
K. pneumoniae O3[d]	Core OS	O-PS/core OS	5/5	3–4	0.5 h: 5/5
H. alvei 1192 (OS1-TS1)	–	–	4/4	0–1	0.5 h: 1/4 24 h: 4/4
H. alvei 1222 (R4)	–	–	5/5	0–1	0.5 h: 0/5 24 h: 5/5
E. coli O55	–[e]	–[e]	0/4	0	0.5 h: 0/4 24 h: 4/4

[a]*Mice were sensitized with 100 µg of muramyldipetide (i.p.) and 4 h later injected with 100 µg of LPS (i.v.). Incidence, score, and mortality were recorded within 0.5 and 1 h after LPS injection.*
[b]*Incidence and mortality are shown as number/total.*
[c]*The scoring of anaphylaxis-like endotoxic shock was as follows: 1, staggering; 2, crawling and prostration; 3, prostration and weak convulsions; 4, prostration and strong convulsions (16).*
[d]*The O-PS of this LPS is composed of mannose homopolymer.*
[e]*Determined only by inhibition of murine MBL–LPS O55 interaction in ELISA with LPS O55.*
LPS, lipopolysaccharide; MBL, mannose-binding lectin.

spp., and *E. anguillimortifera* representing different O-serotypes (O-PS structure) (Table S1 in Supplementary Material). Among 145 LPS tested, as much as approximately 57% were recognized by hMBL within fast-migrating fractions (corresponding to R-LPS built up of lipid A-core OS), whereas the reaction with slow-migrating fractions (S-LPS containing O-PS) was found in approximately 10% only. Accordingly, hMBL interacted with 34 (approximately 87%) out of 39 *H. alvei* LPS within the core OS region of LPS. Moreover, we also showed that highly purified *H. alvei* hexaacylated lipid A is recognized neither by human nor murine MBL. However, such interactions were previously suggested by Ono et al. (58) and Shiratsuchi et al. (59) for commercially available *E. coli* lipid A. This discrepancy may result from impurities of bacterial origin in the commercial preparations or the presence of MBL-binding motifs other than in the lipid A region of LPS (residuals of complete LPS after lipid A isolation by LPS hydrolysis).

Clinical isolates of Gram-negative bacteria are commonly of smooth type and therefore synthesize a highly heterogeneous pool of LPS, consisting of long-chain S-LPS, shorter S-LPS, and R-LPS unsubstituted by O-PS. We found that *H. alvei* PCM 1209 core OS within R-LPS forms exposed on the bacterial surface is accessible for hMBL (**Figure 6**). SPR analysis (**Figure 5A**) clearly demonstrated that PCM 1209 O-PS is not the MBL target. The core OS accessibility may depend on natural LPS heterogeneity (coexistence of R-LPS and S-LPS in smooth strains), and is hindered by core OS substitution with O-PS. It may be influenced by growth phase or environmental conditions. Generally, expression of R-LPS containing hMBL-binding motifs decreased with the culture progression (from lag to stationary phase) (**Figure 6**). Moreover, the immune response against O-PS may cause selective pressure on bacteria to lose the ability to express it (phase variation) (60, 61).

The LPS core OS region is relatively conservative and usually composed of an inner core and an outer core built up of Kdo and Hep residues and hexoses and hexosamines, respectively. For example, among *Salmonella* spp. strains one prevailing core type was described (Ra). Using mutants with defects in LPS core OS synthesis it was demonstrated that Hep residues in the inner core region are recognized by human and murine MBL due to their accessibility in truncated and incomplete core OS (12). Even though the inner core is common for the majority of enterobacterial LPS and represents MBL-binding motifs, our results indicated also outer core structures as natural MBL ligands. Hep and Hep-Kdo motifs were detected also in the latter region, for example, in *P. vulgaris* O25 and *K. pneumoniae* O3, O1, O2, O4, and O5 LPS (28, 33) as well as in numerous *H. alvei* strains (expressing DS, TS1, and TS2) (**Figure 1**). The lectin blotting (**Figure 5C**) and SPR analysis (**Figure 5D**) revealed recombinant MBL binding to DS-decorated *H. alvei* PCM 1200 OS1 and OS1 alone. Moreover, interaction of MBL with purified Hep-Kdo-containing motifs was also evidenced (**Figure 5D**), and determined by Hep residue (but not Kdo) according to the previous reports (12, 62). In spite of *manno* configuration, Kdo residues (even terminal) might be excluded as an MBL ligand, since deep rough mutants (Re) of *S. enterica* ser. Typhimurium or *Yersinia enterocolitica* O3, expressing LPS consisting of lipid A and one, two or three Kdo residues were not recognized (12, 63). Thus, Hep and D-GlcNAc present in outer core regions are the main MBL targets. Any steric obstacles within these motifs hinder MBL access, as was demonstrated for TS-OS1 core type of *H. alvei.* In TS1, the DS motif is substituted by terminal Gal residue that prevented hMBL binding to *H. alvei* PCM 1192 (**Figure 5C**).

Our results indicate a crucial role for MBL-binding motifs within the outer core OS in the recognition of *H. alvei* LPS by human and murine MBL, induction of an anaphylactoid reaction and rapid death in MDP-sensitized mice. Previously, it was demonstrated that such events were induced by several LPS of smooth bacteria with O-PS that were homopolymers of mannose (*K. pneumoniae* O3 and O5), able to activate complement *via* the LP (16). Among six *H. alvei* LPS with different O-serotypes tested, the intravenous injection of DS-containing LPS (PCM 1200, 1209, and 1190) led to development of severe symptoms of an anaphylactoid reaction and resulted in the death of animals within 30 min. Furthermore, *H. alvei* PCM 1212 (synthesizing Ra core type, with D-GlcNAc residue in the outer core region) is as toxic for mice as the aforementioned LPS. By contrast, *H. alvei* PCM 1192 LPS with outer core OS1 substituted with TS1 (preventing MBL binding) was not active. Interestingly, in the case of PCM 1200, 1212, and 1190 LPS, MBL-A was able to recognize not only the core OS (Ra or OS1-DS type) but also the O-PS region. Moreover, MBL-A showed the highest affinity to O-PS of *H. alvei* PCM 1200 LPS, which was found to be the most toxic (**Table 2**). Our results demonstrated that MBL-binding motifs in outer core region are sufficient to induce an anaphylactoid reaction in mice; however, the presence of S-LPS in the heterogeneous LPS preparation was mandatory. It might be suggested that similar to SP-D exhibiting O-PS-stabilized reactivity with common core OS of *K. pneumoniae*, *E. coli*, and *S. enterica* ser. Minnesota LPS, the O-PS–MBL interaction may also stabilize residual interactions of the collectin with the core OS region (54, 64).

The data presented here have extended the repertoire of LPS recognized by MBL, including rough forms present in endotoxin preparations from smooth bacteria (**Figure 1**). Generally, D-GlcNAc or Hep residues in the outer core were common ligands for the lectin. Those structures may be accessible to MBL *in vivo* not only when LPS O-PS is relatively short but also when endotoxin is released due to bacterial cell damage (for example, after treatment of host with antibiotics). We demonstrated also that the O-PS structure might augment immune responses when recognized by MBL (the example of PCM 1200). We believe that clarifying MBL specificity/affinity may contribute to a better understanding of the role of the LP in Gram-negative infections in general, including those leading to sepsis or endotoxic shock. Species of the family *Enterobacteriaceae* are responsible for 40–50% of hospital-acquired infections leading to sepsis and septic shock. Over half of cases in the USA is connected with bacteria of the genera *Klebsiella*, *Escherichia*, *Proteus* or *Enterobacter*, and mortality is in the range of 20–50%. In some cases of invasive infections caused, for example, by *K. pneumoniae*, *E. coli*, or *Proteus* spp., MBL/ficolin-dependent complement activation by common core oligosaccharide regions or MHP might contribute to the severity of infections and sepsis. Although interaction of MBL (or other PAMPs) with LPS is generally beneficial for the host, it may be harmful under certain conditions. Upon antibiotic treatment, aggregates of endotoxin (mixed S- and R-LPS) are released into the bloodstream and activate a host immune response (49). Furthermore, R-LPS was reported to exhibit higher potency in cell activation through the TLR-4/MD-2 receptor (65). Although MBL deficiency has been associated with susceptibility to infections (especially in children or immunocompromised subjects), its contribution to life-threatening events (like post-operative SIRS) has also been proven (66). Our results contribute to a better understanding of MBL–LPS interaction. They also support further development of therapeutic strategies against sepsis based on complement inhibition or complement-related replacement therapies.

AUTHOR CONTRIBUTIONS

JL, AS, AM-K, MC, and CL conceived and planned the experiments. AM-K, AM, AS, and JL carried out the experiments with prevailing role of AM-K and AS. JL, MH, AM, and CL prepared OS1- or TS1-specific rabbit antisera. AM-K, AM, and JL isolated some *H. alvei* LPS. AR and MS isolated and provided the collection of *Proteus* spp. LPS. AM-K, JL, AS, and MC contributed to the interpretation of the results. JL, AS, MC, and AM-K took the lead in writing the manuscript. All the authors approved the manuscript and provided critical feedback.

ACKNOWLEDGMENTS

This work was supported by Wroclaw Research Centre EIT+ within the project "Biotechnologies and advanced medical technologies"—BioMed (POIG.01.01,02-02-003/08) co-financed by the European Regional Development Fund (Operational Programme Innovative Economy, 1.1.2) and the Polish Ministry of Science and Higher Education (project No. N40108432/1944). Publication of the results was supported by Wroclaw Centre of Biotechnology, programme The Leading National Research Centre (KNOW) for years 2014–2018. Wojciech Jachymek and Tomasz Niedziela from the Ludwik Hirszfeld Institute of Immunology and Experimental Therapy, Wroclaw, Poland are acknowledged for their assistance during anaphylaxis-like endotoxic shock induction *in vivo*. Dr. Yuichi Endo from Fukushima Medical University, Fukushima, Japan is kindly acknowledged for rabbit anti-murine ficolin-A Ab. We are very grateful to Dr. David C. Kilpatrick for critical reading of the manuscript and helpful discussion.

REFERENCES

1. De Pascale G, Cutuli SL, Pennisi MA, Antonelli M. The role of mannose-binding lectin in severe sepsis and septic shock. *Mediators Inflamm* (2013) 2013:625803. doi:10.1155/2013/625803
2. Hansen S, Thiel S, Willis A, Holmskov U, Jensenius JC. Purification and characterization of two mannan-binding lectins from mouse serum. *J Immunol* (2000) 164:2610–8. doi:10.4049/jimmunol.164.5.2610
3. Liu H, Jensen L, Hansen S, Petersen SV, Takahashi K, Ezekowitz AB, et al. Characterization and quantification of mouse mannan-binding lectins (MBL-A

and MBL-C) and study of acute phase responses. *Scand J Immunol* (2001) 53: 489–97. doi:10.1046/j.1365-3083.2001.00908.x
4. Uemura K, Saka M, Nakagawa T, Kawasaki N, Thiel S, Jensenius JC, et al. L-MBP is expressed in epithelial cells of mouse small intestine. *J Immunol* (2002) 169:6945–50. doi:10.4049/jimmunol.169.12.6945
5. Wagner S, Lynch NJ, Walter W, Schwaeble WJ, Loos M. Differential expression of the murine mannose-binding lectins A and C in lymphoid and nonlymphoid organs and tissues. *J Immunol* (2003) 170:1462–5. doi:10.4049/jimmunol.170.3.1462
6. Lahtinen P, Brzezinska A, Skurnik M. Temperature and growth phase regulate the transcription of the O-antigen gene cluster of *Yersinia enterocolitica* O:3. *Adv Exp Med Biol* (2003) 529:289–92. doi:10.1007/0-306-48416-1_55
7. Loos M, Bitter-Suermann D, Dierich M. Interaction of the first (C1), the second (C2) and the fourth (C4) component of complement with different preparations of bacterial lipopolysaccharides and with lipid A. *J Immunol* (1974) 112:935–40.
8. Morrison DC, Kline LF. Activation of the classical and properdin pathways of complement by bacterial lipopolysaccharides (LPS). *J Immunol* (1977) 118:362–8.
9. Roumenina LT, Popov KT, Bureeva SV, Kojouharova M, Gadjeva M, Rabheru S, et al. Interaction of the globular domain of human C1q with *Salmonella typhimurium* lipopolysaccharide. *Biochim Biophys Acta* (2008) 1784:1271–6. doi:10.1016/j.bbapap.2008.04.029
10. Swierzko A, Lukasiewicz J, Cedzynski M, Maciejewska A, Jachymek W, Niedziela T, et al. New functional ligands for ficolin-3 among lipopolysaccharides of *Hafnia alvei*. *Glycobiology* (2012) 22:267–80. doi:10.1093/glycob/cwr119
11. Parej K, Kocsis A, Enyingi C, Dani R, Oroszlan G, Beinrohr L, et al. Cutting edge: a new player in the alternative complement pathway, MASP-1 is essential for LPS-induced, but not for zymosan-induced, alternative pathway activation. *J Immunol* (2018) 200:2247–52. doi:10.4049/jimmunol.1701421
12. Devyatyarova-Johnson M, Rees IH, Robertson BD, Turner MW, Klein NJ, Jack DL. The lipopolysaccharide structures of *Salmonella enterica* serovar Typhimurium and *Neisseria gonorrhoeae* determine the attachment of human mannose-binding lectin to intact organisms. *Infect Immun* (2000) 68:3894–9. doi:10.1128/IAI.68.7.3894-3899.2000
13. Dumestre-Perard C, Doerr E, Colomb MG, Loos M. Involvement of complement pathways in patients with bacterial septicemia. *Mol Immunol* (2007) 44:1631–8. doi:10.1016/j.molimm.2006.08.008
14. Swierzko A, Kirikae T, Kirikae F, Hirata M, Cedzynski M, Ziolkowski A, et al. Biological activities of lipopolysaccharides of *Proteus* spp. and their interactions with polymyxin B and an 18-kDa cationic antimicrobial protein (CAP18)-derived peptide. *J Med Microbiol* (2000) 49:127–38. doi:10.1099/0022-1317-49-2-127
15. Takada H, Hirai H, Fujiwara T, Koga T, Ogawa T, Hamada S. Bacteroides lipopolysaccharides (LPS) induce anaphylactoid and lethal reactions in LPS-responsive and -nonresponsive mice primed with muramyl dipeptide. *J Infect Dis* (1990) 162:428–34. doi:10.1093/infdis/162.2.428
16. Shibazaki M, Kawabata Y, Yokochi T, Nishida A, Takada H, Endo Y. Complement-dependent accumulation and degradation of platelets in the lung and liver induced by injection of lipopolysaccharides. *Infect Immun* (1999) 67:5186–91.
17. Vinogradov E, Frirdich E, MacLean LL, Perry MB, Petersen BO, Duus JO, et al. Structures of lipopolysaccharides from *Klebsiella pneumoniae*. Elucidation of the structure of the linkage region between core and polysaccharide O chain and identification of the residues at the non-reducing termini of the O chains. *J Biol Chem* (2002) 277:25070–81. doi:10.1074/jbc.M202683200
18. Zhao L, Ohtaki Y, Yamaguchi K, Matsushita M, Fujita T, Yokochi T, et al. LPS-induced platelet response and rapid shock in mice: contribution of O-antigen region of LPS and involvement of the lectin pathway of the complement system. *Blood* (2002) 100:3233–9. doi:10.1182/blood-2002-01-0252
19. Swierzko AS, Cedzynski M, Kirikae T, Nakano M, Klink M, Kirikae F, et al. Role of the complement-lectin pathway in anaphylactoid reaction induced with lipopolysaccharide in mice. *Eur J Immunol* (2003) 33:2842–52. doi:10.1002/eji.200323949
20. Takada H, Galanos C. Enhancement of endotoxin lethality and generation of anaphylactoid reactions by lipopolysaccharides in muramyl-dipeptide-treated mice. *Infect Immun* (1987) 55:409–13.
21. Janda JM, Abbott SL. The genus *Hafnia*: from soup to nuts. *Clin Microbiol Rev* (2006) 19:12–8. doi:10.1128/CMR.19.1.12-28.2006
22. Bobko E, Tyras M, Jachymek W. New complete structure of *Hafnia alvei* clinical isolate strain PCM 2670 semi-rough lipopolysaccharide. *Carbohydr Res* (2013) 374:67–74. doi:10.1016/j.carres.2013.03.029
23. Lukasiewicz J, Jachymek W, Niedziela T, Kenne L, Lugowski C. Structural analysis of the lipid A isolated from *Hafnia alvei* 32 and PCM 1192 lipopolysaccharides. *J Lipid Res* (2010) 51:564–74. doi:10.1194/jlr.M001362
24. Lukasiewicz J, Niedziela T, Jachymek W, Kenne L, Lugowski C. Two Kdo-heptose regions identified in *Hafnia alvei* 32 lipopolysaccharide: the complete core structure and serological screening of different *Hafnia* O serotypes. *J Bacteriol* (2009) 191:533–44. doi:10.1128/JB.00891-08
25. Romanowska E, Katzenellenbogen E, Jachymek W, Niedziela T, Bogulska M, Lugowski C. Non-typical lipopolysaccharide core regions of some *Hafnia alvei* strains: structural and serological studies. *FEMS Immunol Med Microbiol* (1999) 24:63–71. doi:10.1111/j.1574-695X.1999.tb01266.x
26. Lukasiewicz J, Jachymek W, Niedziela T, Dzieciatkowska M, Lakomska J, Miedzybrodzki R, et al. Serological characterization of anti-endotoxin serum directed against the conjugate of oligosaccharide core of *Escherichia coli* type R4 with tetanus toxoid. *FEMS Immunol Med Microbiol* (2003) 37:59–67. doi:10.1016/S0928-8244(03)00104-4
27. Jachymek W, Petersson C, Helander A, Kenne L, Lugowski C, Niedziela T. Structural studies of the O-specific chain and a core hexasaccharide of *Hafnia alvei* strain 1192 lipopolysaccharide. *Carbohydr Res* (1995) 269:125–38. doi:10.1016/0008-6215(94)00348-J
28. Vinogradov E, Cedzynski M, Ziolkowski A, Swierzko A. The structure of the core region of the lipopolysaccharide from *Klebsiella pneumoniae* O3 – 3-Deoxy-alpha-D-manno-octulosonic acid (alpha-Kdo) residue in the outer part of the core, a common structural element of *Klebsiella pneumoniae* O1, O2, O3, O4, O5, O8, and O12 lipopolysaccharides. *Eur J Biochem* (2001) 268:1722–9. doi:10.1046/j1432-1327.2001.02047
29. Kijewska M, Kuc A, Kluczyk A, Waliczek M, Man-Kupisinska A, Lukasiewicz J, et al. Selective detection of carbohydrates and their peptide conjugates by ESI-MS using synthetic quaternary ammonium salt derivatives of phenylboronic acids. *J Am Soc Mass Spectrom* (2014) 25:966–76. doi:10.1007/s13361-014-0857-4
30. Katzenellenbogen E, Gamian A, Romanowska E. Trisaccharide core fragment occurring in lipopolysaccharides of some *Hafnia alvei* strains. *Carbohydr Lett* (1998) 3:223–30.
31. Jachymek W, Lugowski C, Romanowska E, Witkowska D, Petersson C, Kenne L. The structure of a core oligosaccharide component from *Hafnia alvei* strain 32 and 1192 lipopolysaccharides. *Carbohydr Res* (1994) 251:327–30. doi:10.1016/0008-6215(94)84295-7
32. Katzenellenbogen E, Gamian A, Romanowska E, Dabrowski U, Dabrowski J. 3-Deoxy-octulosonic acid-containing trisaccharide fragment of an unusual core type of some *Hafnia alvei* lipopolysaccharides. *Biochem Biophys Res Commun* (1993) 194:1058–64. doi:10.1006/bbrc.1993.1929
33. Vinogradov E, Cedzynski M, Rozalski A, Ziolkowski A, Swierzko A. The structure of the carbohydrate backbone of the core-lipid A region of the lipopolysaccharide from *Proteus vulgaris* serotype O25. *Carbohydr Res* (2000) 328:533–8. doi:10.1016/S0008-6215(00)00134-8
34. Petersson C, Niedziela T, Jachymek W, Kenne L, Zarzecki P, Lugowski C. Structural studies of the O-specific polysaccharide of *Hafnia alvei* strain PCM 1206 lipopolysaccharide containing D-allothreonine. *Eur J Biochem* (1997) 244:580–6. doi:10.1111/j.1432-1033.1997.00580.x
35. Palusiak A, Maciejewska A, Lugowski C, Rozalski A. The amide of galacturonic acid with lysine as an immunodominant component of the lipopolysaccharide core region from *Proteus penneri* 42 strain. *Acta Biochim Pol* (2014) 61:129–32.
36. Cuatrecasas P, Wilchek M, Anfinsen CB. Selective enzyme purification by affinity chromatography. *Proc Natl Acad Sci U S A* (1968) 61:636–43. doi:10.1073/pnas.61.2.636
37. Srere PA, Mattiasson B, Mosbach K. An immobilized three-enzyme system: a model for microenvironmental compartmentation in mitochondria. *Proc Natl Acad Sci U S A* (1973) 70:2534–8. doi:10.1073/pnas.70.9.2534
38. Westphal O, Jann K. Bacterial lipopolysacharides: extraction with phenol-water and further applications of the procedure. *Methods Carbohydr Chem* (1965) 5:83–9.
39. Palusiak A, Dzieciatkowska M, Sidorczyk Z. Application of two different kinds of sera against the *Proteus penneri* lipopolysaccharide core region in search of epitopes determining cross-reactions with antibodies. *Arch Immunol Ther Exp (Warsz)* (2008) 56:135–40. doi:10.1007/s00005-008-0012-7

40. Yi EC, Hackett M. Rapid isolation method for lipopolysaccharide and lipid A from gram-negative bacteria. *Analyst* (2000) 125:651–6. doi:10.1039/b000368i
41. Man-Kupisinska A, Bobko E, Gozdziewicz TK, Maciejewska A, Jachymek W, Lugowski C, et al. Fractionation and analysis of lipopolysaccharide-derived oligosaccharides by zwitterionic-type hydrophilic interaction liquid chromatography coupled with electrospray ionisation mass spectrometry. *Carbohydr Res* (2016) 427:29–37. doi:10.1016/j.carres.2016.03.024
42. Tsai CM, Frasch CE. A sensitive silver stain for detecting lipopolysaccharides in polyacrylamide gels. *Anal Biochem* (1982) 119:115–9. doi:10.1016/0003-2697(82)90673-X
43. Cedzynski M, Szemraj J, Swierzko AS, Bak-Romaniszyn L, Banasik M, Zeman K, et al. Mannan-binding lectin insufficiency in children with recurrent infections of the respiratory system. *Clin Exp Immunol* (2004) 136:304–11. doi:10.1111/j.1365-2249.2004.02453.x
44. Swierzko AS, Szala A, Sawicki S, Szemraj J, Sniadecki M, Sokolowska A, et al. Mannose-binding lectin (MBL) and MBL-associated serine protease-2 (MASP-2) in women with malignant and benign ovarian tumours. *Cancer Immunol Immunother* (2014) 63:1129–40. doi:10.1007/s00262-014-1579-y
45. Presanis JS, Hajela K, Ambrus G, Gal P, Sim RB. Differential substrate and inhibitor profiles for human MASP-1 and MASP-2. *Mol Immunol* (2004) 40:921–9. doi:10.1016/j.molimm.2003.10.013
46. Petersson C, Jachymek W, Kenne L, Niedziela T, Lugowski C. Structural studies of the O-specific chain of *Hafnia alvei* strain PCM 1190 lipopolysaccharide. *Carbohydr Res* (1997) 298:219–27. doi:10.1016/S0008-6215(96)00311-4
47. Katzenellenbogen E, Zatonsky GV, Kocharova NA, Rowinski S, Gamian A, Shashkov AS, et al. Structure of the O-specific polysaccharide of *Hafnia alvei* PCM 1196. *Carbohydr Res* (2001) 330:523–8. doi:10.1016/S0008-6215(01)00003-9
48. Petersen SV, Thiel S, Jensen L, Steffensen R, Jensenius JC. An assay for the mannan-binding lectin pathway of complement activation. *J Immunol Methods* (2001) 257:107–16. doi:10.1016/S0022-1759(01)00453-7
49. Ulmer AJ, Rietschel ET, Zahringer U, Heine A. Lipopolysaccharide: structure, bioactivity, receptors, and signal transduction. *Trends Glycosci Glycotechnol* (2002) 14:53–68. doi:10.4052/tigg.14.53
50. Hasunuma R, Morita H, Tanaka S, Ryll R, Freudenberg MA, Galanos C, et al. Differential clearance and induction of host responses by various administered or released lipopolysaccharides. *J Endotoxin Res* (2001) 7:421–9. doi:10.1179/096805101101533025
51. Pupo E, Lindner B, Brade H, Schromm AB. Intact rough- and smooth-form lipopolysaccharides from *Escherichia coli* separated by preparative gel electrophoresis exhibit differential biologic activity in human macrophages. *FEBS J* (2013) 280:1095–111. doi:10.1111/febs.12104
52. Charchaflieh J, Wei J, Labaze G, Hou YJ, Babarsh B, Stutz H, et al. The role of complement system in septic shock. *Clin Dev Immunol* (2012) 2012:407324. doi:10.1155/2012/407324
53. Michalski M, Swierzko A St, Lukasiewicz J, Man-Kupisinska A, Karwaciak I, Przygodzka P, et al. Ficolin-3 activity towards the opportunistic pathogen, *Hafnia alvei*. *Immunobiology* (2015) 220:117–23. doi:10.1016/j.imbio.2014.08.012
54. Sahly H, Ofek I, Podschun R, Brade H, He Y, Ullmann U, et al. Surfactant protein D binds selectively to *Klebsiella pneumoniae* lipopolysaccharides containing mannose-rich O-antigens. *J Immunol* (2002) 169:3267–74. doi:10.4049/jimmunol.169.6.3267
55. Jensenius H, Klein DC, van Hecke M, Oosterkamp TH, Schmidt T, Jensenius JC. Mannan-binding lectin: structure, oligomerization, and flexibility studied by atomic force microscopy. *J Mol Biol* (2009) 391:246–59. doi:10.1016/j.jmb.2009.05.083
56. Kjaer TR, Jensen L, Hansen A, Dani R, Jensenius JC, Dobo J, et al. Oligomerization of mannan-binding lectin dictates binding properties and complement activation. *Scand J Immunol* (2016) 84:12–9. doi:10.1111/sji.12441
57. Jensen PH, Weilguny D, Matthiesen F, McGuire KA, Shi L, Hojrup P. Characterization of the oligomer structure of recombinant human mannan-binding lectin. *J Biol Chem* (2005) 280:11043–51. doi:10.1074/jbc.M412472200
58. Ono K, Nishitani C, Mitsuzawa H, Shimizu T, Sano H, Suzuki H, et al. Mannose-binding lectin augments the uptake of lipid A, *Staphylococcus aureus*, and *Escherichia coli* by Kupffer cells through increased cell surface expression of scavenger receptor A. *J Immunol* (2006) 177:5517–23. doi:10.4049/jimmunol.177.8.5517
59. Shiratsuchi A, Watanabe I, Ju JS, Lee BL, Nakanishi Y. Bridging effect of recombinant human mannose-binding lectin in macrophage phagocytosis of *Escherichia coli*. *Immunology* (2008) 124:575–83. doi:10.1111/j.1365-2567.2008.02811.x
60. Lukacova M, Barak I, Kazar J. Role of structural variations of polysaccharide antigens in the pathogenicity of Gram-negative bacteria. *Clin Microbiol Infect* (2008) 14:200–6. doi:10.1111/j.1469-0691.2007.01876.x
61. Maldonado RF, Sa-Correia I, Valvano MA. Lipopolysaccharide modification in Gram-negative bacteria during chronic infection. *FEMS Microbiol Rev* (2016) 40:480–93. doi:10.1093/femsre/fuw007
62. Brade L, Brade H, Fischer W. A 28 kDa protein of normal mouse serum binds lipopolysaccharides of gram-negative and lipoteichoic acids of gram-positive bacteria. *Microb Pathog* (1990) 9:355–62. doi:10.1016/0882-4010(90)90069-3
63. Kasperkiewicz K, Swierzko AS, Bartlomiejczyk MA, Cedzynski M, Noszczynska M, Duda KA, et al. Interaction of human mannose-binding lectin (MBL) with *Yersinia enterocolitica* lipopolysaccharide. *Int J Med Microbiol* (2015) 305:544–52. doi:10.1016/j.ijmm.2015.07.001
64. Kuan SF, Rust K, Crouch E. Interactions of surfactant protein D with bacterial lipopolysaccharides. Surfactant protein D is an *Escherichia coli*-binding protein in bronchoalveolar lavage. *J Clin Invest* (1992) 90:97–106. doi:10.1172/JCI115861
65. Huber M, Kalis C, Keck S, Jiang Z, Georgel P, Du X, et al. R-form LPS, the master key to the activation of TLR4/MD-2-positive cells. *Eur J Immunol* (2006) 36:701–11. doi:10.1002/eji.200535593
66. Pagowska-Klimek I, Swierzko AS, Michalski M, Glowacka E, Szala-Pozdziej A, Sokolowska A, et al. Activation of the lectin pathway of complement by cardiopulmonary bypass contributes to the development of systemic inflammatory response syndrome after paediatric cardiac surgery. *Clin Exp Immunol* (2016) 184:257–63. doi:10.1111/cei.12763

15

The Lectin Pathway of Complement in Myocardial Ischemia/Reperfusion Injury—Review of its Significance and the Potential Impact of Therapeutic Interference by C1 Esterase Inhibitor

*Anneza Panagiotou[1], Marten Trendelenburg[1,2] and Michael Osthoff[1,2]**

[1] *Division of Internal Medicine, University Hospital Basel, Basel, Switzerland,* [2] *Department of Biomedicine, University Hospital Basel, University of Basel, Basel, Switzerland*

***Correspondence:**
Michael Osthoff
michael.osthoff@usb.ch

Acute myocardial infarction (AMI) remains a leading cause of morbidity and mortality in modern medicine. Early reperfusion accomplished by primary percutaneous coronary intervention is pivotal for reducing myocardial damage in ST elevation AMI. However, restoration of coronary blood flow may paradoxically trigger cardiomyocyte death secondary to a reperfusion-induced inflammatory process, which may account for a significant proportion of the final infarct size. Unfortunately, recent human trials targeting myocardial ischemia/reperfusion (I/R) injury have yielded disappointing results. In experimental models of myocardial I/R injury, the complement system, and in particular the lectin pathway, have been identified as major contributors. In line with this, C1 esterase inhibitor (C1INH), the natural inhibitor of the lectin pathway, was shown to significantly ameliorate myocardial I/R injury. However, the hypothesis of a considerable augmentation of myocardial I/R injury by activation of the lectin pathway has not yet been confirmed in humans, which questions the efficacy of a therapeutic strategy solely aimed at the inhibition of the lectin pathway after human AMI. Thus, as C1INH is a multiple-action inhibitor targeting several pathways and mediators simultaneously in addition to the lectin pathway, such as the contact and coagulation system and tissue leukocyte infiltration, this may be considered as being advantageous over exclusive inhibition of the lectin pathway. In this review, we summarize current concepts and evidence addressing the role of the lectin pathway as a potent mediator/modulator of myocardial I/R injury in animal models and in patients. In addition, we focus on the evidence and the potential advantages of using the natural inhibitor of the lectin pathway, C1INH, as a future therapeutic approach in AMI given its ability to interfere with several plasmatic cascades. Ameliorating myocardial I/R injury by targeting the complement system and other plasmatic cascades remains a valid option for future therapeutic interventions.

Keywords: C1 esterase inhibitor, complement system, complement inhibition, ischemia/reperfusion injury, mannose-binding lectin, myocardial infarction, inflammation

INTRODUCTION

Ischemic heart disease is still a major cause of morbidity and mortality worldwide. In the United States, more than 700,000 episodes of acute myocardial infarctions (AMIs) are diagnosed annually (1). AMI is the consequence of rupture or erosion of a vulnerable atherosclerotic plaque in the coronary arteries subsequently leading to total or partial occlusion and tissue ischemia. In patients with total occlusion, emergency reperfusion of ischemic myocardial tissue is the cornerstone of therapy to salvage ischemic tissue from permanent damage. However, abrupt restoration of coronary blood flow with reperfusion of ischemic myocardium may itself trigger additional injury, which is known as ischemia/reperfusion (I/R) injury and may lead to the death of previously viable cardiac tissue (2). Estimates from previous experimental studies suggest that I/R injury may account for a significant (up to 50%) proportion of the final infarct size (3). Several mechanisms and mediators of I/R injury have been previously identified including oxidative stress, inflammation, and endogenous salvage kinase pathways (4). Despite promising results in experimental and early phase human studies (5, 6), interventional strategies targeting cardiac I/R injury have not been successful including the phase 3 trials of cyclosporine or pexelizumab before percutaneous coronary intervention in patients with AMI (7, 8).

Regarding inflammation as one mediator of I/R injury, experimental and clinical studies have shown that reperfusion after transient ischemia results in activation of endothelial cells, the contact and the complement system and attraction of neutrophils to the site of infarction (9, 10). The complement system is a major component of innate immunity, which is involved in both recognition and response to pathogens (11). It is further implicated in an increasing number of homeostatic and disease processes such as the immune complex catabolism, the clearance of dead and dying cells and the modulation of adaptive immune responses (12). Three pathways can activate the complement cascade: the classical, the alternative, and the lectin pathway. After initiation, these three pathways converge at the level of cleavage and activation of complement component C3, which subsequently leads to the generation of the anaphylatoxins (C3a, C5a) and the membrane attack complex (MAC; C5b-9). This review focuses on the role of the lectin pathway in myocardial I/R injury and the potential benefit of therapeutic application of its natural inhibitor, C1 esterase inhibitor (C1INH). In particular, we will focus on the potential advantages of C1INH as a promising candidate for future trials of salvage strategies of hypoxic myocardial tissue after AMI.

THE LECTIN PATHWAY OF COMPLEMENT

The lectin pathway can be activated by the pattern-recognition receptors (PRR), mannose-binding lectin (MBL), ficolin-1, ficolin-2, ficolin-3, collectin 10 (CL-10), and collectin 11 (CL-11 or CL-K1). These glycoproteins bind to carbohydrate patterns, acetyl groups, or immunoglobulin M exposed on microorganisms or dying host cells (13, 14). In plasma, lectin pathway PRR complex together with MBL-associated serine proteases (MASPs)-1, -2, -3, and two non-protease peptides, sMAP (Map19) and MBL/ficolin-associated protein-1 (MAP-1 or Map44). Whereas MAP-1 was shown to be a natural inhibitor of the lectin pathway (15), the exact function of sMAP is still unknown. After binding of the PRR to their target structures, MASP-1 is activated which in turn activates MASP-2, which is required for generating the C3 convertase (C4b2a) (16). The C3 convertase cleaves C3 into the opsonin C3b and the anaphylatoxin C3a, initiating the formation of an additional anaphylatoxin (C5a) and the MAC (C5b-9). Whereas the function of MASP-2 is strictly limited to the activation of the lectin pathway, several proteolytic functions have been observed for MASP-1, such as cleavage of fibrinogen, factor XIII, prothrombin and thrombin-activated fibrinolysis inhibitor (coagulation cascade), cleavage of kininogen (kallikrein-kinin cascade), and activation of protease-activated receptors on endothelial cells (neutrophil attraction) (17). Although the proteolytic activity of MASP-1 toward these proteins is much lower compared with the primary cleaving or activating enzymes of these proteins or compared with the primary lectin and classical pathway target proteins of MASP-1, it may still be of relevance *in vivo*. For example, a prolonged bleeding time and decreased arterial thrombogenesis was observed in a MASP-1 knock-out rodent model (18, 19). In the context of AMI, activation of the lectin pathway of complement after AMI may impact on I/R injury not only through activation of the complement cascade but also *via* promotion of clot formation (coagulation and fibrinolytic system) and of inflammation (kallikrein-kinin cascade, activation of endothelial cells, and attraction of neutrophils). Hence, inhibition of the lectin pathway, particularly at the level of MASP-1/-2 seems to be advantageous over downstream inhibition of the complement.

C1 ESTERASE INHIBITOR

The most important natural inhibitor of the lectin pathway of complement is C1INH. C1INH, a member of the serpin superfamily of serine protease inhibitors, is an acute-phase protein that has manifold targets and biological functions. Although the primary function of serpins involves the inhibition of proteases, they are also implicated in additional biological interactions, such as the inhibition of leukocyte rolling and interactions with endothelial cells and microorganisms (20). For example, treatment with C1INH was shown to limit the activation of endothelial cells and their subsequent transition into a procoagulatory and antifibrinolytic state after I/R injury (21). Proteases that are inactivated by C1INH include C1r, C1s (classical pathway of complement), MASP-1 and MASP-2 (lectin pathway), factor XII and plasma kallikrein (contact system), factor XI and thrombin (coagulation system), and plasmin and tissue plasminogen activator (fibrinolytic system) (22, 23) (**Figure 1**). Binding of C1INH to any of its target proteases leads to tight complexes which are subsequently cleared from the circulation and can be summarized as suicide inhibition (9). Decreased plasmatic antigenic levels of C1INH result in uncontrolled production of vasoactive peptides, which leads to the characteristic episodes of local soft tissue swelling observed in hereditary angioedema (HAE) (24).

Regarding the complement system, MASP-1 and -2 seem to be the major target of C1INH with less effective inhibition of the classical pathway (25). Interestingly, the lectin pathway and in particular MASP-1 have been recently implicated in the

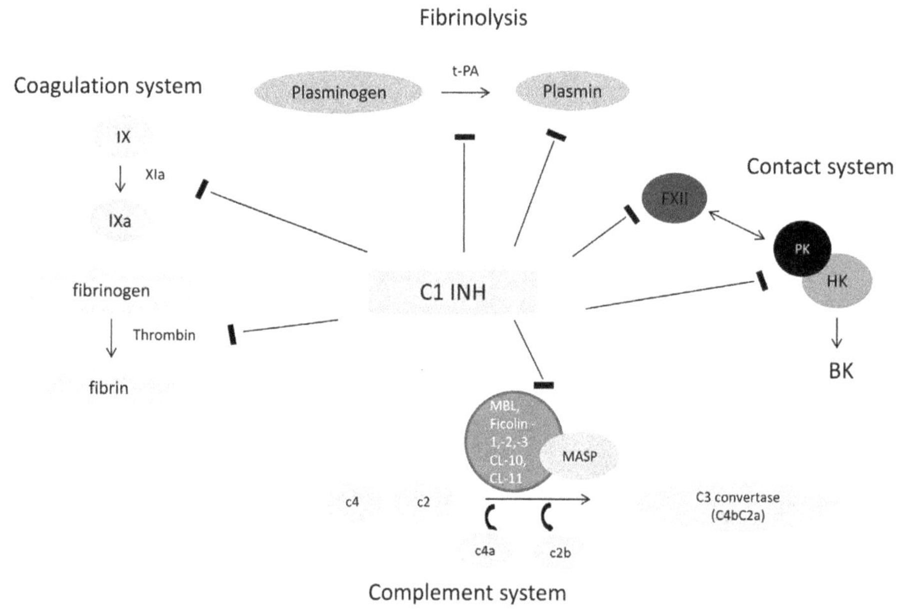

FIGURE 1 | Interaction of C1INH with plasmatic cascades. Abbreviations: HK, high molecular weight kininogen; FXII, factor XII (Hageman factor); PK, prokallikrein; BK, bradykinin; t-PA, tissue plasminogen activator; MAC, membrane attack complex.

pathophysiology of HAE, which underscores the central role of C1INH in controlling the activation of the lectin pathway. C1INH deficiency seems to cause uncontrolled activation of MASP-1, which may aggravate HAE (26).

Currently, three C1INH preparations are approved for the treatment and/or prevention of HAE, two plasma-derived, pasteurized, and nanofiltered (pdC1-INH, Berinert® and Cinryze®), and one recombinant product [rhC1-INH, Conestat alfa (Ruconest®), derived from the breast milk of transgenic rabbits]. Conestat alfa shares an identical protein structure with plasma-derived C1INH, but has a different glycosylation pattern of the amino-terminal domain of the protein (containing abundant oligomannose residues), which is responsible for a markedly shorter half-life compared with plasma-derived C1INH (3 vs. 30 h) (27). In fact, the unique glycosylation pattern introduced by the production of Conestat alfa in the mammary gland of transgenic rabbits may have additional, yet undiscovered consequences. For example, artificial variation of the glycosylation pattern of pdC1INH was previously shown to selectively impact on its target proteases with little impact on C1s inhibition in contrast to its interaction with kallikrein (28). Moreover, an important regulatory function of the amino-terminal domain of C1INH has been identified preventing inhibition of MASP-1-mediated alternative pathway activation (29), which may be influenced by the glycosylation pattern of C1INH. Although comparable inhibition for most target proteases was demonstrated (including C1s, factor XIa, XIIa, and Kallikrein) (30), Conestat alfa seems to target MBL and activation of the lectin pathway more effectively compared with plasma-derived preparations (31). This may be related to the fact that oligomannose-type glycans on average account for 15% of the total amount of glycans of Conestat alfa (compared with less than 1% in pdC1INH) (32), which may expedite the targeting and subsequent inhibition of MBL-MASP-1/MASP-2 complex by Conestat alfa.

Despite the rather broad interference with several cascades and targets, major adverse events or unique toxicities have not been demonstrated in previous studies, with the exception of a potential risk of allergic reactions in patients with rabbit dander allergy receiving Conestat alfa. Previous concerns of an increased thrombotic risk of pdC1INH (33) have not been confirmed in recent trials and registry data of both, pdC1INH and rhC1INH (34, 35). Common side effects described in trials include headache, nausea, and diarrhea. Currently, C1INH is evaluated in interventional clinical trials in the context of transplantation, acute antibody-mediated rejection after transplantation, and contrast-induced nephropathy.

THE LECTIN PATHWAY IN EXPERIMENTAL MYOCARDIAL I/R INJURY

Many animals and a limited number of human studies support the concept, that activation of the complement system and in particular the lectin pathway contributes to tissue injury observed after reperfusion of ischemic myocardial tissue (**Table 1**). Collard et al. were the first to report lectin pathway-dependent local activation of the complement system after myocardial I/R injury (36). Co-localized deposition of MBL and C3 in rat hearts was detected following myocardial I/R but not after sham surgery or myocardial ischemia only. Shortly thereafter, the same group demonstrated in a rat model of myocardial I/R injury that selective inhibition of MBL-A decreased infarct size and limited tissue injury and C3 deposition (37). In addition, infiltration of reperfused myocardial tissue by neutrophils was attenuated. Walsh et al. were the first to demonstrate the crucial involvement

TABLE 1 | Experimental studies investigating the role of the lectin pathway in murine myocardial I/R.

Reference	Intervention/setting	I/R model	Species	Effect
Collard et al. (36)	n/a	30 min LAD occlusion, 30 min reperfusion 60 min LAD occlusion	Rat	I/R: strong C3 and MBL staining throughout ischemic area Ischemia only: minimal C3 or MBL deposition
Jordan et al. (37)	Anti-MBL-A mAbs (P7E4, 14C3.74)	30 min LAD occlusion, 4 h reperfusion Pretreatment with mAbs (5 min before ischemia)	Rat	P7E4: ↓ local C3 deposition, infarct size, accumulation of PMN and expression of pro-inflammatory genes 14C3.74: no effect
Walsh et al. (38)	MBL−/− C1q−/− C2/fB−/− fD−/− C1q/fD−/− Anti-C5 mAb	30 min LAD occlusion, 3 h reperfusion pretreatment with mAb (5 min before ischemia) Reconstitution with C2 or rhMBL	Mouse	MBL−/−, C2−/−, anti-C5 mAb: ↓ infarct size, effect lost after reconstitution with rhMBL or C2 C1q−/−, C1q/fD−/−, fD−/−: no effect; co-localization of MBL and C3 in ischemic area
Busche et al. (40)	Streptozotocin-induced diabetic MBL−/−	15 or 30 min LAD occlusion, 4 h reperfusion	Mouse	↓ hyperglycemia induced myocardial remodeling and loss of cardiac progenitor cells ↓ cardiac tissue injury and local PMN infiltration after I/R injury
Busche et al. (41)	sIgM/MBL−/−	30 min LAD occlusion, 4 h reperfusion reconstitution with MBL null, sIgM null, or sIgM/MBL null plasma	Mouse	↓ cardiac tissue injury, loss of ventricular function, local C3 deposition and PMN infiltration; effect lost after reconstitution with MBL null, sIgM null or sIgM/MBL null plasma
Schwaeble et al. (42)	MASP-2−/− C4−/−	30 min LAD occlusion, 2 h reperfusion	Mouse	MASP-2−/−: ↓ infarct size and cardiac tissue injury C4−/−: no effect
Pavlov et al. (15)	MBL−/− MAP-1	45 min LAD occlusion, 4 h reperfusion pretreatment with rhMBL and/or MAP-1	Mouse	MAP1: ↓ loss of ventricular function, infarct size and local C3 deposition; prevention of occlusive arterial thrombogenesis MBL−/−: ↓ loss of ventricular function and infarct size
Pavlov et al. (44)	hMBL2 expressing mouse Anti-MBL2 mAb	45 min LAD occlusion, 4 h reperfusion treatment with mAb at or 15 and 30 min after reperfusion	Mouse	↓ loss of ventricular function, infarct size (time dependent protection) and myocardial fibrin deposition; prevention of occlusive arterial thrombogenesis
Clark et al. (43)	Anti-MASP-2 mAb	30 min LAD occlusion, 2 h reperfusion pretreatment with mAbs (12–18 h before ischemia)	Mouse	↓ infarct size

fB, factor B; fD, factor D; I/R, ischemia and reperfusion; LAD, left anterior descending artery; mAbs, monoclonal antibodies; MBL, mannose-binding lectin; rhMBL, recombinant human MBL; PMN, polymorphonuclear leukocytes; sIgM, secreted immunoglobin.

of the lectin pathway when compared with the classical and alternative pathway in myocardial I/R injury (38), an important finding, which contradicted earlier studies that had implicated the classical pathway as the most important mediator of tissue injury after I/R (39). According to Walsh et al., myocardial I/R injury was strongly attenuated in MBL knock-out mice, whereas mice with an intact lectin pathway but lacking C1q, the PRR of the classical pathway, or factor D of the alternative pathway were not protected. Reconstitution with recombinant MBL abrogated the protective effect. These results were replicated in a mouse model of diabetes with two weeks of hyperglycemia followed by myocardial I/R injury (40).

As a previous study had suggested a sequence of binding of IgM to stressed endothelial cells followed by complement activation of the lectin pathway, the same group studied myocardial I/R injury in reconstitution experiments using mice lacking natural IgM and MBL (41). Interestingly, both, MBL and IgM were found to be required for increased myocardial C3 deposition, neutrophil infiltration, and loss of left ventricular function after reperfusion of ischemic myocardial tissue. Hence, binding of natural IgM to neoepitopes in ischemic tissue was suggested as a prerequisite for subsequent MBL-mediated complement activation and tissue injury.

Schwaeble et al. investigated myocardial tissue injury in MASP-2 and C4-deficient mouse models, i.e., in the absence of any residual lectin (MASP-2) and presumably of any classical/lectin pathway activity (C4), and further downstream after binding of MBL or other lectin pathway PRR to stressed and injured cardiomyocytes (42). Lack of MASP-2 but not of C4 led to significantly less I/R-induced myocardial damage, which suggests that MASP-2-mediated activation of the lectin pathway is a major requirement for the inflammatory myocardial tissue damage after I/R. Activation of the two other complement pathways does not seem to be sufficient in the absence of any lectin pathway activity. Importantly, the authors identified a MASP-2-dependent, C4-independent route of complement activation, which likely also involves MASP-1 (29). This finding highlights the importance of inhibiting the activation of the complement system as far upstream as possible. In line, treatment of mice with an anti-MASP-2 monoclonal antibody (mAb) administered 12–18 h before coronary artery occlusion and reperfusion led to significantly smaller infarct sizes (15 vs. 26% in isotype control treated animals) (43). Similarly, treatment with MAP-1, an endogenous lectin pathway inhibitor, which displaces MASP-2 from the MASP-MBL/ficolin-3 complex and inhibits MBL- and ficolin-3-dependent complement activation *in vitro*, was associated with a decreased infarct size and C3 deposition in both, wild-type (WT) and MBL-supplemented MBL knock-out mice (15).

Finally, Pavlov et al. confirmed the concept of targeting MBL to attenuate myocardial I/R injury in a humanized mouse model (44). These humanized mice produce functional human MBL while lacking murine MBL-A and -B. Inhibition of human MBL by a monoclonal anti-human MBL antibody preserved cardiac function after myocardial I/R, attenuated myocardial fibrin deposition, and prevented ferric chloride-induced arterial thrombogenesis.

Summarizing the evidence from experimental models, the lectin pathway was shown to be crucially involved in mediating myocardial I/R injury. Conceptually, myocardial I/R injury seems to be initiated by binding of natural IgM to neoepitopes on stressed or dying cardiomyocytes with subsequent binding of MBL to IgM and activation of MASP-1/-2 during reperfusion. The latter is a major requirement for subsequent complement-mediated inflammation including formation of the membrane-attack complex, induction of apoptosis, and attraction of neutrophils. The significance of other lectin pathway PRR in acute myocardial I/R injury remains to be determined.

THE LECTIN PATHWAY IN HUMAN MYOCARDIAL I/R INJURY

Inter-individual serum concentrations of lectin pathway PRR and proteases show a considerable degree of variability in humans (45). In particular, the distribution of MBL plasma levels is huge and ranges from undetectable to approximately 10 μg/ml secondary to well-characterized exon and promoter polymorphisms in the MBL2 gene (46). Very low (<0.1 μg/ml, resembling a knock-out setting in murine models) and low (<0.5 μg/ml) MBL levels are found in approximately 10 and 30% of the population worldwide, respectively. Several studies have investigated associations of lectin pathway protein levels, in particular MBL, with outcome after AMI to confirm the evidence from murine studies (**Table 2**).

In a pilot study of 74 patients with ST elevation myocardial infarction (STEMI) and successful reperfusion, sufficient plasma MBL levels (defined as >0.8 μg/ml) were independently associated with a significant cardiac dysfunction [defined as left ventricular ejection fraction (LVEF) <35%] (47). In line with the concept of downstream complement activation following binding of MBL to stressed endothelial cells and/or cardiomyocytes and subsequent consumption of complement components, plasmatic sC5b-9 levels were significantly lower in patients with cardiac dysfunction. In the largest analysis to date, MBL levels were investigated in 890 patients with STEMI receiving placebo in the setting of a randomized controlled trial of the C5 inhibitor pexelizumab (48). In this study, MBL deficiency was defined as a level ≤0.1 μg/ml. Interestingly, 30-day mortality was markedly lower in MBL deficient patients (0.8 vs. 5.5%), whereas creatine kinase levels, a marker of myocardial injury and infarction size, and complement activation product levels were similar in the two groups. The authors speculate that the observed reduction in mortality was mainly driven by protection from fatal arrhythmias in MBL-deficient patients, a well-appreciated consequence of reperfusion

TABLE 2 | Analysis of lectin pathway proteins in patients with AMI.

Reference	Study type	Condition	Included patients	Analyzed complement proteins	Relevant findings
Haahr-Pedersen et al. (47)	Observational	Acute STEMI	74	Plasma MBL and sC5b-9	↑ risk of cardiac dysfunction (LVEF < 35%) in patients with MBL ≥ 0.8 μg/ml and sC5b-9 ≤ 160 μg/ml
Trendelenburg et al. (48)	*Post hoc* analysis of RCT	Acute STEMI	890	Serum MBL	↓ 30-day mortality in patients with MBL deficiency (≤0.1 μg/ml); no association with cardiac tissue injury
Schoos et al. (50)	Observational	Acute STEMI	55	Plasma MBL, ficolin-2 and -3, MAP-1	↑ left ventricular dilatation/remodeling in patients with high ficolin-2 and combined ficolin-2/MBL or ficolin-2/MAP-1 baseline levels; no association with infarct size
Zhang et al. (51)	Observational	AMI (STEMI and NSTEMI)	AMI: 29 Healthy controls: 50 Stable CAD: 27	Plasma MASP-2 levels	↓ MASP-2 levels in patients with AMI compared with healthy individuals or stable CAD patients
Frauenknecht et al. (52)	Observational	AMI	AMI: 49 Healthy controls: 50 Stable CAD: 104	Plasma MASP-1, -2, -3, and MAP-1	↓ MASP-2 and ↑ MASP-1 levels in patients with AMI compared with healthy individuals or stable CAD patients; no difference in MASP-3 and MAP-1 levels
Holt et al. (53)	*Post hoc* analysis of RCT	Acute STEMI	STEMI: 192 Healthy controls: 140	Plasma MAP-1, MASP-1, MASP-3	↑ MASP-1,-3 and MAP-1 levels in STEMI patients compared with healthy individuals; no association with infarct size

CAD, coronary artery disease; LVEF, left ventricular ejection fraction; MBL, mannose-binding lectin; NSTEMI, non ST-elevation myocardial infarction; RCT, randomized controlled trial; STEMI, ST elevation myocardial infarction; AMI, acute myocardial infarction.

injury (49). However, these results have not yet been confirmed in a cohort of STEMI patients undergoing percutaneous coronary interventions with contemporary stents and antithrombotic therapy.

In a small cohort of 55 STEMI patients, Schoos et al. investigated the association of ficolin-2/-3, MBL, and MAP-1 levels with left ventricular remodeling and infarct size as assessed by cardiac magnetic resonance imaging after percutaneous coronary intervention and at 6-month follow-up (50). Ficolin-2 levels significantly increased from admission to day 4 in contrast to other lectin pathway proteins, which may indicate consumption of ficolin-2 during STEMI. Higher baseline ficolin-2 levels were associated with left ventricular dilatation after STEMI. A similar finding was observed for the combination of higher ficolin-2 and MBL levels or higher ficolin-2 and lower MAP-1 levels indicating that the overall activation of the lectin pathway (rather than higher or lower levels of a single lectin pathway protein or protease) may be the key parameter influencing left ventricular dilatation after STEMI. However, lectin pathway proteins were not associated with infarct size, left ventricular function, or remodeling after 6 months, similar to the lack of association between MBL and infarct size observed in the larger study of Trendelenburg et al. (48). Zhang et al. investigated the role of MASP-2 in myocardial ischemia in the setting of AMI and separately in open heart surgery (51). For the purposes of this article, we only report the results of 29 AMI patients being described in this study. MASP-2 levels determined within two days after admission were almost 50% lower compared with healthy individuals or patients with stable coronary artery disease (CAD). This may be consistent with activation of the lectin pathway during AMI with subsequent consumption of MASP-2, similar to the previously cited observation of reduced ficolin-2 levels on admission. Although follow-up samples were lacking, it seems unlikely that genetically determined lower MASP-2 levels were already present before the AMI or that a temporary change in MASP-2 levels triggered the AMI in these patients.

In another study, lower MASP-2 and higher MASP-1 levels were observed in patients with myocardial infarction compared with patients with stable CAD and healthy controls (only MASP-1) (52), whereas MAP-1 levels were similar in these groups. However, the sample size was limited (n = 49 AMI patients) and protein levels were not associated with the severity of cardiovascular disease. Finally, levels of MAP-1, MASP-1, and -3 were analyzed in 192 AMI patients and 140 healthy controls (53). Whereas protease levels were significantly higher in AMI patients compared with healthy controls, they did not correlate with final infarct size or LVEF at 30 days. Importantly, results were in agreement with the previous study by Holt et al. only with regards to elevated MASP-1 levels but not with regards to observed MAP-1 levels. Again, follow-up samples were not available, and hence it remains to be determined if the observed changes in lectin pathway proteins are the consequence or the cause of the initial AMI event.

In summary, results from the cited studies indicate a potential involvement of the lectin pathway of complement in human myocardial I/R injury. In particular, levels of the PRR ficolin-2 and the activating protease MASP-2 were significantly lower in AMI patients on admission, whereas the levels of the endogenous inhibitor MAP-1 were higher (in only one of two studies), which may indicate activation of the lectin pathway during AMI with consumption of MASP-2 and ficolin-2. With regards to the observed increased MASP-1 concentrations in AMI patients, it remains to be determined if this is a result of an acute-phase reaction or if higher levels of MASP-1 may itself trigger an AMI event under certain circumstances given its clot promoting activity (54).

Importantly, associations of lectin pathway proteins with myocardial dysfunction, infarct size, and outcome were mostly lacking with the exception of an association of higher MBL levels and a higher net activation of the lectin pathway with mortality and ventricular dilatation after STEMI, respectively. However, involvement of MBL as a major initiator of the lectin pathway has not been demonstrated at the tissue level after human myocardial I/R injury to date. Future studies are required to investigate in more detail if PRR or protease levels are indeed associated with outcome after AMI and are causally involved in I/R injury in humans.

In general, evidence for the involvement of the lectin pathway in humans is much weaker than in animal studies, which is related to the limited samples size in most studies, a lack of analysis of a contemporary cohort of patients, and that most individual lectin pathway proteins have only been analyzed in a single study (with the exception of MBL, MASP-1, and MAP-1) and results have not yet been confirmed in subsequent studies. Although the significant variation of MBL levels in humans permits an analysis of complement-deficient patients in analogy to the analysis of knock-out compared with WT animals, this requires large cohorts. Evolutionary, other PRR may have evolved as a consequence of MBL deficiency and may compensate and in the case of I/R injury augment tissue injury independent of MBL. Unfortunately, experimental data regarding the significance of ficolins or collectins in myocardial I/R injury are lacking.

C1INH IN EXPERIMENTAL MYOCARDIAL I/R INJURY

The complement system was thought to play a major role in initiating an inflammatory response secondary to ischemia and reperfusion following studies 30 years ago (55). In particular, the classical pathway had initially been implicated in reperfusion damage of the heart (56, 57). To inhibit the classical pathway and subsequent complement activation at an early step, several studies examined the effects of treatment with C1INH on myocardial tissue damage, long before the central role of C1INH in the inhibition of the lectin pathway on the one hand and the pivotal role of the lectin pathway in myocardial I/R injury on the other hand was discovered (**Table 3**).

In a feline model of myocardial infarction, administration of pdC1INH before reperfusion led to a 65% reduction in cardiac tissue injury, and a markedly attenuated increase of creatine kinase compared with treatment with buffered saline solution (39). In addition, neutrophil activity/accumulation in the reperfused myocardial tissue was significantly reduced, which may be related to thc interaction of C1INH with activated endothelial cells or a reduction in locally generated leukocyte chemo-attractants such as C3a and C5a. The latter was subsequently confirmed in a pig

TABLE 3 | Effect of C1INH in murine models of myocardial I/R injury.

Reference	Intervention/ setting	I/R model	Species	Effect
Buerke et al. (39)	pdC1INH	90 min LAD occlusion, 4.5 h reperfusion 75 IU/kg pdC1INH 10 min before reperfusion	Feline	↓ infarct size cardiac, tissue injury and PMN infiltration
Murohara et al. (59)	pdC1INH sCR1	20 min LAD occlusion, 24 h reperfusion 75 IU/kg pdC1INH or sCR1 1 min before reperfusion	Rat	C1INH: ↓ cardiac tissue injury and PMN infiltration sCR1: non significant decrease in cardiac tissue injury and PMN infiltration
Horstick et al. (58)	pdC1INH	60 min LAD occlusion, 2 h reperfusion Intracoronary application of 20 IU/kg pdC1INH at reperfusion	Swine	↓ infarct size, tissue injury, and local C3a production
Buerke et al. (60)	pdC1INH	20 min LAD occlusion, 24 or 48 h reperfusion 10, 50, or 100 IU/kg pdC1INH 2 min before reperfusion	Rat	100 IU/kg: ↓ tissue injury, PNM accumulation, local expression of adhesion molecules 50 and 10 IU/kg: less or no effect, respectively
Horstick et al. (33)	pdC1INH	60 min LAD occlusion, 2 h reperfusion 40, 100, or 200 IU/kg pdC1INH 10 min before reperfusion	Swine	40 IU/kg: ↓ infarct size, tissue injury and local C3a and C5a production 100 IU/kg: no effect 200 IU/kg: severe coagulopathy leading to death
Buerke et al. (70)	C1s-INH-248 pdC1INH	60 min LAD occlusion, 3 h reperfusion 100 or 200 IU/kg pdC1INH or 0.1–1 mg/kg C1s-INH-248 5 min before reperfusion	Rabbit	C1s-INH-248: ↓ infarct size, tissue injury and PNM accumulation (dose dependent) C1INH: ↓ infarct size (smaller effect than C1s-INH-248)
Schreiber et al. (71)	pdC1INH	2 h LAD occlusion with cardiopulmonary bypass after 1 h, 2 h reperfusion Approximately 15 IU/kg pdC1INH into aortic root at reperfusion	Swine	No effect on ventricular function or infarct size
Fu et al. (63, 64)	pdC1INH	30 min LAD occlusion, 3–72 h reperfusion 40 IU/kg pdC1INH before ischemia	Rat	↓ myocardial apoptosis, local C3 expression, PNM accumulation and tissue injury
Lu et al. (65)	C1INH iC1INH C1INH–/– C3–/–	30 or 60 min LAD occlusion, 4 h reperfusion 400 IU/kg 5 min before reperfusion	Mouse	C1INH and iC1INH in WT mice: ↓ infarct size, tissue injury and PMN accumulation C1INH in C1INH–/– and C3–/– mice: similar effect as in WT mice

pdC1INH, plasma-derived C1 esterase inhibitor; iC1INH, inactive C1INH; C1s-INH-248, selective C1s inhibitor; PMN, polymorphonuclear leukocytes; cardiac CK, cardiac creatine kinase; LAD, left anterior descending artery; LAD left anterior descending artery; sCR1, soluble complement receptor 1; WT, wild-type.

model of myocardial I/R injury (58) administering pdC1INH as an intracoronary bolus before reperfusion. Local C3a production, which markedly increased after reperfusion, was significantly attenuated in the C1INH group compared with the placebo group indicating that C1INH may indeed suppress local complement activation. In a rat model of myocardial infarction, Murohara et al. sought to investigate the differential role of the classical and alternative complement pathway in myocardial I/R (59). Rats were treated with either pdC1INH or an alternative pathway inhibitor (soluble complement receptor 1) immediately before reperfusion. Interestingly, C1INH treatment was associated with a significantly attenuated creatine kinase release and neutrophil accumulation in ischemic myocardial tissue, whereas targeted inhibition of the alternative pathway was clearly inferior in this model. Finally, Buerke et al. confirmed the cardioprotective effect of different doses of plasma-derived C1INH in a rat model (60). Release of creatine kinase and local accumulation of neutrophils was attenuated in a step-wise fashion depending on the dose of C1INH with the greatest effect observed for the highest dose (100 U/kg). In addition, expression of adhesion molecules in the affected vascular endothelium was markedly reduced after administration of C1INH, which may explain the decreased local accumulation of neutrophils (61).

As a consequence of serious thromboembolic events in 13 newborns and babies who had received 500 IU/kg of pdC1INH to prevent capillary leakage after cardiopulmonary bypass operation, Horstick et al. investigated the effect of systemic administration of different doses of plasma-derived C1INH in the same pig model as had been previously used (33). In contrast to their previous model, pdC1INH was administered intravenously 10 min before reperfusion (40, 100, or 200 IU/kg) and without concurrent heparin. Experiments with 200 IU/kg were terminated after the first three pigs had developed severe coagulation disorders. Interestingly, while 40 IU/kg of C1INH reduced infarction size to a similar degree as in the previous model (>50%), there was a lack of beneficial effect with higher doses. The severe adverse events associated with the higher dose may be related to the significant inhibition of bradykinin release and of activators of the fibrinolytic system. The latter may have been prevented by co-administration of heparin, a principal anticoagulation agent in human STEMI patients (62).

In a rat model of AMI, Fu et al. observed a reduced C3 expression and apoptosis in the affected myocardial area associated with the administration of pdC1INH (63, 64). Interestingly, the amino-terminal domain of C1INH was implicated in the anti-apoptotic effect and not the protease activity.

As C1INH is a multi-action multiple-target inhibitor, it is difficult to identify the most important pathway or target protease inhibited by C1INH and responsible for the observed beneficial effect in myocardial I/R injury. While results from previous studies consistently demonstrated a clear benefit of C1INH in myocardial I/R injury, which was at least partly attributable to its inhibitory effect on complement activation, three studies have left more questions than answers with regards to the mechanism of action of C1INH and its effectiveness in cardioprotection after myocardial I/R injury. In particular, the study by Lu et al. questioned the importance of the complement system in mediating myocardial I/R injury in comparison to other mechanisms such as neutrophil influx (65). In their mouse model, a large dose of pdC1INH (400 IU/kg) or inactive C1INH (iC1INH) was administered intravenously 5 min before coronary reperfusion. iC1INH was generated by trypsin incubation, which results in the loss of its reactive center (66) and hence its ability to inhibit target proteases such as C1s. Interestingly, both C1INH and iC1INH similarly reduced myocardial damage and myocardial neutrophil influx in WT mice. In addition, C1INH treatment was effective even in C3 knock-out mice. These data are consistent with a mainly complement-independent cardioprotective mechanism of action of C1INH with the exception of its potential influence on protease-independent actions of the PRR of the lectin pathway [such as direct induction of apoptosis (67)] or its influence on lectin proteases *via* its glycosylated amino-terminal domain. The authors speculate that C1INH mainly acts *via* the inhibition of neutrophil influx across endothelial cells interacting with selectin ligands, which may be mediated by its sugar moieties rather than its proteolytic function. Two aspects warrant further comments. First, the dose of both preparations of C1INH used in the study was very high compared with previous animal models, which may be associated with additional modes of action, particularly in the case of iC1INH. Second, while the authors' dismissed a reaction of iC1INH with C1s of the classical pathway, their work does not fully exclude a residual protease activity of MASP-1/-2 after trypsin digestion. This may be of importance, as activation of MASP-1 in particular may mediate inflammatory actions independent of downstream complement activation (68). The beneficial effect of C1INH in the C3 knock-out model may be mediated by a similar mechanism, i.e., inhibition of MASP-1 and its pro-inflammatory, complement cascade-independent function. Third, previous work has identified C1INH functions that are independent of its proteolytic activity and mediated by its glycosylated, amino-terminal nonserpin domain, such as its interaction with the endotoxin lipopolysaccharide (69) or with selectins on endothelial cells (20). Similar nonserpin actions of C1INH on lectin pathway PRR and proteases have not yet been examined or described, but may contribute to the effect observed in the study by Lu et al. (65).

Similarly, Buerke et al. investigated the effect of a C1s-specific C1INH preparation (C1s-INH-248) in a rabbit model of myocardial I/R injury (70). This novel molecule is a specific inhibitor of the classical pathway of the complement system but does not inhibit MASP-1, kallikrein, and activated factors XII and XI. C1s-INH-248 was associated with attenuated myocardial injury as demonstrated by diminished plasma creatine kinase activity and local neutrophil accumulation. In addition, C1s-INH-248 was more effective than pdC1INH administered at doses up of 200 IU/kg. The authors speculated that cardioprotective effects of C1s-INH-248 may be related to the inhibition of the classical pathway and of the interaction of neutrophils with endothelial cells, and that the lectin pathway does not play a dominant role in their model. Again, the authors do not provide evidence of a total lack of interference of this C1s-specific C1INH with functions of the lectin pathway (in particular with MASP-2).

Finally, Schreiber et al. observed a lack of effect of intracoronary application of C1INH in a pig model of acute myocardial ischemia followed by urgent coronary bypass grafting (71). In contrast to all previous studies, C1INH did not reduce infarct size or release of creatine kinase, which may be explained by several ways. First, the dose of C1INH administered was rather low compared with previous studies (approximately 11–15 IU/kg). Second, C1INH was only administered locally and 60 min after induction of CPB. CPB is well known to systemically trigger activation of the complement system (72, 73), and hence late and local administration of C1INH was probably not able to prevent systemic (and even local) complement activation. In addition, evidence of an epicardial shunt was found which again may have impacted on the limited effect of locally applied C1INH. Ideally, C1INH should be administered before institution of CPB in models of coronary bypass grafting, as this would be practicable in the human setting, too.

In summary, significant cardioprotection by C1INH was evident in all but one experimental myocardial I/R injury studies. Limitations include the use of different doses, routes of administration, and AMI models with different durations of ischemia and reperfusion. However, due to its manifold actions, the exact mechanism of C1INH being responsible for the observed attenuated injury remains to be elucidated. Apart from the inhibition of complement activation, attenuated infiltration, and accumulation of neutrophils in ischemic tissue and a reduction of endothelial cell activation may be the dominant modes of action of C1INH. Unfortunately, experimental studies examining the impact of C1INH administration on the lectin pathway of complement and its consequences in myocardial I/R models are lacking. This is of importance, as a link between the lectin pathway of complement and activation of endothelial cells and subsequent recruitment of leukocytes has been previously demonstrated (16, 17, 68), and protease-independent actions of the PRR of the lectin pathway [such as direct induction of apoptosis (67) or amplification of inflammation *via* the alternative pathway] may play a role in myocardial I/R injury. A limitation of modified C1INH preparation as used in previous studies is that the difference in its function compared with original C1INH has not been comprehensively elucidated, in particular toward its effect on the lectin pathway and regarding a potential unwanted modification in the amino-terminal glycosylation.

C1INH IN HUMAN MYOCARDIAL I/R INJURY

Although multiple experimental studies have demonstrated the beneficial effect of complement inhibition in general and of C1INH in particular, no complement inhibitor is currently approved for the treatment of AMI or other I/R injuries. Interventions specifically and exclusively targeting the lectin pathway of complement are lacking in humans, whereas the effect of C1INH has been already investigated in three clinical trials and one case series (**Table 4**). Similar to the above-mentioned experimental studies, only pdC1INH was used. Bauernschmitt et al. were the first to report on the experience of pdC1INH treatment in three patients undergoing emergency coronary artery bypass grafting (CABG) after failed percutaneous coronary intervention (74). All three patients developed severe postoperative myocardial dysfunction which impaired weaning from CPB. Termination of CPB in all three patients was associated with the administration of a single dose of pdC1INH, which led to improved left ventricular function and hemodynamic stabilization.

In an open-label, dose-escalation study, de Zwaan et al. treated 22 patients with acute STEMI with pdC1INH during 48 h (75). The majority of patients had received antifibrinolytic therapy at least 1–2.5 h before C1INH administration, and only three patients underwent acute percutaneous coronary intervention. Drug-related adverse events were not observed, but creatine kinase and troponin T levels were reduced in comparison to a historical control population.

In a randomized, open-label study 28 patients undergoing emergency CABG after STEMI were treated with pdC1INH at aortic unclamping followed by another bolus dose 6 h later, and were compared with 29 similar patients receiving placebo and 10 patients undergoing elective CABG without evidence of recent STEMI (76). Again, drug-related adverse events were not observed. Administration of C1INH prevented the significant decline in C1INH activity (indicating consumption of C1INH) observed in placebo and control patients, whereas there was no difference in complement fragments. Interestingly, postoperative troponin T increase was only attenuated in patients receiving C1INH and surgical revascularization less than 6 h after symptom onset but not in patients with a longer ischemic interval.

In the largest study to date, Fattouch et al. randomized 80 patients with STEMI undergoing emergency CAGB to treatment with C1INH or placebo in a double-blind manner (77). C1INH was administered as an intravenous bolus before aortic unclamping followed by an intravenous infusion of 500 IU over 3 h after surgery. C1INH treatment resulted in significantly lower troponin T levels, an attenuated increase in complement activation fragments (C3a and C4a) and a shorter intensive care unit stay. Again, a significant decline of C1INH activity was only prevented in the active comparator group, and adverse events related to C1INH were not observed.

In summary, clinical studies of pdC1INH in human myocardial I/R suggest, that treatment of pdC1INH is safe and potentially effective in this setting. Of note, there is a lack of studies investigating C1INH in patients with AMI undergoing contemporary management with drug-eluting stents and state-of-the-art antithrombotic therapy. Mortality of AMI has significantly declined over the last decades as a result of modern drug and interventional treatment (78) and thus a potential benefit of pdC1INH as demonstrated in studies more than 10 years ago may not imply a similar positive effect in contemporary AMI patients. In addition, adverse drug reactions of C1INH administration must be meticulously evaluated in future studies given the potential of an increased bleeding but also thrombotic risk in the era of potent antithrombotic therapy and drug-eluting stents.

DISCUSSION

Acute myocardial infarction remains a leading cause of morbidity and mortality worldwide despite early and successful reperfusion strategies, which have been shown to significantly limit the size of the myocardial infarct and improve clinical outcomes. Although its existence remains controversial, reperfusion injury after restoration of blood flow has been regarded as a critical contributor to myocardial damage paradoxically limiting the beneficial effects

TABLE 4 | Effect of C1INH in clinical trials of AMI.

Reference	Study type	Condition	Included patients	Treatment	Relevant findings
Bauernschmitt et al. (74)	Case series	Emergency CABG after myocardial infarction	3	pdC1-INH 2,000 IU before CPB weaning	Hemodynamic stabilization and improved ventricular function
de Zwaan et al. (75)	Open-label, dose-escalation study	STEMI	STEMI: 22 Historical controls: 18	pdC1-INH 50 or 100 IU/kg loading dose continuous infusion of 1.25–2 IU/kg/h for 48 h	↓ troponin T and creatine kinase levels compared with historical control cohort
Thielmann et al. (76)	Randomized, open-label study	STEMI followed by emergency CABG	57	pdC1-INH 40 IU/kg loading dose before aortic unclamping 20 IU/kg 6 h after surgery	↓ decline in C1INH activity and troponin T increase (only when treated less than 6 h after symptom onset)
Fattouch et al. (77)	Randomized, double-blind study	STEMI followed by emergency CABG	80	pdC1-INH 500 IU loading dose 10 min before aortic unclamping Continuous infusion of 500 IU over 3 h	↓ decline in C1INH levels, increase in C3a, C4a, and toponin I levels, length of stay in ICU and hospital, duration of mechanical ventilation ↑ cardiac contractile function

CABG, coronary artery bypass grafting; CPB, cardiopulmonary bypass; ICU, intensive care unit; pdC1INH, plasma-derived C1 esterase inhibitor; STEMI, ST elevation myocardial infarction; AMI, acute myocardial infarction.

of myocardial reperfusion. With respect to the modulation of the complement response, several complement inhibitors targeting different proteins of the complement cascade have been successfully investigated in experimental models of myocardial I/R injury (79). These models have underscored the potential of attenuating myocardial tissue damage and ventricular remodeling by complement inhibition. However, with the exception of a single randomized placebo-controlled phase 3 trial, there is a lack of high-quality clinical studies of complement inhibition in human AMI (8). In addition, single-target interventions such as inhibition of C5 are probably inadequate to address the manifold inflammatory reactions *via* several cascades and pathways after AMI. For example, pexelizumab only attenuated the increase in C5 and interleukin-6 levels but had no impact on the increase and decrease of several other pro- and anti-inflammatory proteins, respectively (80).

FUTURE PERSPECTIVES

Based on the data as outlined above, we would like to suggest two potential strategies of complement inhibition for future clinical trials that are not mutually exclusive.

The first strategy involves targeted inhibition of the lectin pathway of complement. As the activity of the lectin pathway essentially depends on MASP-2 as the central enzyme (81), selective inhibition of MASP-2 shortly after myocardial ischemia and before reperfusion seems like an obvious next step. However, several caveats have to be considered apart from the availability of a suitable anti-MASP-2 antibody for future clinical trials.

MASP-2 inhibition, although effective in the above mentioned animal model, may be partially bypassed by the function of at least two lectin pathway proteins, such as MBL and MASP-1. For example, targeted MAPS-2 inhibition will not impact on several pro-inflammatory functions of MASP-1 such as endothelial cell activation (82) and the promotion of clot formation (54) *via* cleavage of thrombin substrates and the activation of platelets (68). Most importantly, evidence regarding the significance of the lectin pathway in human AMI is still premature and limited. Hence, a strategy that again only targets a single protein of the complement system (although further upstream in the complement cascade as in the pexelizumab trials) may be of limited or uncertain benefit in clinical trials of AMI. The complement system has also been implicated as a mediator of regenerative processes after myocardial tissue injury (83), and hence it is imperative to study the effect of short-term complement inhibition on outcomes after at least 30 days.

Treatment with C1INH may be regarded as a potential solution to this challenge. There are several advantages of using C1INH compared with isolated MASP-2 inhibition but also some caveats. In contrast to the previously mentioned strategies of complement inhibition, C1INH is a multiple-target, multiple-action inhibitor. Myocardial I/R injury is not mediated or caused by a single protein or even pathway, rather the opposite is true, i.e., several pathways are activated simultaneously and act in parallel. In addition, the relative contribution of each involved protein and pathway to the net damage is unknown and may vary in the line with the significant heterogeneity of AMI itself and of the diverse patient populations that suffer from AMI.

Evidence from multiple experimental studies mentioned in the present review point to a relevant and protective effect of C1INH in myocardial I/R injury. Moreover, results from small clinical trials, though conducted more than 10 years ago, seem to confirm findings from animal models. Similarly important as effectiveness is the fact that adverse drug reactions of C1INH administration were not reported in the setting of human AMI (75–77) and of acute rejection following renal transplantation (84–86).

Potential disadvantages of C1INH include unwanted effects when interfering with the coagulation and the fibrinolysis system at the same time. As a matter of fact, thromboembolic complications were noted in neonates receiving high-dose C1INH during cardiopulmonary bypass surgery and in an animal model of myocardial I/R injury (33). However, there was no safety signal in the above-mentioned clinical trials of C1INH.

When designing clinical trials of C1INH in AMI several aspects and pitfalls have to be addressed such as the required duration of treatment. In the previous pexelizumab trial in STEMI patients, complement inhibition was sustained for at least 24 h with its activity having returned to baseline after 48 h. However, elevated serum complement levels have been demonstrated during the first 10 days after AMI (87).

The second question is which type of C1INH should be investigated in future clinical trials of AMI. PdC1INH seems to be the obvious choice since it has been utilized in every experimental and human myocardial I/R injury study to date. Another advantage is its significantly longer half-life compared with Conestat alfa (30 vs. 3 h) (88). However, Conestat alfa significantly decreased ischemic damage when administered up to 18 h after induction of cerebral ischemia and reperfusion, whereas pd1INH was only effective when given at the time of reperfusion (31, 89). Similarly, the formation of plasmatic functional MBL/MASP-2 complexes after transient cerebral ischemia was attenuated only in mice receiving Conestat alfa but not pdC1INH.

Another important aspect involves the requirement of inhibiting target proteases and non-protease targets at the site of acute inflammation. To maximize effectiveness and minimize adverse reactions, an ideal C1INH preparation should exert its inhibitory function preferably or exclusively in ischemic and/or reperfused myocardial tissue similar to the concept of targeting cancer cells by mAbs. In contrast to cancer, the speed of inactivation is also crucial in I/R injury, as for example MBL-MASP-1/-2 complexes clustered together on ischemic endothelial or myocardial cells may escape inactivation by C1INH long enough to activate downstream effector molecules.

Whereas the protein structure is identical, the glycosylation pattern of Conestat alfa at the amino-terminal domain is markedly different from pdC1INH preparations (32). In particular, exposed mannose residues are significantly more prevalent in Conestat alfa compared with pdC1INH (15 vs. <1%), which may influence the binding preference toward lectins and in particular to MBL. Indeed, Gesuete et al. demonstrated high-affinity binding of Conestat alfa to MBL but not of pdC1INH (31). Although this may not directly influence the degree of inhibition by its serpin domain, it may potentially impact on the speed and location of inhibition in the human body. By binding to MBL, Conestat alfa may be hijacked to the primary site of inflammation, where it may immediately inhibit its target proteases before they are able to activate downstream effector molecules. By contrast, pdC1INH is certainly able to limit random complement activation in plasma but may allow considerable escape of inactivation of complement complexes at the tissue level. Interestingly, Conestat alfa remained confined on the ischemic endothelial wall in co-localization to MBL, whereas pdC1INH was also found in the area around the ischemic vessels (31).

However, due to the lack of comparative studies of pdC1INH vs. Conestat alfa in myocardial I/R injury it is premature to draw any definitive conclusions about any difference in efficacy of the two preparations in the setting of AMI.

SUMMARY AND CONCLUSION

In this review, we have summarized current concepts and evidence addressing the role of the lectin pathway as a potent regulator of myocardial I/R injury in murine models and the human setting. As it still remains to be determined if administration of a complement inhibitor after myocardial ischemia and before reperfusion is effective, we may have to leave the beaten path and "should strike out on new paths" (John D. Rockefeller, 1839–1937) avoiding single-target interventions and investigate pleiotropic compounds such as the natural inhibitor of the lectin pathway, C1INH, that also interferes with other important pro-inflammatory pathways. Given the evidence from several animal models and previous small clinical trials and the lack of major concerns regarding adverse events, there is ample reason to embark on larger clinical trials with C1INH in STEMI patients. In our opinion, ameliorating myocardial I/R injury by targeting the lectin pathway of complement remains a valid option for future therapeutic interventions.

AUTHOR CONTRIBUTIONS

All authors listed have made a substantial, direct, and intellectual contribution to the work including drafting and critical revising the article and approved it for publication.

FUNDING

This work was financially supported by a research grant from the Fondation Machaon, Switzerland (a not for-profit private foundation) to MO.

REFERENCES

1. Mozaffarian D, Benjamin EJ, Go AS, Arnett DK, Blaha MJ, Cushman M, et al. Executive summary: heart disease and stroke statistics – 2016 update: a report from the American Heart Association. *Circulation* (2016) 133(4):447–54. doi:10.1161/CIR.0000000000000366
2. Banz Y, Rieben R. Role of complement and perspectives for intervention in ischemia-reperfusion damage. *Ann Med* (2012) 44(3):205–17. doi:10.3109/07853890.2010.535556
3. Yellon DM, Hausenloy DJ. Myocardial reperfusion injury. *N Engl J Med* (2007) 357(11):1121–35. doi:10.1056/NEJMra071667
4. Allen LA, Turer AT, Dewald T, Stough WG, Cotter G, O'Connor CM. Continuous versus bolus dosing of furosemide for patients hospitalized for heart failure. *Am J Cardiol* (2010) 105(12):1794–7. doi:10.1016/j.amjcard.2010.01.355
5. Piot C, Croisille P, Staat P, Thibault H, Rioufol G, Mewton N, et al. Effect of cyclosporine on reperfusion injury in acute myocardial infarction. *N Engl J Med* (2008) 359(5):473–81. doi:10.1056/NEJMoa071142
6. Mahaffey KW, Van de Werf F, Shernan SK, Granger CB, Verrier ED, Filloon TG, et al. Effect of pexelizumab on mortality in patients with acute myocardial infarction or undergoing coronary artery bypass surgery: a systematic overview. *Am Heart J* (2006) 152(2):291–6. doi:10.1016/j.ahj.2006.03.027
7. Cung TT, Morel O, Cayla G, Rioufol G, Garcia-Dorado D, Angoulvant D, et al. Cyclosporine before PCI in patients with acute myocardial infarction. *N Engl J Med* (2015) 373(11):1021–31. doi:10.1056/NEJMoa1505489
8. Armstrong PW, Granger CB, Adams PX, Hamm C, Holmes D Jr, O'Neill WW, et al. Pexelizumab for acute ST-elevation myocardial infarction in patients undergoing primary percutaneous coronary intervention: a randomized controlled trial. *JAMA* (2007) 297(1):43–51. doi:10.1001/jama.297.1.43
9. Wouters D, Wagenaar-Bos I, van Ham M, Zeerleder S. C1 inhibitor: just a serine protease inhibitor? New and old considerations on therapeutic applications of C1 inhibitor. *Expert Opin Biol Ther* (2008) 8(8):1225–40. doi:10.1517/14712598.8.8.1225
10. Diepenhorst GM, van Gulik TM, Hack CE. Complement-mediated ischemia-reperfusion injury: lessons learned from animal and clinical studies. *Ann Surg* (2009) 249(6):889–99. doi:10.1097/SLA.0b013e3181a38f45
11. Walport MJ. Complement. Second of two parts. *N Engl J Med* (2001) 344(15):1140–4. doi:10.1056/NEJM200104123441506
12. Carroll MC. The complement system in regulation of adaptive immunity. *Nat Immunol* (2004) 5(10):981–6. doi:10.1038/ni1113
13. Alawieh A, Elvington A, Tomlinson S. Complement in the homeostatic and ischemic brain. *Front Immunol* (2015) 6:417. doi:10.3389/fimmu.2015.00417
14. Hansen SW, Ohtani K, Roy N, Wakamiya N. The collectins CL-L1, CL-K1 and CL-P1, and their roles in complement and innate immunity. *Immunobiology* (2016) 221(10):1058–67. doi:10.1016/j.imbio.2016.05.012
15. Pavlov VI, Skjoedt MO, Siow Tan Y, Rosbjerg A, Garred P, Stahl GL. Endogenous and natural complement inhibitor attenuates myocardial injury and arterial thrombogenesis. *Circulation* (2012) 126(18):2227–35. doi:10.1161/CIRCULATIONAHA.112.123968
16. Kjaer TR, Thiel S, Andersen GR. Toward a structure-based comprehension of the lectin pathway of complement. *Mol Immunol* (2013) 56(3):222–31. doi:10.1016/j.molimm.2013.05.007
17. Jani PK, Schwaner E, Kajdacsi E, Debreczeni ML, Ungai-Salanki R, Dobo J, et al. Complement MASP-1 enhances adhesion between endothelial cells and neutrophils by up-regulating E-selectin expression. *Mol Immunol* (2016) 75:38–47. doi:10.1016/j.molimm.2016.05.007
18. Takahashi K, Chang WC, Takahashi M, Pavlov V, Ishida Y, La Bonte L, et al. Mannose-binding lectin and its associated proteases (MASPs) mediate coagulation and its deficiency is a risk factor in developing complications from infection, including disseminated intravascular coagulation. *Immunobiology* (2011) 216(1–2):96–102. doi:10.1016/j.imbio.2010.02.005
19. La Bonte LR, Pavlov VI, Tan YS, Takahashi K, Takahashi M, Banda NK, et al. Mannose-binding lectin-associated serine protease-1 is a significant contributor to coagulation in a murine model of occlusive thrombosis. *J Immunol* (2012) 188(2):885–91. doi:10.4049/jimmunol.1102916
20. Cai S, Dole VS, Bergmeier W, Scafidi J, Feng H, Wagner DD, et al. A direct role for C1 inhibitor in regulation of leukocyte adhesion. *J Immunol* (2005) 174(10):6462–6. doi:10.4049/jimmunol.174.10.6462
21. Zhang S, Shaw-Boden J, Banz Y, Bongoni AK, Taddeo A, Spirig R, et al. Effects of C1 inhibitor on endothelial cell activation in a rat hind limb ischemia-reperfusion injury model. *J Vasc Surg* (2018). doi:10.1016/j.jvs.2017.10.072
22. Davis AE III, Lu F, Mejia P. C1 inhibitor, a multi-functional serine protease inhibitor. *Thromb Haemost* (2010) 104(5):886–93. doi:10.1160/TH10-01-0073
23. Beinrohr L, Dobo J, Zavodszky P, Gal P. C1, MBL-MASPs and C1-inhibitor: novel approaches for targeting complement-mediated inflammation. *Trends Mol Med* (2008) 14(12):511–21. doi:10.1016/j.molmed.2008.09.009

24. Carugati A, Pappalardo E, Zingale LC, Cicardi M. C1-inhibitor deficiency and angioedema. *Mol Immunol* (2001) 38(2–3):161–73. doi:10.1016/S0161-5890(01)00040-2
25. Nielsen EW, Waage C, Fure H, Brekke OL, Sfyroera G, Lambris JD, et al. Effect of supraphysiologic levels of C1-inhibitor on the classical, lectin and alternative pathways of complement. *Mol Immunol* (2007) 44(8):1819–26. doi:10.1016/j.molimm.2006.10.003
26. Hansen CB, Csuka D, Munthe-Fog L, Varga L, Farkas H, Hansen KM, et al. The levels of the lectin pathway serine protease MASP-1 and its complex formation with C1 inhibitor are linked to the severity of hereditary angioedema. *J Immunol* (2015) 195(8):3596–604. doi:10.4049/jimmunol.1402838
27. Davis B, Bernstein JA. Conestat alfa for the treatment of angioedema attacks. *Ther Clin Risk Manag* (2011) 7:265–73. doi:10.2147/TCRM.S15544
28. Ghannam A, Sellier P, Fain O, Martin L, Ponard D, Drouet C. C1 inhibitor as a glycoprotein: the influence of polysaccharides on its function and autoantibody target. *Mol Immunol* (2016) 71:161–5. doi:10.1016/j.molimm.2016.02.007
29. Parej K, Kocsis A, Enyingi C, Dani R, Oroszlan G, Beinrohr L, et al. Cutting edge: a new player in the alternative complement pathway, MASP-1 is essential for LPS-induced, but not for zymosan-induced, alternative pathway activation. *J Immunol* (2018) 200(7):2247–52. doi:10.4049/jimmunol.1701421
30. van Veen HA, Koiter J, Vogelezang CJ, van Wessel N, van Dam T, Velterop I, et al. Characterization of recombinant human C1 inhibitor secreted in milk of transgenic rabbits. *J Biotechnol* (2012) 162(2–3):319–26. doi:10.1016/j.jbiotec.2012.09.005
31. Gesuete R, Storini C, Fantin A, Stravalaci M, Zanier ER, Orsini F, et al. Recombinant C1 inhibitor in brain ischemic injury. *Ann Neurol* (2009) 66(3):332–42. doi:10.1002/ana.21740
32. Koles K, van Berkel PH, Pieper FR, Nuijens JH, Mannesse ML, Vliegenthart JF, et al. N- and O-glycans of recombinant human C1 inhibitor expressed in the milk of transgenic rabbits. *Glycobiology* (2004) 14(1):51–64. doi:10.1093/glycob/cwh010
33. Horstick G, Berg O, Heimann A, Gotze O, Loos M, Hafner G, et al. Application of C1-esterase inhibitor during reperfusion of ischemic myocardium: dose-related beneficial versus detrimental effects. *Circulation* (2001) 104(25):3125–31. doi:10.1161/hc5001.100835
34. Crowther M, Bauer KA, Kaplan AP. The thrombogenicity of C1 esterase inhibitor (human): review of the evidence. *Allergy Asthma Proc* (2014) 35(6):444–53. doi:10.2500/aap.2014.35.3799
35. Relan A, Bakhtiari K, van Amersfoort ES, Meijers JC, Hack CE. Recombinant C1-inhibitor: effects on coagulation and fibrinolysis in patients with hereditary angioedema. *BioDrugs* (2012) 26(1):43–52. doi:10.2165/11599490-000000000-00000
36. Collard CD, Vakeva A, Morrissey MA, Agah A, Rollins SA, Reenstra WR, et al. Complement activation after oxidative stress: role of the lectin complement pathway. *Am J Pathol* (2000) 156(5):1549–56. doi:10.1016/S0002-9440(10)65026-2
37. Jordan JE, Montalto MC, Stahl GL. Inhibition of mannose-binding lectin reduces postischemic myocardial reperfusion injury. *Circulation* (2001) 104(12):1413–8. doi:10.1161/hc3601.095578
38. Walsh MC, Bourcier T, Takahashi K, Shi L, Busche MN, Rother RP, et al. Mannose-binding lectin is a regulator of inflammation that accompanies myocardial ischemia and reperfusion injury. *J Immunol* (2005) 175(1):541–6. doi:10.4049/jimmunol.175.1.541
39. Buerke M, Murohara T, Lefer AM. Cardioprotective effects of a C1 esterase inhibitor in myocardial ischemia and reperfusion. *Circulation* (1995) 91(2):393–402. doi:10.1161/01.CIR.91.2.393
40. Busche MN, Walsh MC, McMullen ME, Guikema BJ, Stahl GL. Mannose-binding lectin plays a critical role in myocardial ischaemia and reperfusion injury in a mouse model of diabetes. *Diabetologia* (2008) 51(8):1544–51. doi:10.1007/s00125-008-1044-6
41. Busche MN, Pavlov V, Takahashi K, Stahl GL. Myocardial ischemia and reperfusion injury is dependent on both IgM and mannose-binding lectin. *Am J Physiol Heart Circ Physiol* (2009) 297(5):H1853–9. doi:10.1152/ajpheart.00049.2009
42. Schwaeble WJ, Lynch NJ, Clark JE, Marber M, Samani NJ, Ali YM, et al. Targeting of mannan-binding lectin-associated serine protease-2 confers protection from myocardial and gastrointestinal ischemia/reperfusion injury. *Proc Natl Acad Sci U S A* (2011) 108(18):7523–8. doi:10.1073/pnas.1101748108
43. Clark JE, Dudler T, Marber MS, Schwaeble W. Cardioprotection by an anti-MASP-2 antibody in a murine model of myocardial infarction. *Open Heart* (2018) 5(1):e000652. doi:10.1136/openhrt-2017-000652
44. Pavlov VI, Tan YS, McClure EE, La Bonte LR, Zou C, Gorsuch WB, et al. Human mannose-binding lectin inhibitor prevents myocardial injury and arterial thrombogenesis in a novel animal model. *Am J Pathol* (2015) 185(2):347–55. doi:10.1016/j.ajpath.2014.10.015
45. Sallenbach S, Thiel S, Aebi C, Otth M, Bigler S, Jensenius JC, et al. Serum concentrations of lectin-pathway components in healthy neonates, children and adults: mannan-binding lectin (MBL), M-, L-, and H-ficolin, and MBL-associated serine protease-2 (MASP-2). *Pediatr Allergy Immunol* (2011) 22(4):424–30. doi:10.1111/j.1399-3038.2010.01104.x
46. Garred P, Larsen F, Seyfarth J, Fujita R, Madsen HO. Mannose-binding lectin and its genetic variants. *Genes Immun* (2006) 7(2):85–94. doi:10.1038/sj.gene.6364283
47. Haahr-Pedersen S, Bjerre M, Flyvbjerg A, Mogelvang R, Dominquez H, Hansen TK, et al. Level of complement activity predicts cardiac dysfunction after acute myocardial infarction treated with primary percutaneous coronary intervention. *J Invasive Cardiol* (2009) 21(1):13–9.
48. Trendelenburg M, Theroux P, Stebbins A, Granger C, Armstrong P, Pfisterer M. Influence of functional deficiency of complement mannose-binding lectin on outcome of patients with acute ST-elevation myocardial infarction undergoing primary percutaneous coronary intervention. *Eur Heart J* (2010) 31(10):1181–7. doi:10.1093/eurheartj/ehp597
49. Bonnemeier H, Wiegand UK, Giannitsis E, Schulenburg S, Hartmann F, Kurowski V, et al. Temporal repolarization inhomogeneity and reperfusion arrhythmias in patients undergoing successful primary percutaneous coronary intervention for acute ST-segment elevation myocardial infarction: impact of admission troponin T. *Am Heart J* (2003) 145(3):484–92. doi:10.1067/mhj.2003.174
50. Schoos MM, Munthe-Fog L, Skjoedt MO, Ripa RS, Lonborg J, Kastrup J, et al. Association between lectin complement pathway initiators, C-reactive protein and left ventricular remodeling in myocardial infarction-a magnetic resonance study. *Mol Immunol* (2013) 54(3–4):408–14. doi:10.1016/j.molimm.2013.01.008
51. Zhang M, Hou YJ, Cavusoglu E, Lee DC, Steffensen R, Yang L, et al. MASP-2 activation is involved in ischemia-related necrotic myocardial injury in humans. *Int J Cardiol* (2013) 166(2):499–504. doi:10.1016/j.ijcard.2011.11.032
52. Frauenknecht V, Thiel S, Storm L, Meier N, Arnold M, Schmid JP, et al. Plasma levels of mannan-binding lectin (MBL)-associated serine proteases (MASPs) and MBL-associated protein in cardio- and cerebrovascular diseases. *Clin Exp Immunol* (2013) 173(1):112–20. doi:10.1111/cei.12093
53. Holt CB, Thiel S, Munk K, Ostergaard JA, Botker HE, Hansen TK. Association between endogenous complement inhibitor and myocardial salvage in patients with myocardial infarction. *Eur Heart J Acute Cardiovasc Care* (2014) 3(1):3–9. doi:10.1177/2048872613507004
54. Jenny L, Dobo J, Gal P, Pal G, Lam WA, Schroeder V. MASP-1 of the complement system enhances clot formation in a microvascular whole blood flow model. *PLoS One* (2018) 13(1):e0191292. doi:10.1371/journal.pone.0191292
55. Crawford MH, Grover FL, Kolb WP, McMahan CA, O'Rourke RA, McManus LM, et al. Complement and neutrophil activation in the pathogenesis of ischemic myocardial injury. *Circulation* (1988) 78(6):1449–58. doi:10.1161/01.CIR.78.6.1449
56. Rossen RD, Swain JL, Michael LH, Weakley S, Giannini E, Entman ML. Selective accumulation of the first component of complement and leukocytes in ischemic canine heart muscle. A possible initiator of an extra myocardial mechanism of ischemic injury. *Circ Res* (1985) 57(1):119–30. doi:10.1161/01.RES.57.1.119
57. Rossen RD, Michael LH, Kagiyama A, Savage HE, Hanson G, Reisberg MA, et al. Mechanism of complement activation after coronary artery occlusion: evidence that myocardial ischemia in dogs causes release of constituents of myocardial subcellular origin that complex with human C1q in vivo. *Circ Res* (1988) 62(3):572–84. doi:10.1161/01.RES.62.3.572
58. Horstick G, Heimann A, Gotze O, Hafner G, Berg O, Bohmer P, et al. Intracoronary application of C1 esterase inhibitor improves cardiac function and reduces myocardial necrosis in an experimental model of ischemia and reperfusion. *Circulation* (1997) 95(3):701–8. doi:10.1161/01.CIR.95.3.701
59. Murohara T, Guo JP, Delyani JA, Lefer AM. Cardioprotective effects of selective inhibition of the two complement activation pathways in myocardial

ischemia and reperfusion injury. *Methods Find Exp Clin Pharmacol* (1995) 17(8):499–507.
60. Buerke M, Prufer D, Dahm M, Oelert H, Meyer J, Darius H. Blocking of classical complement pathway inhibits endothelial adhesion molecule expression and preserves ischemic myocardium from reperfusion injury. *J Pharmacol Exp Ther* (1998) 286(1):429–38.
61. Hack CE, de Zwaan C, Hermens WT. Safety of C1-inhibitor for clinical use. *Circulation* (2002) 106(18):e132; author reply e132. doi:10.1161/01.CIR.0000035928.78148.CB
62. Ibanez B, James S, Agewall S, Antunes MJ, Bucciarelli-Ducci C, Bueno H, et al. 2017 ESC guidelines for the management of acute myocardial infarction in patients presenting with ST-segment elevation: the task force for the management of acute myocardial infarction in patients presenting with ST-segment elevation of the European Society of Cardiology (ESC). *Eur Heart J* (2018) 39(2):119–77. doi:10.1093/eurheartj/ehx393
63. Fu J, Lin G, Zeng B, Wu Z, Wu Y, Chu H, et al. Anti-ischemia/reperfusion of C1 inhibitor in myocardial cell injury via regulation of local myocardial C3 activity. *Biochem Biophys Res Commun* (2006) 350(1):162–8. doi:10.1016/j.bbrc.2006.09.023
64. Fu J, Lin G, Wu Z, Ceng B, Wu Y, Liang G, et al. Anti-apoptotic role for C1 inhibitor in ischemia/reperfusion-induced myocardial cell injury. *Biochem Biophys Res Commun* (2006) 349(2):504–12. doi:10.1016/j.bbrc.2006.08.065
65. Lu F, Fernandes SM, Davis AE III. The effect of C1 inhibitor on myocardial ischemia and reperfusion injury. *Cardiovasc Pathol* (2013) 22(1):75–80. doi:10.1016/j.carpath.2012.05.003
66. Pemberton PA, Harrison RA, Lachmann PJ, Carrell RW. The structural basis for neutrophil inactivation of C1 inhibitor. *Biochem J* (1989) 258(1):193–8. doi:10.1042/bj2580193
67. van der Pol P, Schlagwein N, van Gijlswijk DJ, Berger SP, Roos A, Bajema IM, et al. Mannan-binding lectin mediates renal ischemia/reperfusion injury independent of complement activation. *Am J Transplant* (2012) 12(4):877–87. doi:10.1111/j.1600-6143.2011.03887.x
68. Megyeri M, Mako V, Beinrohr L, Doleschall Z, Prohaszka Z, Cervenak L, et al. Complement protease MASP-1 activates human endothelial cells: PAR4 activation is a link between complement and endothelial function. *J Immunol* (2009) 183(5):3409–16. doi:10.4049/jimmunol.0900879
69. Liu D, Gu X, Scafidi J, Davis AE III. N-linked glycosylation is required for c1 inhibitor-mediated protection from endotoxin shock in mice. *Infect Immun* (2004) 72(4):1946–55. doi:10.1128/IAI.72.4.1946-1955.2004
70. Buerke M, Schwertz H, Seitz W, Meyer J, Darius H. Novel small molecule inhibitor of C1s exerts cardioprotective effects in ischemia-reperfusion injury in rabbits. *J Immunol* (2001) 167(9):5375–80. doi:10.4049/jimmunol.167.9.5375
71. Schreiber C, Heimisch W, Schad H, Brkic A, Badiu C, Lange R, et al. C1-INH and its effect on infarct size and ventricular function in an acute pig model of infarction, cardiopulmonary bypass, and reperfusion. *Thorac Cardiovasc Surg* (2006) 54(4):227–32. doi:10.1055/s-2006-923947
72. Kirklin JK, Westaby S, Blackstone EH, Kirklin JW, Chenoweth DE, Pacifico AD. Complement and the damaging effects of cardiopulmonary bypass. *J Thorac Cardiovasc Surg* (1983) 86(6):845–57.
73. Stiller B, Sonntag J, Dahnert I, Alexi-Meskishvili V, Hetzer R, Fischer T, et al. Capillary leak syndrome in children who undergo cardiopulmonary bypass: clinical outcome in comparison with complement activation and C1 inhibitor. *Intensive Care Med* (2001) 27(1):193–200. doi:10.1007/s001340000704
74. Bauernschmitt R, Bohrer H, Hagl S. Rescue therapy with C1-esterase inhibitor concentrate after emergency coronary surgery for failed PTCA. *Intensive Care Med* (1998) 24(6):635–8. doi:10.1007/s001340050629
75. de Zwaan C, Kleine AH, Diris JH, Glatz JF, Wellens HJ, Strengers PF, et al. Continuous 48-h C1-inhibitor treatment, following reperfusion therapy, in patients with acute myocardial infarction. *Eur Heart J* (2002) 23(21):1670–7. doi:10.1053/euhj.2002.3191
76. Thielmann M, Marggraf G, Neuhauser M, Forkel J, Herold U, Kamler M, et al. Administration of C1-esterase inhibitor during emergency coronary artery bypass surgery in acute ST-elevation myocardial infarction. *Eur J Cardiothorac Surg* (2006) 30(2):285–93. doi:10.1016/j.ejcts.2006.04.022
77. Fattouch K, Bianco G, Speziale G, Sampognaro R, Lavalle C, Guccione F, et al. Beneficial effects of C1 esterase inhibitor in ST-elevation myocardial infarction in patients who underwent surgical reperfusion: a randomised double-blind study. *Eur J Cardiothorac Surg* (2007) 32(2):326–32. doi:10.1016/j.ejcts.2007.04.038
78. Smolina K, Wright FL, Rayner M, Goldacre MJ. Determinants of the decline in mortality from acute myocardial infarction in England between 2002 and 2010: linked national database study. *BMJ* (2012) 344:d8059. doi:10.1136/bmj.d8059
79. Gorsuch WB, Chrysanthou E, Schwaeble WJ, Stahl GL. The complement system in ischemia-reperfusion injuries. *Immunobiology* (2012) 217(11):1026–33. doi:10.1016/j.imbio.2012.07.024
80. Martel C, Granger CB, Ghitescu M, Stebbins A, Fortier A, Armstrong PW, et al. Pexelizumab fails to inhibit assembly of the terminal complement complex in patients with ST-elevation myocardial infarction undergoing primary percutaneous coronary intervention. Insight from a substudy of the assessment of pexelizumab in acute myocardial infarction (APEX-AMI) trial. *Am Heart J* (2012) 164(1):43–51. doi:10.1016/j.ahj.2012.04.007
81. Chen CB, Wallis R. Two mechanisms for mannose-binding protein modulation of the activity of its associated serine proteases. *J Biol Chem* (2004) 279(25):26058–65. doi:10.1074/jbc.M401318200
82. Jani PK, Kajdacsi E, Megyeri M, Dobo J, Doleschall Z, Futosi K, et al. MASP-1 induces a unique cytokine pattern in endothelial cells: a novel link between complement system and neutrophil granulocytes. *PLoS One* (2014) 9(1):e87104. doi:10.1371/journal.pone.0087104
83. Wysoczynski M, Solanki M, Borkowska S, van Hoose P, Brittian KR, Prabhu SD, et al. Complement component 3 is necessary to preserve myocardium and myocardial function in chronic myocardial infarction. *Stem Cells* (2014) 32(9):2502–15. doi:10.1002/stem.1743
84. Viglietti D, Gosset C, Loupy A, Deville L, Verine J, Zeevi A, et al. C1 inhibitor in acute antibody-mediated rejection nonresponsive to conventional therapy in kidney transplant recipients: a pilot study. *Am J Transplant* (2016) 16(5):1596–603. doi:10.1111/ajt.13663
85. Montgomery RA, Orandi BJ, Racusen L, Jackson AM, Garonzik-Wang JM, Shah T, et al. Plasma-derived C1 esterase inhibitor for acute antibody-mediated rejection following kidney transplantation: results of a randomized double-blind placebo-controlled pilot study. *Am J Transplant* (2016) 16(12):3468–78. doi:10.1111/ajt.13871
86. Vo AA, Zeevi A, Choi J, Cisneros K, Toyoda M, Kahwaji J, et al. A phase I/II placebo-controlled trial of C1-inhibitor for prevention of antibody-mediated rejection in HLA sensitized patients. *Transplantation* (2015) 99(2):299–308. doi:10.1097/TP.0000000000000592
87. Earis JE, Marcuson EC, Bernstein A. Complement activation after myocardial infarction. *Chest* (1985) 87(2):186–90. doi:10.1378/chest.87.2.186
88. Farrell C, Hayes S, Relan A, van Amersfoort ES, Pijpstra R, Hack CE. Population pharmacokinetics of recombinant human C1 inhibitor in patients with hereditary angioedema. *Br J Clin Pharmacol* (2013) 76(6):897–907. doi:10.1111/bcp.12132
89. De Simoni MG, Rossi E, Storini C, Pizzimenti S, Echart C, Bergamaschini L. The powerful neuroprotective action of C1-inhibitor on brain ischemia-reperfusion injury does not require C1q. *Am J Pathol* (2004) 164(5):1857–63. doi:10.1016/S0002-9440(10)63744-3

16

Lectin Pathway Mediates Complement Activation by SARS-CoV-2 Proteins

Youssif M. Ali[1,2], Matteo Ferrari[1], Nicholas J. Lynch[1], Sadam Yaseen[3], Thomas Dudler[3], Sasha Gragerov[3], Gregory Demopulos[3], Jonathan L. Heeney[1] and Wilhelm J. Schwaeble[1]*

[1] Department of Veterinary Medicine, School of Biological Sciences, University of Cambridge, Cambridge, United Kingdom, [2] Department of Microbiology and Immunology, Faculty of Pharmacy, Mansoura University, Mansoura, Egypt, [3] Omeros Corporation, Seattle, WA, United States

Correspondence:
Youssif M. Ali
myima2@cam.ac.uk

Early and persistent activation of complement is considered to play a key role in the pathogenesis of COVID-19. Complement activation products orchestrate a proinflammatory environment that might be critical for the induction and maintenance of a severe inflammatory response to SARS-CoV-2 by recruiting cells of the cellular immune system to the sites of infection and shifting their state of activation towards an inflammatory phenotype. It precedes pathophysiological milestone events like the cytokine storm, progressive endothelial injury triggering microangiopathy, and further complement activation, and causes an acute respiratory distress syndrome (ARDS). To date, the application of antiviral drugs and corticosteroids have shown efficacy in the early stages of SARS-CoV-2 infection, but failed to ameliorate disease severity in patients who progressed to severe COVID-19 pathology. This report demonstrates that lectin pathway (LP) recognition molecules of the complement system, such as MBL, FCN-2 and CL-11, bind to SARS-CoV-2 S- and N-proteins, with subsequent activation of LP-mediated C3b and C4b deposition. In addition, our results confirm and underline that the N-protein of SARS-CoV-2 binds directly to the LP- effector enzyme MASP-2 and activates complement. Inhibition of the LP using an inhibitory monoclonal antibody against MASP-2 effectively blocks LP-mediated complement activation. FACS analyses using transfected HEK-293 cells expressing SARS-CoV-2 S protein confirm a robust LP-dependent C3b deposition on the cell surface which is inhibited by the MASP-2 inhibitory antibody. In light of our present results, and the encouraging performance of our clinical candidate MASP-2 inhibitor Narsoplimab in recently published clinical trials, we suggest that the targeting of MASP-2 provides an unsurpassed window of therapeutic efficacy for the treatment of severe COVID-19.

Keywords: complement system, lectin pathway, SARS-CoV-2, COVID-19, innate immunity

INTRODUCTION

Coronaviruses (CoVs) are single-stranded RNA viruses causing life threatening respiratory infection in humans and other species. The CoV genome encodes four main structural proteins, spike (S), membrane (M), envelope (E), and nucleocapsid (N), as well as other accessory proteins that facilitate replication and entry into cells. The transmembrane bound spike protein (S), consists of two subunits S1 and S2 that cover the surface of CoVs and serve as receptor binding entry proteins for infection. The nucleocapsid protein complexes with the viral RNA and plays a major role in viral replication as well as viral pathogenesis. M and E are two transmembrane proteins, which are responsible for viral assembly (1). In 2019, a pandemic respiratory infection caused by corona virus was reported and identified as coronavirus disease 2019 (COVID-19), the etiological agent of which is a β-coronavirus called severe acute respiratory syndrome coronavirus 2 (SARS-CoV-2). The clinical manifestation of SARS-CoV-2 infection include fever, cough, fatigue, myalgia, and pneumonia, that may develop into acute respiratory distress syndrome (ARDS), necessitating respiratory support, as well as disseminated intravascular coagulopathy and kidney failure (2, 3).

The complement system (CS) is an integral part of the innate and the adaptive immune systems. The CS is composed of more than 30 plasma and cell-resident components that form a first defence-line against infection and provides an essential scavenger system to eliminate injured, apoptotic or aberrant cells. Complement activation products modulate inflammation and direct the innate and the adaptive immune response. The CS is activated *via* three pathways, which funnel into a shared terminal activation route. The classical pathway (CP) is initiated through the binding of a recognition subcomponent, specifically complement component 1q (C1q). Two C1q-associated serine protease zymogens, C1r and C1s, form a C1s-C1r-C1r-C1s hetero-tetramer, which sits within the calix of the C1q macromolecule. The C1r/C1s zymogen complex is converted into active form when at least two arms of the C1q macromolecule bind to the Fc region of immune complexes. Activation of C1s leads to the cleavage of C4 to C4a and C4b, with the latter binding to C2. C4b-bound C2 is then cleaved by C1s to create the C3 convertase C4b2a, which cleaves the abundant complement component C3 into the anaphylatoxin C3a and the major fragment C3b (4). The Lectin pathway (LP) is initiated by multimolecular pattern-recognition complexes that bind to immune complexes and pathogen-associated molecular patterns (PAMPs). Six different LP recognition subcomponents can form LP activation complexes by binding dimers of three different mannan-binding lectin-associated serine proteases (i.e., MASP-1, MASP-2 and MASP-3). The recognition subcomponents comprise multimers of homotrimeric chains, which can bind directly to their cognate ligands present on pathogens, or to aberrant glycosylation patterns on apoptotic, necrotic, malignant, or damaged host cells (5, 6). The LP recognition subcomponents in humans are: mannan-binding lectin-2 (MBL-2), collectin-11 (CL-11), heterocomplexes of CL-11 and CL-10 and three different ficolins (ficolins 1, 2, and 3), two of which can also form heterocomplexes (ficolins 2 and 3). MASP-2 is the key enzyme of the LP; only MASP-2 can cleave C4 efficiently, whereas both MASP-2 and MASP-1 can cleave C2. In the absence of MASP-2, complement can no longer be activated by the LP activation route because the C3 and C5 convertase complexes C4b2a and C4b2a (C3b)n cannot be formed (7, 8). In addition, MASP-2 was shown to cleave C3 directly, forming a novel C4-bypass activation route. This C4-bypass route was shown to be important in the innate immune defence (9). The alternative pathway (AP) fulfils its surveillance function through a constant low-rate activation (C3 tick-over) and provides an efficient amplification loop of C3 activation. The C3 activation product C3b can bind to zymogen complement factor B (FB), forming a complex that can in turn convert more C3 into C3a and C3b if C3b-bound FB is cleaved by a serine protease called FD (10).

Complement activation was reported to be associated with development of acute respiratory distress syndrome (ARDS) and respiratory failure during viral pneumonia (11, 12). A direct link between complement activation and pathogenesis of Corona virus infection was established using C3-deficient mice infected with SARS-CoV. C3-deficient mice showed significantly less severe respiratory inflammation, decreased infiltration of neutrophils and inflammatory monocytes, and lower levels of cytokines and chemokines in both the lungs and sera compared to wild-type control mice (13). The involvement of complement-mediated pathology and lung injury during SARS-CoV-2 infection was revealed by a histopathological study of post-mortem biopsies taken from COVID-19 patients. The presence of thrombotic microangiopathies (TMAs) and the deposition of complement activation products, including C5b-9, C3d, C4d and the LP effector enzyme MASP-2 implied the involvement of LP and CP activation in severe COVID-19 (14). In this study, we address the involvement of the lectin activation pathway of complement in the response against recombinant SARS-CoV-2 proteins and which can trigger activation of the complement system.

MATERIALS AND REAGENTS

Recombinant S and N proteins of SARS-CoV-2 expressed in mammalian cell lines were purchased from R & D systems, UK. The pEVAC plasmids expressing the coding sequences for S protein were kindly provided by DIOSynVax Ltd Cambridge, UK. Recombinant truncated MASP-2, containing the 2 CCP domains and the serine protease domain, was expressed previously described (9).

HG4, a monospecific fully humanised antibody against MASP-2 that inhibits LP-mediated C4 cleavage was kindly provided by Omeros Corporation, Seattle, USA. Pre-pandemic, non-immune NHS, was pooled from 4 healthy donors. The mean levels of key lectin pathway components in the pool were: MBL, 1.43μg/ml; FCN2, 2.9μg/ml; CL-11, 0.39μg/ml; and MASP-2, 0.4μg/ml.

Transfection of HEK 293T Cells

HEK 293T cells were cultured in Dulbecco's Modified Eagle's Medium (DMEM) supplemented with 10% Foetal bovine serum albumin (FBS), 2 mM glutamine and 10 U/mL penicillin, 10 µg/mL streptomycin (Gibco). Cells were maintained in a CO_2 incubator at 37°C. HEK 293T cells were seeded in 6-well plates with cell density of 1×10^6 cells/mL. Next day, cells were transfected with 1 µg of plasmid DNA for each well using the Fugene transfection kit (Promega) according to the manufacturer's protocol. Cells transfected with empty pEVAC vector were used as a control. 48 hours after transfection, cells were harvested for flow cytometer analysis.

FACS Analysis

Transfected HEK 293T cells were washed twice using Hank's balanced salt solution with C^{2+} and Mg^{2+} ($HBSS^{++}$) and resuspended in $HBSS^{++}$ to a final concentration of 10^7 cell/mL. 10^6 cells were opsonised with 2.5% NHS in $HBSS^{++}$ for 30 minutes at 37°C with or without 100 nM of HG4. Cells transfected with empty vector were used as a negative control. After opsonization, cells were washed twice with $HBSS^{++}$ buffer, and bound C3b was detected using FITC-conjugated rabbit anti-human C3c (Dako). Fluorescence intensity was measured with The Attune NxT Flow Cytometer (Invitrogen).

Solid Phase Binding Assays

Nunc MaxiSorp microtiter ELISA plates were coated with 10 µg/mL of purified recombinant SARS-CoV-2 proteins S and N in coating buffer (10 mM Tris-HCl, 140 mM NaCl, pH 7.4). Control wells were coated with 10 µg/mL mannan (a control for MBL binding), 10 µg/mL zymosan (a control for CL-11 binding) or 10 µg/mL N-acetylated BSA (a control for L-ficolin binding). Immune complexes formed by incubation of BSA with rabbit anti-BSA were prepared. The ELISA plates were coated with 1 µg/mL BSA-anti-BSA immune complex as a control ligand for C1q binding. The following day, wells were blocked for 2 hours at room temperature with 250 µL of 1% (w/v) BSA in TBS buffer (10 mM Tris-HCl, 140 mM NaCl, pH 7.4), then washed three times with 250 µL of TBS with 0.05% Tween 20 and 5 mM $CaCl_2$ (wash buffer). Serial dilutions of serum in 100 µL of wash buffer were added to the wells and the plates were then incubated for 90 minutes at room temperature. Plates were washed as above and bound proteins were detected using rabbit anti-human L-ficolin, mouse anti-human CL-11 or mouse anti-human MBL mAbs. HRP conjugated goat anti-rabbit IgG followed by the colorimetric substrate (15).

Complement Deposition Assays

To measure C3 and C4 activation, Nunc MaxiSorp microtiter plates were coated with 100 µL of 10 µg/mL mannan (Promega), or 100 µL of 10 µg/mL SARS-CoV-2 proteins in coating buffer. After overnight incubation, wells were blocked with 1% BSA in TBS then washed with wash buffer. Serum samples were diluted in BBS (4 mM barbital, 145 mM NaCl, 2 mM $CaCl_2$, 1 mM $MgCl_2$, pH 7.4), starting at 5%, then added to the plates and incubated for 1.5 hours at 37°C. The plates were washed again, and bound C3b or C4b were detected using rabbit anti-human C3c (Dako) or rabbit anti-human C4c (Dako) followed by HRP conjugated goat anti-rabbit IgG followed by the colorimetric substrate TMB (15).

Complement Inhibition Assay

The activity of HG4 against MASP-2 was tested using C4b deposition assay. 2.5% NHS containing different concentrations of Hg4 in BBS were added to an ELISA plate coated with mannan as previously described. Control wells received no antibodies. The plate was incubated at 37°C for 15 min, then washed. Bound C4b were detected using rabbit anti human C4c (Dako, Denmark) followed by an HRP conjugated goat anti- rabbit IgG (Sigma, USA). Bound antibody was detected using the Colorimetric substrate TMB.

MASP-2 Binding Assay With SARS-CoV-2 Proteins

An ELISA plate was coated with 100 µL of 10 µg/mL SARS-CoV-2 proteins in coating buffer. Wells were blocked with 1% BSA in TBS then washed with wash buffer. Wells coated with BSA only were used as a negative control. Serial concentrations of recombinant MASP-2 in BBS, starting from 1µg/mL, were added to the plate and incubated at room temperature. After 1 hour, the plate was washed and MASP-2 binding to SARS-CoV-2 proteins was detected using monoclonal antibodies against MASP-2 followed by HRP-conjugated rabbit anti-human IgG and the chromogenic substrate ELISA Colorimetric TMB Reagent (Sigma). In a parallel experiment, 1µg of rMASP-2 in 100 µL BBS was incubated with wells coated with SARS-CoV-2 proteins for 1 hour at 37°C. After three washing steps using wash buffer, 2.5 µg of purified C4 (Comptech, USA) in 100 µL BBS were added to each well. Purified C4 added to wells coated with BSA was used as a negative control. After 1-hour incubation at 37°C, supernatants were collected from each well and boiled with 4X SDS loading dye. C4 cleavage mediated *via* MASP-2 was detected using SDS-PAGE and Coomassie bule staining under reducing conditions.

RESULTS

Recognition Molecules of LP Bind to SARS-CoV-2 Proteins

A series of solid-phase binding ELISA were performed to identify LP recognition molecules present in NHS that bind SARS-CoV-2 proteins. MBL, FCN2 and CL-11 bind to S and N proteins, indicating possible activation of the complement system *via* the LP. Interestingly, no C1q binding with SARS-CoV-2 proteins was observed using non-immune NHS, suggesting that the classical pathway is not activated in the absence of specific antibody (**Figure 1**).

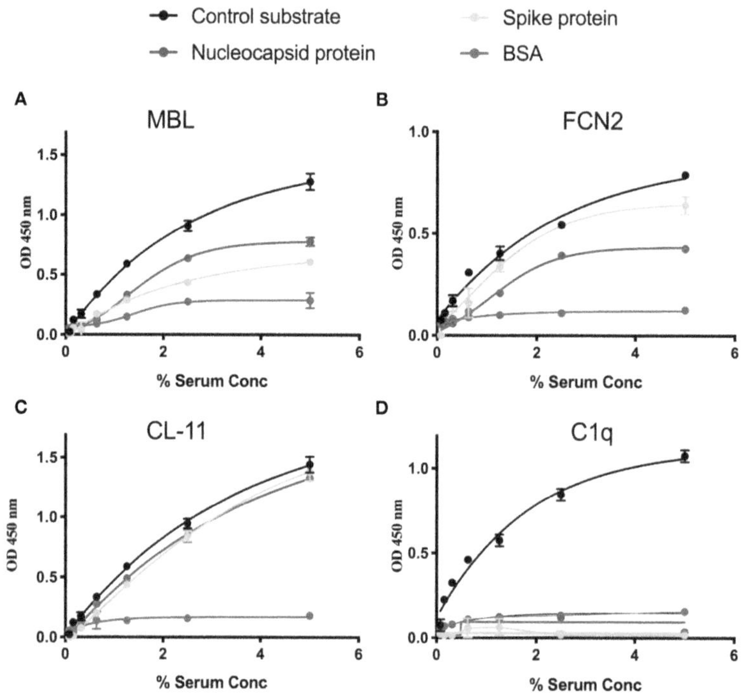

FIGURE 1 | Binding of LP recognition molecules and C1q to SARS-CoV-2 proteins. A microtitre ELISA plate was coated with either S, N or control ligands (mannan for MBL, N-acetyl BSA for FCN2, zymosan for CL-11 or immune complexes for C1q). Following incubation with blocking buffer and washing steps, serial dilutions of NHS, starting at 5% were added to detect binding of LP recognition molecules and C1q from NHS to SARS-CoV-2 proteins. Human MBL **(A)**, FCN2 **(B)**, Cl-11 **(C)** and C1q **(D)** were assayed by ELISA. A significant binding of LP recognition molecules to S and N proteins was clearly observed. No C1q binding to any of the viral proteins was detected. Results are means of duplicates ± SD.

The Lectin Pathway Drives Complement Deposition on SARS-CoV-2

We measured complement C3b and C4b deposition on SARS-CoV-2 proteins immobilised on microtiter plates. When serial dilutions of pre-pandemic NHS were incubated on the plates, there was a dose-dependent and saturable deposition of C3b and C4b, indicative of LP activation, and comparable with the control substrates. Essentially no C3b or C4b deposition was detected on wells that were just blocked with BSA ($p<0.01$, 2-way ANOVA vs. the control) (**Figures 2A, B**).

HG4 Inhibits LP Mediated C4b Deposition

The ability of the fully humanised monoclonal antibody HG4 to inhibit LP functional activity was assessed using a C4b deposition

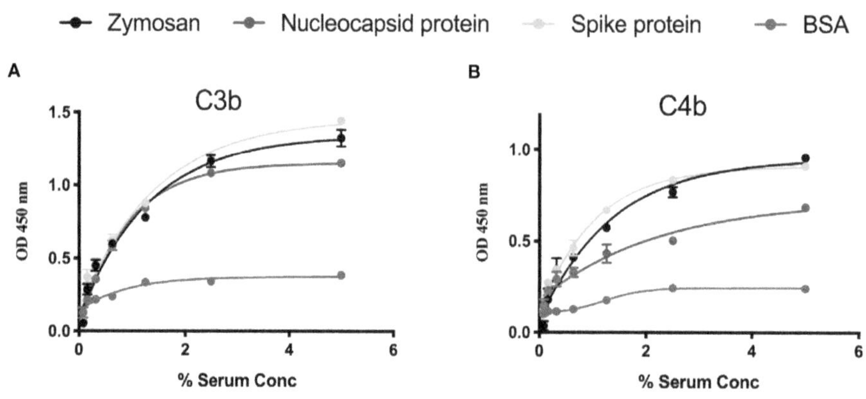

FIGURE 2 | Detection of C3b and C4b deposition on SARS-CoV-2 proteins. An ELISA plate was coated with SARS-CoV-2 proteins (S or N) or zymosan and incubated with serial dilutions of NHS (starting at 5%) for 1 h at 37°C. C3b or C4b deposition were detected using antibodies against human C3c or C4c. High levels of C3b **(A)** and C4b **(B)** deposition were observed on surface immobilised SARS-CoV-2 proteins.

inhibition assay. Our results showing that HG4 significantly inhibits LP functional activity with an IC50 around 0.74 nM (**Figure 3**).

MASP-2 Binds Directly to N Protein and Promotes MASP-2-Mediated C4 Cleavage

The ability of MASP-2 to bind directly to SARS-CoV-2 N protein was tested using ELISA. A significant binding of rMASP-2 to N protein was detected. To further confirm the functional significance of this finding, ELISA wells coated with N-protein or BSA were incubated with 1µg of rMASP-2 for 1 hour at 37°C. After washing, 2.5 µg of purified C4 in BBS was then added to the wells and incubated at 37°C. After 1 hour, the supernatant was removed from the wells and the degree of C4 cleavage was analysed using SDS-PAGE. C4 cleavage was observed when purified C4 was incubated with N protein and rMASP-2 but not with BSA and rMASP-2. This experiment clearly showed that MASP-2 binds to N protein and promotes LP-mediated C4 cleavage. Interestingly, inhibition of MASP-2 activity using HG4 completely blocks LP-mediated C4 cleavage (**Figure 4**).

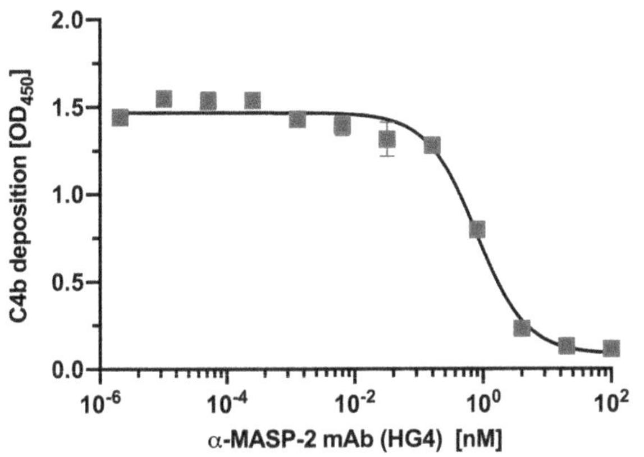

FIGURE 3 | HG4 inhibits lectin pathway mediated C4b deposition. A microtiter ELISA plate was coated with mannan and blocked with BSA. Different concentrations of HG4 antibody were mixed with 2% NHS and incubated on the plate. Bound C4b was detected using anti C4c antibodies.

Evaluation of HEK 293 T Cells Expressing SARS-CoV-2 Surface Proteins as a Model to Detect COVID-19-Related Complement Activation

To analyse complement activation on SARS-CoV-2 S protein using a model that mimics the natural surface expression in cells infected with SARS-CoV-2, we employed transiently transfected HEK 293T cells. In this model, a transient high level of expression of S protein on the surface of HEK 293T cells was achieved after transfection with the mammalian expression vector pEVAC containing the coding sequences for SARS-CoV-2 S protein. Cells expressing viral protein were incubated with NHS or pooled serum from convalescent patients, followed by detection of bound human antibodies by incubation with goat anti-human IgG Alexa fluor 647 antibodies. Fluorescence intensity was measured with The Attune NxT Flow Cytometer (Invitrogen). The level of anti-S protein antibody bound to HEK 293T cells was approximately 100 fold higher when using convalescent human serum compared to non-immune NHS (**Figure 5**). In a parallel experiment, C1q binding to HEK293 cells expressing S protein was not observed when using NHS (data not shown).

Inhibition of LP Impairs Complement C3b Deposition on SARS-CoV-2 Proteins

To evaluate complement C3b deposition on the surface of HEK 293T cells expressing S protein, cells were incubated with 2.5% NHS, and complement C3b deposition was detected using FACS analysis. A significantly higher level of complement C3b deposition was detected on cells expressing S protein compared to non-transfected cells. Inhibition of lectin pathway using HG4

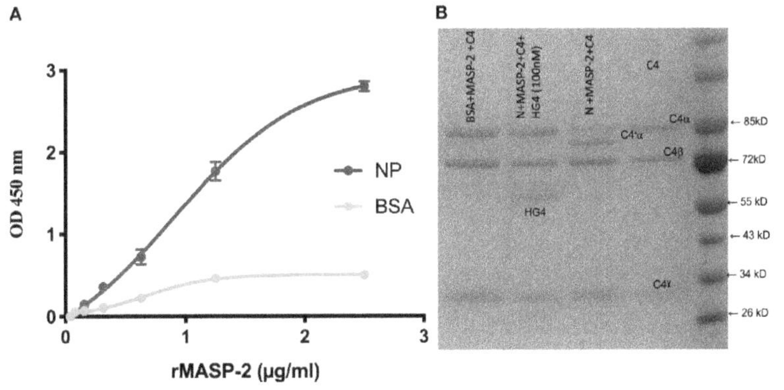

FIGURE 4 | MASP-2 binds directly to SARS-Cov-2 N-protein and mediates complement C4 activation. **(A)** Microtiter plates were coated with 2.5µg/well N-protein or BSA as a control. Residual binding sites were blocked using 1% BSA. Serial dilutions of rMASP-2 were added, and binding was detected using an anti-MASP-2 mAb. MASP-2 bound to the NP protein in a concentration-dependent and saturable manner **(A)**. **(B)** In a parallel experiment, 1µg of rMASP-2 in barbital buffered saline (BBS) was added to wells coated with NP or BSA. After 1 hr at 37°C, wells were washed and 1µg of purified human C4 was added to each well. After 1 hr incubation at 37°C, the supernatant was collected and separated on SDS-PAGE. The results showed that rMASP-2 binds directly to NP and cleaves C4. Addition of HG4 (a mAb that inhibits MASP-2) inhibited MASP-2 mediated C4 cleavage. Purified C4 was run on the gel as a control.

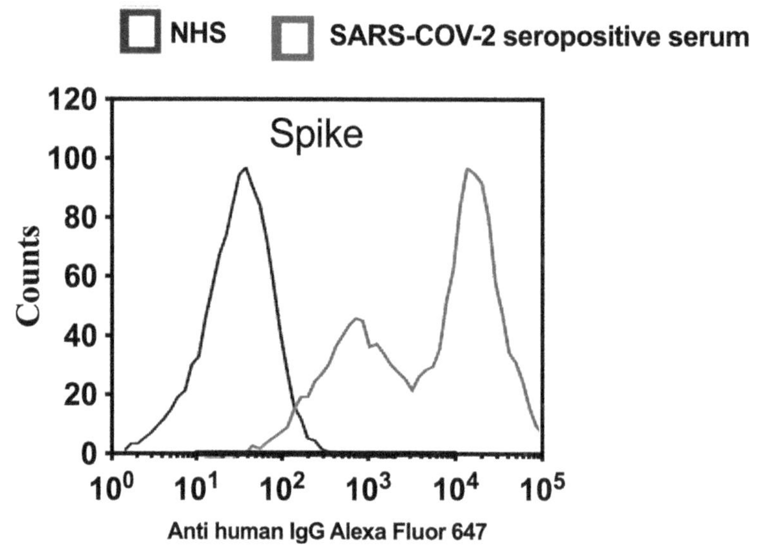

FIGURE 5 | Transfection of HEK 293T promotes high levels of expression of SARS-CoV-2 surface proteins. The expression levels of S protein on the surface of HEK 293 T cells were measured using serum from convalescent SARS-CoV-2 PCR positive patients or NHS (PCR negative) followed by anti-human IgG Alexa fluor 647 antibodies. Significant high levels of IgG binds to S were observed on the surface of HEK T293 cells.

significantly decreased complement C3b deposition from NHS (**Figure 6**).

DISCUSSION

SARS-CoV-2 is an emerging virus with a very high infectivity that causes life-threatening complications with mild to severe long-term morbidity and mortality, especially in patients with underlying medical conditions (16). The immunopathology differentiating mild from severe disease is not as yet sufficiently well understood to identify the windows of therapeutic opportunities for treatment (13, 17, 18). Excessive activation of complement, initiated in part by viral invasion of endothelial cells, causes collateral tissue injury (12). This work demonstrates that the LP recognition molecules MBL, FCN-2 and CL-11 bind to S

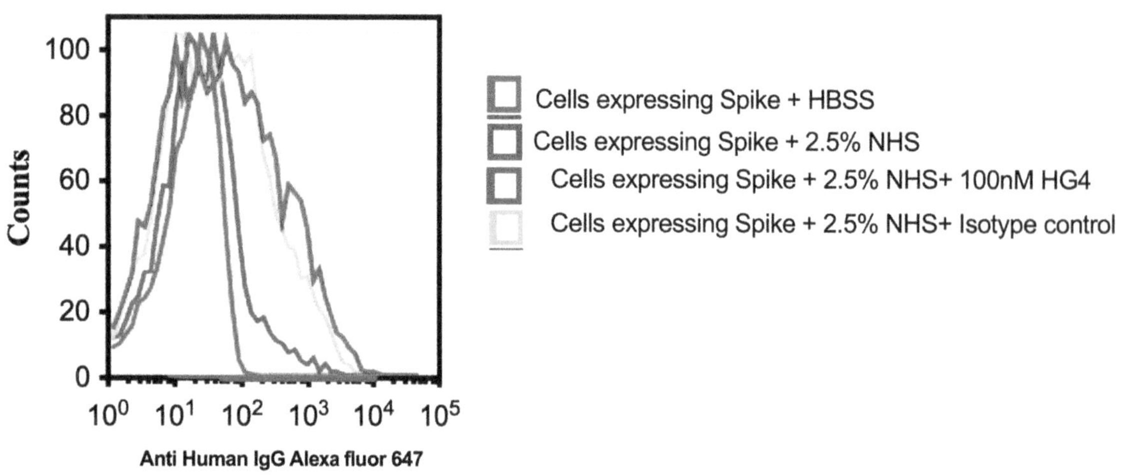

FIGURE 6 | Inhibition of LP impairs complement C3b deposition on SARS-CoV-2 surface proteins. HEK 293T cells expressing SARS-CoV-2 S protein were used. Cells were incubated with 2.5% NHS with 100nM HG4 or an isotype control antibody at 37C for 30 min. Cells were washed and C3b deposition was detected using rabbit anti human C3b followed by goat anti rabbit FITC labelled antibodies. A significant C3b deposition was detected on HEK 293T cells expressing S protein. Inhibition of MASP-2 using HG4 significantly impairs complement C3b deposition on the surface of HEK 293T cells expressing S protein.

and N proteins of SARS-CoV-2 with subsequent activation of LP-mediated C3b and C4b deposition. These findings clearly show the activation of the LP on SARS-CoV-2 surface proteins and N protein, confirming the central role of LP activation in the immunopathogenesis of COVID-19. Tissue damage consistent with complement-mediated microvascular injury has been observed in the lung and/or skin of patients with severe COVID-19, with significant deposition of the LP effector enzyme MASP-2, a hallmark of profound activation of the LP (14). Furthermore, extensive deposition of MASP-2 in the capillaries and venules of small bowel thrombotic microvascular injury in COVID-19 has also been reported, and endothelial complement staining patterns colocalized with staining of SARS-CoV-2 membrane and spike proteins (19). Our work also shows direct binding of MASP-2 to the N protein of SARS-CoV-2 with subsequent LP-mediated C4 cleavage into C4b and C4a, confirming the previous finding of Gao et al., who reported direct activation of MASP-2 on the SARS-CoV-2 N protein and showed that MASP-2-deficient mice are protected from disease (20). Since we used a truncated zymogen form of MASP-2, containing the CCP1, CCP2 and serine protease domains, our results also narrow down the N-protein binding site to these C terminal domains. Our *in vitro* study confirms that inhibition of MASP-2 blocks complement activation *via* the LP. Interestingly, Narsoplimab, a fully humanized immunoglobulin gamma 4 (IgG4) monoclonal antibody against MASP-2 that inhibits LP functional activity, has been used successfully in treatment of critically ill, mechanical ventilation-dependent COVID-19 patients. Patients who received Narsoplimab recovered and survived, demonstrating corresponding improvement/normalization of laboratory markers of inflammation (21). Many other complement inhibitors and anti-inflammatory drugs have been re-purposed and evaluated in COVID-19 clinical trials but, to date, none of those other agents have yielded a breakthrough in the treatment of severe COVID-19 (22–27). While vaccination is reducing hospitalisation, there is a fear of possible reduction in the efficacy against the new variants, which are responsible for severe cases of COVID-19 in younger age groups. Therapeutic approaches utilizing passive immunity (e.g., convalescent plasma, mono- and polyclonal antibodies), have also been disappointing, demonstrating no meaningful efficacy in severe COVID-19 and, possibly, adding to selection pressure on SARS-CoV-2. There remains a need to pursue aggressively and apply therapeutic strategies that block the COVID-19 immunopathological events and endothelial pathology, all of which appear to remain consistent across viral variants, with the objective of increasing access to any effective treatment(s) for acute as well as long-term post-COVID pathology. As an alternative to tackling the virus itself, protection from emerging new mutant viral strains could be achieved by tackling the immune physiological events that turn SARS-CoV-2 infections into generalised endothelial disease and ARDS in those susceptible to moderate-to-severe COVID-19. More research is needed to fully understand the disease processes triggered by SARS-CoV-2 at a molecular level.

The present study provides new insights into the direct triggers by SARS-CoV-2 at the protein level of LP activation in the early phase of COVID-19, and the role of the LP in types of long-haul COVID-19 are currently under investigation.

AUTHOR CONTRIBUTIONS

YA and MF designed and performed the experiments. YA, MF, NL, JH, and WS wrote and revised the manuscript. SY, TD, SG, and GD provided essential reagents and revised the manuscript. All authors contributed to the article and approved the submitted version.

FUNDING

This work was supported by National Institute for Health Research Grant G107217, awarded to WS.

REFERENCES

1. Astuti I, Ysrafil. Severe Acute Respiratory Syndrome Coronavirus 2 (SARS-CoV-2): An Overview of Viral Structure and Host Response. *Diabetes Metab Syndr* (2020) 14:407–12. doi: 10.1016/j.dsx.2020.04.020
2. Elharrar X, Tr Y, Dols AM, Touchon F, Martinez S, Prud'homme E, et al. Use of Prone Positioning in Nonintubated Patients With COVID-19 and Hypoxemic Acute Respiratory Failure. *JAMA* (2020) 323:2336–8. doi: 10.1001/jama.2020.8255
3. Hirsch JS, Ng JH, Ross DW, Sharma P, Shah HH, Barnett RL, et al. Acute Kidney Injury in Patients Hospitalized With COVID-19. *Kidney Int* (2020) 98:209–18. doi: 10.1016/j.kint.2020.05.006
4. Almitairi JOM, Venkatraman Girija U, Furze CM, Simpson-Gray X, Badakshi F, Marshall JE, et al. Structure of the C1r-C1s Interaction of the C1 Complex of Complement Activation. *Proc Natl Acad Sci USA* (2018) 115:768–73. doi: 10.1073/pnas.1718709115
5. Schwaeble W, Dahl MR, Thiel S, Stover C, Jensenius JC. The Mannan-Binding Lectin-Associated Serine Proteases (MASPs) and MAp19: Four Components of the Lectin Pathway Activation Complex Encoded by Two Genes. *Immunobiology* (2002) 205:455–66. doi: 10.1078/0171-2985-00146
6. Fujita T. Evolution of the Lectin-Complement Pathway and its Role in Innate Immunity. *Nat Rev Immunol* (2002) 2:346–53. doi: 10.1038/nri800
7. Iwaki D, Fujita T. Production and Purification of Recombinants of Mouse MASP-2 and sMAP. *J Endotoxin Res* (2005) 11:47–50. doi: 10.1179/096805105225006704
8. Skjoedt MO, Hummelshoj T, Palarasah Y, Honore C, Koch C, Skjodt K, et al. A Novel Mannose-Binding Lectin/Ficolin-Associated Protein is Highly Expressed in Heart and Skeletal Muscle Tissues and Inhibits Complement Activation. *J Biol Chem* (2010) 285:8234–43. doi: 10.1074/jbc.M109.065805
9. Yaseen S, Demopulos G, Dudler T, Yabuki M, Wood CL, Cummings WJ, et al. Lectin Pathway Effector Enzyme Mannan-Binding Lectin-Associated Serine Protease-2 can Activate Native Complement C3 in Absence of C4 and/or C2. *FASEB J* (2017) 31:2210–9. doi: 10.1096/fj.201601306R
10. Lachmann PJ. The Amplification Loop of the Complement Pathways. *Adv Immunol* (2009) 104:115–49. doi: 10.1016/S0065-2776(08)04004-2

11. de Nooijer AH, Grondman I, Janssen NAF, Netea MG, Willems L, van de Veerdonk FL, et al. Complement Activation in the Disease Course of Coronavirus Disease 2019 and Its Effects on Clinical Outcomes. *J Infect Dis* (2021) 223:214–24. doi: 10.1093/infdis/jiaa646
12. Holter JC, Pischke SE, de Boer E, Lind A, Jenum S, Holten AR, et al. Systemic Complement Activation is Associated With Respiratory Failure in COVID-19 Hospitalized Patients. *Proc Natl Acad Sci USA* (2020) 117:25018–25. doi: 10.1073/pnas.2010540117
13. Gralinski LE, Sheahan TP, Morrison TE, Menachery VD, Jensen K, Leist SR, et al. Complement Activation Contributes to Severe Acute Respiratory Syndrome Coronavirus Pathogenesis. *mBio* (2018) 9:e01753–18. doi: 10.1128/mBio.01753-18
14. Magro C, Mulvey JJ, Berlin D, Nuovo G, Salvatore S, Harp J, et al. Complement Associated Microvascular Injury and Thrombosis in the Pathogenesis of Severe COVID-19 Infection: A Report of Five Cases. *Transl Res* (2020) 220:1–13. doi: 10.1016/j.trsl.2020.04.007
15. Ali YM, Sim RB, Schwaeble W, Shaaban MI. Enterococcus Faecalis Escapes Complement-Mediated Killing *via* Recruitment of Complement Factor H. *J Infect Dis* (2019) 220:1061–70. doi: 10.1016/j.immuni.2020.05.002
16. Vabret N, Britton GJ, Gruber C, Hegde S, Kim J, Kuksin M, et al. Immunology of COVID-19: Current State of the Science. *Immunity* (2020) 52:910–41. doi: S1074-7613(20)30183-7
17. Java A, Apicelli AJ, Liszewski MK, Coler-Reilly A, Atkinson JP, Kim AH, et al. The Complement System in COVID-19: Friend and Foe? *JCI Insight* (2020) 5:10.1172/jci.insight.140711. doi: 10.1172/jci.insight.140711
18. Risitano AM, Mastellos DC, Huber-Lang M, Yancopoulou D, Garlanda C, Ciceri F, et al. Complement as a Target in COVID-19? *Nat Rev Immunol* (2020) 20:343–4. doi: 10.1038/s41577-020-0320-7
19. Plotz B, Castillo R, Melamed J, Magro C, Rosenthal P, Belmont HM. Focal Small Bowel Thrombotic Microvascular Injury in COVID-19 Mediated by the Lectin Complement Pathway Masquerading as Lupus Enteritis. *Rheumatol (Oxford)* (2021) 60:e61–3. doi: 10.1093/rheumatology/keaa627
20. Ting G, Mingdong H, Xiaopeng Z, Hongzhen L, Lin Z, Hainan L, et al. Highly Pathogenic Coronavirus N Protein Aggravates Lung Injury by MASP-2-Mediated Complement Over-Activation. *medRxiv* [Preprint] (2020). doi: 10.1101/2020.03.29.20041962
21. Rambaldi A, Gritti G, Mico MC, Frigeni M, Borleri G, Salvi A, et al. Endothelial Injury and Thrombotic Microangiopathy in COVID-19: Treatment With the Lectin-Pathway Inhibitor Narsoplimab. *Immunobiology* (2020) 225:152001. doi: 10.1016/j.imbio.2020.152001
22. Della-Torre E, Della-Torre F, Kusanovic M, Scotti R, Ramirez GA, Dagna L, et al. Treating COVID-19 With Colchicine in Community Healthcare Setting. *Clin Immunol* (2020) 217:108490. doi: 10.1016/j.clim.2020.108490
23. Diurno F, Numis FG, Porta G, Cirillo F, Maddaluno S, Ragozzino A, et al. Eculizumab Treatment in Patients With COVID-19: Preliminary Results From Real Life ASL Napoli 2 Nord Experience. *Eur Rev Med Pharmacol Sci* (2020) 24:4040–7. doi: 10.26355/eurrev_202004_20875
24. Ho TC, Wang YH, Chen YL, Tsai WC, Lee CH, Chuang KP, et al. Chloroquine and Hydroxychloroquine: Efficacy in the Treatment of the COVID-19. *Pathogens* (2021) 10:217. doi: 10.3390/pathogens10020217
25. Jean SS, Hsueh PR. Old and Re-Purposed Drugs for the Treatment of COVID-19. *Expert Rev Anti Infect Ther* (2020) 18:843–7. doi: 10.1080/14787210.2020.1771181
26. Mastaglio S, Ruggeri A, Risitano AM, Angelillo P, Yancopoulou D, Mastellos DC, et al. The First Case of COVID-19 Treated With the Complement C3 Inhibitor AMY-101. *Clin Immunol* (2020) 215:108450. doi: 10.1016/j.clim.2020.108450
27. Mastellos DC, Pires da Silva BGP, Fonseca BAL, Fonseca NP, Auxiliadora-Martins M, Mastaglio S, et al. Complement C3 vs C5 Inhibition in Severe COVID-19: Early Clinical Findings Reveal Differential Biological Efficacy. *Clin Immunol* (2020) 220:108598. doi: 10.1016/j.clim.2020.108598

17

CR4 Signaling Contributes to a DC-Driven Enhanced Immune Response Against Complement-Opsonized HIV-1

Marta Bermejo-Jambrina[1,2], Michael Blatzer[3], Paula Jauregui-Onieva[1], Teodor E. Yordanov[4], Paul Hörtnagl[5], Taras Valovka[4,6], Lukas A. Huber[4], Doris Wilflingseder[1] and Wilfried Posch[1]**

[1] Institute of Hygiene and Medical Microbiology, Medical University of Innsbruck, Innsbruck, Austria, [2] Department of Experimental Immunology, Amsterdam Infection and Immunity Institute, Academic Medical Center, University of Amsterdam, Amsterdam, Netherlands, [3] Experimental Neuropathology Unit, Infection and Epidemiology Department, Institute Pasteur, Paris, France, [4] Institute of Cell Biology, Biocenter, Medical University of Innsbruck, Innsbruck, Austria, [5] Central Institute for Blood Transfusion and Immunological Department, Innsbruck, Austria, [6] Department of Pediatrics I, Medical University of Innsbruck, Innsbruck, Austria

***Correspondence:**
Doris Wilflingseder
doris.wilflingseder@i-med.ac.at
Wilfried Posch
wilfried.posch@i-med.ac.at

Dendritic cells (DCs) possess intrinsic cellular defense mechanisms to specifically inhibit HIV-1 replication. In turn, HIV-1 has evolved strategies to evade innate immune sensing by DCs resulting in suboptimal maturation and poor antiviral immune responses. We previously showed that complement-opsonized HIV-1 (HIV-C) was able to efficiently infect various DC subsets significantly higher than non-opsonized HIV-1 (HIV) and therefore also mediate a higher antiviral immunity. Thus, complement coating of HIV-1 might play a role with respect to viral control occurring early during infection via modulation of DCs. To determine in detail which complement receptors (CRs) expressed on DCs was responsible for infection and superior pro-inflammatory and antiviral effects, we generated stable deletion mutants for the α-chains of CR3, CD11b, and CR4, CD11c using CRISPR/Cas9 in THP1-derived DCs. We found that CD11c deletion resulted in impaired DC infection as well as antiviral and pro-inflammatory immunity upon exposure to complement-coated HIV-1. In contrast, sole expression of CD11b on DCs shifted the cells to an anti-inflammatory, regulatory DC type. We here illustrated that CR4 comprised of CD11c and CD18 is the major player with respect to DC infection associated with a potent early pro-inflammatory immune response. A more detailed characterization of CR3 and CR4 functions using our powerful tool might open novel avenues for early therapeutic intervention during HIV-1 infection.

Keywords: HIV-1, dendritic cell, complement, CD11c, CD11b

INTRODUCTION

Dendritic cells (DCs) play a pivotal role in the defense against invading pathogens, acting as the most potent antigen-presenting cells (APCs) of the innate immune system (1–3). They reside in the peripheral tissue, where they capture antigens and present them to naïve T cells in the lymph nodes. Hence, DCs orchestrate immune responses, serving as critical links between innate and adaptive immunity. DCs are among the first cells to encounter HIV-1 at mucosal sites (2, 4). At the same time, HIV-1 spontaneously activates the classical complement (C-) pathway (5), even in seminal fluid (6), through direct binding of C1q to the viral surface. Therefore, complement-opsonized HIV-1 (HIV-C) accumulates at mucosal sites early during HIV-1 infection (7, 8). HIV-1 poorly replicates in DCs due to the activity of SAMHD1 [Sterile Alpha Motif (SAM) domain and histidine/aspartic acid (HD) domain containing protein 1] and effectively evades DC-mediated antiviral immunity (9). When SAMHD1 restriction of HIV-1 was abrogated by degradation of HIV-2/SIVsm viral protein Vpx, DCs demonstrated a potent type I IFN response, maturation and co-stimulatory function (10). Further, phosphorylation of the T592 residue of SAMHD1 in DCs after exposure to HIV-C overcame this restriction mechanism and initiated an effective antiviral immune response (9). The low-Beside hiding from DC-mediated immunity by low-level infection, the virus additionally exploits DCs as shuttles to promote its own dissemination (11, 12).

In previous studies we demonstrated that HIV-C has the ability to bypass SAMHD1 restriction in DCs, which resulted in more pronounced maturation and significantly higher co-stimulatory capacity compared to DCs exposed to non-opsonized HIV (9).

Additionally, complement coating of HIV-1 further activated highly functional HIV-1 specific cellular immunity as well as pro-inflammatory and type I IFN responses (9, 13, 14). Thus, enhanced DC infection was associated with an increased quality and quantity of virus-specific immune responses (9, 10, 15, 16). We could also show that HIV-C interacts with the abundantly expressed CR3 and CR4 on immature DCs (iDCs), whereas non-opsonized HIV binds via gp120 to DC-SIGN (9, 17). Taken together, these already published results clearly indicate that triggering CR3 and CR4 by HIV-C influences infection of DCs and strongly shapes immunity driven by DCs.

Here, we analyzed in detail the specific roles of CR3 and CR4 in modulating the immune response of HIV-1-infected DCs by generating knock-out (KO) cell lines lacking CD11b, CD11c, and CD18, respectively. For this we performed CRISPR/Cas9 to generate stable and irreversible deletions of these receptors in THP1 monocytes. Furthermore, we optimized the differentiation protocol to generate THP1 derived DCs and to use these THP1-differentiated DCs (THP1-DCs), comprising an iDC phenotype, as an operative model for primary DC infection. After detailed comparison of THP1-DCs with primary DCs at phenotypic and phagocytic properties, we characterized the specific tasks of CR3 and CR4 on THP1-KO DCs with respect to HIV-1 infection and antiviral immune induction using differentially opsonized HIV-1. Here we identified CR4 as potent inducer of early antiviral immunity. Further, the importance of CR3 and CR4 fine-tuning on DCs with respect to controlling viremia during the acute phase of HIV-1 infection by CR4 or down-modulating type I IFNs during chronic phase by CR3 was highlighted.

MATERIALS AND METHODS

Ethics Statement

Written informed consent was obtained from all participating blood donors by the Central Institute for Blood Transfusion and Immunological Department, Innsbruck, Austria. The use of anonymized leftover specimens for research on host/pathogen interactions was approved by the Ethics Committee of the Medical University of Innsbruck (ECS 1166/2018, PI: DW).

Generation of Human Monocyte-Derived DCs and THP1-DCs

Blood for the monocyte isolation was received by the Central Institute for Blood Transfusion and Immunological Department, Innsbruck, Austria. Briefly, PBMCs (peripheral blood mononuclear cells) were isolated from blood of healthy donors (8, 16) obtained by a density gradient centrifugation using a Ficoll Paque Premium (GE Healthcare) gradient. After washing, $CD14^+$ monocytes were isolated from PBMCs using anti-human CD14 Magnetic Beads (BD) – the purity of the isolated cells was at least 98%. Monocytes were stimulated by addition of IL-4 (200 U/ml) and GM-CSF (300 U/ml) for 5 days to generate iDCs, which were used for all further experiments. Non-stimulated iDCs were used as controls for all experiments using DCs. THP1-WT and KO DCs were generated from the respective THP1 cells by addition of IL-4 (200 U/ml), GM-CSF (300 U/ml) and TNF-α (10 ng/ml) for 5 days.

Genome Editing Using CRISPR/Cas9-Mediated Depletion of CD11b, CD11c, and CD18

For CRISPR/Cas9-mediated depletion, three guide RNA (gRNA) targeting sequences for CD11b, CD11c, and CD18 as depicted in **Table 1** were selected using an online prediction tool—CRISPR Design; Zhang Lab (18). Out of the three constructs, only one clone for each target [CD11b (5′-GCCGTAGGTTGGATCCAAACAGG-3′), CD11c (5′-GTAGAGGCCACCCGTTTGGTTGG-3′) and CD18 (5′-TGGCCGGTGTCGCSGCGSSTGG-3′)] was used for further analyses. gRNAs were cloned into a lentiCRISPRv2 vector via *Bsm*BI restriction sites. lentiCRISPRv2 was a gift from F. Zhang (Massachusetts Institute of Technology, Cambridge, MA, United States; Addgene plasmid 52961 (19).

Lentiviral Transduction

Lentiviral plasmids were co-transfected with Lipofectamine LTX (Invitrogen, cat 15338100) together with pMDG, psPAX2 and lentiCRISPRv2 into the HEK293T producer cell line. Supernatants containing viral particles were harvested 48 and 72 h post transfection, filtered using a 0.2 μm filter and directly used to transduce target THP1 cells with 5 μg/ml Polybrene (Sigma-Aldrich, cat TR-1003-G). After 7 days, transduced cells were selected using puromycin (5 μg/ml, Sigma-Aldrich, cat SBR00017). After selection, the depletion efficiency of CD11b, CD11c, and CD18 was analyzed by flow cytometry. Single-cell clones of the specific KO cells were generated after FACS

TABLE 1 | CRISPR/Cas9 gRNA sequences used to produces the THP-1 CD11b KO, THP-1 CD11c KO, and THP-1 CD18 KO.

Number	Target gene	Sequence
1	CD11b exon5	GCCGTAGGTTGGATCCAAACAGG
2	CD11b exon6	TCATCCGCCGAAAGTCATGTGGG
3	CD11b exon6	TTCATCCGCCGAAAGTCATGTGG
4	CD11c exon3	GTAGAGGCCACCCGTTTGGTTGG
5	CD11c exon3	ACTGGTAGAGGCCACCCGTTTGG
6	CD11c exon4	GACATGTTCACGGCCTCCGGGGG
7	CD18 exon3	GCCGGGAATGCATCGAGTCGGGG
8	CD18 exon3	TGCCGGGAATGCATCGAGTCGGG
9	CD18 exon4	TGGCCGGGTGTCGCAGCGAATGG

Indicated sequences target different exons of the CD11b, CD11c, and CD18 genes. One clone out of the three was used for further analyses.

sorting by the Core Facility FACS Sorting at the Medical University of Innsbruck.

Virus Production

Primary isolates as 92BR030 (subtype B/B, R5-tropic) and the laboratory strain BaL were obtained by the National Institutes of Health AIDS (available through World Health Organization depositories). Virus was propagated in PHA-L and IL-2 stimulated PBMCs. 93BR020 (subtype B/F, X4/R5-tropic) and the laboratory strain NL43 both from National Institutes of Health AIDS (available through World Health Organization depositories) were produced in the M8166 cell line. HEK293T cells were transfected with YU- 2-, and R9Bal (kindly provided by Prof. Thomas Hope, Northwestern University) plasmids using the $CaCl_2$ method (9). Vpx expression construct pcDNA3.1Vpx SIVmac239-Myc was used to obtain Vpx-carrying HIV virus preparations (20). Viral supernatants were collected on several days post infection (dpi) and cleared by filtration through 0.22 μm pore-size filters and concentrated by ultracentrifugation at 20,000 rpm for 90 min at 4°C (Beckham Coulter). The virus pellet was re-suspended in RPMI1640 without supplements and stored in small aliquots at −80°C to avoid multiple thawing. One aliquot was taken to determine the virus concentration by p24 ELISA (21) and the 50% tissue culture infective dose of the viral stock.

Opsonization of Viral Stocks

To mimic opsonization *in vitro*, purified HIV-1 and VLP stocks were incubated for 1 h at 37°C with human complement (C) serum (Quidel) in a 1:10 dilution. As negative control the virus was incubated under the same conditions in commercially available C3-deficient serum (Sigma) or in culture medium. After opsonization, the virus was thoroughly washed to remove unbound components, pelleted by ultracentrifugation (20,000 rpm/90 min/4°C), re-suspended in culture medium without supplements and virus concentrations were determined using p24 ELISA. The opsonization pattern was analyzed using a virus capture assay (VCA) described below.

Virus Capture Assay

The opsonization pattern was determined by virus capture assay (VCA) as described (8). Briefly, 96-well high-binding plates were coated with anti-human C3c, C3d, or IgG antibodies. Mouse IgG antibody was used as a control for background binding. Plates were then incubated overnight at 4°C with the differentially opsonized virus preparations (10 ng p24/well) at 4°C. After extensive washing, virus was lysed and p24 ELISA was performed to confirm the opsonization pattern.

p24 ELISA

p24 ELISA was performed as described (21). Antibodies used for p24 ELISA were kindly provided by Polymun Scientific, Vienna, Austria.

DC Infection

Cells were infected in triplicates using differentially opsonized HIV-1 as described before (8, 17). Briefly, cells (1×10^5/100 μl) were incubated for 3 h with HIV or HIV-C (25 ng p24/ml) or left uninfected and virus concentrations from supernatants were measured on several dpi. To confirm productive infection by HIV-1 and not cell-associated virus, we thoroughly washed the cells after overnight incubation with different viruses and cultured the cells at 37°C/5% CO_2. By ELISA we measured the p24 concentrations of the supernatants following spinning down the plate to pellet cells on several dpi. The following antibodies were used for blocking experiments (all anti-human): LEAF purified CD11b-Antibody (Biolegend, San Diego, CA, United States), LEAF purified CD11c-Antibody (Biolegend, San Diego, CA, Untied States).

Immunoblot Analyses of Phosphorylated Proteins

THP1-DCs were starved in RPMI 1640 containing 0.5% FCS and 1% L-Glutamine for 3 h. Starving of cells was performed to set their phosphorylation to background levels. Following starvation, THP1-DCs were incubated with the differentially opsonized HIV-1 particles. After 4 h co-incubation, cells were lysed with RIPA Buffer (Sigma-Aldrich) containing protease and phosphates inhibitors and EDTA (Thermo Fisher Scientific) for 20 min at 4°C. The protein content was determined by BCA (Thermo Fisher Scientific). Lysates were separated using 10% SDS-PAGE gels, transferred to PVDF membranes and incubated with anti-human a-tubulin as loading control as well as anti-human phospho-IRF3 (1:1000, Cell Signaling Technology) and developed with the Lass 4000 Image Quant. For this, the peak values of the target protein were divided by the peak values of the loading control before doing a relative comparison. Quantification was performed using values from three to six different experiments.

Relative Quantification by Real-Time RT-PCR

THP1-DCs (WT and KOs) were infected with the differentially opsonized HIV-1 particles at different time-points from 1–12 h at 37°C with a p24 concentration of 350 ng/mL for

0.5 × 10^6 cells. Cells were lysed with RLT Buffer (Qiagen) and total RNA was purified according to the manufacturer's instructions. RNA was then quantified (NanoVue) and reverse transcribed into cDNA (iScript Reverse Transcription Supermix for RT-qPCR, BioRad). The cDNA was then used for multiplex qPCR (iQ Multiplex Powermix, BioRad) amplification, using PrimePCR^{TM} Probes for IL-10, IL-6, IL-1B, and IL23A (all from BioRad Laboratories). The RT-qPCR was run in the BioRad CFX96 Real Time PCR System. The cycling conditions were as follows: 3 min at 95°C, 44 cycles: 15 s at 95°C, 60 s at 60°C. For mRNA expression of IFNB1 real-time PCR using Sybr green qPCR (EvaGreen, BioRad) amplification and gene-specific primer pairs (BioRad) were used. The cycling conditions were: 30 s at 95°C, 39 cycles: 5 s at 95°C, 10 s at 60°C with a melt curve 65–95°C with an increment of 0.5°C for 5 s. A GAPDH (human) PCR using specific primer/probe pairs (BioRad) served as internal control to quantify the relative gene expression of target genes. Data were analyzed with the BioRad CFX Manager Software ($\Delta\Delta$CT method) and values were exported to GraphPad Prism.

Cytokine Analyses by ELISA

THP1-DCs were plated in a 12-well tissue culture-plate at 0.5 × 10^6 cells/well. Cells were infected with R5-tropic virus (R9Bal) for 12, 24, and 48 h. Supernatants were collected and inactivated with Igepal 5% (1:2). The amounts of IL-1β were measured by ELISA (eBioscience).

Multicolor FACS Analyses

Differentiation of THP1 into DCs exposed to cytokine cocktail (IL-4, GM-CSF, TNF-α) was analyzed by using anti-human CD11b-PE, CD11c-AlexaFluor488, CD18-APC, HLA-ABC-PerCP/Cy5.5, HLA-DR-APC-Cy7, DC-SIGN-PE, CD86-FITC, CD83-APC, CD1a-FITC, CD4-APC, CCR-PerCP/Cy5.5 and CXCR4-PE as described (16) on a FACS Verse flow cytometer (BD Biosciences). Data were analyzed using FACS DIVA software (BD Biosciences).

Statistical Analysis

Differences were analyzed by using GraphPad Prism software (GraphPad Software Inc.) and one-way ANOVA with Bonferroni post-test for multiple comparisons or Unpaired Student's t test depending on the analyses performed.

RESULTS

WT THP1-DCs and KO THP1-DCs Resemble Primary DCs Regarding Their Phenotypic and Phagocytic Capacities

To characterize CR3 and CR4 with respect to DC modulation upon exposure to differentially opsonized HIV-1, we generated CD11b-, CD11c-, and CD18 KO THP1-DCs. Since THP1 monocytes constitute an immortalized cell line and are of tumorigenic origin derived from the peripheral blood of a one-year-old male with acute monocytic leukemia, we wanted to make sure to generate an appropriate model for KO DCs. Therefore, we first characterized by multi-parameter flow cytometric analyses in detail WT-THP1 cells after optimized differentiation to DCs for their expression of characteristic DC markers, CR3 and CR4 and HIV-1 receptor and co-receptors CD4, CCR5, and CXCR4.

We found that THP1-DCs differentiated *in vitro* into a functional DC-like phenotype (**Figure 1A** and **Supplementary Figure S1** >monocyte-derived iDCs, moDCs), expressing high levels of both CRs, CR3, and CR4, as analyzed by the expression of CD11b, CD11c, and CD18. HLA-ABC, HLA-DR, and DC-SIGN were also found to be expressed on WT-THP1 DCs, and also on moDCs as illustrated by Posch et al. (9) and in **Supplementary Figure S1**. No expression of CD1a was detected. Importantly, low levels of CD83 and CD86 were indicative of an iDC state and displayed a mature phenotype upon LPS stimulation (not shown). The profile of characteristic markers CD11b, CD11c, CD18, DC-SIGN, CD83, CD86, CD4, CXCR4, and HLA-DR on immature moDCs is illustrated in **Supplementary Figure S1**. Entry of HIV-1 into target cells requires formation of a complex between the viral envelope protein gp120, the primary receptor CD4 and a chemokine co-receptor (CCR5, CXCR4). We found that THP1-DCs expressed similar amounts of CD4, CCR5, and CXCR4 as primary DCs.

THP1-DCs further illustrated a similar phagocytic capacity as their primary counterparts (**Figure 1B**). Phagocytosis of non- and complement-opsonized beads (Beads, Beads-C) was low in THP1 monocytes, while WT THP1-DCs demonstrated a similar phagocytosis of Beads/Beads-C compared to monocyte-derived DCs.

Next we investigated the expression of CD11b, CD11c, and CD18 on KO THP1-DCs generated by CRISPR-Cas9 technology. CD11b expression on single-cell clones of CD11b KO THP1-DCs was reduced to 0.81% compared to 63.43% on WT THP1-DCs (**Figure 2A**). CD11c was only slightly affected on CD11b KO THP1-DCs (**Supplementary Figure S2**). Expression of CD11c on CD11c KO THP1-DCs was also reduced from 50.53% on WT THP1-DCs to 0.81% (**Figure 2A**), while CD11b was expressed on CD11c KO THP1-DCs (**Supplementary Figure S2**). In contrast, CD18 KO resulted in significant down-modulation of CD11b as well as CD11c (**Supplementary Figure S2**) and in addition, also CD11a disappeared from the surface of CD18 KO THP1-DCs, but not on CD11b- and CD11c KO THP1-DCs (**Supplementary Figure S3**). Phagocytosis of the various KO THP1-DCs revealed that in CD11b KO cells the levels of Beads or Beads-C internalized slightly decreased compared to WT THP1-DCs (**Figure 2B**), while CD11c KO had a highly decreased phagocytosis of Beads-C, but not Beads (**Figure 2B**). KO CD18 severely reduced the amounts of Beads ingested and completely abrogated internalization of Beads-C (**Figure 2B**). We further focused on CD11b- and CD11c KO THP1-DCs throughout the manuscript and CD18 KO-THP1 DCs were used in some experiments as controls. Phenotypic and phagocytic characterization of WT and KO THP1-DCs revealed these cells as a good DC model to study

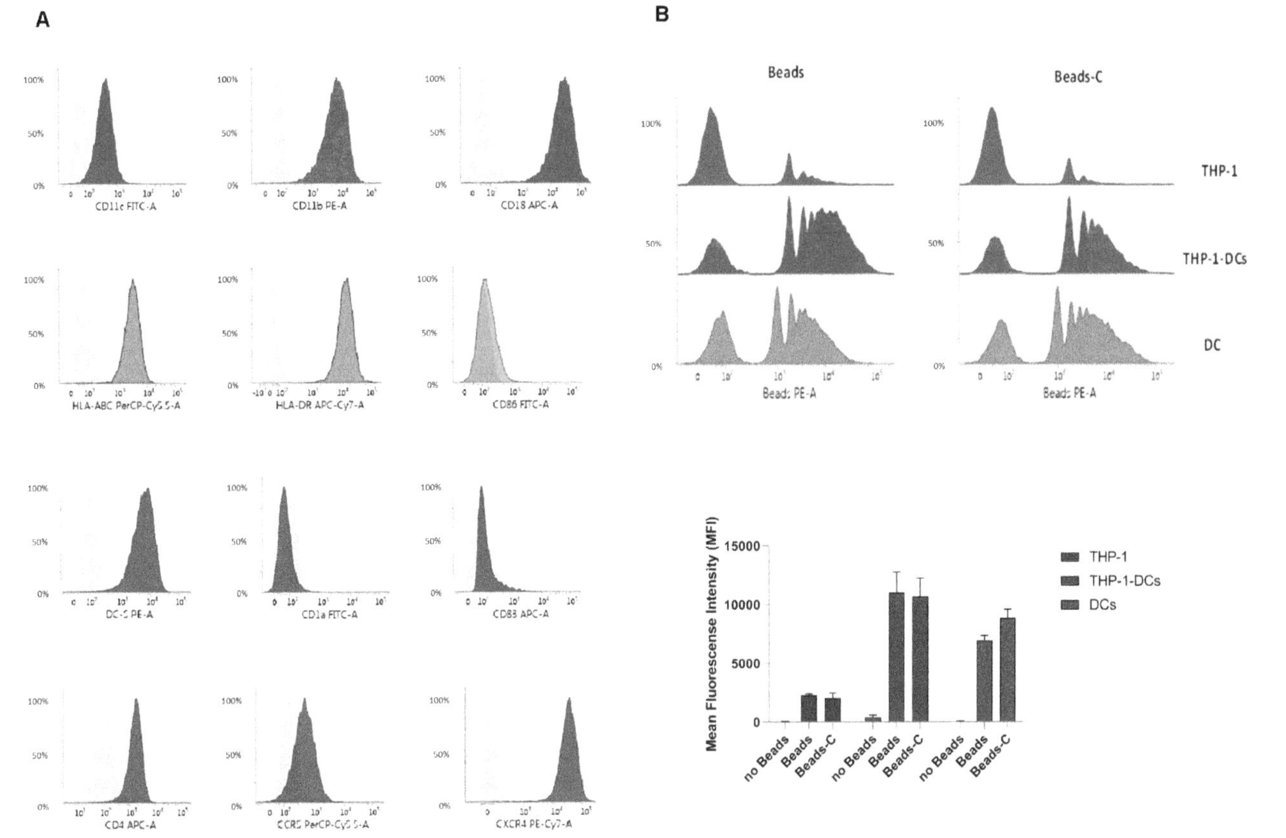

FIGURE 1 | THP1 monocytes can be differentiated into functional DCs. **(A)** WT THP1 cells were differentiated into DCs and expression of characteristic DC markers CD11c, CD11b, CD18, HLA-ABC, HLA-DR, CD86, DC-SIGN, CD1a, CD83, and HIV-1 receptors CD4, CCR5, and CXCR4 was analyzed using flow cytometry. A representative flow cytometry analysis is shown out of five independent experiments. **(B)** Phagocytosis of non- and complement-opsonized Beads (Beads, Beads-C) was analyzed in WT THP1 monocytes (blue), WT THP1-DCs (red), and monocyte-derived DCs (green). THP1-DCs (red) exerted similar phagocytosis capacities with respect to Beads and Beads-C compared to monocyte-derived DCs (green), while THP1 monocytes had a very low phagocytic activity (blue). Panel **(B)** illustrates a FACS analysis from one representative experiment (upper panel) and data from three independent experiments are summarized in panel **(B)** (lower panel).

distinct roles of CR3 and CR4 during the very early steps of HIV-1 infection.

CR4 Plays a Major Role With Respect to HIV-C Infection of DCs

Efficient antiviral T cell responses are initiated when DCs are productively infected by HIV-1 after their resistance to infection is bypassed (10, 13). In contrast, the inability of DCs to become infected is supposed to be an evasion strategy for HIV-1 survival. As previously shown by our group and also herein in **Supplementary Figure S4**, DCs are efficiently infected by complement-opsonized HIV-1 (HIV-C), while only low-level productive infection was mediated by HIV-1 (HIV) (8, 9). To unravel the specific roles of CR3 and CR4 with respect to productive DC infection, we first analyzed infection of WT THP1-DCs after exposure to HIV or HIV-C. As previously demonstrated, virus concentrations of WT THP1-DCs were similar to the ones obtained in primary DCs (13). Thus, low-level productive infection was only monitored in WT THP1-DCs exposed to HIV, whereas infection was significantly enhanced using HIV-C (**Figure 3A**). Non-infected and therefore immature THP1-DCs were used as negative controls (**Figure 3A**, uninfected or UI). Consistently with Posch et al. (9) using monocyte-derived DCs (moDCs), we could also illustrate that infection of WT THP1-DCs with Vpx-carrying HIV illustrated a similar pattern compared to HIV-C by enhancing productive infection compared to non-opsonized HIV. In addition, complement opsonization of HIV-Vpx (HIV-C Vpx) improved infection even more (**Figure 3B**). Since same infection patterns could be displayed in THP1-DCs, moDCs and BDCA1$^+$ DCs (9), we continued the next steps using WT THP1-DCs and their CD11b- and CD11c KO THP1-DCs counterparts to characterize in detail the specific roles of CR3 and CR4 during HIV-1 infection. We found that infection of CD11b- or CD11c KO THP1-DCs with non-opsonized HIV (HIV, **Figure 3C**) or non-opsonized Vpx-carrying HIV (HIV-Vpx, **Figure 3D**) was similar to infection levels of WT THP1 DCs. Vpx-carrying HIV-1 mediated a more than fivefold enhanced infection compared to the low-level productive infection induced by non-opsonized HIV-1. In contrast, infection

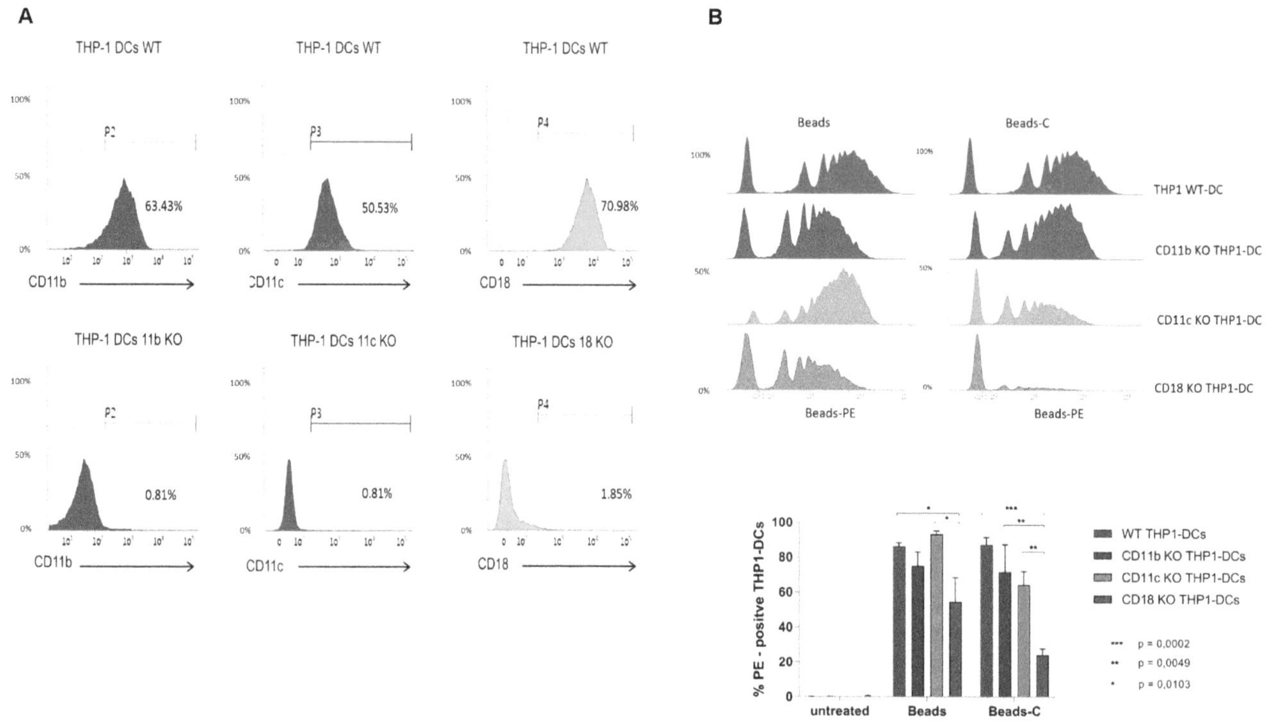

FIGURE 2 | CD11b-, CD11c-, and CD18 KO THP1 DCs comprise a novel tool to decrypt distinct functions of CR3 and CR4. **(A)** CD11b, CD11c, or CD18 were stably deleted by using the CRISPR/Cas9 genome editing technology. Top panel: WT THP1 cells differentiated to DCs were used as controls for monitoring expression of CD11b (blue), CD11c (red), and CD18 (green). Bottom panel: CD11b KO THP1-DCs do not express CD11b (blue), CD11c KO THP1-DCs are devoid of CD11c (red), and no CD18 is expressed on CD18 KO THP1-DCs (green). A representative flow cytometric analysis from one out of five experiments is illustrated. **(B)** Phagocytosis of C-opsonized Beads is hampered in CD11c- (yellow) and CD18 KO (green) THP1-DCs compared to WT (red) and CD11b KO (blue) THP1-DCs. Lowest phagocytosis using non-opsonized Beads was monitored in CD18 KO THP1 DCs (green). A representative flow cytometric analysis out of three independent experiments is depicted.

of WT- or CD11b KO THP1-DCs with complement-opsonized HIV (HIV-C, **Figure 3C**) was significantly enhanced similar to moDCs (**Supplementary Figure S4A**). This was also the case for complement-opsonized Vpx-carrying HIV (HIV-C Vpx, **Figure 3D**).

In contrast, CD11c KO-THP1 DCs showed similar p24 levels between HIV and HIV-C or HIV-Vpx and HIV-C Vpx (**Figures 3C,D**, yellow), and productive infection using HIV-C or HIV-C Vpx was significantly reduced when compared to CD11b KO or WT THP1-DCs (**Figures 3C,D**, HIV-C, yellow vs. blue and red bars). Uninfected iDCs and LPS-exposed THP1-DCs were used as controls. Using blocking antibodies against CD11b and CD11c and moDCs revealed similar results as the THP1 KO DC models. While CD11b blocking significantly enhanced productive DC infection upon exposure to HIV-C, blocking CD11c significantly decreased productive infection as seen also in CD11c KO THP1 DCs (**Supplementary Figure S4B**). This reduction was in part rescued when combining the CD11b/CD11c blocking Abs (**Supplementary Figure S4B**), highlighting the cross-talk of these two receptors.

These experiments demonstrated that THP1-DCs represent a valid model for DC infection, due to the similar infection kinetics observed in WT THP1-DCs compared to primary DCs and also because complement opsonization of HIV-1 significantly enhanced productive DC infection. Furthermore, our data revealed that CR3 is not involved in infection of DCs by HIV-C, since CD11b KO THP1-DCs or CD11b blocking using a blocking anti-human CD11b mAb showed a significant HIV-C-mediated enhancement of DC infection (**Figure 3** and **Supplementary Figure S4B**). In contrast, deleting CD11c (CR4) had a severe effect on DC infection, which caused a low-level productive DC infection with complement-opsonized HIV-1, comparable to the low-level infection observed using non-opsonized HIV-1 (**Figure 3** and **Supplementary Figure S4B**). To summarize, abrogation of CR3 does not impact productive infection with HIV-C, while CR4 KO results in low-level DC infection comparable to HIV.

CR4 KO Diminishes Antiviral Signaling Pathways and Mediates an Anti-inflammatory DC Type

To determine, whether CR4 KO also impacts the antiviral and inflammatory DC profile induced by HIV-C, we studied antiviral signaling pathway IRF3 and type I IFN expression, IL-1β production and mRNA level expression of IL6, IL10, and IL23A.

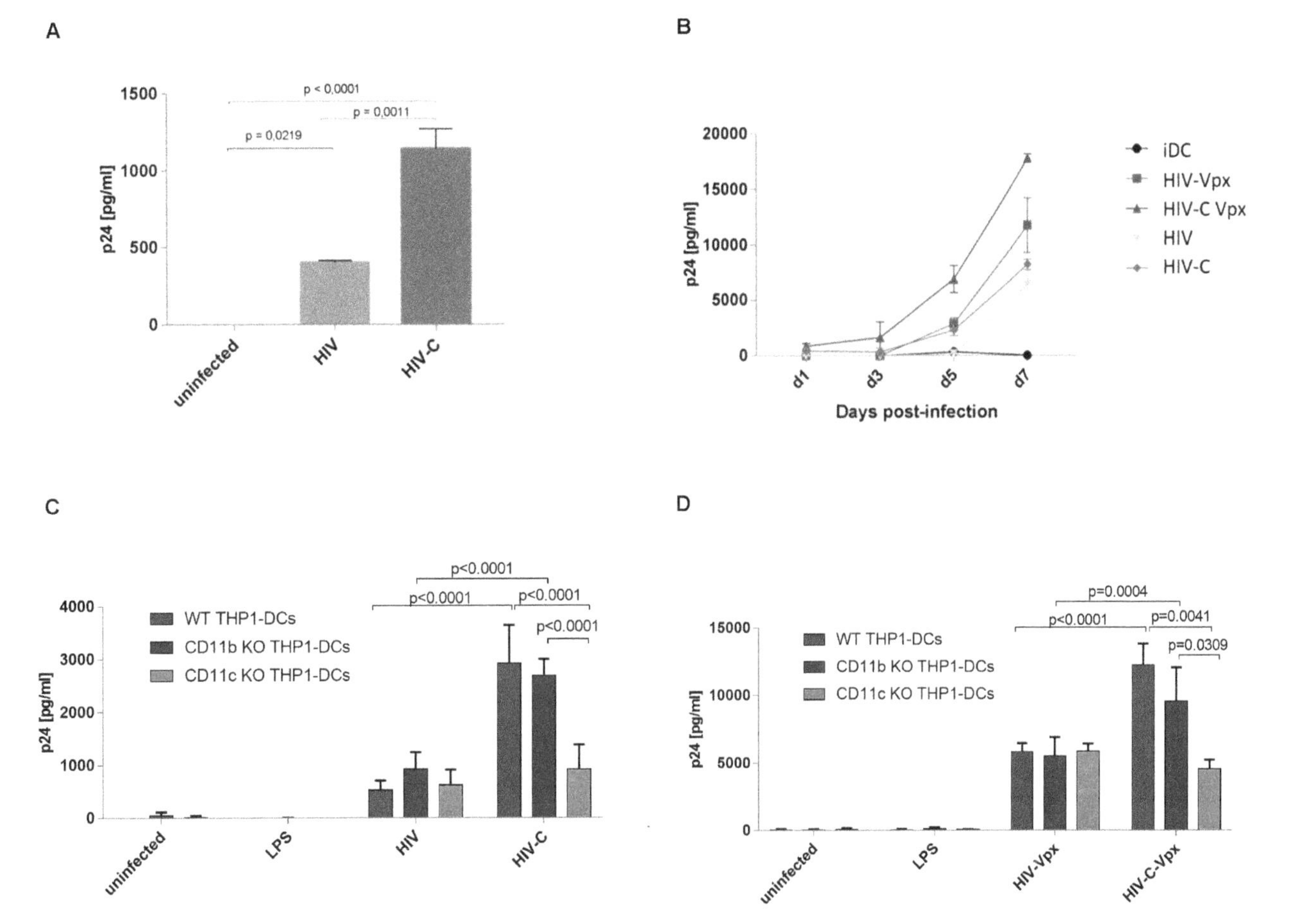

FIGURE 3 | Complement-opsonized HIV-1 effectively infects WT- and CD11b KO THP1-DCs, while productive HIV-1 infection is impaired in CD11c KO THP1-DCs. **(A,B)** Upon infection of WT THP1 DCs with HIV or HIV-C (25 ng p24/ml) a significantly enhanced productive infection was monitored using HIV-C. Means ± SD from three independent experiments in duplicates are depicted in **(A)**. Differences were analyzed using Unpaired Student's *t*-test. In **(B)** a time-course of WT THP1-DC infection exposed to HIV (lime), HIV-C (orange), HIV-Vpx (green), and HIV-Vpx-C (red) is illustrated. Experiments were repeated three times in duplicates. **(C,D)** WT- (red), CD11b KO (blue), and CD11c KO (yellow) THP1-DCs were infected with HIV or HIV-C (C) and HIV-Vpx or HIV-C-Vpx. Uninfected and LPS-incubated THP1-DCs served as controls. Infection experiments were performed in three independent experiments performed in triplicates. Differences were analyzed using GraphPad Prism and one-way ANOVA with Bonferroni post-test.

Antiviral signaling pathways involving TANK Binding Kinase 1 (TBK1) and Interferon regulatory factor 3 (IRF3) are associated with induction of an early type I IFN response. Upon analyzing IRF3 phosphorylation after exposure of DCs to HIV or HIV-C (**Figure 4A**), we found significantly increased activation levels in CD11b KO THP1-DCs upon stimulation with both, HIV- and HIV-C (**Figure 4A**). Stimulation of CD11c KO THP1-DCs with HIV, too, increased IRF3 phosphorylation, while in HIV-C-exposed CD11c KO THP1-DCs the levels were significantly decreased compared to CD11b KO THP1-DCs and reduced in comparison to WT THP1-DCs (**Figure 4A**). This enhanced activation of pIRF3 in CD11b KO THP1-DCs by HIV-C was further associated with a significantly increased expression of type I interferon IFNB, but not in case of HIV-exposed DCs (**Figure 4B**). In contrast, CD11c KO cells did not show any change on IFNB mRNA expression levels compared to WT- and CD11b KO-THP1 DCs (**Figure 4B**).

Next, we studied pro-inflammatory cytokine induction as measured by IL-1β production and IL6, IL10, and IL23A mRNA levels, since in monocyte- and blood-derived DCs we previously found that HIV-C significantly increased production of Th17-polarizing cytokines, such as IL-1β, IL-6, and IL-23, while IL-10 expression was even decreased (14). Strikingly, we found a significantly increased IL-1β secretion in HIV-C-exposed WT THP1-DCs compared to HIV-loaded or iDCs (**Figure 5A**, WT), corroborating what has already been published in primary DCs. CD11b KO THP1-DCs mediated an augmented IL-1β production, upon exposure to non-opsonized HIV, similar to HIV-C-loaded WT- and CD11b KO THP1-DCs (**Figure 5A**, CD11b and WT). In contrast, CR4 KO significantly decreased IL-1β levels secreted in HIV-C-exposed CD11c KO THP1-DCs (**Figure 5A**, CD11c). IL6 and IL23A mRNA expression were significantly enhanced in WT THP1-DCs upon exposure to HIV-C as described in primary DCs (14). In case of CD11c KO THP1-DCs, IL23A was significantly reduced in HIV-C-exposed

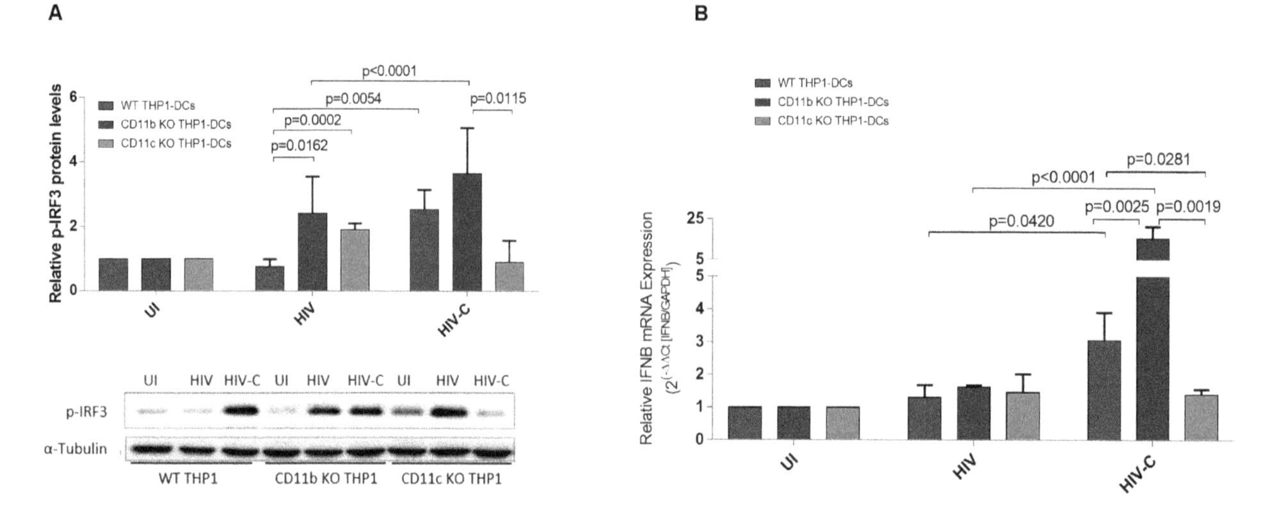

FIGURE 4 | Antiviral signaling pathways are impeded in CD11c-deleted THP1 DCs. **(A)** Relative p- p-IRF3 protein levels were assessed in WT- (red), CD11b KO (blue), and CD11c KO (yellow) THP1-DCs. Experiments were repeated four times independently and a summary as well as a representative immunoblot are depicted. UI, uninfected. **(B)** RT-PCR analyses of type I IFN (IFNB) levels in WT-, CD11b KO-, and CD11c KO-THP1 DCs after infection with HIV or HIV-C (BaL, YU-2). Non-infected iDC were used as controls. Data are mean ± SD from four different donors in duplicates. Differences were analyzed by using one-way ANOVA with Bonferroni post-test.

DCs to levels mediated by HIV (**Figure 5C**). In addition, IL6 mRNA expression was reduced, although not significantly, as for CD11c KO THP1-DCs (**Figure 5B**). A different picture was observed for IL-10 expression, since this cytokine was expressed at similar levels in all treatments (iDCs, HIV, HIV-C) using WT-, CD11b-, and CD18 KO-THP1 DCs (**Figure 5D**, WT, CD11b). In contrast, CD11c KO-THP1 DCs significantly increased expression of this anti-inflammatory cytokine upon exposure to HIV-C, but not HIV (**Figure 5D**, CD11c). Thereby, abolishing CD11c on DCs diminishes the antiviral profile in DCs, while IL-10-producing DCs (DC-10) were induced by knocking out CR4. These data point to a role of CR3 (CD11b/CD18) as regulator of dampening immune responses and CR4 (CD11c/CD18) as inducer of pro-inflammatory and antiviral immune responses.

DISCUSSION

Integrins are crucial components linking intra- and extracellular environments and thereby coordinating vital features of cellular behavior, such as adhesion, cell contact formation, signaling, immune activation. Among an array of PRRs, DCs abundantly express integrin receptors CR3 (CD11b/CD18) and CR4 (CD11c/CD18), composed of α-M (CD11b) or α-X (CD11c) and the common β2-subunit CD18. Emerging evidence suggests that integrins play an important role in immune activation and inflammation. We recently showed that complement-opsonized HIV-1 (HIV-C) overcomes restriction in DCs by efficiently activating SAMHD1 phosphorylation, and this was associated with a higher DC maturation and co-stimulatory potential, aberrant type I interferon and signaling as well as a stronger induction of pro-inflammatory and cellular immune responses (9, 14). This was not the case for non-opsonized HIV-1 (HIV), which was restricted by SAMHD1 in DCs. Therefore, we here defined in more detail the involvement of the α integrins CD11b and CD11c in this increased DC activation during HIV-1 infection, when the virus was C-opsonized. With this purpose, we generated stable CD11b- and CD11c-KO THP1 DCs using CRISPR/Cas9 technology and characterized them in detail with respect to their similarity to primary monocyte-derived DCs.

Coating of HIV-1 with complement (C-) fragments and binding of HIV-C to CRs might contribute to protecting virus particles from immediate and extensive degradation in intracellular compartments as illustrated for non-opsonized HIV-1 (22). We and others (8, 9, 17, 23, 24) found a significant enhancement of productive DC infection by HIV-C associated with the above mentioned improved antiviral immune responses as well as an adjuvant role with respect to induction of HIV-specific CTLs. This C-mediated, significantly enhanced productive HIV-1 infection was also detected in WT THP1-DCs. After detailed evaluation of WT THP1-DCs on additional characteristics exerted by primary DCs, we proved this cell line to be a suitable model, since similar expression of specific receptors were confirmed. In addition, WT THP1-DCs showed same HIV-1 infection kinetics as primary DCs, since HIV-1 subverts complement for productive infection compared to non-opsonized HIV-1 (9, 13). This complement-mediated enhancement in DC infection was further confirmed using Vpx-carrying HIV and HIV-C Vpx preparations. Productive infection of primary DCs was shown to be limited due to the restriction of SAMHD1, which is not counteracted by non-opsonized HIV-1. However, our group previously illustrated that bypassing SAMHD1 by phosphorylation through HIV-C in iDCs significantly enhanced productive HIV-1 infection and subsequent antiviral humoral and cellular immunity *in vitro* (9).

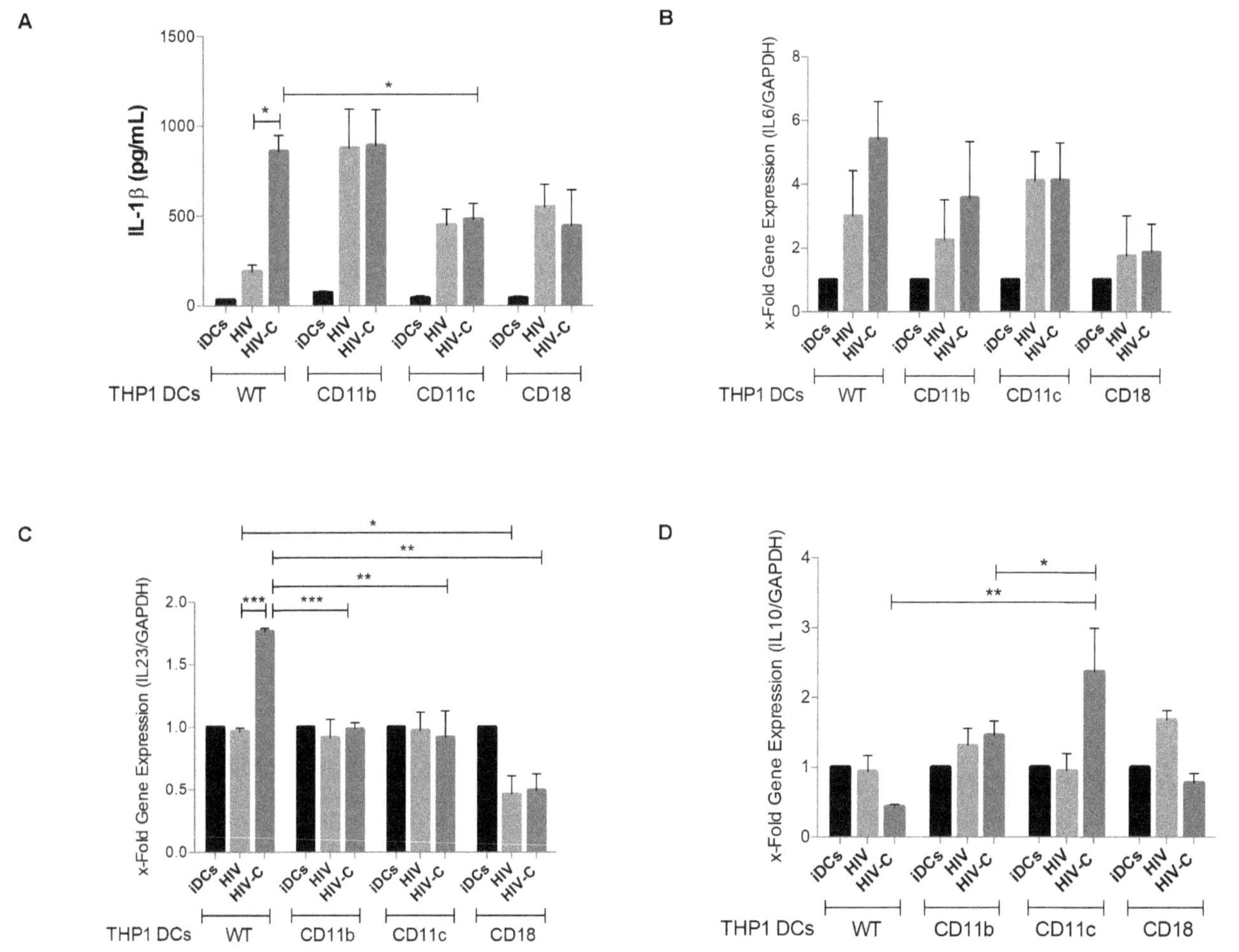

FIGURE 5 | CD11c deletion significantly modifies the cytokine profile by decreasing IL-1β production and IL23 expression, while up-regulating IL10 levels. IL-1β production **(A)**, IL6 **(B)**, IL23A **(C)**, and IL10 **(D)** expression levels were analyzed in WT-, CD11b KO-, CD11c KO-, and CD18 KO THP1-DCs as indicated following infection with HIV or HIV-C. UI cells served as controls. Experiments were repeated thrice in duplicates and RT-PCR analyses were performed. Differences were analyzed by using GraphPad Prism software and one-way ANOVA with Bonferroni post-test. *$p < 0.01$, **$p < 0.001$, ***$p < 0.0001$.

Despite significantly higher SAMHD1 levels in THP1 monocytes (11), HIV-C- and Vpx-mediated effects were also seen in WT THP1-DCs, which proves them to be a valuable model for studying functions of CR3 and CR4 in relation to HIV-1 infection in more detail.

To characterize the KO CD11b and CD11c cells, we infected WT-, CD11b-, and CD11c KO-THP1 DCs using HIV and HIV-C. In CD11b KO-THP1 DCs, HIV-C mediated a significantly enhanced productive infection similar to primary DCs and WT-THP1 DCs. However, the considerably augmented productive infection was lost in CD11c KO-THP1 DCs or upon blocking CD11c on moDCs and infection levels were comparable to the low-level productive infection mediated by HIV. Complement-mediated effects in presence of Vpx were also lost in CD11c KO THP1-DCs only, but not in CD11b KO THP1-DCs. Similar results to CD11c KO THP1-DCs were observed in CD18 KO cells, devoid of both CR3 and CR4.

Our data represent the first evidence of the major role of CR4 in DC infection with complement-opsonized HIV-1, and is in controversy to findings from Tjomsland et al. (25), who illustrated that blocking CR3 significantly decreased infection of emigrating DCs from cervical mucosal tissues. These authors used a combination of blocking antibodies against CD11b and CD18, which could cause CR3 and CR4 blocking due to the shared integrin beta chain-2 (CD18) of both CRs. Thus, effects seen in this study might not rely on CR3 blocking, but probably on blocking CR4-mediated signaling.

IRF3 and IRF7 are the main regulators of type I IFN expression (26). IRF3, localized in the cytoplasm in a latent form, gets activated by phosphorylation via TBK1 or IKKε and translocates to the nucleus. Once in the nucleus, IRF3 dimerizes with NFκB and activating transcription factor 2 (ATF2)–c-jun to recruit CREB-binding protein to the IFNB promoter to form a functional beta interferon "enhanceosome" (27). We found this IRF3/NFκB "enhanceosome" also in primary DCs exposed to HIV-C (9) and within this study we unraveled the CR responsible for this axis using the CD11b/CD11c KO THP1-DCs. In line with the results obtained from the infection analyses, we detected that the p-IRF3 signaling is significantly disrupted upon CD11c KO, but intact in WT- and CD11b KO-THP1 DCs. Disturbance of IRF3 activation was associated with a significantly impaired *IFNB* mRNA level expression in CD11c KO THP1-DCs. These results confirm the findings, that abolishment of IFN-β was observed in DCs deficient of *Irf3* upon LPS stimulation or significantly impaired upon Poly(I:C) treatment (28) and also upon virus infection of *Irf3*$^{-/-}$ mouse embryonic fibroblasts (MEFs) (29). Additionally, these activated cascades contribute to the type I IFN positive feedback loop. We observed in WT THP1-DCs that type I *IFNB* mRNA significantly increased in HIV-C infection, leading to a better antiviral response. These findings are consistent with our other study (9) finding elevated levels of *IFNB* mRNA and ISGs in HIV-C exposed primary DCs. Our findings differ from results published by Ellegård et al. (30), who showed that complement opsonization of HIV-1 resulted in a decreased antiviral immune response in DCs. In contrast to that finding, the authors illustrated in line with our data, that DCs are infected to significantly higher levels when the virus was complement-opsonized (30, 31). Furthermore, they illustrated considerably enhanced IRF3 activation in DCs upon HIV-C treatment, which point to induction of an efficient antiviral immune response by DCs. Nonetheless the authors concluded that complement-opsonized HIV dampens immune responses via DCs compared to non-opsonized HIV-1. In contrast, we found, enhanced productive infection of DCs exposed to HIV-C also increases IRF3 activation and phosphorylation of TBK1 only in WT-THP1-DCs and CD11b KO THP1-DCs, but not CD11c KO THP1-DCs. In addition, CD11b KO resulted in an overshooting type I IFN response.

Since CD11b plays a key role in phagocytosis of apoptotic cells, ligation of this member of the heterodimeric β2 integrin family results in production of anti-inflammatory cytokines such as TGF-β or IL-10 (32). At the same time ligation of CD11b negatively regulates pro-inflammatory signals via e.g., TLRs or FcγR (33–35). Our data confirm this anti-inflammatory, IL-10-inducing role of CD11b, which does not only seem to negatively regulate TLR or FcγR signaling pathways (32), but also signaling pathways initiated via CD11c. A role for anti-inflammatory signaling via CD11b was also observed in CD11c KO THP1-DCs that solely express CR3, since in these cells significantly increased IL-10 expression levels were detected similar to DC-10, a human subset of tolerogenic DCs endowed with the ability to spontaneously release IL-10 as described by Comi et al. (36).

Our results nicely reflect the distinct roles of CD11b and CD11c with respect to inflammatory or antiviral host responses, but also point to the importance of balanced levels regarding either elevated, overshooting induction of antiviral signaling pathways (CD11b KO) or dampening via pIRF3/IFNB reduction and IL-10 induction (CD11c KO). Our results in WT- and CD11b KO THP1-DCs showed an enhanced antiviral type I IFN signaling pathway, comparable to the one seen in primary DCs, e.g., BDCA1^{+} DCs (9). The contradictory data seen in our experiments compared to Ellegard et al. (30) might rely on diverse monocyte isolation and differentiation protocols or cell sources to work on and thereby differential expression levels of either CR3 or CR4 on generated DCs.

Our data suggest an important and distinct role for β2 integrins, CR3 and CR4, in myeloid cells. Beyond initial binding of complement-opsonized particles, myeloid cells encounter ligands within the extracellular matrix while en route to their intended targets. Here, these ligands are modified by local inflammatory mediators (37). Dependent on interaction with either CR3 or CR4, inflammatory cytokine production is restricted to minimize damage of the host via CD11b, while CD11c seems to take action with respect to efficient antiviral immune responses in a type I interferon autocrine-paracrine manner. Cooperation of the NFκB-dependent pathway leading to inflammatory cytokine secretion and the IFN-dependent pathway mediating type I IFN and ISGs was also described upon TLR7/8 triggering in DCs (38) and this type I IFN autocrine-paracrine loop seems to also play an important role in CR4-signaling, which has to be confirmed in more detail. Nevertheless, specific targeting of either CD11b or CD11c might be an innovative tool to regulate pro- and anti-inflammatory processes during infectious diseases such as HIV-1.

AUTHOR CONTRIBUTIONS

DW and WP: conceptualization and funding acquisition. MB-J, MB, PJ-O, TY, TV, LH, WP, and DW: investigation. DW, WP, and MB-J: writing – original draft. DW, MB-J, MB, TV, LH, and WP: writing – review and editing. DW: project administration. All authors contributed to the article and approved the submitted version.

FUNDING

This work was funded by the Austrian National Bank (OeNB) Jubiläumsfonds: 17614 to WP and the Austrian Science Fund (FWF): W11 and P-33510B to DW.

ACKNOWLEDGMENTS

We thank our technicians Karolin Thurnes and Christina Witting for their valuable help and support regarding this manuscript, and also Profs. Oliver Keppler, Nathaniel Landau, and Thomas J. Hope for providing reagents and virus plasmids. We also thank Prof. Sieghart Sopper from the FACS Sort Core Facility of the Medical University of Innsbruck and Polymun Scientific, Donaustrasse 99, Klosterneuburg, Austria who provided all reagents for p24 ELISA. The reagents ARP118 (HIV-BaL) and ARP177.8 (HIV-92UG037) were obtained from the Centre for AIDS Reagents, NIBSC HPA UK, supported by the EC FP6/7 Europrise Network of Excellence, and NGIN consortia and the Bill and Melinda Gates GHRC-CAVD Project and were donated by Dr. S. Gartner, Dr. M. Popovic, Dr. R. Gallo [Courtesy of the NIH AIDS Research and Reference Reagent Program (BaL)], and the WHO UN AIDS Network for HIV-isolation and characterization (92UG037).

REFERENCES

1. Fernandez NC, Lozier A, Flament C, Ricciardi-Castagnoli P, Bellet D, Suter M, et al. Dendritic cells directly trigger NK cell functions: cross-talk relevant in innate anti-tumor immune responses in vivo. *Nat Med.* (1999) 5:405–11. doi: 10.1038/7403
2. Steinman RM, Hemmi H. Dendritic cells: translating innate to adaptive immunity. *Curr Top Microbiol Immunol.* (2006) 311:17–58. doi: 10.1007/3-540-32636-7_2
3. Steinman RM. Decisions about dendritic cells: past, present, and future. *Annu Rev Immunol.* (2012) 30:1–22. doi: 10.1146/annurev-immunol-100311-102839
4. Shen R, Richter HE, Smith PD. Early HIV-1 target cells in human vaginal and ectocervical mucosa. *Am J Reprod Immunol.* (2011) 65:261–7. doi: 10.1111/j.1600-0897.2010.00939.x
5. Ebenbichler CF, Thielens NM, Vornhagen R, Marschang P, Arlaud GJ, Dierich MP. Human immunodeficiency virus type 1 activates the classical pathway of complement by direct C1 binding through specific sites in the transmembrane glycoprotein gp41. *J Exp Med.* (1991) 174:1417–24. doi: 10.1084/jem.174.6.1417
6. Bouhlal H, Chomont N, Haeffner-Cavaillon N, Kazatchkine MD, Belec L, Hocini H. Opsonization of HIV-1 by semen complement enhances infection of human epithelial cells. *J Immunol.* (2002) 169:3301–6. doi: 10.4049/jimmunol.169.6.3301
7. Stoiber H, Soederholm A, Wilflingseder D, Gusenbauer S, Hildgartner A, Dierich MP. Complement and antibodies: a dangerous liaison in HIV infection? *Vaccine.* (2008) 26(Suppl. 8):I79–85. doi: 10.1016/j.vaccine.2008.11.050
8. Wilflingseder D, Banki Z, Garcia E, Pruenster M, Pfister G, Muellauer B, et al. IgG opsonization of HIV impedes provirus formation in and infection of dendritic cells and subsequent long-term transfer to T cells. *J Immunol.* (2007) 178:7840–8. doi: 10.4049/jimmunol.178.12.7840
9. Posch W, Steger M, Knackmuss U, Blatzer M, Baldauf H-M, Doppler W, et al. Complement-opsonized HIV-1 overcomes restriction in dendritic cells. *PLoS Pathog.* (2015) 11:e1005005. doi: 10.1371/journal.ppat.1005005
10. Manel N, Hogstad B, Wang Y, Levy DE, Unutmaz D, Littman DR. A cryptic sensor for HIV-1 activates antiviral innate immunity in dendritic cells. *Nature.* (2010) 467:214–7. doi: 10.1038/nature09337
11. Laguette N, Sobhian B, Casartelli N, Ringeard M, Chable-Bessia C, Segeral E, et al. SAMHD1 is the dendritic- and myeloid-cell-specific HIV-1 restriction factor counteracted by Vpx. *Nature.* (2011) 474:654–7. doi: 10.1038/nature10117
12. Lahouassa H, Daddacha W, Hofmann H, Ayinde D, Logue EC, Dragin L, et al. SAMHD1 restricts the replication of human immunodeficiency virus type 1 by depleting the intracellular pool of deoxynucleoside triphosphates. *Nat Immunol.* (2012) 13:223–8. doi: 10.1038/ni.2236
13. Banki Z, Posch W, Ejaz A, Oberhauser V, Willey S, Gassner C, et al. Complement as an endogenous adjuvant for dendritic cell-mediated induction of retrovirus-specific CTLs. *PLoS Pathog.* (2010) 6:e1000891. doi: 10.1371/journal.ppat.1000891
14. Wilflingseder D, Schroll A, Hackl H, Gallasch R, Frampton D, Lass-Florl C, et al. Immediate T-helper 17 polarization upon triggering CD11b/c on HIV-exposed dendritic cells. *J Infect Dis.* (2015) 212:44–56. doi: 10.1093/infdis/jiv014
15. Manel N, Littman DR. Hiding in plain sight: how HIV evades innate immune responses. *Cell.* (2011) 147:271–4. doi: 10.1016/j.cell.2011.09.010
16. Posch W, Cardinaud S, Hamimi C, Fletcher A, Muhlbacher A, Loacker K, et al. Antibodies attenuate the capacity of dendritic cells to stimulate HIV-specific cytotoxic T lymphocytes. *J Allergy Clin Immunol.* (2012) 130:1368–74.e2. doi: 10.1016/j.jaci.2012.08.025
17. Pruenster M, Wilflingseder D, Banki Z, Ammann CG, Muellauer B, Meyer M, et al. C-type lectin-independent interaction of complement opsonized HIV with monocyte-derived dendritic cells. *Eur J Immunol.* (2005) 35:2691–8. doi: 10.1002/eji.200425940
18. Hsu PD, Scott DA, Weinstein JA, Ran FA, Konermann S, Agarwala V, et al. DNA targeting specificity of RNA-guided Cas9 nucleases. *Nat Biotechnol.* (2013) 31:827–32. doi: 10.1038/nbt.2647
19. Sanjana NE, Shalem O, Zhang F. Improved vectors and genome-wide libraries for CRISPR screening. *Nat Methods.* (2014) 11:783–4. doi: 10.1038/nmeth.3047
20. Baldauf HM, Pan XY, Erikson E, Schmidt S, Daddacha W, Burggraf M, et al. SAMHD1 restricts HIV-1 infection in resting CD4(+) T cells. *Nat Med.* (2012) 18:1682–7. doi: 10.1038/nm.2964
21. Purtscher M, Trkola A, Gruber G, Buchacher A, Predl R, Steindl F, et al. A broadly neutralizing human monoclonal antibody against gp41 of human immunodeficiency virus type 1. *AIDS Res Hum Retroviruses.* (1994) 10:1651–8. doi: 10.1089/aid.1994.10.1651
22. Moris A, Nobile C, Buseyne F, Porrot F, Abastado JP, Schwartz O. DC-SIGN promotes exogenous MHC-I-restricted HIV-1 antigen presentation. *Blood.* (2004) 103:2648–54. doi: 10.1182/blood-2003-07-2532
23. Bajtay Z, Speth C, Erdei A, Dierich MP. Cutting edge: productive HIV-1 infection of dendritic cells via complement receptor type 3 (CR3, CD11b/CD18). *J Immunol.* (2004) 173:4775–8.
24. Bouhlal H, Chomont N, Requena M, Nasreddine N, Saidi H, Legoff J, et al. Opsonization of HIV with complement enhances infection of dendritic cells and viral transfer to CD4 T cells in a CR3 and DC-SIGN-dependent manner. *J Immunol.* (2007) 178:1086–95.
25. Tjomsland V, Ellegard R, Kjolhede P, Wodlin NB, Hinkula J, Lifson JD, et al. Blocking of integrins inhibits HIV-1 infection of human cervical mucosa immune cells with free and complement-opsonized virions. *Eur J Immunol.* (2013) 43:2361–72. doi: 10.1002/eji.201243257
26. Taniguchi T, Ogasawara K, Takaoka A, Tanaka N. IRF family of transcription factors as regulators of host defense. *Annu Rev Immunol.* (2001) 19:623–55. doi: 10.1146/annurev.immunol.19.1.623
27. Falvo JV, Parekh BS, Lin CH, Fraenkel E, Maniatis T. Assembly of a functional beta interferon enhanceosome is dependent on ATF-2-c-jun heterodimer orientation. *Mol Cell Biol.* (2000) 20:4814–25. doi: 10.1128/mcb.20.13.4814-4825.2000
28. Sakaguchi S, Negishi H, Asagiri M, Nakajima C, Mizutani T, Takaoka A, et al. Essential role of IRF-3 in lipopolysaccharide-induced interferon-beta gene expression and endotoxin shock. *Biochem Biophys Res Commun.* (2003) 306:860–6. doi: 10.1016/s0006-291x(03)01049-0
29. Sato M, Suemori H, Hata N, Asagiri M, Ogasawara K, Nakao K, et al. Distinct and essential roles of transcription factors IRF-3 and IRF-7 in response to viruses for IFN-alpha/beta gene induction. *Immunity.* (2000) 13:539–48.
30. Ellegard R, Crisci E, Burgener A, Sjowall C, Birse K, Westmacott G, et al. Complement opsonization of HIV-1 results in decreased antiviral and inflammatory responses in immature dendritic cells via CR3. *J Immunol.* (2014) 193:4590–601. doi: 10.4049/jimmunol.1401781
31. Tjomsland V, Ellegard R, Burgener A, Mogk K, Che KF, Westmacott G, et al. Complement opsonization of HIV-1 results in a different intracellular processing pattern and enhanced MHC class I presentation by dendritic cells. *Eur J Immunol.* (2013) 43:1470–83. doi: 10.1002/eji.201242935
32. Amarilyo G, Verbovetski I, Atallah M, Grau A, Wiser G, Gil O, et al. iC3b-opsonized apoptotic cells mediate a distinct anti-inflammatory response and transcriptional NF-kappaB-dependent blockade. *Eur J Immunol.* (2010) 40:699–709. doi: 10.1002/eji.200838951
33. Faridi MH, Khan SQ, Zhao W, Lee HW, Altintas MM, Zhang K, et al. CD11b activation suppresses TLR-dependent inflammation and autoimmunity in systemic lupus erythematosus. *J Clin Invest.* (2017) 127:1271–83. doi: 10.1172/JCI88442
34. Means TK, Luster AD. Integrins limit the Toll. *Nat Immunol.* (2010) 11:691–3. doi: 10.1038/ni0810-691
35. Han C, Jin J, Xu S, Liu H, Li N, Cao X. Integrin CD11b negatively regulates TLR-triggered inflammatory responses by activating Syk and promoting degradation of MyD88 and TRIF via Cbl-b. *Nat Immunol.* (2010) 11:734–42. doi: 10.1038/ni.1908

36. Comi M, Amodio G, Gregori S. Interleukin-10-producing DC-10 is a unique tool to promote tolerance via antigen-specific T regulatory type 1 cells. *Front Immunol.* (2018) 9:682. doi: 10.3389/fimmu.2018.00682
37. dair-Kirk TLA, Senior RM. Fragments of extracellular matrix as mediators of inflammation. *Int J Biochem Cell Biol.* (2008) 40:1101–10. doi: 10.1016/j.biocel.2007.12.005
38. Gautier G, Humbert M, Deauvieau F, Scuiller M, Hiscott J, Bates EE, et al. A type I interferon autocrine-paracrine loop is involved in Toll-like receptor-induced interleukin-12p70 secretion by dendritic cells. *J Exp Med.* (2005) 201:1435–46. doi: 10.1084/jem.20041964

18

Complement Alternative and Mannose-Binding Lectin Pathway Activation is Associated with COVID-19 Mortality

Federica Defendi[1], Corentin Leroy[2,3], Olivier Epaulard[4,5], Giovanna Clavarino[1], Antoine Vilotitch[2], Marion Le Marechal[4], Marie-Christine Jacob[1], Tatiana Raskovalova[1], Martine Pernollet[1], Audrey Le Gouellec[5,6], Jean-Luc Bosson[5], Pascal Poignard[7,8], Matthieu Roustit[9,10], Nicole Thielens[7], Chantal Dumestre-Pérard[1,7†] and Jean-Yves Cesbron[1†]*

[1] Laboratoire d'Immunologie, Institut de Biologie et Pathologie, Centre Hospitalier Universitaire Grenoble Alpes, Grenoble, France, [2] Cellule d'Ingénierie des Données, Centre Hospitalier Universitaire Grenoble Alpes, Grenoble, France, [3] Centre d'Investigation Clinique de l'Innovation et de la Technologie (CIC-IT), Centre Hospitalier Universitaire Grenoble Alpes, Grenoble, France, [4] Service des Maladies Infectieuses et Tropicales, Centre Hospitalier Universitaire Grenoble Alpes, Grenoble, France, [5] Université Grenoble Alpes, TIMC-IMAG, Grenoble, France, [6] Laboratoire de Biochimie, Institut de Biologie et Pathologie, Centre Hospitalier Universitaire Grenoble Alpes, Grenoble, France, [7] Université Grenoble Alpes, CNRS, CEA, Institut de Biologie Structurale (IBS), Grenoble, France, [8] Laboratoire de Virologie, Institut de Biologie et Pathologie, Centre Hospitalier Universitaire Grenoble Alpes, Grenoble, France, [9] Département de Pharmacologie Clinique INSERM CIC 1406, Centre Hospitalier Universitaire Grenoble Alpes, Grenoble, France, [10] Université Grenoble Alpes, UMR 1042-HP2, INSERM, Grenoble, France

Correspondence:
Federica Defendi
fdefendi@chu-grenoble.fr

†These authors have contributed equally to this work

Background: The SARS-CoV-2 infection triggers excessive immune response resulting in increased levels of pro-inflammatory cytokines, endothelial injury, and intravascular coagulopathy. The complement system (CS) activation participates to this hyperinflammatory response. However, it is still unclear which activation pathways (classical, alternative, or lectin pathway) pilots the effector mechanisms that contribute to critical illness. To better understand the immune correlates of disease severity, we performed an analysis of CS activation pathways and components in samples collected from COVID-19 patients hospitalized in Grenoble Alpes University Hospital between 1 and 30 April 2020 and of their relationship with the clinical outcomes.

Methods: We conducted a retrospective, single-center study cohort in 74 hospitalized patients with RT-PCR-proven COVID-19. The functional activities of classical, alternative, and mannose-binding lectin (MBL) pathways and the antigenic levels of the individual components C1q, C4, C3, C5, Factor B, and MBL were measured in patients' samples during hospital admission. Hierarchical clustering with the Ward method was performed in order to identify clusters of patients with similar characteristics of complement markers. Age was included in the model. Then, the clusters were compared with the patient clinical features: rate of intensive care unit (ICU) admission, corticoid treatment, oxygen requirement, and mortality.

Results: Four clusters were identified according to complement parameters. Among them, two clusters revealed remarkable profiles: in one cluster (n = 15), patients exhibited activation of alternative and lectin pathways and low antigenic levels of MBL, C4, C3, Factor B, and C5 compared to all the other clusters; this cluster had the higher proportion of patients who died (27%) and required oxygen support (80%) or ICU care (53%). In contrast, the second cluster (n = 19) presented inflammatory profile with high classical pathway activity and antigenic levels of complement components; a low proportion of patients required ICU care (26%) and no patient died in this group.

Conclusion: These findings argue in favor of prominent activation of the alternative and MBL complement pathways in severe COVID-19, but the spectrum of complement involvement seems to be heterogeneous requiring larger studies.

Keywords: COVID-19, complement, alternative pathway, MBL, lectin pathway

INTRODUCTION

The severe acute respiratory syndrome coronavirus 2 (SARS-CoV-2) infection drives sustained inflammatory response considered to be a major cause of disease severity and death in patients with COVID-19 (1). Growing evidence suggests that the complement system (CS) activation instigates this dysregulated inflammatory reaction in COVID-19: elevated levels of the anaphylatoxin C5a have been reported to be proportional to disease severity (2); the membrane attack complex concentration has been linked with respiratory failure and systemic inflammation in infected patients (3); and deposits of mannose-binding lectin (MBL) and MBL-associated protease MASP-2 have been found in the microvasculature of critical patients with SARS CoV-2 infection (4). On the other hand, patients treated with complement blockers (anti-C5a mAb [eculizumab] or C3-inhibitor) exhibited a drop in inflammatory markers and significant clinical improvement (5–9). However, it is still not fully understood which of the three complement activation pathways (classical, alternative, or lectin pathway) drives the effector mechanisms that contribute to the tissue injury. To address these questions, we performed extensive analysis of CS activation pathways and components in samples collected from hospitalized COVID-19 patients and their relationship with the clinical outcomes.

METHODS

Study Participants

This retrospective, single center study included 74 patients with RT-PCR-proven COVID-19 admitted to Grenoble Alpes University Hospital from April 1 to 30, 2020. Samples were collected during hospitalization in infectious/pneumology/internal medicine department or intensive care unit (ICU) of our hospital. The study was performed in accordance with the Declaration of Helsinki, Good Clinical Practice guidelines, and CNIL (Commission Nationale de l'Informatique et des Libertés) methodology reference. Patients were informed and consent was obtained, according to French law. Demographic, clinical characteristics (oxygen requirements, ICU admission, mortality, steroid treatment) and laboratory data were collected from electronic clinical records and included in an anonymized database. Patients were classified as severe on the basis of oxygen requirement (>2 L O_2/min), ICU admission, limitation of therapeutic effort (LTE), and mortality, according to (10).

Complement Testing

Peripheral blood samples were collected in citrate anticoagulated or without anticoagulant tubes for hemolytic and functional assays or antigenic level measurement, respectively. Total hemolytic assays for classical pathway (CP, TH50c) and alternative pathway (AP, TH50a) were assessed as previously published (11); 100% lysis is defined by the TH50c/TH50a of the control sample. Reference values (TH50c: 86–126%; TH50a: 84–150%) were established by testing samples from 50 blood donors.

Antigenic levels of C1q, C4, C3, C5, and Factor B proteins in the serum samples were measured using a laser nephelometer BNII (Dade Behring, GmbH, Marburg, Germany). Reference intervals (RI; C1q: 154–258 mg/L; C4: 100–380 mg/L; C3: 880–1650 mg/L; C5: 120–220 mg/L; Factor B: 216–504 mg/L) were obtained by testing samples from 50 blood donors.

Determination of MBL protein concentration and function was realized by an enzyme-linked immunosorbent assay (ELISA) as described previously (12). The characterization of MBL protein expression deficiency was established by the combination of three assays: ELISA for antigen and functional MBL and hemolytic activity of C4 (C4H) (13) normal values of C1q confirmed the absence of CP activation. Low values of antigenic (<100 μg/L) (14) and functional MBL associated with a normal value of C4H defined patients with MBL protein expression deficiency. Low levels of antigenic and functional MBL associated with decreased value of C4H identified patients

Abbreviations: AP, alternative pathway; COVID-19, coronavirus disease 19; CP, classical pathway; CS, Complement system; C4H, C4 hemolytic activity; LTE, limitation of the therapeutic effort; LP, lectin pathway; MBL, mannose-binding lectin; RI, reference interval.

with MBL pathway activation. Reference values for MBL protein concentration and function and C4H were determined from 50 blood donors (MBL antigen: 30–3000 µg/L; MBL function: 35–115%; C4H: 70–130%).

Statistical Analysis

Statistical analysis was performed using hierarchical ascendant clustering (HAC) in order to identify groups of COVID-19 patients with similar characteristics ("clusters") in terms of complement variables: TH50c, TH50a, C1q, C4, C3, C5, Factor B, and MBL antigen. Age was included in the model (**Supplementary Methods**).

The biological significance of the clusters was analyzed by comparing the values of every complement parameter between the clusters. The ANOVA F-test was performed for variables with a Gaussian distribution, and the Kruskal-Wallis test for the variables with other distribution. Mean (standard deviation [sd]) or median (interquartile range [IQR]) were presented for the parametric or non-parametric variables, respectively. For the markers with a significant difference between the clusters, specific cluster by cluster tests were performed using Student or Wilcoxon tests to identify the cluster significantly different from the others. Post-hoc analysis with the Fisher's exact test was used to test specific difference between the clusters.

RESULTS

Table 1 details the main demographic and clinical characteristics of our cohort. The median age of patients was 72 years (IQR: 62;82; range: 32–96); more than half of patients were men (58%). Of the 74 patients, 43 (58%) were severe, 8 (11%) died, 23 (31%) were admitted in the ICU, 3 (4%) were with LTE, and 23 (31%) required treatment by corticoids.

The results of complement proteins and activation pathways analysis performed in samples collected during hospitalization are summarized in **Table 2**.

Four clusters of individuals were identified in the studied cohort by HAC analysis according to the complement data (**Supplementary Figure S1**). The comparison between the clusters (cluster 2 against others and/or cluster 4 against others) is presented in **Figure 1** and **Table 3**. There was no statistically significant difference among the four clusters for sex, age, CRP, severity, ICU admission, O_2 requirement, or corticoid treatment (**Table 4**).

For patients of the first cluster (n = 20; 27%), the complement profile was overall without anomalies (TH50c: 128%; TH50a: 132%; C1q: 201 mg/L; C4: 368 mg/L; C3: 1440 mg/L; C5: 216 mg/L; Factor B: 474 mg/L; MBL antigen: 900 µg/L; MBL function: 110%; C4H: 125%; **Table 3**). A large percentage of patients in this cluster was severe (n = 14; 70%) and required corticoid treatment (n = 10; 50%) (**Table 4**).

Patients of cluster 2 (n = 19; 26%) exhibited an inflammatory profile: high values of CP, LP, and C4 activities (TH50c: 145%; MBL function: 117%; C4H: 118%) and increased antigenic levels of C3 (1795 mg/L), C5 (278 mg/L), Factor B (586 mg/L), and MBL (1025 µg/L) were observed in this cluster compared to other clusters (**Table 3**). The majority of patients of the second cluster were men (men/women: 14/5). Interestingly, none of the patients died in this cluster (**Table 4**).

In cluster 3 (n = 20; 27%), most complement markers were within reference interval (TH50c: 118%; TH50a: 122%; C1q: 216 mg/L; C4: 317 mg/L; C3: 1150 mg/L; C5: 199 mg/L; Factor B: 437 mg/L; MBL antigen: 725 µg/L; C4H: 104%); only MBL function was decreased (43%) (**Table 3**). The third cluster was characterized by the lowest rate of ICU admission (20%) and by the lowest rate of patients having required corticoid treatment (10%); the rate of mortality was also low in this cluster (10%) (**Table 4**).

TABLE 1 | Patient characteristics.

Clinical and biological characteristics	
n	74
Age: median (IQR) (min-max), years	72 (62;82) (32–96)
Sex: men/women	43/31
CRP: mean (sd), mg/L	71 (66.4)
CRP: median (IQR), mg/L	59 (22-92)
Prognosis/outcome, n (%)	
Severe COVID-19[1], n (%)	43 (58)
Mortality	8 (11)
ICU admission	23 (31)
Limitation of therapeutic effort, n (%)	3 (4)
Corticosteroid treatment, n (%)	23 (21)
Oxygen support:	
>2 L O_2/min	39 (53)
≤2 L O_2/min	13 (18)

[1]Severe COVID-19 defined as: O_2 > 2 L/min, ICU [intensive care unit] admission, LTE [limitation of the therapeutic effort], decease.

TABLE 2 | Complement parameters.

	RI	Mean	sd	Min	Lower quart	Median	Upper quart	Max
TH50c (%)	86–126	124	30	67	101	121	142	234
TH50a (%)	84–150	122	70	23	71	102	155	317
C1q (mg/L)	154–258	208	48	71	195	212	234	336
C4 (mg/L)	100–380	318	114	57	249	327	402	551
C3 (mg/L)	880–1650	1339	357	603	1050	1355	1550	2210
Factor B (mg/L)	216–504	466	148	182	345	465	581	828
C5 (mg/L)	120–220	225	52	142	186	214	260	367
MBL antigen (µg/L)	30–3000	1344	1586	20	270	775	1750	9000
MBL function (%)	35–115	94	79	0	22	66	178	200
C4 hemolytic activity (%)	70–130	106	51	5	76	100	132	251

RI, reference interval.

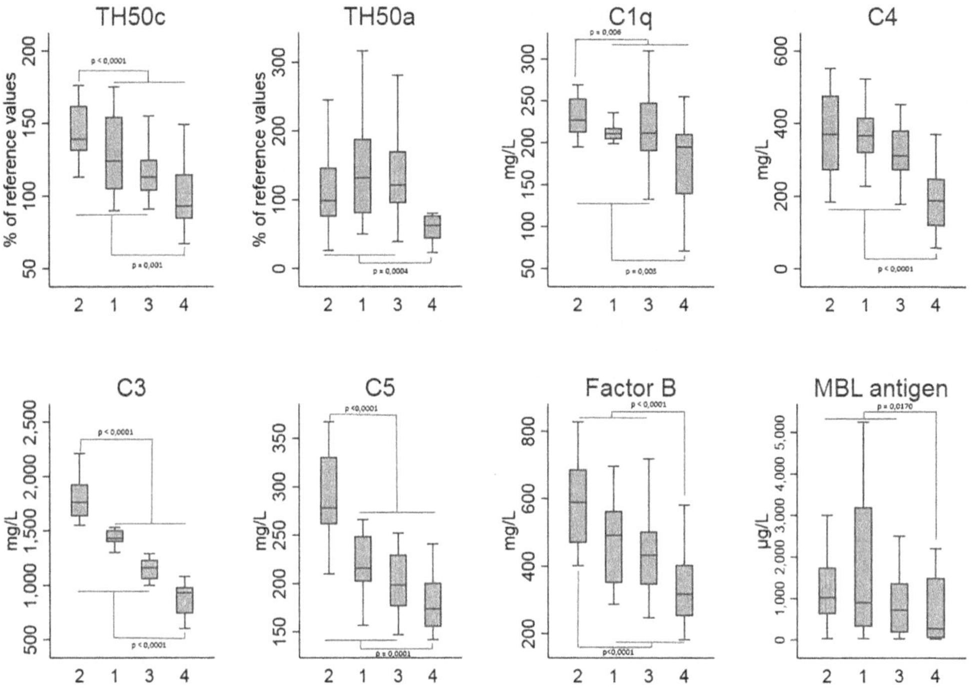

FIGURE 1 | Boxplots representing the complement parameters of the four clusters of patients. Statistical analysis by hierarchical ascendant clustering discriminates the 74 patients with COVID-19 of the cohort in four distinct clusters according to complement variables: TH50c, TH50a, C1q, C4, C3, C5, Factor B, and MBL antigen. Age was included in the model. Boxplots represent the median and 25th to 75th percentiles, the whiskers denote the maximum and minimum values, and the horizontal bars indicate the medians. Outside values were excluded.

Finally, the fourth cluster (n = 15; 20%) (**Tables 3**, **4**; **Supplementary Table S1**) was specifically characterized by significant activation of alternative (TH50a: 62%; p = 0.0004 against other clusters) and lectin (MBL antigen: 270 µg/L: p = 0.0170 against other clusters) complement pathways. Decreased MBL concentration was associated with reduced MBL function (13%) and C4H (67%) confirming the MBL pathway activation. TH50c was also decreased compared to the other clusters (101%; p = 0.001), but remained in the RI (86–126%). Interestingly, in this cluster, 13 patients (87%) exhibited AP activation and 7 patients (47%) exhibited MBL pathway activation; 6 (40%) patients presented simultaneously AP and MBL pathway activation (**Supplementary Table S1**). A large percentage of patients of the fourth cluster was severe (73%) and required ICU admission (53%) and corticoid treatment (47%) (**Table 4**). Among the 11 severe patients, 10 exhibited AP activation; 6 exhibited MBL pathway activation, and 5 presented at the same time AP and MBL pathway activation (**Supplementary Table S1**). Of note, cluster 4 was characterized by a higher mortality rate (27% versus 10%, 0% and 10% in clusters 1, 2, and 3, respectively; p = 0.048) (**Table 4**). Among the four patients who died, three presented AP activation, two exhibited MBL pathway activation, and two patients showed concurrent activation of alternative and MBL pathways (**Supplementary Table S1**). Regarding the four other patients who died, all presented a normal complement profile except patient 1 who exhibited an MBL deficiency (**Supplementary Table S2**).

DISCUSSION

SARS-CoV-2 infection triggers an innate immune response including CS activation which is a key weapon both implicated in disease resolution and organ damage depending on the time of infection (15).

Recent studies addressing the role of complement in the pathogenesis of COVID-19 have shown a relationship between respiratory failure, intravascular coagulopathy, and complement overactivation in COVID-19 patients (3, 16). There are several lines of evidence for local deposition of complement proteins and activation products in lung, skin, and other tissues showing activation of the three pathways, CP, LP, and AP (17–21). Furthermore, systemic complement activation and consumption were related to severe COVID-19 and predictive of in-hospital mortality (22). However, despite *in vitro* lines of evidence suggesting that the SARS-CoV-2 spike proteins activate the AP (23), it remains incompletely understood which complement activation pathways contribute to critical illness in COVID-19.

Concerning the possible involvement of MBL in coronavirus infection, it has been described so far for SARS-CoV in several

TABLE 3 | Clusters of COVID-19 patients according to complement parameters.

Number	RI	Cluster 1 20	Cluster 2 19	Cluster 3 20	Cluster 4 15	p-value	p-value comparison 2 by 2
TH50c % mean (sd)	86–126	128.1 (27.1)	145.2 (27.3)	117.5 (22.7)	100.6 (24.8)	<0.0001[1]	p = 0.001 cluster 4 against others; p < 0.0001 cluster 2 against others
TH50a % median (IQR)	84–150	132 (80;189)	99 (75;147)	122 (95;171)	62 (43;77)	0.003[2]	p = 0.0004 cluster 4 against others
C1q mg/L mean (sd)	154–258	201.4 (40.1)	234.3 (32.5)	215.9 (52.2)	175.2 (52.4)	0.003[1]	p = 0.003 cluster 4 against others: p = 0.006 cluster 2 against others
C4 mg/L mean (sd)	100–380	367.8 (77.8)	374.7 (112.9)	317.1 (79.5)	182.3 (85.1)	<0.0001[1]	p < 0.0001 cluster 4 against others
C3 mg/L mean (sd)	880–1650	1440 (66.7)	1795.3 (189.8)	1149.5 (99.0)	878.1 (149.9)	<0.0001[1]	p < 0.0001cluster 2 against others; cluster 4 against others
Factor B mg/L mean (sd)	216–504	473.5 (134.0)	585.6 (122.6)	436.9 (110.5)	345 (134.8)	<0.0001[1]	p < 0.0001 cluster 2 against others; cluster 4 against others
C5 mg/L median (IQR)	120–220	216 (202;249)	278 (261;331)	199 (177;230)	174 (155;201)	<0.0001[2]	p < 0.0001 cluster 2 against others; p = 0.0001 cluster 4 against others
MBL antigen µg/L median (IQR)	30–3000	900 (318;3200)	1025 (625;1750)	725 (171;1375)	270 (42;1500)	0.0374[2]	p = 0.0170 cluster 4 against others
MBL function* % median (IQR)	35–115	110 (24;187)	117 (62;200)	43 (28;181)	13 (0;168)	0.0558[2]	
C4 hemolytic activity* % mean (sd)	70–130	125 (8.1)	117.3 (50.8)	104.1 (40.8)	66.6 (49.0)	0.004[1]	p = 0.001 cluster 4 against others

Mean (sd) or median (IQR) were presented for the parametric or non-parametric variables, respectively. RI, reference interval.
**Post-hoc analysis was performed for this parameter. [1] Fisher ANOVA test. [2] Kruskal-Wallis test.*

studies. Among those, two *in vitro* studies demonstrated binding of MBL to SARS-CoV or viral particles pseudotyped with SARS-CoV spike protein and activation of the lectin complement pathway (24, 25). More recently, Ali and *al* showed binding of LP recognition molecules to S- and N- proteins of SARS-CoV-2, as also robust LP activation on the surface of HEK 293 cells expressing SARS-CoV-2 S protein (26).

One of the limitation of the study is that it reports data about the original variant of the virus, while the delta variant is now a majority among the infected patients. The crucial mutations leading to delta variant concern the S1 subunit (intimately involved in the initiation of infection) for which we have no data concerning its molecular interaction with complement components. However, the replication rate of delta strain is much higher. It would therefore be interesting to compare our results with samples collected from patients infected with the delta variant of the virus.

Using an original, unsupervised statistical approach by hierarchical clustering on complement and clinical parameters, this study reveals for the first time the association between AP and LP activation, and the mortality in COVID-19 patients (cluster 4). Our data are in line with Ma et al. showing increased AP components in COVID-19 patients with worse prognosis (27) and with Sinkovits et al. relating significant association between AP activity and COVID-19 severity (22).

Furthermore, our results provide additional evidence for an association between MBL pathway activation and mortality, supported by the data of Eriksson et al. (4). In contrast, Sinkovits et al. reported that the LP activity showed no difference between severity groups (22). Our data are consistent with recent reports describing deposits of MBL and MASP2 in affected tissues of COVID-19 patients and *in vitro* MBL pathway activation by recombinant SARS-CoV2 proteins (17, 28). Collectively, these findings are consistent with the CS implication in the pathogenesis of severe COVID-19 infection. As consequences of unrestrained complement activation, the strong pro-inflammatory C5a-C5aR axis promotes neutrophil/monocyte infiltration and the "cytokine storm" driving lung inflammation and injury, responsible for complications in hospitalized COVID-19 patients (2).

If complement activation is evident from our results and associated with the severity of the disease, the spectrum of involvement of the complement cascade in COVID-19 seems to be heterogeneous and depending on patients: notably, complement activation could be deleterious in some ones and expression of the severity of the disease in other ones. A recent review summarizes the current knowledge about modulating complement cascade as therapeutic approach in COVID-19 patients (29). In brief, despite nonconclusive studies, the available data suggested favorable outcomes in a small number of patients with severe COVID-19 treated either with C1 inhibitor, MASP-2 monoclonal antibodies, compstatin-based complement C3 inhibitor, anti-C5 drugs, or C5a-C5aR1 antagonists. Clinical trials of complement inhibitors in COVID-19 are ongoing (NCT04288713, NCT04414631, NCT04395456). However, awaiting final results from the clinical trials, the potential benefits from complement inhibition in COVID-19 remain to be elucidated.

TABLE 4 | Overall comparison of clinical and biological characteristics between the clusters.

	Cluster 1	Cluster 2	Cluster 3	Cluster 4	p-value global test
Number	**20**	**19**	**20**	**15**	
Men, n (%)	12 (60%)	14 (74%)	8 (40%)	9 (60%)	0.2109[1]
Age, (years) mean, sd	70 (15)	69 (14)	72 (14)	73 (14)	0.6265[2]
CRP, (mg/L) mean (sd) (n=73)	89.4 (84.89)	82.1 (70.77)	47.8 (44.08)	63.7 (53.86)	0.2598[2]
Severe COVID-19[3], n (%)	14 (70%)	9 (47.37%)	9 (45%)	11 (73.33%)	0.1912[1]
ICU admission, n (%)	6 (30%)	5 (26.32%)	4 (20%)	8 (53.33%)	0.199[1]
Oxygen requirement, n (%)	18 (90%)	13 (68.42%)	11 (55%)	12 (80%)	0.774[1]
Mortality, dead, n (%)	2 (10%)	0 (0%)	2 (10%)	4 (26.67%)	0.048[4]
Corticoid requirement, n (%)	10 (50%)	4 (21.05%)	2 (10%)	7 (46.67%)	0.0181[1]

Reference values: CRP < 10 mg/L.
[1]Fisher exact test. [2] Kruskal-Wallis test. [3] Severe COVID-19 defined as: O_2 > 2 L/min, ICU [intensive care unit] admission, LTE [limitation of the therapeutic effort], decease. [4] Post-hoc analysis with Fisher exact test.

Interestingly, we found high incidence of MBL expression deficiency in patients of our cohort (16%, established as described in Methods), all clusters combined. Further studies based on MBL genotyping would be of interest to support biochemical data. MBL deficiency is fairly common, affecting approximately 5–10% of individuals and usually associated with increased susceptibility to bacterial infections of the upper respiratory in young children (30).

Our results highlight the dichotomous nature of the complement MBL pathway: on one hand, MBL appears to contribute to the pathogenesis of disease because it mediates complement activation that is related to clinical deterioration of patients; on the other hand, MBL could have a protective role against SARS-CoV-2 infection by promoting phagocytosis and virus lysis or neutralization. Further *in vitro* studies using pseudoviral particles or the SARS-CoV-2 virus are necessary to check the latter hypothesis.

In summary, our study suggests that alternative and lectin pathways assessment might be useful as biomarker of disease severity. Extensive investigations of complement pathways have to be performed on a larger cohort of patients with SARS-CoV-2 infection to help rationalize therapeutic choices.

AUTHOR CONTRIBUTIONS

Study conception: FD, CD-P, and J-YC. Immunological determinations: FD, CD-P, M-CJ, TR, and MP. Methodology: MR. Statistical analysis: CL, AV, and J-LB. Collection of patients' samples and clinical information: OE and MM. Funding acquisition: FD, CD-P, NT, OE, GC, AG, and PP. Writing original draft: FD and CD-P. Review manuscript: J-YC and NT. All authors contributed to the article and approved the submitted version.

FUNDING

This work was supported by funding from the Université Grenoble Alpes (projects COMPLEC-COV and BIOMARCOVID).

ACKNOWLEDGMENTS

The authors are grateful for the excellent work from the staff of technicians at Complement Laboratory of Grenoble-Alpes University Hospital: Marion Allegret-Cadet, Véronique Bergerot, Nadège Fondraz, Marie-Anne Pasquier and from Pierre Audoin for help in project conception.

REFERENCES

1. Mehta P, McAuley DF, Brown M, Sanchez E, Tattersall RS, Manson JJ. HLH Across Speciality Collaboration, UK. COVID-19: Consider Cytokine Storm Syndromes and Immunosuppression. *Lancet* (2020) 395:1033–4. doi: 10.1016/S0140-6736(20)30628-0
2. Carvelli J, Demaria O, Vély F, Batista L, Benmansour NC, Fares J, et al. Association of COVID-19 Inflammation With Activation of the C5a-C5aR1 Axis. *Nature* (2020) 588:146–50. doi: 10.1038/s41586-020-2600-6
3. Holter JC, Pischke SE, de Boer E, Lind A, Jenum S, Holten AR, et al. Systemic Complement Activation is Associated With Respiratory Failure in COVID-19 Hospitalized Patients. *Proc Natl Acad Sci USA* (2020) 117:25018–25. doi: 10.1073/pnas.2010540117
4. Eriksson O, Hultström M, Persson B, Lipcsey M, Ekdahl KN, Nilsson B, et al. Mannose-Binding Lectin Is Associated With Thrombosis and Coagulopathy in Critically Ill COVID-19 Patients. *Thromb Haemost* (2020) 120:1720–4. doi: 10.1055/s-0040-1715835
5. Diurno F, Numis FG, Porta G, Cirillo F, Maddaluno S, Ragozzino A, et al. Eculizumab Treatment in Patients With COVID-19: Preliminary Results From Real Life ASL Napoli 2 Nord Experience. *Eur Rev Med Pharmacol Sci* (2020) 24:4040–7. doi: 10.26355/eurrev_202004_20875
6. Laurence J, Mulvey JJ, Seshadri M, Racanelli A, Harp J, Schenck EJ, et al. Anti-Complement C5 Therapy With Eculizumab in Three Cases of Critical COVID-19. *Clin Immunol* (2020) 219:108555. doi: 10.1016/j.clim.2020.108555
7. Peffault de Latour R, Bergeron A, Lengline E, Dupont T, Marchal A, Galicier L, et al. Complement C5 Inhibition in Patients With COVID-19 - A Promising Target? *Haematologica* (2020) 105:2847–50. doi: 10.3324/haematol.2020.260117
8. Annane D, Heming N, Grimaldi-Bensouda L, Frémeaux-Bacchi V, Vigan M, Roux A-L, et al. Eculizumab as an Emergency Treatment for Adult Patients With Severe COVID-19 in the Intensive Care Unit: A Proof-of-Concept Study. *EClinicalMedicine* (2020) 28:100590. doi: 10.1016/j.eclinm.2020.100590
9. Mastaglio S, Ruggeri A, Risitano AM, Angelillo P, Yancopoulou D, Mastellos DC, et al. The First Case of COVID-19 Treated With the Complement C3 Inhibitor AMY-101. *Clin Immunol* (2020) 215:108450. doi: 10.1016/j.clim.2020.108450

10. WHO. *COVID-19 Therapeutic Trial Synopsis* World Health Organisation. (2020). Novel Coronavirus. Available at: https://www.who.int/publications/i/item/covid-19-therapeutic-trial-synopsis [Accessed June 9, 2020].
11. Dumestre-Pérard C, Lamy B, Aldebert D, Lemaire-Vieille C, Grillot R, Brion J-P, et al. Aspergillus Conidia Activate the Complement by the Mannan-Binding Lectin C2 Bypass Mechanism. *J Immunol* (2008) 181:7100–5. doi: 10.4049/jimmunol.181.10.7100
12. Dumestre-Perard C, Ponard D, Arlaud GJ, Monnier N, Sim RB, Colomb MG. Evaluation and Clinical Interest of Mannan Binding Lectin Function in Human Plasma. *Mol Immunol* (2002) 39:465–73. doi: 10.1016/s0161-5890(02)00119-0
13. Dumestre-Perard C, Ponard D, Drouet C, Leroy V, Zarski J-P, Dutertre N, et al. Complement C4 Monitoring in the Follow-Up of Chronic Hepatitis C Treatment. *Clin Exp Immunol* (2002) 127:131–6. doi: 10.1046/j.1365-2249.2002.01729.x
14. Garred P, Madsen HO, Hofmann B, Svejgaard A. Increased Frequency of Homozygosity of Abnormal Mannan-Binding-Protein Alleles in Patients With Suspected Immunodeficiency. *Lancet* (1995) 346:941–3. doi: 10.1016/S0140-6736(95)91559-1
15. Kim AHJ, Wu X, Atkinson JP. The Beneficial and Pathogenic Roles of Complement in COVID-19. *Cleve Clin J Med* (2020) 88:1–4. doi: 10.3949/ccjm.87a.ccc065
16. de Nooijer AH, Grondman I, Janssen NAF, Netea MG, Willems L, van de Veerdonk FL, et al. RCI-COVID-19 Study Group. Complement Activation in the Disease Course of Coronavirus Disease 2019 and Its Effects on Clinical Outcomes. *J Infect Dis* (2021) 223:214–24. doi: 10.1093/infdis/jiaa646
17. Magro C, Mulvey JJ, Berlin D, Nuovo G, Salvatore S, Harp J, et al. Complement Associated Microvascular Injury and Thrombosis in the Pathogenesis of Severe COVID-19 Infection: A Report of Five Cases. *Transl Res* (2020) 220:1–13. doi: 10.1016/j.trsl.2020.04.007
18. Prendecki M, Clarke C, Medjeral-Thomas N, McAdoo SP, Sandhu E, Peters JE, et al. Temporal Changes in Complement Activation in Haemodialysis Patients With COVID-19 as a Predictor of Disease Progression. *Clin Kidney J* (2020) 13:889–96. doi: 10.1093/ckj/sfaa192
19. Macor P, Durigutto P, Mangogna A, Bussani R, D'Errico S, Zanon M, et al. Multi-Organ Complement Deposition in COVID-19 Patients. *medRxiv* (2021) 9:1–15. doi: 10.1101/2021.01.07.21249116
20. Satyam A, Tsokos MG, Brook OR, Hecht JL, Moulton VR, Tsokos GC. Activation of Classical and Alternative Complement Pathways in the Pathogenesis of Lung Injury in COVID-19. *Clin Immunol* (2021) 226:108716. doi: 10.1016/j.clim.2021.108716
21. Pfister F, Vonbrunn E, Ries T, Jäck H-M, Überla K, Lochnit G, et al. Complement Activation in Kidneys of Patients With COVID-19. *Front Immunol* (2020) 11:594849. doi: 10.3389/fimmu.2020.594849
22. Sinkovits G, Mező B, Réti M, Müller V, Iványi Z, Gál J, et al. Complement Overactivation and Consumption Predicts In-Hospital Mortality in SARS-CoV-2 Infection. *Front Immunol* (2021) 12:663187. doi: 10.3389/fimmu.2021.663187
23. Yu J, Yuan X, Chen H, Chaturvedi S, Braunstein EM, Brodsky RA. Direct Activation of the Alternative Complement Pathway by SARS-CoV-2 Spike Proteins is Blocked by Factor D Inhibition. *Blood* (2020) 136:2080–9. doi: 10.1182/blood.2020008248
24. Zhou Y, Lu K, Pfefferle S, Bertram S, Glowacka I, Drosten C, et al. A Single Asparagine-Linked Glycosylation Site of the Severe Acute Respiratory Syndrome Coronavirus Spike Glycoprotein Facilitates Inhibition by Mannose-Binding Lectin Through Multiple Mechanisms. *J Virol* (2010) 84:8753–64. doi: 10.1128/JVI.00554-10
25. Ip WKE, Chan KH, Law HKW, Tso GHW, Kong EKP, Wong WHS, et al. Mannose-Binding Lectin in Severe Acute Respiratory Syndrome Coronavirus Infection. *J Infect Dis* (2005) 191:1697–704. doi: 10.1086/429631
26. Ali YM, Ferrari M, Lynch NJ, Yaseen S, Dudler T, Gragerov S, et al. Lectin Pathway Mediates Complement Activation by SARS-CoV-2 Proteins. *Front Immunol* (2021) 12:2645–52. doi: 10.3389/fimmu.2021.714511
27. Ma L, Sahu SK, Cano M, Kuppuswamy V, Bajwa J, McPhatter J, et al. Increased Complement Activation is a Distinctive Feature of Severe SARS-CoV-2 Infection. *Sci Immunol* (2021) 6:1–18. doi: 10.1126/sciimmunol.abh2259
28. Gao T, Hu M, Zhang X, Li H, Zhu L, Dong Q, et al. Highly Pathogenic Coronavirus N Protein Aggravates Lung Injury by MASP-2-Mediated Complement Over-Activation. *medRxiv* [preprint]. doi: 10.1101/2020.03.29.20041962v3.
29. Fodil S, Annane D. Complement Inhibition and COVID-19: The Story So Far. *Immunotargets Ther* (2021) 10:273–84. doi: 10.2147/ITT.S284830
30. Heitzeneder S, Seidel M, Förster-Waldl E, Heitger A. Mannan-Binding Lectin Deficiency — Good News, Bad News, Doesn't Matter? *Clin Immunol* (2012) 143:22–38. doi: 10.1016/j.clim.2011.11.002

Permissions

All chapters in this book were first published by Frontiers; hereby published with permission under the Creative Commons Attribution License or equivalent. Every chapter published in this book has been scrutinized by our experts. Their significance has been extensively debated. The topics covered herein carry significant findings which will fuel the growth of the discipline. They may even be implemented as practical applications or may be referred to as a beginning point for another development.

The contributors of this book come from diverse backgrounds, making this book a truly international effort. This book will bring forth new frontiers with its revolutionizing research information and detailed analysis of the nascent developments around the world.

We would like to thank all the contributing authors for lending their expertise to make the book truly unique. They have played a crucial role in the development of this book. Without their invaluable contributions this book wouldn't have been possible. They have made vital efforts to compile up to date information on the varied aspects of this subject to make this book a valuable addition to the collection of many professionals and students.

This book was conceptualized with the vision of imparting up-to-date information and advanced data in this field. To ensure the same, a matchless editorial board was set up. Every individual on the board went through rigorous rounds of assessment to prove their worth. After which they invested a large part of their time researching and compiling the most relevant data for our readers.

The editorial board has been involved in producing this book since its inception. They have spent rigorous hours researching and exploring the diverse topics which have resulted in the successful publishing of this book. They have passed on their knowledge of decades through this book. To expedite this challenging task, the publisher supported the team at every step. A small team of assistant editors was also appointed to further simplify the editing procedure and attain best results for the readers.

Apart from the editorial board, the designing team has also invested a significant amount of their time in understanding the subject and creating the most relevant covers. They scrutinized every image to scout for the most suitable representation of the subject and create an appropriate cover for the book.

The publishing team has been an ardent support to the editorial, designing and production team. Their endless efforts to recruit the best for this project, has resulted in the accomplishment of this book. They are a veteran in the field of academics and their pool of knowledge is as vast as their experience in printing. Their expertise and guidance has proved useful at every step. Their uncompromising quality standards have made this book an exceptional effort. Their encouragement from time to time has been an inspiration for everyone.

The publisher and the editorial board hope that this book will prove to be a valuable piece of knowledge for researchers, students, practitioners and scholars across the globe.

List of Contributors

Eija Nissilä, Pipsa Hakala, Katarzyna Leskinen, Angela Roig, Shahan Syed, T. Sakari Jokiranta, Karita Haapasalo, Päivi Saavalainen and Seppo Meri
Department of Bacteriology and Immunology, and Research Programs Unit, Immunobiology, University of Helsinki, Helsinki, Finland

Kok P. M. Van Kessel, Carla J. C. De Haas and Jos A. G. Van Strijp
Medical Microbiology, University Medical Center Utrecht, Utrecht, Netherlands

Jari Metso and Matti Jauhiainen
Minerva Foundation Institute for Medical Research, Helsinki, Finland

Angeliki Chroni
Institute of Biosciences and Applications, National Center for Scientific Research "Demokritos," Athens, Greece

Katariina Öörni
Wihuri Research Institute, Helsinki, Finland

Thomas Vorup-Jensen
Biophysical Immunology Laboratory, Department of Biomedicine, Aarhus University, Aarhus, Denmark
Interdisciplinary Nanoscience Center, Aarhus University, Aarhus, Denmark

Rasmus Kjeldsen Jensen
Department of Molecular Biology and Genetics—Structural Biology, Aarhus University, Aarhus, Denmark

Pilar Sánchez-Corral
Complement Research Group, Hospital La Paz Institute for Health Research (IdiPAZ), La Paz University Hospital, Center for Biomedical Network Research on Rare Diseases (CIBERER), Madrid, Spain

Richard B. Pouw
Department of Pharmaceutical Sciences, University of Basel, Basel, Switzerland

Margarita López-Trascasa
Complement Research Group, Hospital La Paz Institute for Health Research (IdiPAZ), La Paz University Hospital, Center for Biomedical Network Research on Rare Diseases (CIBERER), Madrid, Spain
Department of Medicine, Universidad Autónoma de Madrid, Madrid, Spain
MTA-SE Research Group of Immunology and Hematology, Hungarian Academy of Sciences and Semmelweis University, Budapest, Hungary

Simon Freeley and John Cardone
School of Immunology and Microbial Sciences, King's College London, London, United Kingdom

Sira C. Günther
School of Immunology and Microbial Sciences, King's College London, London, United Kingdom
Institut für Medizinische Virologie, University of Zurich, Zurich, Switzerland

Erin E. West
Laboratory of Molecular Immunology and Immunology Center, National Heart, Lung and Blood Institute, Bethesda, MD, United States

Thomas Reinheckel
Faculty of Medicine, Institute of Molecular Medicine and Cell Research, Albert-Ludwigs University Freiburg, and German Cancer Consortium (DKTK), Freiburg, Germany

Colin Watts
Division of Cell Signaling & Immunology, School of Life Sciences, University of Dundee, Dundee, United Kingdom

Claudia Kemper
School of Immunology and Microbial Sciences, King's College London, London, United Kingdom
Laboratory of Molecular Immunology and Immunology Center, National Heart, Lung and Blood Institute, Bethesda, MD, United States
Institute for Systemic Inflammation Research, University of Lübeck, Lübeck, Germany

Martin V. Kolev
Laboratory of Molecular Immunology and Immunology Center, National Heart, Lung and Blood Institute, Bethesda, MD, United States

Barbro Persson and Bo Nilsson
Rudbeck Laboratory C5:3, Department of Immunology, Genetics and Pathology, Uppsala University, Uppsala, Sweden

Camilla Mohlin and Kerstin Sandholm
Centre of Biomaterials Chemistry, Linnaeus University, Kalmar, Sweden

Lillemor Skattum
Section of Microbiology, Immunology and Glycobiology, Department of Laboratory Medicine, Clinical Immunology and Transfusion Medicine, Lund University, Lund, Sweden

Kristina N. Ekdahl
Rudbeck Laboratory C5:3, Department of Immunology, Genetics and Pathology, Uppsala University, Uppsala, Sweden
Centre of Biomaterials Chemistry, Linnaeus University, Kalmar, Sweden

Barbro Persson and Bo Nilsson
Rudbeck Laboratory C5:3, Department of Immunology, Genetics and Pathology, Uppsala University, Uppsala, Sweden

Camilla Mohlin and Kerstin Sandholm
Centre of Biomaterials Chemistry, Linnaeus University, Kalmar, Sweden

Mariana Gaya da Costa and Marc A. Seelen
Division of Nephrology, Department of Internal Medicine, University of Groningen, University Medical Center Groningen, Groningen, Netherlands

Felix Poppelaars
Division of Nephrology, Department of Internal Medicine, University of Groningen, University Medical Center Groningen, Groningen, Netherlands
Department of Obstetrics and Gynecology, Martini Hospital, Groningen, Netherlands

Cees van Kooten
Department of Nephrology, University of Leiden, Leiden University Medical Center, Leiden, Netherlands

Tom E. Mollnes
Department of Immunology, Oslo University Hospital and University of Oslo, Oslo, Norway
Research Laboratory, Bodø Hospital, and K.G. Jebsen TREC, University of Tromsø, Tromsø, Norway
Centre of Molecular Inflammation Research, Norwegian University of Science and Technology, Trondheim, Norway

William Tse and Janina Ratajczak
Stem Cell Institute at James Graham Brown Cancer Center, University of Louisville, Louisville, KY, United States

Reinhard Würzner
Department of Hygiene, Microbiology and Public Health, Medical University of Innsbruck, Innsbruck, Austria

Leendert A. Trouw
Department of Rheumatology, Leiden University Medical Center, Leiden, Netherlands
Department of Immunohematology and Blood Transfusion, Leiden University Medical Center, Leiden, Netherlands

Lennart Truedsson
Department of Laboratory Medicine, Section of Microbiology, Immunology and Glycobiology, Lund University, Lund, Sweden

Mohamed R. Daha
Division of Nephrology, Department of Internal Medicine, University of Groningen, University Medical Center Groningen, Groningen, Netherlands
Department of Nephrology, University of Leiden, Leiden University Medical Center, Leiden, Netherlands

Anja Roos
Department of Medical Microbiology and Immunology, St. Antonius Hospital, Nieuwegein, Netherlands

Michele Mutti, Katharina Ramoni, Gábor Nagy, Eszter Nagy and Valéria Szijártó
Arsanis Biosciences, Vienna, Austria

Mariusz Z. Ratajczak and Magda Kucia
Stem Cell Institute at James Graham Brown Cancer Center, University of Louisville, Louisville, KY, United States
Department of Regenerative Medicine, Center for Preclinical Research and Technology, Warsaw Medical University, Warsaw, Poland

Mateusz Adamiak
Department of Regenerative Medicine, Center for Preclinical Research and Technology, Warsaw Medical University, Warsaw, Poland

Francesco Tedesco
Immunorheumatology Research Laboratory, Istituto Auxologico Italiano, IRCCS, Milan, Italy

Wieslaw Wiktor-Jedrzejczak
Department of Hematology Warsaw Medical University, Warsaw, Poland

Rafael Bayarri-Olmos, Nikolaj Kirketerp-Moller, Laura Pérez-Alós, Mikkel-Ole Skjoedt and Peter Garred
Laboratory of Molecular Medicine, Department of Clinical Immunology, Faculty of Health and Medical Sciences, Rigshospitalet, University of Copenhagen, Copenhagen, Denmark

Richard B. Pouw and Anna E. van Beek
Department of Immunopathology, Sanquin Research and Landsteiner Laboratory of the Academic Medical Center, University of Amsterdam, Amsterdam, Netherlands
Department of Pediatric Hematology, Immunology and Infectious Diseases, Emma Children's hospital, Academic Medical Center, Amsterdam, Netherlands

Karsten Skjodt
Department of Cancer and Inflammation Research, University of Southern Denmark, Odense, Denmark

Mieke C. Brouwer and Diana Wouters
Department of Immunopathology, Sanquin Research and Landsteiner Laboratory of the Academic Medical Center, University of Amsterdam, Amsterdam, Netherlands

Mihály Józsi
MTA-ELTE "Lendület" Complement Research Group, Department of Immunology, ELTE Eötvös Loránd University, Budapest, Hungary

Soren W. K. Hansen, Josephine B. Aagaard, Karen B. Bjerrum, Karsten Skjoedt, Anna L. Sørensen, Jonas H. Graversen and Maiken L. Henriksen
Institute of Cancer and Inflammation Research, University of Southern Denmark, Odense, Denmark

Eva K. Hejbøl, Ole Nielsen and Henrik D. Schrøder
Department of Pathology, Odense University Hospital, Odense, Denmark

Anna E. van Beek
Department of Immunopathology, Sanquin Research and Landsteiner Laboratory of the Academic Medical Centre, University of Amsterdam, Amsterdam, Netherlands
Department of Pediatric Hematology, Immunology and Infectious Diseases, Emma Children's Hospital, Academic Medical Centre, Amsterdam, Netherlands

Angela Kamp, Simone Kruithof, Diana Wouters, Ilse Jongerius and Theo Rispens
Department of Immunopathology, Sanquin Research and Landsteiner Laboratory of the Academic Medical Centre, University of Amsterdam, Amsterdam, Netherlands

Ed J. Nieuwenhuys and Kyra A. Gelderman
Sanquin Diagnostic Services, Amsterdam, Netherlands

József Dobó, Andrea Kocsis and Péter Gál
Institute of Enzymology, Research Centre for Natural Sciences, Hungarian Academy of Sciences, Budapest, Hungary

Mischa P. Keizer
Department of Immunopathology, Sanquin Blood Supply, Division Research and Landsteiner Laboratory of the Academic Medical Center, University of Amsterdam, Amsterdam, Netherlands
Department of Pediatric Hematology, Immunology and Infectious Diseases, Emma Children's Hospital, AMC, University of Amsterdam, Amsterdam, Netherlands

Angela Kamp, Gerard van Mierlo and Diana Wouters
Department of Immunopathology, Sanquin Blood Supply, Division Research and Landsteiner Laboratory of the Academic Medical Center, University of Amsterdam, Amsterdam, Netherlands

Taco W. Kuijpers
Department of Pediatric Hematology, Immunology and Infectious Diseases, Emma Children's Hospital, AMC, University of Amsterdam, Amsterdam, Netherlands
Department of Blood Cell Research, Sanquin Blood Supply, Division Research and Landsteiner Laboratory of the AMC, University of Amsterdam, Amsterdam, Netherlands

Seline A. Zwarthoff, Evelien T. M. Berends, Sanne Mol, Maartje Ruyken, Piet C. Aerts, Carla J. C. de Haas, Suzan H. M. Rooijakkers and Ronald D. Gorham Jr.
Department of Medical Microbiology, University Medical Center Utrecht, Utrecht University, Utrecht, Netherlands

Cecilie E. Hertz, Rafael Bayarri-Olmos, Nikolaj Kirketerp-Møller, Katrine Pilely, Mikkel-Ole Skjoedt and Peter Garred
Laboratory of Molecular Medicine, Department of Clinical Immunology Section, Rigshospitalet, Faculty of Health and Medical Sciences, University of Copenhagen, Copenhagen, Denmark

Sander van Putten
Finsen Laboratory, Rigshospitalet, Biotech Research and Innovation Center (BRIC), Faculty of Health and Medical Sciences, University of Copenhagen, Copenhagen, Denmark

Youssif M. Ali
Department of Veterinary Medicine, School of Biological Sciences, University of Cambridge, Cambridge, United Kingdom
Department of Microbiology and Immunology, Faculty of Pharmacy, Mansoura University, Mansoura, Egypt

Matteo Ferrari, Nicholas J. Lynch, Jonathan L. Heeney and Wilhelm J. Schwaeble
Department of Veterinary Medicine, School of Biological Sciences, University of Cambridge, Cambridge, United Kingdom

Marta Bermejo-Jambrina
Institute of Hygiene and Medical Microbiology, Medical University of Innsbruck, Innsbruck, Austria
Department of Experimental Immunology, Amsterdam Infection and Immunity Institute, Academic Medical Center, University of Amsterdam, Amsterdam, Netherlands

Sadam Yaseen, Thomas Dudler, Sasha Gragerov and Gregory Demopulos
Omeros Corporation, Seattle, WA, United States

Michael Blatzer
Experimental Neuropathology Unit, Infection and Epidemiology Department, Institute Pasteur, Paris, France

Paula Jauregui-Onieva, Doris Wilflingseder and Wilfried Posch
Institute of Hygiene and Medical Microbiology, Medical University of Innsbruck, Innsbruck, Austria

Teodor E. Yordanov and Lukas A. Huber
Institute of Cell Biology, Biocenter, Medical University of Innsbruck, Innsbruck, Austria

Paul Hörtnagl
Central Institute for Blood Transfusion and Immunological Department, Innsbruck, Austria

Taras Valovka
Institute of Cell Biology, Biocenter, Medical University of Innsbruck, Innsbruck, Austria
Department of Pediatrics I, Medical University of Innsbruck, Innsbruck, Austria

Federica Defendi, Giovanna Clavarino, Marie-Christine Jacob, Tatiana Raskovalova, Martine Pernollet and Jean-Yves Cesbron
Laboratoire d'Immunologie, Institut de Biologie et Pathologie, Centre Hospitalier Universitaire Grenoble Alpes, Grenoble, France

Corentin Leroy
Cellule d'Ingénierie des Données, Centre Hospitalier Universitaire Grenoble Alpes, Grenoble, France
Centre d'Investigation Clinique de l'Innovation et de la Technologie (CIC-IT), Centre Hospitalier Universitaire Grenoble Alpes, Grenoble, France

Olivier Epaulard
Service des Maladies Infectieuses et Tropicales, Centre Hospitalier Universitaire Grenoble Alpes, Grenoble, France
Université Grenoble Alpes, TIMC-IMAG, Grenoble, France

Antoine Vilotitch
Cellule d'Ingénierie des Données, Centre Hospitalier Universitaire Grenoble Alpes, Grenoble, France

Marion Le Marechal
Service des Maladies Infectieuses et Tropicales, Centre Hospitalier Universitaire Grenoble Alpes, Grenoble, France

Audrey Le Gouellec
Université Grenoble Alpes, TIMC-IMAG, Grenoble, France
Laboratoire de Biochimie, Institut de Biologie et Pathologie, Centre Hospitalier Universitaire Grenoble Alpes, Grenoble, France

Jean-Luc Bosson
Université Grenoble Alpes, TIMC-IMAG, Grenoble, France

Pascal Poignard
Université Grenoble Alpes, CNRS, CEA, Institut de Biologie Structurale (IBS), Grenoble, France
Laboratoire de Virologie, Institut de Biologie et Pathologie, Centre Hospitalier Universitaire Grenoble Alpes, Grenoble, France

Matthieu Roustit
Département de Pharmacologie Clinique INSERM CIC 1406, Centre Hospitalier Universitaire Grenoble Alpes, Grenoble, France
Université Grenoble Alpes, UMR 1042-HP2, INSERM, Grenoble, France

Nicole Thielens
Université Grenoble Alpes, CNRS, CEA, Institut de Biologie Structurale (IBS), Grenoble, France

Chantal Dumestre-Pérard
Laboratoire d'Immunologie, Institut de Biologie et Pathologie, Centre Hospitalier Universitaire Grenoble Alpes, Grenoble, France
Université Grenoble Alpes, CNRS, CEA, Institut de Biologie Structurale (IBS), Grenoble, France

Index

Printed in the USA
CPSIA information can be obtained
at www.ICGtesting.com
JSHW052312231023
50683JS00006BA/80

9 781646 466061